Advances in
PARASITOLOGY

Control of Human Parasitic Diseases

VOLUME 61

Advances in
PARASITOLOGY

Control of Human Parasitic Diseases

Guest Editor

DAVID H. MOLYNEUX

Lymphatic Filariasis Support Centre
Liverpool School of Tropical Medicine
Liverpool, UK

VOLUME 61

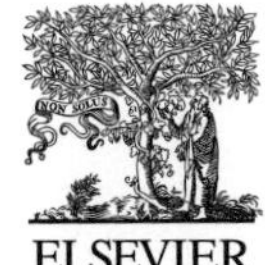

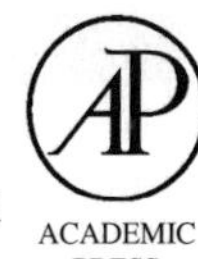

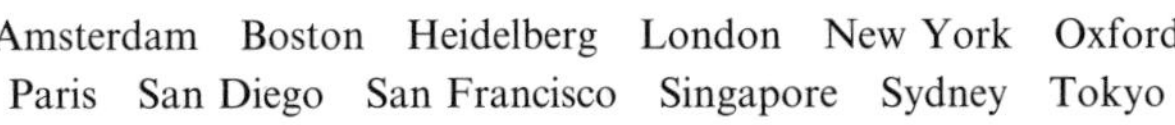

ELSEVIER   Amsterdam Boston Heidelberg London New York Oxford
Paris San Diego San Francisco Singapore Sydney Tokyo

ACADEMIC PRESS

Academic Press is an imprint of Elsevier
84 Theobald's Road, London WC1X 8RR, UK
Radarweg 29, PO Box 211, 1000 AE Amsterdam, The Netherlands
The Boulevard, Langford Lane, Kidlington, Oxford OX5 1GB, UK
30 Corporate Drive, Suite 400, Burlington, MA 01803, USA
525 B Street, Suite 1900, San Diego, CA 92101-4495, USA

First edition 2006

ISBN-13: 978-0-12-031761-5
ISBN-10: 0-12-031761-3
ISSN: 0065-308X

For information on all Academic Press publications
visit our website at books.elsevier.com

Printed and bound in The United Kingdom

06 07 08 09 10   10 9 8 7 6 5 4 3 2 1

Working together to grow
libraries in developing countries

www.elsevier.com | www.bookaid.org | www.sabre.org

ELSEVIER   BOOK AID International   Sabre Foundation

CONTRIBUTORS TO VOLUME 61

M. ALBONICO, *Ivo de Carneri Foundation, Via IV Marzo 14, 10122 Torino, Italy*

J. ALVAR, *Department for Control of Neglected Tropical Diseases, World Health Organization, 20 Avenue Appia CH-1211 Geneva 27, Switzerland*

B.A. BOATIN, *TDR, World Health Organization, 20 Avenue Appia, CH-1211, Geneva 27, Switzerland*

P.S. CRAIG, *Cestode Zoonoses Research Group, Biomedical Sciences Institute & School of Environment and Life Sciences, University of Salford, Salford, Greater Manchester M5 4WT, UK*

S.L. CROFT, *Drugs for Neglected Diseases Initiative (DNDi), 1 Place Saint Gervais, CH-1201 Geneva, Switzerland*

D.W.T. CROMPTON, *Institute of Biomedical and Life Sciences, University of Glasgow, Glasgow G12 8QQ, UK*

D. ENGELS, *Coordinator, Preventative Chemotherapy and Transmission Control, Department of Control of Neglected Tropical Diseases, World Health Organization, 20 Avenue Appia, CH-1211 Geneva 27, Switzerland*

A. FENWICK, *Schistosomiasis Control Initiative, Department of Infectious Disease Epidemiology, Imperial College, London W2 1PG, UK*

E.M. FÈVRE, *Centre for Infectious Diseases, Royal (Dick) School of Veterinary Studies, University of Edinburgh, Easter Bush, Roslin, Midlothian EH25 9RG, UK*

ISSN: 0065-308X
DOI: 10.1016/S0065-308X(05)61015-9

J. HILL, *Child and Reproductive Health Group, Liverpool School of Tropical Medicine, Pembroke Place, Liverpool L3 5QA, UK*

D.R. HOPKINS, *The Carter Center, 453 Freedom Parkway, Atlanta, GA 30307, USA*

J. JANNIN, *World Health Organization, 20 Avenue Appia, CH-1211 Geneva 27, Switzerland*

E. LARRIEU, *Veterinary Faculty, University of La Pampa, General Pico, Calle 5y116, (6360), La Pampa Province, Argentina*

J. LINES, *Malaria Knowledge Programme, London School of Hygiene and Tropical Medicine, Keppel Street, London WC1E 7HT, UK*

I. MAUDLIN, *Centre for Infectious Diseases, Royal (Dick). School of Veterinary Studies, University of Edinburgh, Easter Bush, Roslin, Midlothian EH25 9RG, UK*

D.H. MOLYNEUX, *Lymphatic Filariasis Support Centre, Liverpool School of Tropical Medicine, Pembroke Place, Liverpool L3 5QA, UK*

A. MONTRESOR, *World Health Organization, 63 Tran Hung Dao Street, Mail P.O. Box 52, Hanoi, Viet Nam*

J. NAKAGAWA, *Japan International Cooperation Agency, Apdo. postal 1752, Tegucigalpa, M.D.C., Honduras*

P. OLLIARO, *UNICEF/UNDP/WB/WHO Special Programme for Research & Training in Tropical Diseases (TDR), World Health Organization, 20 Avenue Appia, CH-1211 Geneva 27, Switzerland*

E.A. OTTESEN, *Lymphatic Filariasis Support Centre, Task Force for Child Survival and Development, 750 Commerce Drive, Decatur, GA 30030, USA*

K. PICOZZI, *Centre for Infectious Diseases, Royal (Dick) School of Veterinary Studies, University of Edinburgh, Easter Bush, Roslin, Midlothian EH25 9RG, UK*

F.O. RICHARDS, *The Carter Center, One Copenhill, Atlanta, GA 30307, USA*

D. ROLLINSON, *Wolfson Wellcome Biomedical Laboratories, Department of Zoology, The Natural History Museum, Cromwell Road, London SW7 5BD, UK*

M. ROWLAND, *Gates Malaria Partnership, London School of Hygiene and Tropical Medicine, Keppel Street, London WC1E 7HT, UK*

E. RUIZ-TIBEN, *Dracunculiasis Eradication, The Carter Center, 453 Freedom Parkway, Atlanta, GA 30307, USA*

L. SAVIOLI, *Department of Control of Neglected Tropical Diseases (NTD), WHO, 20 Avenue Appia, 1211 Geneva 27, Switzerland*

V. SOUTHGATE, *Wolfson Wellcome Biomedical Laboratories, Department of Zoology, The Natural History Museum, Cromwell Road, London SW7 5BD, UK*

S. WARD, *Liverpool School of Tropical Medicine, Pembroke Place, Liverpool L3 5QA, UK*

S.C. WELBURN, *Centre for Infectious Disease, Royal (Dick) School of Veterinary Studies, University of Edinburgh, Easter Bush, Roslin, Midlothian EH25 9RG, UK*

A.L. WILLINGHAM III, *WHO/FAO Collaborating Center for Parasitic Zoonoses, Royal Veterinary and Agricultural University, Frederikserg, Denmark and Human Health Impacts Operating Project, People, Livestock and the Environment Thematic Programme, International Livestock Research Institute, Nairobi, Kenya*

P. WINSTANLEY, *Department of Pharmacology & Therapeutics, University of Liverpool, Liverpool L69 3GE, UK*

Y. YAMAGATA, *Institute for International Cooperation, Japan International Cooperation Agency, 10-5 Ichigaya Honmura-cho, Shinjuku-ku, Tokyo 162-8433, Japan*

Foreword

Jeffrey D. Sachs

The parasitic diseases covered in this enormously useful and timely volume continue to inflict massive suffering, mortality, and economic distress throughout the low-income world, especially in the tropics. Thirteen high-quality and up-to-date chapters describe not only the epidemiology, complex life cycles, and pathogenesis of these diseases, but also the powerful technologies that make possible their effective control, if not eradication. The chapters also document that these strategies—many of them with extremely low cost and very high efficacy—are not reaching the poorest people who are afflicted with these diseases. This book is therefore not only a unique state-of-the-art sourcebook on parasitic disease control, but also a major prod to policy action.

Control of Human Parasitic Diseases comes at a time of potential policy breakthrough. After decades of substantial neglect by the wealthy countries, human parasitic diseases are back in policy focus. The major donor countries have in recent years repeatedly pledged to take stepped-up action against these diseases at G8 Summits, UN gatherings, World Health Assemblies, and other important venues. New financing is finally being mobilized through areas such as the Global Fund to Fight AIDS, TB, and Malaria, the World Bank, as well as from private foundations and bilateral donors. The threats of emerging diseases, such as SARS and avian flu, are drawing global attention to the urgency, possibility, and practical challenges of disease control.

ADVANCES IN PARASITOLOGY VOL 61
ISSN: 0065-308X
DOI: 10.1016/S0065-308X(05)61020-2

The Millennium Development Goals (MDGs) provide an important shared global framework and timetable for action. Several of the authors of this book have played a special role in promoting support for the MDGs, including Professor David Molyneux, whose lucid overview chapter provides an especially fitting introduction to the themes of the entire volume. This book comes at a crucial time, and through its excellent coverage, can play an important role in spurring science-based action.

Jeffrey D. Sachs is Director of the Earth Institute at Columbia University and Director of the UN Millennium Project. He is also Special Advisor to UN Secretary General Kofi Annan on the Millennium Development Goals.

Preface

This special volume of *Advances in Parasitology* is perhaps the most practical, covering the latest developments in methods of control of parasitic infections, including both prophylactic and curative chemotherapy and other preventive methods. The range of infections covered is wide—malaria, human trypanosomiasis (African and South American), leishmaniasis, dracunculiasis, soil-transmitted helminths, onchocerciasis, lymphatic filariasis, cystic echinococcosis, taeniasis and neurocysticercosis, and schistosomiasis.

The guest editor, David Molyneux of the Liverpool School of Tropical Medicine (UK), has brought together a panel of international experts from Europe, North and South America, Asia, and Africa to contribute to a volume which will surely prove to be an invaluable source of information on this most pressing of topics—the control of global parasitic disease.

John Baker
Ralph Muller
David Rollinson

ISSN: 0065-308X
DOI: 10.1016/S0065-308X(05)61019-6

Contents

Control of Human Parasitic Diseases: Context and Overview

David H. Molyneux

Malaria Chemotherapy

Peter Winstanley and Stephen Ward

Insecticide-Treated Nets

Jenny Hill, Jo Lines and Mark Rowland

ISSN: 0065-308X
DOI: 10.1016/S0065-308X(05)61016-0

Control of Chagas Disease

Yoichi Yamagata and Jun Nakagawa

Human African Trypanosomiasis: Epidemiology and Control

E.M. Fèvre, K. Picozzi, J. Jannin, S.C. Welburn and I. Maudlin

Chemotherapy in the Treatment and Control of Leishmaniasis

Jorge Alvar, Simon Croft and Piero Olliaro

Dracunculiasis (Guinea Worm Disease) Eradication

Ernesto Ruiz-Tiben and Donald R. Hopkins

Intervention for the Control of Soil-Transmitted Helminthiasis in the Community

Marco Albonico, Antonio Montresor, D.W.T. Crompton and Lorenzo Savioli

Control of Onchocerciasis

Boakye A. Boatin and Frank O. Richards, Jr

Lymphatic Filariasis: Treatment, Control and Elimination

Eric A. Ottesen

Control of Cystic Echinococcosis/Hydatidosis: 1863–2002

P.S. Craig and E. Larrieu

Control of *Taenia solium* Cysticercosis/Taeniosis

Arve Lee Willingham and Dirk Engels

Implementation of Human Schistosomiasis Control: Challenges and Prospects

Alan Fenwick, David Rollinson and Vaughan Southgate

Colour Plate Section can be found at the back of this book

Control of Human Parasitic Diseases: Context and Overview

David H. Molyneux

Lymphatic Filariasis Support Centre, Liverpool School of Tropical Medicine, Pembroke Place, Liverpool, L3 5QA, UK

ABSTRACT

The control of parasitic diseases of humans has been undertaken since the aetiology and natural history of the infections was recognized and the deleterious effects on human health and well-being appreciated by policy makers, medical practitioners and public health specialists. However, while some parasitic infections such as malaria

ADVANCES IN PARASITOLOGY VOL 61
ISSN: 0065-308X
DOI: 10.1016/S0065-308X(05)61001-9

have proved difficult to control, as defined by a sustained reduction in incidence, others, particularly helminth infections can be effectively controlled. The different approaches to control from diagnosis, to treatment and cure of the clinically sick patient, to control the transmission within the community by preventative chemotherapy and vector control are outlined. The concepts of eradication, elimination and control are defined and examples of success summarized. Overviews of the health policy and financing environment in which programmes to control or eliminate parasitic diseases are positioned and the development of public–private partnerships as vehicles for product development or access to drugs for parasite disease control are discussed. Failure to sustain control of parasites may be due to development of drug resistance or the failure to implement proven strategies as a result of decreased resources within the health system, decentralization of health management through health-sector reform and the lack of financial and human resources in settings where per capita government expenditure on health may be less than $US 5 per year. However, success has been achieved in several large-scale programmes through sustained national government investment and/or committed donor support. It is also widely accepted that the level of investment in drug development for the parasitic diseases of poor populations is an unattractive option for pharmaceutical companies. The development of partnerships to specifically address this need provides some hope that the intractable problems of the treatment regimens for the trypanosomiases and leishmaniases can be solved in the not too distant future. However, it will be difficult to implement and sustain such interventions in fragile health services often in settings where resources are limited but also in unstable, conflict-affected or post-conflict countries. Emphasis is placed on the importance of co-endemicity and polyparasitism and the opportunity to control parasites susceptible to cost-effective and proven chemotherapeutic interventions for a package of diseases which can be implemented at low cost and which would benefit the poorest and most marginalized groups. The ecology of parasitic diseases is discussed in the context of changing ecology, environment, sociopolitical developments and climate change. These drivers of global change will affect the epidemiology of parasites over the coming decades, while in many of the most endemic and impoverished countries parasitic infections will be accorded lower priority as resourced stressed health systems cope with the burden of the higher-profile killing diseases viz., HIV/AIDS, TB and malaria. There is a need for more holistic thinking about the interactions between parasites and other infections. It is clear that as the prevalence and awareness of HIV has increased, there is a growing recognition of a host of complex interactions that determine disease outcome in individual patients. The competition for resources in the health as well as other social sectors will be a continuing challenge; effective parasite control will be dependent on how such resources are accessed and deployed to effectively address well-defined problems some of which are readily amenable to successful interventions with proven methods. In the health sector, the problems of the HIV/AIDS and TB pandemics and the problem of the emerging burden of chronic non-communicable diseases will be significant competitors for these limited resources as parasitic infections aside from malaria tend to be chronic disabling problems of the poorest who have limited access to scarce health services and are representative of the poorest quintile. Prioritization and advocacy for parasite control in the national and international political environments is the challenge.

1. CONTROL OF PARASITIC DISEASES

1.1. Concepts of Control, Elimination and Eradication

A distinction must be made between the terms 'control', 'elimination' and 'eradication'; the latter term is often used inappropriately and it should be employed with caution. The International Task Force for Disease Eradication (ITFDE) was established in 1988 to evaluate systematically the potential for eradication of candidate diseases and to identify specific barriers to eradication. The criteria used to assess the feasibility of eradication are provided in Table 1. The Task Force was reconstituted in 2001 to evaluate the current situation. The IT-FDE defined eradication as 'reduction of the world-wide incidence of a disease to zero as a result of deliberate efforts obviating the

Table 1 Criteria for assessing eradicability of diseases or conditions (Dowdle and Hopkins, 1998)

Scientific feasibility

Epidemiologic vulnerability (e.g. absence of non-human reservoir; ease of spread; natural cyclical decline in prevalence; naturally induced immunity; ease of diagnosis; and duration of any relapse potential)

Effective, practical intervention available (e.g. vaccine or other primary preventive, curative treatment, and means of eliminating vector). Ideally, intervention should be effective, safe, inexpensive, long lasting and easily deployed

Demonstrated feasibility of elimination (e.g. documented elimination from island or other geographic unit)

Political will/popular support

Perceived burden of the disease (e.g. extent, deaths, other effects; true burden may not be perceived; the reverse of benefits expected to accrue from eradication; relevance to rich and poor countries)

Expected cost of elimination or eradication (especially in relation to perceived burden from the disease)

Synergy of eradication efforts with other interventions (e.g. potential for added benefits or savings or spin-off effects)

---

necessity for further control measures'. The original ITFDE reviewed more than 90 diseases, 30 of them in depth, and concluded that dracunculiasis, rubella, poliomyelitis, mumps, lymphatic filariasis and cysticercosis could probably be eradicated using existing technology. The term 'elimination' is increasingly being used to replace the term 'eradication', which should be only used in Global terms. The Dahlem conference held in Berlin in 1997 (Dowdle and Hopkins, 1998) also considered these issues in some detail and introduced the term extinction to classify an organism that did not exist on the planet contrasting with smallpox, which had been eradicated as a cause of disease but stocks had been retained in secure laboratories. The use of the term elimination is now regarded as referring to the removal of the organism from a defined geographical region ("local eradication"), which creates problems for quantification of achievement towards the goal. The accepted position being that the disease is not eradicated but no longer requires ongoing investment in control and is maintained at a level when the problem is no longer a significant health burden. A new concept has also been introduced through World Assembly Resolutions of the "Elimination of a disease as a Public Health problem". The definitions which will be used in this chapter are from Dowdle and Hopkins (1998), WHO (1998) and Molyneux *et al.* (2004):

Control reduction of disease incidence, prevalence, morbidity or mortality to a locally acceptable level as a result of deliberate efforts; continued intervention measures are required to maintain the reduction.

Elimination of disease reduction to zero of the incidence of a specified disease in a defined geographical area as a result of deliberate efforts; continued intervention measures are required.

Elimination of infection reduction to zero of the incidence of infection caused by a specified agent in a defined geographical area as a result of deliberate efforts; continued measures to prevent the re-establishment of transmission are required.

Eradication permanent reduction to zero of the worldwide incidence of infection caused by a specific agent as a result of deliberate efforts; intervention measures are no longer needed.

Extinction the specific infectious agent no longer exists in nature or the laboratory

1.2. Examples of Parasite Elimination and Vector "Eradication"

The classic eradication programme was that of smallpox which achieved its target in 1977. To date, no parasitic disease has been eradicated, although attempts to eradicate Guinea worm are under-way (Hopkins *et al.*, 2002; Ruiz-Tiben and Hopkins, 2006). Never-theless, successful "local eradication" (correctly elimination) has been achieved in some restricted geographical or epidemiological situa-tions. For example, onchocerciasis has been eliminated from several parts of Kenya and from the Nile at Jinja in Uganda, by using DDT to remove the local vectors (*Simulium neavei* and *S. damnosum*, respectively) (Davies, 1994). The Onchocerciasis Control Programme (OCP) in West Africa has achieved the same goal eliminating particular cytoforms of the *S. damnosum* complex using aerial application of insecticides. Local elimination has also been achieved; the malaria vector *Anopheles gambiae* from Brazil in the late 1930s using larviciding measures and house spraying with pyrethrum, a success repeated in early 1940s after the same species had been introduced into Egypt; *Glossina palpalis,* the tsetse fly, the vector of human trypanosomiasis was eliminated from the Island of Principe in 1905 by trapping out flies using sticky back packs on plantation workers; animal trypanosomiasis from parts of North-East Nigeria by ground spraying of tsetse resting sites with persistent doses of DDT; *Aedes aegypti,* the vector of yellow fever, in parts of Central and South America. Local anti-mosquito spraying has eliminated lymphatic filariasis from the Solomon Islands with no evidence that over a 20-year period there has been any resurgence; filariasis due to *Brugia malayi* was eliminated from Sri Lanka through selective treatment with DEC, anti-larval measures (host plants killed by herbiciding), house spraying with DDT as part of the malaria eradication programme and environmental improvements. Chemotherapeutic approaches have eliminated filariasis (due to *Wuchereria bancrofti*) from Japan, South Korea and Taiwan in Asia and Suriname and Trinidad and Tobago in the Americas (WHO, 1992, 1994). Filariasis has also been eliminated as a public health problem in large areas of China where it seems transmission has been stopped for a period of over 10 years (WHO, 2003). Long-term "elimination" programmes have been successful against hydatid disease in Iceland, New Zealand and Cyprus; and malaria was eliminated from Sardinia by DDT spraying as well as in other marginal areas of distribution such as North Africa, Greece and parts of Turkey and the Middle East.

One noticeable feature of these successes is that many examples refer to islands or isolated populations or areas where the parasite is at the edge of its geographical range. Clearly, the advantages of isolation and a greater ability to control animal or human population movements are important. Elimination or global eradication of any disease is difficult to achieve and costs increase per case detected, controlled or averted as the end point is reached.

However, the high cost of eradication or local elimination programmes may be justified as they are time limited, whereas disease control implies a long-term commitment. Any control programme must be cost effective and should reduce the target disease to a level at which costs are sustainable by the local community or by public or private healthcare systems. Control seeks to bring the problems to a level at which the disease is no longer of public health importance with morbidity at an acceptable level within the community, an absence of mortality and, if appropriate, greatly reduced levels of disability. To translate the level of control achieved to eradication or elimination status requires a vastly increased cost per case treated or prevented which, for financial and ecological reasons, may never be feasible or the development of a more effective intervention.

1.3. Components of Control

1.3.1. The Range of Interventions

The spectrum of interventions against parasitic diseases, currently used against parasitic diseases, is summarized in Figure 1 and discussed in detail in the accompanying chapters in the volume.

1.3.2. Control of Animal Reservoir Hosts

Many parasitic diseases are zoonoses, defined as 'those diseases and infections (the agents of) which are naturally transmitted between (other) vertebrate animals and man' (WHO, 1979). A list of recognized parasitic zoonoses is provided by the WHO (1979). Ostfeld and Keesing (2000) provide an up-dated list of vector-borne infections of potential public health importance, while a recent analysis of all emergent and re-emergent infections (Taylor *et al.*, 2001) has identified that 75% of emerging pathogens are zoonotic and that such organisms are more than twice as likely to emerge as non-zoonotic ones. However, viruses and protozoa are more likely to emerge than the macroparasites such as helminths. The important zoonoses for which reservoir host control can have a cost-effective impact are

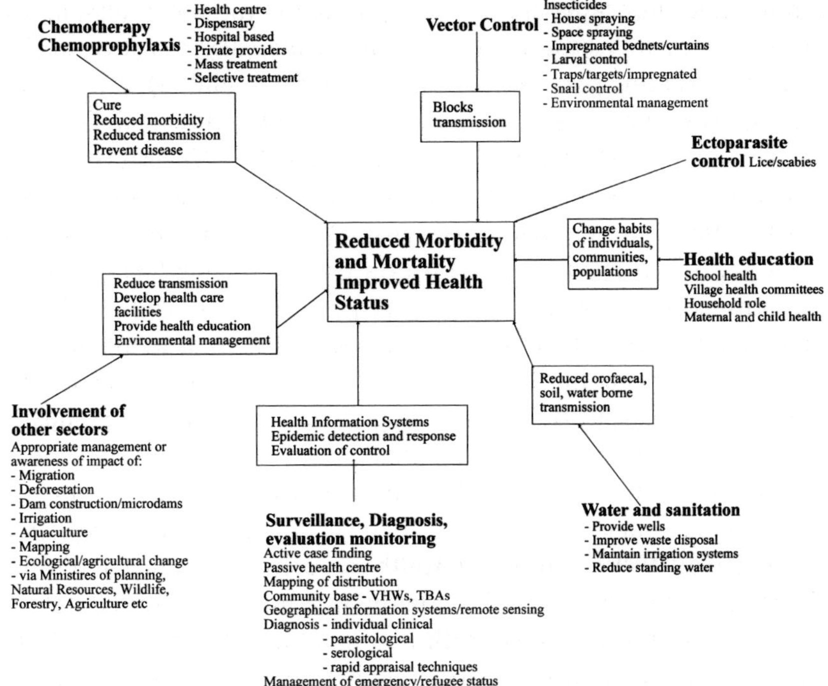

Figure 1   Interventions for the control of parasitic diseases.

leishmaniasis, echinococcosis and cysticercosis; while treatment of cattle with trypanocides in Uganda is a strategy used to reduce the role of cattle as a reservoir of *Trypanosoma rhodesiense* sleeping sickness (Fèvre *et al.*, 2005). However, the presence of an animal reservoir host may be a major impediment to control a disease particularly if the habits and habitats of the animal host prevent the intervention either on the grounds of practicality or for reasons such as protected status of host species e.g. primates or endangered species status. The ITFDE recognizes that the existence of an animal reservoir precludes the likelihood of the eradication of the infection.

1.3.3. *Community Participation in Parasitic Disease Control*

The drive towards primary healthcare following the Alma-Ata declaration of 1978 provoked a greater degree of involvement of communities in healthcare through (1) the use of community leaders to support various programmes; (2) the identification of personnel to undertake health activities on a voluntary basis; and (3) emphasizing the importance of such activities in community well-being. The topic of community participation has been reviewed by Curtis (1991) who provides a series of examples in vector-borne disease control. MacCormack (1991) provides an insight into the underlying principles of sustainable vector control in a community context emphasizing that success in small pilot projects depends on particular characteristics such as leadership; a responsive, well-motivated and well-educated community support; incentives from agencies and insecticide manufacturers; and ease of communication. Following initial success, there is a danger that a 'hot' project will fall into a steady state as enthusiasm and donor support wane while the project life cycle faces inevitable problems. The scaling up of pilot projects to national ones within a primary healthcare context presents additional challenges. For instance, the community may be affected by the replacement of local leaders with national bureaucracy. In establishing a functional link between the communities and the health systems, each group must be trained to understand the social role on the one hand and technical skills on the other. Communities' local knowledge about insects should be exploited to aid in vector control. Appropriate control methods, and the importance of maintaining them, must then be clearly explained to all those involved at the local level.

It must also be established whether unpaid community labour can be sustained over time; although it has been achieved in pilot programmes, doubts exist about longer-term sustainability (Walt, 1988). Much is likely to depend on the community structure and its relationship with those in authority, who are perceived as those most likely to benefit. If, for example, a cost recovery system operates, the volunteers are less able to collect fees from their social superiors. Professional interaction between technicians and volunteers can also fuel conflicts based on perceptions about status.

The outcome of community participation in any project will depend on the numerous complex social interactions existing within the community environment. The interaction between weak and strong groups, and the impact of participation on such group relationships, are of critical importance (Antia, 1988). It is valuable to define the boundaries of the community involved, as individuals tend to identify with a particular locale; this is despite the risk of inherent social instability of villages, resulting from factors such as migration, schooling and marriage. For practical reasons the community is usually defined by a geographical boundary such as an urban neighbourhood or an agricultural village while nomadic groups themselves represent a mobile community.

Communities differ in how they function and are stratified; for example, they may be democratic, autocratic or under military control. In a democratic environment, obtaining consensus may be a slow process, but the likelihood of sustainability will be high. MacCormack concludes that community participation in vector control will be sustainable only if the assessment of the costs to benefits ratio takes account of 'opportunity costs' (the value of activities people would undertake if they had not committed themselves to a particular control activity). Sustainability will be enhanced if activities are linked to the communities' priorities; skills training enhances the communities' well-being; and preventative work links to curative or care outcomes that increase income (Rajagopalan *et al.*, 1987).

Community-based treatments are usually better targeted and tend to involve volunteers, traditional birth attendants (TBAs) and primary healthcare workers. Increasingly, other types of groups are also becoming involved, such as women's groups, faith groups, civil society organizations (CSO) and non-governmental developmental organizations (NGDOs). The NGDO community has become increasingly involved in onchocerciasis control as the programmes in Africa and the Americas have expanded using the donated drug Mectizan® (ivermectin). The momentum for NDGO involvement came from the organizations committed to blindness control who recognized the value of ivermectin as a tool for reducing morbidity associated with onchocercal eye disease (Drameh *et al.*, 2002). NGDOs provide some 25% of the resources required for National Onchocerciasis programmes and 12 international as well as some local NGDOs are active in some 20 countries in Africa through the African Programme for Onchocerciasis Control (APOC) and the countries from the former OCP. The key element of the approach to control is community directed treatment with ivermectin (CDTI), which is regarded as the key driver in ensuring sustainabilitiy of this programme. The progress of the APOC programme is documented in a publication, which highlights the status of these programmes (*Annals of Tropical Medicine and Parasitology, 2002*). Amazigo *et al.* (2002) review the challenges presented by CDTI strategies with an approach based on the principle of community participation but also ensuring empowerment; allowing communities to decide on who should be distributors (CDDs) allowing the planning of ivermectin distribution to be decided by communities e.g. dates, location model of distribution. The replacement of the "Community-directed" approach from a "Community-based" treatment system has been encouraged as the former is likely to be more sustainable, provides community ownership and empowerment and reduces costs to the health system. CDTI enables communities to organize distribution in line with cultural norms and organizational structures—such as kinship and clan structures in Uganda (Katabarwa *et al.*, 2000) while stimulating basic healthcare infrastructure in remote areas (Hopkins, 1998). The experience of the Guinea Worm Eradication programme has led Seim (2005) to identify 10 components to bridge the divide between the systems approach and the disease-specific intervention. He also identifies the criteria for the effective use of volunteers, an approach described as the community-based catalyst to public health. The 10 elements can be summarized as the requirement for a few dedicated individuals, a data manager and a programme manager in each country, the role of a fast non-bureaucratic organization, resident technical advisers, international meetings, regular programme reviews, annual training and retraining of volunteers, network of supervisors, adequate transportation and continuous research for course correction.

1.3.4. Steps in a Control Programme

Components of control are listed under the following headings: (1) situation analysis; (2) definition of objectives and strategy; (3) roles and responsibilities at different levels of health system; (4) planning and resourcing; (5) monitoring and evaluation; and (6) implementation and integration of selected methods of control.

(1) Situation analysis
Stratification of parasitic diseases

Control programmes often involve specific approaches to arrest the transmission of infection (e.g. via vector control) or to prevent or cure a disease. Although such programmes have been successful in the past, integrated approaches are now recognized as being more appropriate for reducing prevalence and incidence. This is important if the strategy is aimed at alleviation of a disease problem in a community or population rather than in an individual. Integrated control is based on coordinated planning and detailed knowledge from many different areas: scientific, technical, inter-sectoral, financing and managerial. An approach termed 'stratification' has been used in malaria control; this means that the strategy is modified according to different epidemiological situations (WHO, 1993). Malaria stratification has been taken a step further by those with particular interests in different environments and geographical regions, a process known as 'microstratification' (Rubio-Palis and Zimmerman, 1997). While stratification has been most widely used in malaria control the concept is equally applicable to other parasitic diseases, for example leishmaniasis (WHO, 1990), onchocerciasis (Boatin *et al.*, 1997), filariasis (WHO, 1992), schistosomiasis and African trypanosomiasis. Molyneux (2005) details in a series of tables, examples of stratification of the epidemiology and its relevance to the planning of control in selected parasitic diseases.

Planning for Control

- Desk study of published and unpublished reports to assess problems in the context of country, region and district.
- Acquisition of information on prevalence and incidence.
- Appraisal of the validity of information.
- Evaluation of current epidemiological situation by passive surveillance at health centers or by use of questionnaires of health workers—for example using the postal system.
- Observation of changes over time and prediction of future change.

- Definition of the structure of health services and their existing capacity, human resources available and needs for training and capacity building.
- The priority afforded to the disease by the government, the MOH, the district management teams and the communities themselves.
- Establishment of linkages to other sectors or organizations in planning for control (e.g. other ministries, development organizations, NGOs).
- The influence of other activities such as development projects on planned programmes.
- Spot surveillance of local prevalence, vectors and, if applicable, animal reservoirs.
- Use of rapid assessment methodologies e.g. for schistosomiasis, onchocerciasis, filariasis or loiasis.
- Assess the available methods for prediction of epidemics using remote sensing or climate prediction available to other sectors, e.g. agriculture, natural resources, environment.
- Establishment of a National Task Force composed of various stakeholder groups to address the problem.

(2) Definition of objectives and strategy

- Analysis of cost effectiveness of different control approaches and options.
- Selection of appropriate methodology and definition of control requirements.
- Establishment of an inventory of personnel and facilities (including estimation of training needs and requirements for equipment and drugs).
- Establishment of feasibility in the context of other health needs.
- Contrasting epidemic ('firefighting') problems when rapid action is required to prevent further transmission (e.g. establish emergency response capacity to address predicted epidemic risk) compared with endemic situations for which a long-term approach and integration are required (Table 2).

(3) Roles and responsibilities of different levels of the health service

Table 2   Role of different levels of the health system in parasitic disease control

---

Community
Identification of suspects/patients
Follow-up of patients
Coordination of any appropriate vector control activities, e.g. bednet distribution to vulnerable
    groups/re-impregnation
Facilitation of cooperation, local logistics for community-directed treatment schemes, e.g. drug
    distribution of ivermectin and albendazole
Communication by Village Health Committees

District
Passive detection and treatment
Parasitological/serological diagnosis
Treatment and clinical care
Follow-up of microscopy

Regional
Active surveillance
Confirmatory diagnosis
Data collection
Technical supervision of vector control
Distribution of reagents and materials for vector control

Ministry and country level
Situation analysis/policy position
National strategy and plan
Establish stakeholder group/National Task Force
Financing
Training needs and responsibility
Health education
Distribution of technical information, equipment, drugs and materials
Purchase of equipment and supplies
Human resource management

---

(4) Planning and resourcing

- Define the expected contribution from the government.
- Develop national plan.
- Evaluate targeted approaches to donors in the context of donor priorities and prevailing national policy.
- Define appropriate timeframes for implementation of plans.
- Define the relationship of the action to overall health plans and budgets.
- Establishment of linkages with appropriate international reference centres for technical support; control of an epidemic may merit application for emergency status to provide rapid funding

(e.g. requests for therapeutic drugs and insecticides from international aid agencies and NGDOs).

- Establishment of drug supply line following identification of sources, initiate quality assurance mechanisms, define tax status of drugs (e.g. donated products).
- Definition of the role of the non-government sector (e.g. private providers, NGOs) in control policy.
- Ensure adequate information exchange about control policy between different bodies and individuals involved in healthcare provision.
- Undertake knowledge, attitudes and practice (KAP) studies as a basis to inform approaches to social mobilization strategies.
- Training (including management training) through courses, instruction of trainers, educational materials and health education programmes.
- Assessment of community acceptability and the perceived priority of any involvement that will require resource input from the communities (e.g. role and views of village health workers (VHWs), volunteers, TBAs, community leaders, school teachers).
- Definition of the management structure of the programme and its relationship with existing management structures.
- Assess capacity available (managerial, financial, technical) and ensure capacity building is embedded in planning.

(5) Monitoring and evaluation

- Assessment of progress towards objectives (prevalence distribution, vector status).
- Establish Sentinel site/baseline data in defined units.
- Definition of appropriate methods for epidemiological evaluation, e.g. parasitological, serological and vector-sampling methods.
- Longitudinal surveys or spot surveys at indicator villages.
- Adjustment of the programme in the light of results.
- Establish process indicators at national and sub-national level.

(6) Implementation and integration of selected methods of control
Chemotherapy and chemoprophylaxis

- Assessment of the availability and quality of drugs and the distribution system.

- Establish relationship between national bodies, donation programmes and NGDO community to define operational relationships, e.g. onchocerciasis, lymphatic filariasis, African trypanosomiasis, schistosomiasis, Trachoma programmes.
- Assessment of, or monitoring for, drug resistance (e.g. East-African network for antimalarial drug resistance).
- Assessment of the role of private providers and control of quality and price (e.g. malaria drug policy).
- Utilization of other systems for distribution (e.g. schools, agricultural extension workers, other health or government workers, NGOs, committees).

Vector and reservoir control

- Availability, cost and appropriateness of insecticides.
- Availability of skills to monitor insecticide resistance.
- Availability and effectiveness of alternative chemicals.
- Capacity for management of the control programme.
- Relationship to other sectors in providing support for environmental control measures.
- Acceptability and feasibility of reservoir control.
- Environmental acceptability of interventions.
- Personal protection, e.g. bednets, sustainability of a bednet programme/retreatment modalities.
- Policy in relation to bednet distribution—vulnerable groups, social marketing.
- Investigate opportunities for integration if appropriate, e.g. malaria and lymphatic filariasis in Africa; dengue and filariasis in the Pacific; leishmaniasis, Chagas disease and malaria via bednets in Latin America.

Environmental management

- Ensuring effective linkages between health and other sectors.
- Assessment of potential impact on other diseases.

Health education, information education communication (IEC), social mobilization

- Media resources, including radio, television and videos.
- Posters and drama sessions oriented around the local environment and traditions.
- Participation of teachers, local leaders, health workers, local medical practitioners, religious leaders.
- Ensure linkage to KAP studies to inform social mobilization strategies.

1.4. Scaling up Control Programmes

Control of a parasitic infection can be focused on the individual, with a view to alleviating pain, reducing disability or avoiding death, while at the same time reducing the parasite load and transmission within a community. Such an approach will be less cost effective than larger-scale control programmes that employ methods such as vector control, reservoir host control or mass drug distribution. Large-scale measures have a public health objective but also provide socioeconomic benefits through improved agricultural productivity, improved cognitive function improved educational prospects, and better nutrition. These benefits accrue as a result of increased and more varied agricultural output and hence diet and enhanced food security. Large scale control will alleviate individual suffering and reduce the community morbidity and mortality thereby providing additional economic opportunities. Control of animal parasitic diseases also has benefits for human populations through increased protein availability and higher income from the sale of higher-quality livestock enhancing both local and national economies. Parasitic disease control programmes vary in scale, but they have generally been targeted at two different types of disease situations (1) the alleviation of an endemic disease in which long-term chronic infections have persisted in communities, e.g. river blindness (onchocerciasis), hydatid disease (*Echinococcus*), schistosomiasis, Guinea worm (dracunculiasis), Chagas disease and filariasis; and (2) the contrasting epidemic situation where rapid intervention is required to prevent widespread morbidity and mortality. Epidemics are frequently predictable, but if health facilities are ill equipped or non-existent, high mortality may occur before control can be instigated despite the technological capacity to predict epidemics of malaria using climate models and remote sensing data (WHO/RBM, 2001).

1.5. Strengthening the Evidence Base

The use of reliable, systematic reviews of evidence of effectiveness to inform policy is becoming recognized as an important contribution to enable resources to be used appropriately. A scientific approach has been developed by systematic reviews of randomized control trials, which provide reliable assessment of the effectiveness of various healthcare interventions. This approach has been promoted, as traditional reviews are unsystematic and do not respect scientific principles or control for biases and random errors. The Cochrane Collaboration approach involves world-wide partners, designed to build on enthusiasm for the process, to minimize duplication, to avoid bias, to maintain an electronic database and to ensure wide access in order to make the information available to decision makers (www.cochrane.org). Molyneux (2005) lists the Cochrane reviews relevant to the control and elimination of parasitic diseases.

2. THE HEALTH POLICY ENVIRONMENT

Disease control, elimination or eradication activities must be implemented in the context of broader health policy issues and the requirements for prioritization, which confront resource constrained health systems. There has been an increased political awareness of health issues in poor populations over the past decade with an increasing commitment to poverty alleviation as the core component of agreed international development targets and millennium development goals (MDGs) (WHO, 2005a). The publication of the report of the Millennium project provided a detailed analysis of the progress towards the attainment of the MDGs (Sachs, 2004; Haines and

Cassels, 2004; Sachs and MacArthur, 2005). In addition, there have also been changes in international organization policy and focus generated by changed leadership. There have been a series of initiatives of the World Health Organization (WHO) which recognize the need for broadly based partnerships for health development such as Roll Back Malaria (RBM), Stop TB (2002) and the 3×5 initiative to respond to the problems of HIV/AIDS and in the NCDs the Tobacco-Free Initiative. The establishment of the Global Fund to specifically address the problems of HIV/AIDS, TB and Malaria (Global Fund to fight AIDS, TB and malaria (GFATM)) following the initiative of the UN Secretary General has raised awareness of the relentless problems of these diseases. However, even the Global Fund resources will have limited impact against the estimated needs of HIV/AIDS, TB and malaria control which is an annual figure of around US$10 billion (www.theglobalfund.org). This is also an open-ended commitment as there is currently little impact on transmission of these diseases (Molyneux *et al.*, 2005); without an impact on incidence these diseases will continue to increase as public health problems, hence the need for efficacious preventative interventions such as stable, easy-to-administer vaccines.

2.1. Health Financing and Sector-Wide Approaches

New approaches to donor funding of health in poor countries the "sector wide approach to financing" (sector-wide approaches (SWAPs)) (Cassels, 1997) has been instituted particularly in African countries to enable a more coordinated approach to financing; this prevents donors from influencing, via special projects, overall national health policy and plans. SWAPs should provide for increased coordination in the health sector, stronger leadership and improved management and delivery systems. As Hutton and Tanner (2004) assert this should reduce duplication, lower transaction costs, increase equity and sustainability and improve effectiveness and efficiency of health-targeted aid. This approach-so-called "basket" funding recognizes that ownership rests with the country, that donors all contribute to the "basket", that, once committed, control of resources is lost, that priorities are established through policy dialogue and that partnership relations are strengthened. The SWAPs approach is also layered onto the increasing decentralization of national budgets to district-level management in many countries. However, the approaches of SWAPs to discourage project or disease-specific funding appears at odds with the approaches of the Global Fund where disease-specific projects and programmes are part of the application process. In addition, Hutton and Tanner (2004) have pointed that there is a limited evidence base, despite some 10 years experience, that SWAP support has impacted on improved health outcomes; such evidence is urgently required. In contrast to disease-specific interventions where strategies are based on effective monitoring of scientific information, to guide the interventions the policies which are designed to strengthen the health system may not achieve the desired outcomes in ever-changing political, social, economic and environmental settings.

Over recent years, large international NGDOs have become increasingly active in disease-control implementation and policy. Medecins Sans Frontierés (MSF), Save the Children (SCF), Oxfam and others have been vociferous on issues of equity and access to drugs often criticizing "vertical" programmes and drug donations. Notwithstanding policy papers introduced by NGDOs, MSF for example has driven the establishment of the Drugs for Neglected Disease initiative (DNDi) which should recognize that in many circumstances drugs for the diseases DNDi targets-the trypanosomiases, and leishmaniases require delivery through disease-specific treatments based on the availability of the necessary medical knowledge and with the requirement for clinical management. While over the last three decades the UNDP/World Bank/World Health Organization Special Programme for Research in Tropical Diseases (TDR) has played a prominent role with many partners in bringing new drugs into widespread use. Such treatment-based interventions respond to clinical need but have a limited impact on transmission-approaches which do not fit easily into the SWAPs, decentralization and health sector reform for diseases such as trypanosomiasis or leishmaniasis.

In attempts to increase resources for health, models have emerged such as the "Bamako Initiative" to raise money through imposing user fees to create revolving funds at the periphery of the health system, insurance systems have been introduced, while macrofinancing to provide overall budget support for the social sector has been promoted through policies such as the Heavily Indebted Poor Countries (HIPC) initiative, Poverty Reduction Strategy Papers (PSRP) and more recently by debt cancellation agreements.

There has been increasing recognition that infectious diseases are more prevalent and inflict a greater burden of disease on the poorest quintile of the population. The poorest 20% however would benefit proportionately more if there was a pro-poor focus in tackling infectious diseases compared with other health interventions (Gwatkin *et al.*, 1999).

2.2. Public–Private Partnerships

There has been a dramatic expansion of the number PPPs in health over the last decade. These developments are summarized by Widdus (2001, 2005) who identifies around 100 such initiatives. The diversity of objectives, financing, governance, legal status and management of these alliances prevents significant generalizations about best practice and how lessons can be learned as most of the alliances/partnerships are disease or product development specific. Widdus (2005) recognizes two main groups of PPPs, those dealing with product development and those concerned with access to medicines or drugs for mass distribution to target populations (Access PPPs). Some partnerships also act as global coordinating mechanisms. Croft (2005) provides case studies of the most prominent product development PPPs. These partnerships have often been funded by long-term commitments from donors, through drug donations, from the private sector and by a recognition that relatively cheap interventions can be sustained by health systems and bring long-term health benefits. Analysis of these partnerships have also been carried out by Buse and Walt (2000a, b) and Buse and Waxman (2001). Table 3 lists partnerships relevant to parasitic disease control. The major characteristic of most PPPs is the interaction between the public, private and civil society (NGDOs, academia) sectors. The establishment of the Bill and

Table 3 Public–private partnerships and alliances in control of parasitic diseases

---

African Programme for Onchocerciasis Control (APOC)
Onchocerciasis Control Programme (OCP) (1974–2002)
Onchocerciasis Elimination Programme in the Americas (OEPA)
Roll Back Malaria Partnership (RBM, WHO, Geneva)
Multilateral Initiative on Malaria (MIM)
Malaria Vaccine Initiative (MVI)
Medicines for Malaria Venture (MMV)
Global Alliance to Eliminate Lymphatic Filariasis (GAELF)
Global School Health Initiative
WHO Partnership for Parasite Control (PPC)
Drugs for Neglected Disease Initiative (DNDi)
Global Alliance for African Human Trypanosomiasis (WHO, Geneva)
Guinea Worm Eradication Programme (Global 2000)
Institute for One World Health (IOWH) (San Francisco, California)
Diseases of the Most Impoverished (DOMI) (Seoul Korea)
Human Hookworm Vaccine Initiative (HHVI) (Washington, DC)
Infectious Diseases Research Institute (Seattle, Washington)

Melinda Gates Foundation as a key player in Global Health has also greatly enhanced the opportunities for research and partnership interaction and development. However, an often understated factor in these relationships is the time required specifically for partnership management to ensure regular communication between partners and enhance the added value of the whole as opposed to the component entities.

2.3. The Global Burden of Parasitic Diseases

The World Development Report (World Bank, 1993), introduced the concept of the Global Burden of Disease expressed as the Disability Adjusted Life Years (DALYs) lost. This measure has been expanded enabling an assessment of likely change in global disease burden between 1990 and 2020 (Murray and Lopez, 1996). These projections suggest that as a proportion of global disease burden only malaria remains a significant burden as a parasitic infection. Malaria falls in Global Burden importance from a ranking of 11th to a predicted 26th over this period. The majority of the projected change in Global burden is in the increased burden of NCDs such as cerebrovascular events, depressive illness, conflict-related conditions, road traffic accidents and cancers (WHO, 2005b). The DALY burden of parasitic disease is projected to remain largely stable, while the surge of NCD burden due to the epidemiological transition, diet and life style change associated with urbanization, substance abuse, environmental degradation, population growth and increased conflict are projected to be proportionally greater contributions. The DALYs burden and overall public health importance of major parasitic disease is given in Table 4. However, a recent meta analysis of disability due to schistosomiasis has demonstrated there is a significant and underestimated burden of subtle morbidity due to anaemia, chronic pain, diarrhoea, reduced exercise tolerance and malnutrition (King *et al.*, 2005). This subtle morbidity is likely to apply to other diseases in the neglected cluster as pointed out by Savioli *et al.* (2005) who call for the reassessment of the overall burden in view of potential gains which can be achieved by reducing this burden through cheap regular delivery of anthelmintics.

The impact of financing and policies in public sectors of developing country economies such as education, agriculture, transport, natural resources has a significant impact on health outcomes; of particular importance will be levels of investment and achievement of education targets in an attempt to provide universal primary education by 2015 in the context of the Millennium Development Goals (WHO, 2005a); the importance of increasing the proportion of females in primary education will be of particular significance in achieving targets of reducing maternal, child and infant mortality. In the agricultural sector productivity, efficiency and diversity will have a major impact on nutrition and food security particularly in regions dependent on rain-fed agriculture at a time of increasingly unpredictable weather patterns and climate uncertainty (Patz *et al.*, 2005).

2.4. "Neglected" Tropical Disease Initiatives and the Integration of Control

2.4.1. Integrated Control

Recent publications argue for the integration of vertical control activities into a more integrated approach (Molyneux and

Table 4 Public health importance of selected human parasitic infections (see Remme *et al.*, 2002; Hotez *et al.*, 2006)

	Population at risk (m)	No. of endemic countries	No. of infected/ prevalence (m)	Estimated deaths mortality/y humans × 1000	Total DALYs (m)
Malaria	2000	90	300–500	1080	46.5
Leishmaniasis	350	82	12	41	2.1
Lymphatic filariasis	750	65	119	No direct mortality	5.8
Guinea worm	140	18	c. 120 000	No direct mortality	
Onchocerciasis	122	34	17.6	No direct mortality	0.5
African trypanosomiasis	50	36	20 000–300 000	50	1.5
Chagas disease	90	19	16	21	7
Schistosomiasis	500–600	74	200	11	4.5
Ascaris			1000		10.5
Trichuris			900		6.4
Hookworm			500		22.1
Entamoeba			500	40–100	NA
Giardia			200		NA
Taeniasis	40		15		NA
Neurocystocercosis			50	50	NA
Food-borne trematodes			500		NA
Fascioliasis	180.25	8	2.39		NA
Clonorchiasis	289.26	6	7.0		NA
Opisthorchiasis	63.6	5	10.3		NA
Paragonimiasis	194.8	5	20.6		NA
Other intestinal flukes		6	1.28		NA

NA = not available

Nantulya, 2004). Four drugs, albendazole, Mectizan®, azithromax and praziquantel, if given to communities once a year would have a significant impact on lymphatic filariasis, onchocerciasis, hookworm, trichuriasis, ascariasis, schistosomiasis and trachoma in areas where the diseases are co-endemic particularly in sub-Saharan Africa and focal regions of the Americas. In much of Africa individuals are polyparasitized; with three gastrointestinal worms, filarial parasites in the skin and/or blood, malaria and intestinal protozoan parasites (Raso *et al.*, 2004; Hotez *et al.*, 2006). These four drugs can be delivered through existing mechanisms and such integrated control approaches have the potential to eliminate morbidity and blindness from these diseases at a fraction of the cost needed to control other diseases (Molyneux *et al.*, 2005).

The Commission for Africa (www.commissionforafrica.org) and the Millennium Project reporting on the progress towards the achievement of the Millennium Development Goals recognized the importance of these neglected infections in their 2005 report. Fenwick *et al.* (2005) calculated that some 500 million people living in communities endemic for these diseases in Africa could be treated with all the four drugs at a cost of $200 million annually, or $0.40 per patient if these resources were allocated as a package, particularly as multinational corporations like Merck Co. Inc., GSK and Pfizer are committed to long-term donations of three of the four drugs, Mectizan®, albendazole and azithromax, respectively. Molyneux *et al.* (2005) have compared these costs with the published costs of treatment of HIV/AIDS, tuberculosis and malaria per person annually. Figures for antiretrovirals alone reach $200, TB costs around the same figure in Africa while malaria can cost the poorest families some 30% of the annual household expenditure in Malawi imposing a huge burden on the poorest families (Ettling *et al.*, 1994). Despite high unit costs, the current curative approaches to the big three diseases are "reactive" strategies. The treatment of individuals infected with HIV/AIDS, TB and malaria fails to significantly reduce transmission while there is significant interaction between the diseases themselves in co-infected patients. In seeking to combat the big three diseases, decision makers, policy makers and donors should consider supporting a programme of "rapid impact interventions", an approach that would bring real benefit to millions suffering disablement, poverty and ill health. This would enable the treatment of poor people more equitably, by providing such polyparasitized populations with effective and cheap interventions that would reduce stigma and disability, as well as reduce morbidity and mortality, thus reaching the MDGs quickly and cost effectively.

2.4.2. Evidence for the Value of Integrated Control

As noted elsewhere there are several major PPPs committed in Africa to elimination or control programme addressing a specific tropical disease. These PPPs often operate in parallel, using drugs deployed over wide areas and among large populations. Currently, four drugs, albendazole, ivermectin (Mectizan), praziquantel and azithromycin (Zithromax) are being used to target more than one hundred million people in around 30 countries (Hotez *et al.*, 2006). Such partnerships have a role in strengthening health systems (Amazigo *et al.*, 2002). The most prominent example being APOC which has established a successful community-directed treatment initiative, providing an entry point for other community-directed health interventions in regions where there is little access to traditional health services (Homeida *et al.*, 2002).

The tropical diseases in Africa exhibit considerable geographical overlap and hence, in many cases, show extensive co-endemicity (Molyneux *et al.*, 2005). There is significant value in exploring whether a drug employed by a vertical programme that targets one condition could also be used to simultaneously impact on some of the others. A significant number of school-aged children in Africa are polyparasitized with three different soil-transmitted helminths (STHs) (*Ascaris*, *Trichuris* and hookworm), early filarial infections and schistosomes, who could be simultaneously treated with three drugs, Mectizan, albendazole and praziquantel (Loukas and Hotez, 2006; Raso *et al.*, 2004). In 2001, the 54th World Health Assembly urged its member states to undertake frequent and periodic deworming with praziquantel together with either albendazole or mebendazole as a means to control and reduce the morbidity in this paediatric age group (www.who.int/wormcontrol) while more recently an editorial highlighted the opportunities of deworming for development (Lancet, 2004), the Millennium project listed regular deworming as one of the quick wins towards the MDGs, while the Commission for Africa recommended "donors should ensure that there is adequate funding for the treatment of parasitic diseases and micronutrient deficiency. Governments and global health partnerships should ensure that this is integrated into public health campaigns by 2006".

The Schistosomiasis Control Initiative, a PPP based in London supporting control in Uganda, Tanzania, Zambia, Mali, Niger and Burkina Faso, adds albendazole to its praziquantel regimen (www.schisto.org). Similarly, the major drugs used for lymphatic filariasis and onchocerciasis control, ivermectin and albendazole (www.filariasis.org), have significant impact on the STH where albendazole is the drug of choice. Ivermectin also has a significant anthelmintic effect on *Ascaris* and *Trichuris* infections, and is the drug of choice for the treatment of human strongyloidiasis.

More recently, selective mass treatment with ivermectin has been shown to also reduce the prevalence of ectoparasitic skin infections such as pediculosis, scabies and tungiasis as well as cutaneous larva migrans (Heukelbach *et al.*, 2004).

2.4.3. *The Cost-Effectiveness of Parasite Control*

The economic rates of return (ERR) when they have been calculated suggest investment in control/elimination of these diseases produces an ERR of between 15–30%, and are capable of delivery on a large scale (Molyneux, 2004). The potential synergies in collateral benefits delivered using the four drugs as mentioned in Section 1.3.1 is appropriate as they often have compatible approaches to delivery. The numbers requiring treatment for each of these infections, the unit drug price (if applicable) and the estimated total delivery costs of treating these chronic-disabling conditions in sub-Saharan Africa. Such interventions, are pro-poor, are based on safe, efficacious drugs that reach a high coverage of the target population, are known to be cost effective, and do not, as yet, have any associated drug resistance (Albonico *et al.*, 2004). They can be delivered through community directed approaches, school health programmes, the World Food Programme, school feeding programme, or NGDO supplementary feeding and nutrition programmes usually on an annual basis (www.wfp.org).

2.4.4. Scaling Up Integrated Control

A number of issues require to be addressed before integrated control of neglected tropical diseases can be implemented on a large scale. For example, the final costs of an integrated package may need to include the costs of drug use monitoring and of developing new tools for neglected disease control. In some areas neither mebendazole nor ivermectin are highly effective against hookworm, the most common STH in Africa, especially when these drugs are used in a single dose (Loukas and Hotez, 2006). Moreover, the rate of post-treatment hookworm infection is high, and there is additional evidence that the efficacy of benzimidazole anthelmintics diminishes even further with frequent and periodic use—there are therefore some concerns about the possibility of emerging resistance, which is now common for STHs that infect livestock (Albonico *et al.*, 2004). Therefore, additional costs must be considered in order to promote ongoing research and development for new neglected diseases control tools.

An equally important challenge will be to determine the actual feasibility of integrating six different vertical control programmes. There are currently disparities between the groups targeted for lymphatic filariasis and onchocerciasis control (treatment is excluded for children under 90 cm and pregnant women in 2nd and 3rd trimester) and the groups targeted for STH and schistosome control (control is primarily aimed at school-aged children, but WHO encourages treatment of pregnant women and children above the age of 12 months). Pilot studies will be necessary to identify common age groups for integrated control. While the partnerships themselves require to cooperate on disease control efforts and integrate their activities to reduce costs and enhance efficiency.

2.4.5. Defining End Points for Integrated Control

In the case of *Ascaris, Trichuris* and schistosome infections, the major goal is a sustainable reduction in worm burden and control of morbidity, while for lymphatic filariasis, onchocerciasis and trachoma, the major goals are to reduce or eliminate transmission resulting in much reduced morbidity in future generations. The externalities of these two goals are considerable and include improved education, and economic productivity. The calculated annual loss of US $1 billion from lymphatic filariasis in India (Ramiah *et al.*, 2000) and $5.3 billion from blinding trachoma while substantial reductions in future wage-earning capacity as a result of chronic hookworm infection in childhood, illustrates the burden and costs of these diseases to poor individuals and communities. An added externality emphasizes the immunosuppressive effects of helminths, and their possible impact on promoting susceptibility to HIV-AIDS, tuberculosis and malaria (Fincham *et al.*, 2003). The control of helminth infections has been suggested as a means to reduce the burden of malaria by reducing the frequency of malaria fevers, the frequency of severe and cerebral malaria, and the prevalence of anaemia (Speigel *et al.*, 2003; Le Hesran *et al.*, 2004; Sockna *et al.*, 2004; Druilhe *et al.*, 2005), although a recent study concludes *S. haematobium* infections are protective against *P. falciparum* in children in Mali (Lyke *et al.*, 2005).

3. PARASITIC DISEASES: NEW AND OLD CHALLENGES

3.1. Emerging Diseases

The problem of emerging diseases (defined by either new infections of humans or re-emerging ones where a rapid increase in incidence of an existing infection or in a new geographical area) has been a significant concern as new viruses such as SARS, Avian influenza and Ebola virus have been identified. In the USA, potential epidemics of West Nile Fever and the recognition of Lyme Disease and Hanta virus have alerted authorities to previously unidentified threats. As a result, considerable additional resources have become available for research on such emerging agents. Recent quantitative analysis of the risk of emergence allied to the nature of the organisms, their mode of transmission and source have been provided by Taylor *et al.* (2001). They note that viruses, bacteria and protozoa are more likely to emerge than macroparasites (e.g. helminths), that around 75% of emergent organisms are from zoonotic sources and that emergences are independent of the mode of transmission. It should be noted however that despite the emphasis in some circles of the importance of such agents they are not predicted to play a significant role in the Global Burden of Disease estimates as a proportion of Global DALYs.

Such conclusions are based on the current definition of species. However, the capacity to identify "species complexes/groups" and the level of intraspecies variation is becoming apparent as a result of molecular analyses. The development of the discipline of molecular epidemiology, which has been applied to vectors and causative parasites, clearly suggests that the absolute numbers of genetically distinct parasites and vectors irrespective of sub-specific variation is much greater than hitherto recognized emphasizing the degree of biodiversity in microorganisms and its importance in the strategies of parasite and vector control (Yameogo *et al.*, 2004).

3.2. Climate Change

The suggestions that Global Climate Change will have a widespread impact on health as mean temperatures rise over the next decades have provoked studies on the projected change in distribution of vector-borne infections (Patz *et al.*, 2005). It is generally agreed from different climate models that the mean rise of temperature over the next 100 years will be of the order of 2–4 °C. The impact of these changes particularly on the distribution of *Plasmodium falciparum* malaria has been projected by various groups (IPCC, 2001; Rogers and Randolph, 2000; Hay *et al.*, 2002) although little consensus is available (Patz *et al.*, 2002; McMichael and Le Sueur, 2002). In addition, the role of El-Niño events have been studied which have been identified with a change in epidemic patterns in different regions of several vector-borne infections (dengue in Indonesia; malaria in most of Africa, Colombia and India) (Bouma *et al.*, 1997).

3.3. Epidemics of Parasitic Diseases

Anthropogenic and environmental changes frequently result in epidemics of parasitic disease. Several reviews have identified the primary drivers of these changes (Molyneux, 1997, 2003; Patz *et al.*, 2004). These are

1. Movements of non-immune populations in areas where transmission occurs; such movements may be of an organized nature, e.g. mobilization of the workforce in Brazil to exploit forest resources has resulted in malaria epidemics. Alternatively, they may occur without formal organization, e.g. movements of workers involved in mining for gold or gems in the Amazon and South East Asia.

2. Climatic changes, e.g. temperature change is considered to be a cause of highland malaria in Kenya and Ethiopia. Unusual levels of rainfall following periods of drought result in epidemics of malaria in East and South Africa.

3. Urbanization results in populations being exposed to new organisms, vectors establish in new habitats and peri-domestic reservoirs act as the source of infection. Health services are grossly inadequate or non-existent and service providers are often only NGDOs or faith groups.

4. Change in vegetation such as the growth of thickets of the plant *Lantana* in Uganda, which provided a habitat for *Glossina fuscipes*, provoking epidemics of Rhodesian sleeping sickness. Another example is deforestation, which has resulted in exposure to leishmaniasis in the Amazon and malaria in South-East Asia (Walsh *et al.*, 1993).

5. Development projects particularly those involving water resource development themselves frequently exacerbate the health problems of the local or incoming population (Birley, 1995; Hunter and Rey, 1993; Erlanger *et al.*, 2005; Keiser *et al.*, 2005).

6. Conflict, civil unrest and associated population disruption have profound impacts on parasitic diseases. Epidemics are frequently associated with such events; those organisms which have a rapid capacity for adaptation and reproduction and are associated with vectors which have characteristics as generalists are more prone to create health problems in conflict environments (Molyneux, 1997, 2003). Table 5 lists recently documented conflict-related changes in parasitic disease epidemiology.

7. Agricultural development projects particularly associated with irrigated agriculture and development of monocultures are associated with changed patterns of insect-borne infections particularly malaria (Ijumba and Lindsay, 2001), leishmaniasis and schistosomiasis (Patz *et al.*, 2004). A recent review (Keiser and Utzinger, 2005) on food-borne trematode infections (*Clonorchis, Opisthorchis, Paragonimus, Fasciola* and *Fasciolopsis*) has suggested that the growth of aquaculture is the major risk factor in the emergence of food-borne trematode diseases as public health problems in particular in South Asia; whilst Lun *et al.* (2005) has emphasized the importance of Clonorchiasis as one of the leading causes of cancers in this region.

Common themes that appear to operate in the above settings are expressed in Tables 6–8 (Molyneux, 2003).

Epidemics are provoked as stated above by ecological, climatic and environmental change, urbanization, human population movement resulting from civil unrest and conflict, reduced surveillance and drug or insecticide resistance. It is recommended by policy makers that health systems are restructured to include: a generalized 'horizontal' pattern of healthcare; insurance systems and user charges; and decentralization of management to district level (or equivalent). Such restructuring reduces the ability of the system to respond to factors that lead to epidemics. It must be borne in mind that the so-called "vertical" parasitic disease control activities, such as onchocerciasis control, lymphatic filariasis, Chagas disease and Guinea worm eradication programmes, have been remarkably successful (Molyneux, 2004) producing economic rates of return of between 15% and 30% which is regarded as being compatible with the best available

Table 5 Conflict-related change in parasitic diseases

Diseases	Changes
Sleeping sickness (African trypanosomiasis)	
Trypanosoma brucei gambiense	Epidemics in Democratic Republic of Congo (DRC) and Angola associated with destruction/disruption of health services (Ekwanzala *et al.*, 1996). Epidemics spread in north-western Uganda following conflict-related migration from Sudan
Trypanosoma b. rhodesiense	Disruption of cotton and coffee production in Busoga during the Amin regime resulted in spread of *Lantana,* providing breeding sites for *Glossina fuscipes* and initiating transmission of acute sleeping sickness in peri-domestic environments, with cattle acting as reservoir hosts; restocking following cattle raiding induced epidemics following importations of infected cattle (Fèvre *et al.*, 2001, 2005)
Visceral Leishmaniasis	Epidemics of *Leishmania donovani* in southern Sudan; a changed ecological situation, associated with an increase in *Phlebotomus orientalis* populations in maturing *Acacia/Balanites* woodland, initially provoked the epidemics, which were left largely uncontrolled because of the civil war, migration of infected populations, and scarcity of treatment centres and availability of drugs (Ashford and Thomson, 1991; Seaman *et al.*, 1992)
Cutaneous Leishmaniasis *Leishmania tropica* *Leishmania major*	Resurgence of *L. tropica* in Afghanistan (Kabul) following an increase in urban population density of non-immunes because of conflict (Ashford *et al.*, 1992)
Refugee camps in Africa	Movement of populations to Khartoum, because of conflict and drought, and establishment of transmission amongst peri-urban reservoir of non-immunes living in shanties.
Malaria	
Refugee camps in Afghanistan and Pakistan	Refugee populations settled at lower altitude, in sites with relatively high rainfall; refugees with inadequate immunity or exposed to different strains of *Plasmodium falciparum*; absence of drugs and no control of *Anopheles*; malaria epidemics in camps (controlled by spraying tents to control *A. stephensi* and *A. culicifacies*), exacerbated by increase in prevalence of *Plasmodium falciparum*

Table 5 (*continued*)

Diseases	Changes
Cambodia	Mass deportation of urban non-immunes to forced labour in rice fields and forests; conscription for construction of defences in border areas where multi-drug-resistant malaria commonly occurs
Onchocercaisis	
Sierra Leone	Weekly aerial larviciding against *Simulium* suspended because of security problems and local conflict. Levels of transmission consequently increased
Guinea Bissau	Civil unrest prevented the distribution of Mectizan with consequent resurgence in incidence (Borsboom *et al.*, 2003). Suspension or reduction of ivermectin distribution because of conflict.
Sudan and Sierra Leone	
DRC, Central African Republic, Liberia and Angola	Planning of programme for community-directed distribution of ivermectin retarded by the collapse of national structures; remaining (passive) distribution by non-governmental donors.
Dracunculasis	
Ghana	Increase in reported cases 1 year after local conflict failed to contain cases from the previous year
Sudan	The civil war prevented adequate case-finding, case-containment, water-supply control and filter distribution (Hopkins *et al.*, 2002)

development investments (Benton and Skinner, 1990). Because of the complexity of the biological systems inherent in parasitic infections, such diseases are not amenable to control by a strictly "horizontal" health system approach.

However, there is an ever-increasing recognition that integration of disease control programmes, particularly those which involve regular chemotherapy, will be cost effective and produce significant synergies, collateral benefits and externality benefits e.g. in improved educational performance and school attendance (Miguel and Kremer, 2001; Molyneux and Nantulya, 2004; Molyneux *et al.*, 2005). These approaches, largely preventative chemotherapy, are extremely low

Table 6 Common themes associated with changing vector-borne parasitic diseases

Epidemics are often associated with generalist vectors (see Table 7)
Animal reservoirs or mixing vessels are associated as food sources for such vectors
Animal reservoirs may be domestic, wild animals or intensively reared species
Reduced biodiversity (often associated with 7 and 8 below) encourages expansion of adaptable generalist vectors and reservoirs
Ratios of *P. vivax:P. falciparum* change with increasing *P. falciparum*
Extractive activities (uncontrolled) generate the development of anti-malaria resistance
Water resource development (dams, microdams, irrigation, aquaculture) generates change in vector-borne disease patterns over variable time frames
Malaria and Japanese encephalitis—Acute
Schistosomiasis/dracunculaisis—Medium
Filariasis—Chronic/long term
Deforestation/reafforestation impacts on vector-borne infections via behaviour of human, reservoirs and vectors through edge/interface effects/fragmentation patterns, degree and type of reafforestation, loss of biodiversity, loss of forest eliminating vector species common pattern of change occurring within different vector complexes

Table 7 Characteristics of generalist vectors

Wide geographical distribution
Species complexes or species groups
Capacity to feed on a range of available hosts
Capacity for zoophily and anthropophily
Ability to exploit peri-domestic and peri-urban settings
Ability to exploit new pre-imaginal habitats
Efficient vectors with high vectorial capacity
No transovarial transmission

cost compared with the costs of treating some of the higher-profile infections such as HIV/AIDS, TB and even malaria. Fenwick *et al.* (2005) calculate the costs of annual chemotherapy for polyparasitized populations of 500 million in sub-Saharan Africa as US$0.40; if this intervention was integrated effectively, a group of diseases could be tackled permanently reducing transmission, in some cases to the point of elimination and reducing morbidity in others. Molyneux *et al.* (2005) compare the costs of this intervention approach with costs of treatment of TB and HIV/AIDS and recommend a different approach by policy makers given the available interventions for these diseases which barely impact on the transmission hence

Table 8 Examples of changes in *Plasmodium falciparum:P. vivax* ratios associated with anthropogenic change (conflict; irrigation; mining)

	Projected changes	Reference
Tajikistan	Health systems disruption, conflict migration, chloroquine resistance in *P. falciparum*	Pitt *et al.* (1998)
Afghanistan/Pakistan	Chloroquine resistance in *P. falciparum*	Rowland and Nosten (2001)
Sri Lanka, Mahaweli	Irrigation on large scale	Amerasinghe and Indrajith (1994)
Thar Desert, Rajasthan, India	Irrigation on large scale. Establishment of A*nopheles culcifacies* efficient *P. falciparum* vector and dominance over *An. stephensi* a poor vector	Tyagi and Chaudhary (1997)
Amazonia, Brazil	New breeding sites for efficient vectors *An. darlingi* through mining, deforestation, road building	Marques (1987)

regrettably there will be increasing incidence with no diminution of the pressure to apply and react to demands for treatment.

It is also important to distinguish between the control of an organism (parasite, vector or ectoparasite) at the level of the individual and at the level of the community. An example of the paradox (individual vs. community) is the conflict between the treatment of individual patients compared with the need to control or eliminate which requires large-scale community involvement.

The changing health policy environment has been emphasized, because it is important to recognize that approaches to control are dependent on an accurate knowledge of the totality of the problem. This requires biological, medical, epidemiological and social science inputs to define the aetiology (causative organisms), the vectors (if vector-borne), the parameters and the mode of transmission (e.g. vector-borne, water-borne, aerosol, orofaecal, venereal). Systems of surveillance, monitoring and evaluation are required to define prevalence and trends of infection and disease. Without such information a control programme cannot be appropriately designed and implemented. Biological information needs to be supplemented by consideration of issues such as logistics; cost effectiveness; potential for integration within existing programmes; past successes or failures; input from governmental sectors other than health (agriculture, forestry, education, water, other natural resources, wildlife); acceptability of an intervention to the target communities; potential for ecological damage; priority rating afforded by the Ministry of Health (MOH); availability of human resources for implementation; and potential of research to provide improved products within a particular timescale.

4. CONCLUSIONS

This chapter provides the broader context and overview in which the specific disease control, elimination or eradication interventions are positioned within Ministries of Health and the underlying principles which govern such activities. Many interventions while strongly supported by government require extensive donor support if they are to succeed while other programmes operate and have been successful by the effective management and resourcing directly from allocated and identified budgets over many years. These have been vertical approaches in middle-income countries to solve particular disease problems and have not been incorporated in the general health programmes at district or sub-district level where the specialist skills are not available. There have been significant successes in driving some infections in local often isolated environments to elimination with only a limited need for future resources for evaluation and monitoring to ensure there is no recrudescence. The individual chapters in this volume provide detailed reviews of diseases and identify progress needs and prospects for control or even eradication. The reality remains that parasites remain a significant and unacceptable burden particularly in the poor and neglected populations of the least-developed countries. The increased global awareness of the problems of the poor and the clear link between poor health and poverty provides the opportunities for these diseases to be more widely recognized. The establishment of the GFATM but particularly the report of the Commission for Africa and the UN Millennium project identified parasitic diseases in Africa as an impediment to development. There is a need for either development research to develop more effective, affordable and accessible drugs or simply to provide access to highly effective drugs, some of which are donated via generous pharmaceutical companies for as long as needed at the cost of simply annual or biannual delivery. These are the "quick wins" or rapid interventions. The challenge in the latter case does not depend on science but on the prioritization of resources towards implementation and the evaluation and assessment of the development impact of such interventions against the overwhelming burden of health needs in the poorest countries.

REFERENCES

Albonico, M., Engels, D. and Savioli, L. (2004). Monitoring drug efficacy and early detection of drug resistance in human soil-transmitted nematodes: a pressing public health agenda for helminth control. *International Journal for Parasitology* **34**, 1205–1210.

Amazigo, U., Brieger, W.R., Katabarwa, M., Akogun, O., Ntep, M., Boatin, B., N'Dyoyo, J., Noma, M. and Seketeli, A. (2002). The challenges of community directed treatment with ivermectin (CDTI) within the African Programme for Onchocerciasis Control (APOC). *Annals of Tropical Medicine and Parasitology* **96**(supplement 1), 41–58.

Amerasinghe, F.P. and Indrajith, N.G. (1994). Post irrigation breeding patterns of surface water mosquitoes in the Mahaweli Project, Sri Lanka and comparisons with preceding developmental phases. *Journal of Medical Entomology* **4**, 516–523.

Annals of Tropical Medicine and Parasitology. (2002). The African Programme for Onchocerciasis (APOC) at mid point: history, achievements and Future Challenges **96**(supplement 1), S3–S106.

Antia, N.H. (1988). The Mandwa Project: an experiment in community participation. *International Journal of Health Services* **18**, 153–164.

Ashford, R.W., Kohestany, K.A. and Karimzad, M.A. (1992). Cutaneous leishmaniasis in Kabul: observations on a prolonged epidemic. *Annals of Tropical Medicine and Parasitology* **86**, 361–371.

Ashford, R.W. and Thomson, M. (1991). Visceral Leishmaniasis in Sudan. A delayed development disaster. *Annals of Tropical Medicine and Parasitology* **85**, 571–572.

Benton, B. and Skinner, E. (1990). Cost benefits of onchocerciasis control. *Acta Leidensia* **59**, 405–411.

Birley, M.H. (1995). *The Health Impact Assessment of Development Projects.* London: HMSO.

Boatin, B., Molyneux, D.H., Hougard, J.-M., Christensen, O., Alley, E.S., Yameogo, L., Seketeli, A. and Dadzie, K.Y. (1997). Patterns of epidemiology and control of onchocerciasis in West Africa. *Journal of Helminthology* **71**, 71–101.

Borsboom, G.J.J.M., Boatin, B., Nagelkerke, N.J.D., Agoua, H., Komlan, L.B., Akpoboua, E., et al. (2003). Impact of ivermectin on onchocerciasis transmission: assessing the empirical evidence that repeated ivermectin mass treatments may lead to elimination/eradication in West Africa. *Filaria Journal* **2**, 8.

Bouma, M., Poveda, G., Rochas, W., Chavasse, D., Quinones, M., Cox, J. and Patz, J. (1997). Predicting high risk years for malaria in Colombia using parameters of El-Nino Southern Oscillation. *Tropical Medicine and International Health* **2**, 1122–1127.

Buse, K. and Walt, G. (2000). Global public–private partnerships: part II—what are the health issues for global governance? *Bulletin of the World Health Organization* **78**, 699–709.

Buse, K. and Waxman, A. (2001). Public–private health partnerships: a strategy for WHO. *Bulletin of the World Health Organization* **79**, 748–754.

Cassels, A. (1997). *A guide to sector-wide approaches for health development: concepts, issues and working arrangements.* Geneva, Switzerland: World Health Organization WHO/ARA/97.12.

Cochrane Reviews. www.cochrane.org/cochrane/revabstr/g070index.htm

Croft, S. (2005). Public–private partnership: from there to here. *Transactions of the Royal Society of Tropical Medicine and Hygiene* **99**, S9–S14.

Curtis, C.F. (1991). *Control of Disease Vectors in the Community.* London: Wolfe 233 pages.

Davies, J.D. (1994). Sixty years of onchocerciasis control: a chronological summary with comments on eradication, reinvasion and insecticide resistance. *Annual Review of Entomology* **39**, 23–45.

Drameh, P.S., Richards, F.O., Cross, C., Etaale, D.E. and Kassalow, J.S. (2002). Ten years of NGDO action against river blindness. *Trends in Parasitology* **18**, 378–380.

Druilhe, P., Tall, A. and Sokhna, C. (2005). Worms can worsen malaria: towards a new means to roll back malaria? *Trends in Parasitology* **21**, 359–362.

Dowdle, W. and Hopkins, D., eds. (1998). *The Eradication of Infectious Diseases. Report of the Dahlem Workshop*, p. 218. Freie Universitat: Wiley, Berlin.

Ekwanzala, M., Pepin, J., Khonde, N., Molisho, S., de Wals, P. (1996). In the heart of darkness: sleeping sickness in Zaire. Lancet **ii** 1427–1430.

Erlanger, T.E., Keiser, J., de Castro, M.C., Bos, R., Singer, B.H., Tanner, M. and Utzinger, J. (2005). Effect of water resource development and management on lymphatic filariasis, and estimates of population at risk. *American Journal of Tropical Medicine and Hygiene* **73**, 523–533.

Ettling, M., McFarlane, D.D., Schultz, L.J. and Chitsulo, L. (1994). Economic impact of malaria in Malawian households. *Tropical Medicine and Parasitology* **45**, 74–79.

Fenwick, A., Molyneux, D. and Nantulya, V. (2005). Achieving the millennium development goals. *Lancet* **365**, 1029–1030.

Fèvre, E.M., Coleman, P.G., Odiit, M., Magona, J.W., Welburn, S.C. and Woolhouse, M.E.J. (2001). The origins of a new *Trypanosoma brucei rhodesiense* sleeping sickness outbreak in eastern Uganda. *Lancet* **358**, 625–628.

Fèvre, E.M., Picozzi, K., Fyfe, J., Waiswa, C., Odiit, M., Coleman, P.G. and Welburn, S.C. (2005). A burgeoning epidemic of sleeping sickness in Uganda. *Lancet* **366**, 745–747.

Fincham, J.E., Markus, M.B. and Adams, V.J. (2003). Could control of soil-transmitted helminthic infection influence the HIV/AIDS pandemic. *Acta Tropica* **86**, 315–333.

Gwatkin, D.R., Guillot, M. and Heuvelin, P. (1999). The burden of disease among the global poor. *Lancet* **354**, 586–589.

Haines, A. and Cassels, A. (2004). Can the millennium development goals be attained. *British Medical Journal* **329**, 394–397.

Hay, S.I., Cox, J., Rogers, D.J., Randolph, S.E., Stern, D.I., Shanks, G.D., Myers, M.F. and Snow, R.W. (2002). Climate change and the resurgence of malaria in the East African highlands. *Nature* **415**, 59.

Heukelbach, J., Winter, B., Wilcke, T., Muehlen, M., Albrecht, S., de Oliveira, F.A., Kerr-Pontest, L.R., Liesenfeld, O. and Feldmeier, H. (2004). Selective mass treatment with ivermectin to control intestinal helminthiases and parasitic skin diseases in a severely infected population. *Bulletin of the World Health Organization* **82**, 563–571.

Homeida, M., Braide, E., Elhassan, E., Amazigo, U.V., Liese, B.L., Benton, B., Noma, M., Etya'ale, D., Dadzie, K.Y., Kale, O.O. and Seketeli, A. (2002). APOC's strategy of community directed treatment with ivermectin (CDTI) and its potential for providing additional health services to the poorest populations. *Annals of Tropical Medicine and Parasitology* **96**, 93–104.

Hopkins, D.R. (1998). Perspectives from the dracunculiasis eradication programme. *Bulletin of the World Health Organization* **76**(suppl 2), 38–41.

Hopkins, D.R., Ruiz-Tiben, E., Diallo, N., Withers, P.C., Jr. and Maguire, J.H. (2002). Dracunculiasis eradication: and now, Sudan. *American Journal of Tropical Medicine and Hygiene* **67**, 415–422.

Hotez, P.J., Ottesen, E., Fenwick, A. and Molyneux, D.H. (2006). The neglected tropical diseases: the ancient afflictions of stigma and poverty and the prospects for their integrated control and elimination. In: *Hot Topics in Infection and Immunity in Children III. Advances in Experimen-*

tal Medicine (A.J. Pollard and A. Finn, eds). New York: Kluwer Academic/Plenum Publishers in press.

Hunter, H.J. and Rey, L. (1993). *Parasitic Diseases in Water Resources Development. The Need for Intersectoral Negotiations.* Geneva: World Health Organization.

Hutton, G. and Tanner, M. (2004). The sector wide approach: a blessing for public health? *Bulletin of the World Health Organization* **82**, 893.

Ijumba, J.N. and Lindsay, S.W. (2001). Impact of irrigation in Africa: paddies paradox. *Medical and Veterinary Entomology* **15**, 1–11.

IPCC (2001). *Climate Change: Synthesis Report, Summary for Policymakers.* In: Watson, R. T. and Core Writing team Editors, (Eds.), Cambridge: Cambridge University Press (published for Intergovernmental Panel on Climate Control).

Katabarwa, N.M., Richards, F.R. and Ndyomugyeni, R. (2000). In rural Ugandan communities the traditional kinship/clan system is vital to the success and sustainment of the African Programme for Onchocerciasis Control. *Annals of Tropical Medicine and Parasitology* **94**, 485–495.

Keiser, J., Castro, M.C., Maltese, M.F., Bos, R., Tanner, M., Singer, B.H. and Utzinger, J. (2005). Effect of irrigation and large dams on the burden of malaria on a global and regional scale. *American Journal of Tropical Medicine and Hygiene* **72**, 392–406.

Keiser, J. and Utzinger, J. (2005). Emerging foodborne trematodiasis. *Emerging Infectious Diseases* **11**, 1507–1514.

King, C., Kickman, K. and Tisch, D.J. (2005). Re-guaging the cost of chronic helminth infections: meta-analysis of disability-related outcomes in endemic schistosomiasis. *Lancet* **365**, 1561–1569.

Lancet. (2004). Thinking beyond deworming. *Lancet* **364**, 1993–1994 [Editorial].

Le Hesran, J.K., Akiana, J., Nidiaye el, H.M., Dia, M., Senghor, P. and Konate, L. (2004). Severe malaria attack is associated with high prevalence of *Ascaris lumbricoides* infection among children in rural Senegal. *Transactions of the Royal Society Tropical Medicine Hygiene* **98**, 397–399.

Loukas, A. and Hotez, P.J. (2006). Chemotherapy of helminth infections, Chapter 41. In: *Goodman &Gilman's The Pharmacological Basis of Therapeutics* (L.L. Brunton, J.S. Lazo and K.P. Parker, eds), 11th Edn, pp. 1073–1093. New York: McGraw-Hill.

Lun, Z.R., Gaser, R.B., Lai, D.H., Li, A.X., Zhu, X.Q., Yu, X.B. and Fang, Y.Y. (2005). Clonorchiasis: a key foodborne zoonosis in China. *Lancet Infectious Diseases* **5**, 312–341.

Lyke, K.E., Dicko, A., Dabo, A., Sangare, L., Kone, A., Loulibaly, D., Guindo, A., Traore, K., Daou, M., Diarra, I., Sztein, M.B., Plowe, C.V. and Doumbo, O.K. (2005). Association of *Schistosma haematobium* infection with protection against acute *Plasmodium falciparum* malaria in

Malian children. *American Journal of Tropical Medicine and Hygiene* **73**, 1124–1130.

MacCormack, C.P. (1991). Appropriate vector control in primary health care, Chapter 13. In: *Control of Disease Vectors in the Community* (C. Curtis, ed.), pp. 221–227. London: Wolfe Publishing.

Marques, A.C. (1987). Human migration and the spread of malaria in Brazil. *Parasitology Today* **3**, 166–170.

McMichael, A.J. and Le Sueur, D. (2002). Climate change: regional warming and malaria resurgence. *Nature* **420**, 627–628.

Miguel, E. and Kremer, M., 2001. Worms: *education and health externalities in Kenya.* Cambridge, MA: National Bureau of Economic Research (NBER). Working Paper No w 8481.

Molyneux, D.H. (1997). Patterns of change in vector-borne diseases. *Annals of Tropical Medicine and Parasitology* **91**, 827–839.

Molyneux, D.H. (2003). Common themes in changing vector borne disease scenarios. *Transactions of the Royal Society of Tropical Medicine and Hygiene* **97**, 129–132.

Molyneux, D.H. (2004). Neglected diseases but unrecognized successes-challenges and opportunities for infectious disease control. *Lancet* **364**, 380–383.

Molyneux, D.H. (2005). Control of parasites, parasitic disease and parasitic infections. In: *Topley, Wilson's Microbiology and Microbial infection*, 10th ed. *Parasitology* (F.E.G. Cox, S.H. Gillespie, D.D. Despommier and D. Wakelin, eds), Chapter 5, pp. 103–147, 889pp. London: Hodder Arnold, ISBN 0340 88568 8.

Molyneux, D.H., Hopkins, D. and Zagaria, N. (2004). Disease eradication, elimination and control: the need for accurate and consistent usage. *Trends in Parasitology* **20**, 347–351.

Molyneux, D.H., Hotez, P.J. and Fenwick, A. (2005). "Rapid Impact interventions"; how a policy of integrated control for Africa's neglected tropical diseases could benefit the poor. *PLoS Medicine* **2**, e336.

Molyneux, D.H. and Nantulya, V. (2004). Linking disease control programmes in rural Africa: a pro poor strategy for reaching the millennium development goals. *British Medical Journal* **328**, 1129–1132.

Murray, C.J.L. and Lopez, A.D. (1996). *The Global Burden of Disease.* Geneva: World Health Organization, Harvard School of Public Health, World Bank.

Ostfeld, R. and Keesing, F. (2000). The function of biodiversity in the ecology of vector-borne zoonotic diseases. *Canadian Journal of Zoology* **78**, 2061–2078.

Patz, J.A., Daszak, P., Tabor, G.M., Aguirre, A.A., Pearl, M., Epstein, J., Wolfe, N.D., Kilpatrick, A.M., Foufopoulos, J., Molyneux, D. and Bradley, D.J. (2004). Working group on land use change and disease emergence. Unhealthy landscapes: policy recommendations on land use change and infectious disease emergence. *Environmental Health Perspectives* **112**, 1092–1098.

Patz, J.A., Campbell-Lendrum, D., Holloway, T. and Foley, J.A. (2005). Impact of regional climate change on human health. *Nature* **438**, 310–317.

Pitt, S., Pearcy, B.E., Stevens, R.H., Sharipov, A., Saraov, K. and Banatvala, N. (1998). War in Tajikistan and re-emergence of *Plasmodium falciparum*. *Lancet* **352**, 1279.

Rajagopalan, P.K., Paniker, K.N. and Das, P.K. (1987). Control of malaria and filariasis in South India. *Parasitology Today* **3**, 233–241.

Ramaiah, K.D., Michael, E., Guyatt, H. and Das, P.K. (2000). The economic burden of lymphatic filariasis in India. *Parasitology Today* **16**, 251–253.

Raso, G., Luginbhuhl, A., Adjoua, C.A., Tian-Bi, N.T., Silue, K.D., Matthys, B., Vounatsou, P., Wang, Y., Dumas, M.E., Holmes, E., Singer, B.H., Tanner, M., N'goran, E.K. and Utzinger, J. (2004). Multiple parasite infections and their relationship to self-reported morbidity in a community of rural Cote d'Ivoire. *International Journal of Epidemiology* **33**, 1092–1102.

Remme, J.H.F., Blas, E., Chitsulo, L., Desjeux, P.M.P., Engers, H.D., Kanyok, T.P., Kayondo, K.J.F., Kioy, D.F., Kumaraswami, V., Lazdins, J.K., Nunn, P.P., Oduola, A., Ridley, R.G., Touré, Y.T., Zicker, F. and Morel, C.M. (2002). Strategic emphases for tropical diseases research: a TDR perspective. *Trends in Parasitology* **18**, 421–426.

Rogers, D.J. and Randolph, S.E. (2000). The global spread of malaria in a future, warmer world. *Science* **289**, 73–76.

Rowland, M. and Nosten, F. (2001). Malaria epidemiology and control in refugee camps and complex emergencies. *Annals of Tropical Medicine and Parasitology* **95**, 741–754.

Rubio-Palis, Y. and Zimmerman, R.H. (1997). Ecoregional classification of malaria vectors in the neotropics. *Journal of Medical Entomology* **34**, 499–510.

Ruiz-Tiben, E. and Hopkins, D.R. (2006). Dracunculiasis (Guinea Worm Disease). In: *Advances in Parasitology*, (D.H. Molyneux, ed.). Vol. 61, Amsterdam: Elsevier.

Sachs, J.D. (2004). Health in the developing world: achieving the millennium development goals. *Bulletin of the World Health Organization* **82**, 947–951.

Sachs, J.D. and MacArthur, J.W. (2005). The millennium project: a plan for meeting the millennium development goals. *Lancet* **365**, 347–353.

Savioli, L., Engels, D. and Endo, H. (2005). Extending the benefits of deworming for development. *Lancet* **365**, 1520–1521.

Seaman, J., Ashford, R.W., Schorscher, J. and Dereure, J. (1992). Visceral leishmaniasis in southern Sudan: status of health villagers in epidemic conditions. *Annals of Tropical Medicine and Parasitology* **86**, 481–486.

Seim, A. (2005). Time for an additional paradigm? The community-based catalyst approach to public health. *Bulletin of the World Health Organization* **83**, 392–394.

Sockna, C., Le Hesran, J.Y., Mbaye, P.A., Akiana, J., Camara, P., Diop, M., Ly, A. and Druilhe, P. (2004). Increase in Malaria attacks among children presenting concomitant infection by *Schistosoma mansoni* in Senegal. *Malaria Journal* **3**, 43.

Spiegel, A., Tall, A., Raphenson, G., Trape, J.-F. and Druilhe, P. (2003). Increased frequency of malaria attacks in subjects co-infected by intestinal worms and *Plasmodium falciparum*. *Transactions of the Royal Society of Tropical Medicine and Hygiene* **97**, 198–199.

Stop TB. (2002). *WHO Report 2002*. Geneva, Switzerland: WHO.

Taylor, L.H., Latham, S.M. and Woolhouse, M.E.J. (2001). Risk factors for human disease emergence. *Proceedings of the Royal Society, Series B* **356**, 983–989.

Tyagi, B.K. and Chaudhary, R.C. (1997). Outbreak of falciparum malaria in the Thar Desert (India) with particular emphasis on physiographic changes brought about by extensive canalization and their impact on vector density and dissemination. *Journal of Arid Environment* **36**, 541–555.

Walsh, J.F., Molyneux, D.H. and Birley, M.H. (1993). Deforestation: effects on vector borne disease. *Parasitology* **106**, 855–875.

Walt, G. (1988). CHWs: are national programmes in crisis? *Health Policy and Planning* **3**, 1–21.

Widdus, R. (2001). Public–private partnerships for health: their main targets, their diversity, and their directions. *Bulletin of the World Health Organization* **79**, 713–720.

Widdus, R. (2005). Public–private partnerships: an overview. *Transactions of the Royal Society of Tropical Medicine and Hygiene* **99**, S1–S8.

World Bank. (1993). *World Development Report. Investing in Health*. Oxford: Oxford University Press.

World Health Organization (WHO). (1979). *"Parasitic Zoonoses", Report of a WHO Expert Committee with the Participation of FAO*, 107pp. WHO Technical Report Series No. 637.

World Health Organization (WHO). (1990). *Control of the Leishmaniases. Report of an WHO Expert Committee*, 158 pp. Technical Report Series No. 793.

World Health Organization (WHO). (1992). *Lymphatic Filariasis: the Disease and its Control. Fifth Report of a WHO Expert Committee*, 77 pp. Technical Report Series No. 821.

World Health Organization (WHO). (1993). *A Global Strategy for Malaria Control*. Geneva: World Health Organization.

World Health Organization (WHO). (1994). *Lymphatic Filariasis Infection and Disease Control Strategies. Report of a Consultative Meeting*. Penang, Malaysia: Division of Control of Tropical.

World Health Organization (WHO). (1998). Global disease elimination and eradication as public health strategies. *Bulletin of the World Health Organization* **76**(suppl. 2), 162.

World Health Organization/Roll Back Malaria WHO/RBM. (2001). *Malaria Early Warning Systems. Concepts, Indicators and Partners. A Framework for Field Research in Africa*. Geneva: World Health Organization 78.

World Health Organization WHO. (2003). *Control of Lymphatic Filariasis in China, The Editorial Board of Control of Lymphatic Filariasis in China*. Manila: World Health Organization, Western Pacific Region 229, ISBN 92 99061 048 4.

World Health Organization WHO. (2005a). *Health and the Millennium Development Goals. 2005 Keep the Promise*. Switzerland: WHO, Geneva 81, ISBN 92 4 156298 6.

World Health Organization WHO. (2005b). *Preventing Chronic Diseases: A Vital Investment*. Geneva, Switzerland: World Health Organization 200.

Yameogo, L., Resh, V. and Molyneux, D.H. (2004). Control of river blindness: case history of biodiversity in a disease control programme. *Ecohealth* **1**, 172–184.

Useful Websites:

www.cochrane.org.
www.commissionforafrica.org pp. 72, 198.
www.filariasis.org.
www.schisto.org.
www.theglobalfund.org.
www.wfp.org.
www.who.int/wormcontrol.

Malaria Chemotherapy

Peter Winstanley[1] and Stephen Ward[2]

[1]*Department of Pharmacology & Therapeutics, University of Liverpool, Liverpool L69 3GE, UK*
[2]*Liverpool School of Tropical Medicine, Pembroke Place, Liverpool, UK*

ABSTRACT

Most malaria control strategies today depend on safe and effective drugs, as they have done for decades. But sensitivity to chloroquine, hitherto the workhorse of malaria chemotherapy, has rapidly declined throughout the tropics since the 1980s, and this drug is now useless in many high-transmission areas. New options for resource-constrained governments are few, and there is growing evidence that

ADVANCES IN PARASITOLOGY VOL 61
ISSN: 0065-308X
DOI: 10.1016/S0065-308X(05)61002-0

the burden from malaria has been increasing, as has malaria mortality in Africa.

In this chapter, we have tried to outline the main pharmacological properties of current drugs, and their therapeutic uses and limitations. We have summarised the ways in which these drugs are employed, both in the formal health sector and in self-medication. We have briefly touched on the limitations of current drug development, but have tried to pick out a few promising drugs that are under development.

Given that *Plasmodium falciparum* is the organism that kills, and that has developed multi-drug resistance, we have tended to focus upon it. Similarly, given that around 90% of global mortality from malaria occurs in Africa, there is the tendency to dwell on this continent. We give no apology for placing our emphasis upon the use of antimalarial drugs in endemic populations rather than their use for prophylaxis in travellers.

1. THE PHARMACOLOGY AND THERAPEUTICS OF ANTIMALARIALS

1.1. The 4-Aminoquinolines

1.1.1. Summary

Chloroquine is probably still the most widely used antimalarial drug in much of Africa, but the extensive spread of resistance has severely limited its usefulness (Dollery, 1999b). It remains effective for, *P. ovale, P. malariae* and most cases of *P. vivax* infections worldwide. Many chloroquine-resistant strains of *P. falciparum* remain sensitive to its congener amodiaquine and the utility of this drug (alone or in combination with other antimalarial drugs) is being studied (Olliaro and Mussano, 2003). The parasite has found it quite difficult to develop resistance to this drug group and it remains of scientific and public health interest.

1.1.2. Mode of Action

It is accepted that high-level drug accumulation within the parasitised red blood cell is central to drug action and several explanations have been put forward to explain this observation. Although there may be contributions to accumulation from a number of processes, binding to haem or ferriprotoporphyrin IX (FPIX) is the predominant driving force (Bray *et al.*, 1998, 1999). Haem, which is cytotoxic, is generated from the degradation of haemoglobin. Under normal circumstances, haem is detoxified by the formation of an inert crystal structure called haemozoin. Chloroquine forms a complex with haem, prevents crystallisation and thereby retains the cytotoxic potential of the haem. All 4-aminoquinolines, including amodiaquine and its active metabolite desethylamodiaquine, appear to act in this way. The superior potency of amodiaquine to chloroquine *in vitro* is probably due to differences in the ability to form complexes with haem within the highly compartmentalised infected red blood cell system.

1.1.3. Mechanisms of Resistance

Chloroquine resistance is characterised by reduced cellular accumulation of drug. This phenotype can be partially reversed by agents such as verapamil, the so-called 'resistance reversing agents' (this is also the case in multi-drug resistant (MDR) cancer cells) (Wellems *et al.*, 1990; Wellems and Plowe, 2001). Early explanations of this phenotype were based on analogies with MDR-based resistance mechanisms; however, these hypotheses could never fully explain the experimental data. The most robust explanation of the chloroquine resistance mechanism has been derived from investigation of the progeny of a genetic cross between a chloroquine-resistant clone of *P. falciparum* and a chloroquine-sensitive clone. Detailed molecular interrogation of these offspring has identified a single gene, PfCRT, which is predictive of chloroquine resistance. This gene encodes a protein which is located at the parasite's digestive food vacuole and which has features suggestive of a role as a transporter. In comparison to chloroquine-sensitive parasites, resistant parasites carry a number of mutations in PfCRT, of which the K76T mutation is predictive of the verapamil-responsive resistance phenotype. Observation with field isolates from a range of geographical settings and transfection studies provides compelling support for the claim that PfCRT is the major chloroquine-resistant gene in *P. falciparum*. It is not clear what the real function of PfCRT is: certainly recent studies suggesting a role in pH modulation are fundamentally flawed. There is evidence that the protein acts as a transporter capable of either directly or indirectly allowing chloroquine movement out of the food vacuole. Recently, a number of reports suggest that predictability of chloroquine resistance is increased if both PfCRT and PfMDR1 are taken into consideration. Interestingly in Malawi, which stopped using chloroquine in 1993, there is evidence that the prevalence of PfCRT has declined from 85% (in 1992) to 13% (in 2000) raising the question 'might chloroquine be a useful—and inexpensive—component of combination therapy?' (Kublin *et al.*, 2003).

Amodiaquine has been shown to have clinical utility even in areas of chloroquine resistance (Bakyaita *et al.*, 2005). However, this assertion is now being brought into question, especially in areas of high-level chloroquine resistance. *In vitro* studies clearly demonstrate cross-resistance between chloroquine and amodiaquine, and the extent of cross-resistance is even greater if you consider the desethyl metabolite (Bray *et al.*, 1996). This data suggests a potential role for PfCRT in amodiaquine sensitivity and this claim is supported by recent transfection studies.

1.1.4. Clinical Pharmacokinetics

- Chloroquine is rapidly absorbed from the gut and from intramuscular or subcutaneous injections (Dollery, 1999b): indeed dangerously high peak plasma concentrations may be reached soon after an injection of 5 mg base/kg, and this has been linked to fatalities. About half of the absorbed chloroquine is cleared unchanged by the kidney, the rest being biotransformed in the liver to desethyl- and bisdesethyl-chloroquine (White *et al.*, 1988). Although clearance is reduced in renal failure, it is not usually necessary to reduce the dose. The terminal elimination half-time is very long (1–2 months).

- Amodiaquine is extensively converted into its equipotent metabolite desethyl-amodiaquine, which is responsible for most of the antimalarial activity: desethyl-amodiaquine achieves much higher concentrations than its parent drug (Winstanley *et al.*, 1987, 1990). Another metabolite, amodiaquine–quinoneimine, has an important role in toxic reactions.

1.1.5. Therapeutic Use

Oral chloroquine is used for the treatment and prophylaxis of *vivax, ovale* and *malariae* malarias. It is still used for uncomplicated *P. falciparum* malaria in semi-immune people, but use in this context is likely to diminish over the next 5-years as it is phased out of public health policy.

Because of the higher efficacy of amodiaquine in much of Africa, this drug is being re-examined usually in combination with an artemisinin-class drug (Olliaro and Mussano, 2003). Children in high-transmission areas are usually treated for malaria several times annually, and there is concern to examine the immunogenicity and adverse effect profile of amodiaquine under such operational use (see below).

1.1.6. Adverse Effects and Adverse Interactions

- Chloroquine is well tolerated but, when plasma concentrations exceed around 250 µg/ml, unpleasant symptoms (such as headache, diplopia, dizziness and nausea) may develop. In black-skinned people, pruritus of the palms, soles and scalp is frequent, and may impact upon adherence.
- In cases of deliberate chloroquine overdose, toxicity is manifested rapidly (sometimes within 30 minutes). The main problems are coma, convulsions, hypotension, respiratory paralysis and cardiac arrest. ECG changes include sinus tachycardia, sinus bradycardia, prolonged QT interval, ventricular tachycardias and asystole. Diazepam and epinephrine may have roles in severe chloroquine poisoning (Riou *et al.*, 1988).
- Continuous weekly chloroquine use (cumulative dose $>100\,g$) may cause retinopathy. However, while such cumulative doses

may be encountered in long-term antimalarial prophylaxis, retinopathy is more usually associated with the higher anti-inflammatory doses used in collagen vascular diseases.

- Rare toxic effects of chloroquine include photo-allergic dermatitis, aggravation of psoriasis, skin pigmentation, leucopenia, bleaching of the hair and aplastic anaemia. Chloroquine can exacerbate epilepsy.

- Amodiaquine caused hepatitis and agranulocytosis in patients taking it for prophylaxis, and the drug is no longer recommended for this indication (Hatton *et al.*, 1986). Amodiaquine–quinoneimine can be generated from amodiaquine both spontaneously, when the drugs are in aqueous solution, and as a result of enzyme activity. The quinoneimine is highly reactive and haptenates proteins, generating antigen to which an immune response may be mounted. Repeated exposure to this antigen may be important in the generation of organ damage.

1.2. Antifolate Drugs and Combinations

1.2.1. Summary

The antifolates are mainly used in fixed-ratio combinations, most commonly sulfadoxine-pyrimethamine (SP), which has been the first-line drug for uncomplicated *P. falciparum* malaria in many parts of Africa (particularly Eastern/Southern Africa where chloroquine resistance developed) for around 5 years (Dollery, 1999d). Unfortunately, resistance to SP is developing rapidly in Africa, as it previously developed elsewhere. Chlorproguanil has recently been launched in fixed ratio with dapsone (CD; Lapdap^{TM}) for malaria treatment. Of the sulfa drugs, sulfadoxine, sulfalene and dapsone are given for their synergistic effects with pyrimethamine or chlorproguanil.

1.2.2. Mode of Action

This large group of drugs interferes with DNA synthesis by depleting the pool of tetrahydrofolate, a cofactor of DNA synthesis. One structurally diverse group of drugs inhibits the enzyme dihydrofolate reductase (DHFR) and has greater affinity with the plasmodial enzyme than with the human enzyme. This group includes pyrimethamine and the biguanides proguanil and chlorproguanil (both of which require biotransformation in the liver to the triazines cycloguanil and chlorcycloguanil for their action on DHFR). Another group of drugs inhibits dihydropteroate synthetase (DHPS), an 'earlier' enzyme of the folate pathway, and one which is lacked by mammals. The group includes the sulfonamides and sulfones. The DHFR-inhibitors have some therapeutic utility if used alone, but this is not the case for the DHPS-inhibitors. In the treatment of malaria, DHFR- and DHPS-inhibitors are used in synergistic combinations. Proguanil has been widely used for malaria prophylaxis, usually when co-administered with chloroquine (the popularity of this combination has fallen over the last 10 years because of deteriorating clinical response).

1.2.3. *Mechanisms of Resistance*

Resistance to DHFR-inhibitors results from specific mutations in the DHFR gene (*dhfr*). Under pressure from SP, a Ser-108 to Asn-108 mutation is the first to appear in the field, and this reduces sensitivity to pyrimethamine around 10-fold (Watkins and Mosobo, 1993). Subsequent further common mutations of Asn-51 to Ile-51 and Cys-59 to Arg-59 enhance resistance, and Ile-164 to Leu-164 provides high-level resistance. Triple mutations of *dhfr* (at positions 108, 51 and 59) are now very common throughout Africa; the *dhfr*-164 mutation has been reported at extremely low frequency in African isolates over the last six years, but it is not clear to what extent this mutation is spreading. Mutations in the DHPS gene (*dhps*) correlate with *in vitro* sulfonamide chemosensitivity. Parasite lines exhibiting high-level resistance commonly carry either a double mutation in *dhps*, altering both Ser-436 and Ala-613, or a single mutation affecting Ala-581 (Plowe *et al.*, 1997). Pyrimethamine and sulfadoxine both have long-elimination half-lives: this equates with a strong selective pressure for resistance, as new infections are ultimately exposed to sub-inhibitory drug concentrations.

1.2.4. Clinical Pharmacokinetics

- Pyrimethamine is well absorbed after oral or intramuscular administration. Elimination half-life in children with malaria averages 81 and 124 hours after oral and intramuscular injection, respectively.

- Proguanil and chlorproguanil, which can only be given orally, reach peak plasma concentrations in 2–4 hours, and have short-elimination half-lives. Most of the antimalarial activity is due to the triazine metabolites, cycloguanil and chlorcycloguanil, respectively, which reach peak concentrations within 4–9 hours (Plowe *et al.*, 1997; Bray *et al.*, 1996). The extent of biguanide metabolism varies considerably: metabolism is catalysed by the cytochrome P450 group (CYP 2C19 and CYP 3A4), which are subject to genetic polymorphism. 'Poor metabolisers' of the biguanides sustain low or undetectable concentrations of the active triazines; clinical trials have failed to show diminished prophylactic efficacy in 'poor metabolisers'.

- The elimination half-life of sulfadoxine is between 100 and 200 hours, that of sulfalene is shorter at about 65 hours. Both drugs undergo limited Phase-II metabolism (to the acetyl and glucuronide derivatives); certain minor Phase-I metabolites may contribute to idiosyncratic toxicity. The degree of acetylation varies among populations as a result of a genetic polymorphism. Dapsone is eliminated quickly in comparison with sulfadoxine, with a mean half-life of about 26 hours.

1.2.5. Therapeutic Use

SP is in frequent use for the treatment of chloroquine-resistant *P. falciparum* malaria in Africa. Dapsone in combination with pyrimethamine (Maloprim) is occasionally used for prophylaxis. A fixed-ratio combination of dapsone with chlorproguanil (as *Lap-dap*[TM]) has been developed for the treatment of chloroquine-resistant *P. falciparum* malaria, and is being developed further as a fixed-ratio combination with artesunate.

Proguanil is formulated alone (for chemoprophylaxis) and also in fixed-ratio combination with atovaquone (Malarone (see below)).

1.2.6. Adverse Effects and Drug Interactions

- Severe allergic reactions to sulfa drugs are well recognised; in the case of such slowly eliminated drugs as sulfadoxine such reactions can be life threatening. Such severe reactions to sulfadoxine are reported in the setting of prophylaxis; their frequency in the setting of treatment is unknown, but current data are reassuring (Centers for Disease Control, 1985).
- Dapsone is associated with a range of concentration-related and idiosyncratic adverse reactions (Dollery, 1999c).
  - Patients with the severer forms of G6PD deficiency may develop severe haemolysis and methaemoglobinaemia. These seem to be less of an issue with the common A-form of G6PD encountered in most of Africa.
  - Allergy to dapsone is recognised, with rash and fever as major clinical features.
  - Patients given pyrimethamine–dapsone twice weekly for malaria prophylaxis developed bone marrow reactions, and Maloprim (which is recommended for only certain geographical areas) is now taken once weekly. The mechanism of this reaction, and the responsible drug (dapsone, pyrimethamine or both) remains unclear.
- Pyrimethamine and the biguanides proguanil and chlorproguanil seem to be associated with little serious toxicity, although folate deficiency may be exacerbated.

1.3. Quinine and Congeners

1.3.1. Summary

Quinine is less potent than chloroquine and has a small therapeutic range (Dollery, 1999e). However, resistance to quinine is uncommon, and parenteral quinine is the drug of first choice for severe malaria.

Oral quinine is used for uncomplicated *P. falciparum* malaria in some countries, but its long and complicated regimen often makes this impracticable.

1.3.2. Mode of Action

Like chloroquine, quinine interferes with parasite metabolism of haem, a toxic product of haemoglobin digestion.

1.3.3. Clinical Pharmacokinetics

The oral bioavailability of quinine is high. After intramuscular injection, the absorption half-time seems to vary with the drug concentration in the injectate, ranging from about 10 to 40 minutes (Winstanley *et al.*, 1993). Areas under the concentration–time curve and maximum plasma concentrations are similar following intramuscular and intravenous administration of quinine. Quinine is extensively bound to plasma proteins, principally to the acute phase-reactant α_1-acid-glycoprotein (AGP). In health, about 80% of the total plasma quinine concentration is bound, but in patients with malaria, AGP concentrations rise and around 90% is bound: this may explain the apparently lower toxicity of high quinine concentrations in patients with malaria, when compared to patients who have taken a deliberate overdose.

Quinine undergoes extensive hepatic metabolism to 3- and 2-hydroxyquinine: less than 20% of the drug is excreted unchanged in urine, and the impact of renal failure on the disposition of quinine does not appear to be great. Dose reductions are not recommended in severe malaria complicated by either hepatic or renal impairment. In adults with malaria, the elimination half-time of quinine is longer than in health.

1.3.4. Therapeutic Use

This is reviewed below.

1.3.5. Adverse Effects and Drug Interactions

- 'Cinchonism' (comprising tinnitus, deafness, headache, nausea and visual disturbance) affects the majority of conscious patients with therapeutic levels and does not warrant dose reduction.
- Potentially life-threatening adverse events include:
  - Hypersensitivity reactions are uncommon, but include rashes, thrombocytopenia, leucopenia, disseminated intravascular coagulation, haemolytic-uraemic syndrome, bronchospasm and pancytopenia.
  - Quinine stimulates the release of insulin and may exacerbate hypoglycaemia.
  - Concentration-related toxicity can be seen with doses as low as 2 g of the anhydrous free base in adults and the fatal dose ranges from 8 to 15 g. In the setting of acute poisoning, visual impairment is common and may be permanent. Serious cardiovascular compromise is less common than oculotoxicity, and is usually seen with higher drug concentrations. At high concentration, quinine can cause coma and seizures. Activated charcoal has been shown to increase the clearance of quinine. Stellate ganglion block confers no benefit.
- Adverse drug interactions include the following:
  - Marked reduction in the clearance of digitalis glycosides.
  - Reduction in the clearance of flecainide.
  - Potentiation of oral anticoagulants.

1.4. The Artemisinin Group

1.4.1. Summary

Artemisinin is a potent antimalarial compound extracted from plant material. Artemether, artesunate and dihydroartemisinin (DHA) are semi-synthetic derivatives of artemisinin that are in common clinical use (Dollery, 1999a). The artemisinin group is used in the management of severe malaria and also, usually in combination with other drugs, uncomplicated *P. falciparum* malaria. 'Artemisinin

Combination Therapy' is now being widely adopted for uncomplicated malaria, and this has recently been noted by an Institute of Medicine report (White, 2004). However, the global supply of artemisinin is currently unequal to this task, which is a matter of concern (Senior, 2005).

1.4.2. Mode of Action

It is thought that haemazoin probably catalyses breakdown of the labile peroxide bridge within the sesquiterpene lactone molecule generating free radicals that alkylate parasite macromolecules. Recent evidence suggests that artemisinins may act by inhibiting PfATP6 outside the parasite's food vacuole (Eckstein-Ludwig *et al.*, 2003). In contrast to other antimalarial drug groups, the artemisinins have marked effects on the circulating forms of the parasite (Murphy *et al.*, 1995), the viability of which decline soon after the start of treatment (Nosten *et al.*, 2004). The artemisinins have gametocytocidal effects on *P. falciparum*, and this may help reduce transmission. Resistance to the artemisinins is not yet encountered in the field.

1.4.3. Clinical Pharmacokinetics

Artemisinin and its derivatives are rapidly hydrolysed *in vivo* to DHA; all artemisinin group drugs have very short-elimination half-lives (White, 1994). Artemether absorption is slower, more variable and with lower biotransformation to DHA when administered by the intramuscular or intravenous routes, in comparison to oral dosage.

1.4.4. Therapeutic Use

The use of artemisinins for severe malaria and as ACT is reviewed in the following sections.

1.4.5. Adverse Effects

- In general, this is a safe and well-tolerated drug group.
- The main current concern centres on reproductive safety. The

embryotoxic effects of this drug class have been known for some time and recent drug development work provides evidence of morphological abnormalities in two mammalian species (rat and rabbit): most concern focusses on long-bone shortening (Clark *et al.*, 2004). These effects are seen at doses and concentrations similar to those used in clinical practice.

- It is reassuring that the artemisinins have been extensively used without apparent teratogenicity for many years in China and SE Asia, and huge numbers of pregnant women have been treated (McGready *et al.*, 2001). Pharmacovigilance systems are not well established in China and SE Asia but, despite this, it is important to note that no spontaneous reports of congenital abnormalities have been generated. Furthermore, published data on nearly 1000 pregnancies (nearly 100 from the first trimester) have shown no evidence of treatment-related, adverse pregnancy outcomes. These results are encouraging, but the numbers of first trimester exposures studied in detail are too small to remove all concern, and pharmacovigilance systems are now being established to increase the data base.

- The WHO has concluded that (1) the artemisinins cannot be recommended for treatment of malaria in the first trimester (but should not be withheld if they are lifesaving for the mother) and (2) they should only be used in later pregnancy when other treatments are considered unsuitable. It is salutary to remember that many women exposed to artemisinins may not know that they are pregnant (inadvertent treatment) and, given the inadequacy of diagnostic facilities, that they may not have malaria.

1.5. A Summary of Other Drugs Used for Malaria

1.5.1. Mefloquine

- Mefloquine acts against the asexual stages of all species of human malaria parasite, but resistant strains of *P. falciparum* are now common in SE Asia (www.rocheuk.com).

- This drug is very slowly eliminated, the half-life ranging from 15 to 33 days; steady state is reached after 8 weeks of weekly dosing (in the setting of prophylaxis).
- Mefloquine is used for prophylaxis and treatment of uncomplicated multi-resistant *P. falciparum* malaria. Mefloquine co-administered with artesunate has proved effective against uncomplicated *P. falciparum* malaria in areas where there is a high level of resistance to mefloquine alone (Nosten *et al.*, 2000).
- Dose-related adverse reactions are common, usually mild and most frequently gastrointestinal. 'Serious' central nervous system (CNS) events, including seizures, are estimated to occur in about 1 in 10 000 prophylactic users which is about the same reported rate as chloroquine. The estimated frequency of non-serious CNS events (including headache, dizziness, insomnia and depression) varies between 1.8% and 7.6% (and is generally higher in females than males); these proportions are similar to those for chloroquine, but about five-fold higher than reported by patients taking no prophylaxis.
- Mefloquine used during pregnancy increases the risk of stillbirth, and the British National Formulary advises that pregnancy should be excluded before mefloquine is started. The manufacturer has recently revised its advice on the relative contraindications of mefloquine.

1.5.2. Atovaquone–Proguanil

- Atovaquone is thought to inhibit mitochondrial respiration. Atovaquone synergises with the biguanide proguanil (and not with proguanil's active triazine metabolite cycloguanil) and is formulated in a fixed ratio tablet (Malarone^{TM}) (Canfield *et al.*, 1995).
- Resistance of *P. falciparum* to atovaquone is selected readily; whether resistance to the combination atovaquone–proguanil will appear when this drug is widely used remains to be seen.
- Atovaquone is poorly and variably absorbed, and is almost entirely eliminated unchanged via the bile into the gut (there is enterohepatic circulation). The elimination half-life is long (50–70 hours).

- Atovaquone–proguanil may be used for the treatment of multi-resistant *P. falciparum* malaria. But it is a very expensive drug, which mainly confines its use to chemoprophylaxis in travellers.

1.5.3. Halofantrine

- Halofantrine is a drug sometimes used for uncomplicated, but multi-resistant *P. falciparum* malaria.
- Its absorption is incomplete and variable (bioavailability increases after fatty food). Halofantrine is eliminated with a terminal half-life of 1–2 days.
- The most important adverse effect is prolongation of the ECG QT and resulting ventricular arrhythmias. The need for electrocardiography, to exclude pre-existing QT prolongation, has greatly limited the usefulness of this drug (Nosten *et al.*, 1993).

1.5.4. Antibiotics

- Certain antibiotics, particularly clindamycin and the tetracyclines, have useful antimalarial activity. They are never used alone but are most frequently added to quinine, in patients who can take oral medication; this practice is most commonly needed in areas of intense drug resistance, where clearance of parasitaemia on quinine may be prolonged.
- Clindamycin has recently been studied in combination with fosmidomycin for the treatment of uncomplicated *P. falciparum* malaria but, in the setting of widespread adoption of ACT, this combination is unlikely to see extensive use at present (Borrmann *et al.*, 2004).

1.5.5. Primaquine

- Hypnozoite stages of *P. vivax* or *ovale* are unaffected by the drugs used to eliminate erythrocytic infection (mainly chloroquine). The 8-aminoquinoline primaquine remains the only drug available to kill this stage (and achieve so-called 'radical cure'), thereby reducing the chance of late relapse.

- Primaquine is given orally once daily, and courses usually last 14 to 21 days, although longer courses may be required for some SE Asian and western Pacific strains.
- Primaquine readily causes haemolysis in patients with G6PD deficiency, and G6PD testing should be done before the drug is used. In patients with the severer forms of G6PD deficiency the risks of primaquine might well exceed the benefits, and it should be remembered that *P. vivax* and *P. ovale* malarias rarely cause life-threatening illness (whereas massive haemolysis may well be life threatening).

2. DEVELOPING NEW ANTIMALARIAL DRUGS

The recent completion of the malaria, mosquito and human genome projects has raised the expectation that we are at the dawn of a new generation of rational antimalarial drug discovery, design and development. It is argued that, by better understanding the complex interactions between molecules within an organism under defined conditions (life cycle stage, drug exposure, etc.) and by comparing key molecules in the host and the pathogen, it should be possible to identify potential chemotherapeutic targets for validation. But it remains a major challenge to distil this mass of information and develop strategies capable of target identification. The most recent crop of new discovery projects are embracing post-genomic technologies although most target simple enzymes in potentially important pathways. The long-term exploitability of such targets and the problems of simple mutation-based resistance mechanisms on the utility of drugs designed against these enzymes remains to be seen. There remain many technical, political and health policy hurdles to be cleared although it is accepted that there will be many more opportunities for rational drug design in the coming years. However, drug development is a slow and expensive process and the provision of sufficient resource to diseases of neglect such as malaria will require a long-term commitment from the funding agencies and the international Pharma industry.

Whatever means are used to identify a potential antimalarial drug and demonstrate its potency *in vitro*, or in animal models, the compound must then be developed into a medicine, during which process its benefits and risks start to be evaluated. Although the ideas underpinning development projects often emanate from academia, almost all drugs require the expertise and facilities of a pharmaceutical company for formal development into a medicine. This is done at high financial risk, thus, although industrial 'research and development' teams are motivated by scientific and medical concerns, resources have traditionally been provided on the expectation of profit. Since antimalarial drugs compete poorly with most other drug categories, there have been few new drugs in the last decade. Things may be changing now: financial contributions from the *Medicine for Malaria Venture* (MMV) together with changing public/shareholder perceptions have succeeded in establishing several development projects with major pharmaceutical companies. MMV is new on the scene, and it would be unrealistic to expect it to have had a chance to impact yet. So the pace of antimalarial drug development is still too slow, even though antimalarial drug resistance is now a major threat to global health. The need for industrial collaborations in antimalarial drug development has never been keener, but maintaining long-term public–private partnerships (and dealing with political agendas in the World Health Organization) is not for the faint-hearted.

3. THE USE OF ANTIMALARIAL DRUGS

3.1. Chemoprophylaxis

Readers will be familiar with the provision of chemoprophylaxis to travellers, but will perhaps be less familiar with the issues relevant to endemic country populations. In summary, only a very small proportion of malaria-endemic populations takes chemoprophylaxis: people are unwilling to use their over-committed resources in this way. Further, risk vs. benefit analyses do not always favour chemoprophylaxis: if one lives permanently in a high-transmission setting, protective immunity reduces the mortality and morbidity of *P. falciparum* malaria after early childhood, whereas the cumulative risks of drug exposure would remain. There are special groups for whom the benefits of chemoprophylaxis probably outweigh the cumulative risks: these include children aged under 5-years who reside in high-transmission areas and patients with haemoglobinopathies (infants and pregnant women merit separate consideration and will be discussed below). In fact few of these 'at risk' patient groups actually receive chemoprophylaxis—in much the same way as few diabetics in malaria-endemic countries receive comprehensive care—for reasons of economics and logistics.

3.2. Intermittent Presumptive Treatment (for Pregnant Women and infants)

In high-transmission regions, immunity to malaria develops in the first few years of life, and older people rarely suffer severe malaria (Day and Marsh, 1991). However, during pregnancy the risks of maternal anaemia, maternal death and low-birth-weight infants are increased by *P. falciparum* infection and are further exacerbated if there is coincident HIV-infection (Nosten *et al.*, 2004). In HIV-negative mothers, risk is greatest in primigravidae, and declines with succeeding pregnancies; in HIV-positive mothers, the risks seem to persist with succeeding pregnancies. Critically, infection is usually asymptomatic and blood slides may be negative, despite placental infection. As a result, when one relies on a case-management approach for febrile illness (which is a rather passive process for health systems, relying on the patient to identify themselves and seek treatment), one would miss the majority of infections. Trials of weekly chloroquine prophylaxis showed an impact on maternal anaemia and birth weight. But compliance with a weekly regimen is poor, and sensitivity to chloroquine has probably declined to a point where this strategy would give little benefit throughout Africa. SP has been studied in pregnant women but, instead of being given at frequent intervals as a form of chemoprophylaxis, SP has been given intermittently, in the assumption of infection, in the second and third trimesters (Shulman *et al.*, 1999). This *Intermittent Presumptive Treatment* (IPT) approach has been shown to improve both maternal and fetal outcomes, and is being introduced operationally. It is important to emphasise two points. (1) It is not known whether the success of IPT relies on the prolonged chemoprophylactic effect of SP (which is eliminated very slowly) or whether IPT is successful simply because of periodic 'clearance' of placental infection. (2) Sensitivity to SP is declining in Africa and it is unclear for how much longer IPT with SP will continue to work. There is no clear successor to SP, but the Gates Foundation has been funding extensive trials in this area over the last couple of years.

A similar concept is also being applied to children less than 12 months old, in whom clinical malaria and severe anaemia are major causes of paediatric hospital admission and death (Schellenberg *et al.*, 2001). Case management (see below) is currently the main strategy but has its limitations: (1) very young children are, effectively, non-immune and may deteriorate within hours of the onset of symptoms; (2) in rural areas, parents may be unable to reach health centres or hospitals in time to prevent death. A randomised trial has been done in infants in a rural area of Tanzania to examine the efficacy of intermittent SP on the rate of malaria and severe anaemia. Children were given SP (or placebo) and iron supplementation at 2, 3 and 9 months of age. SP gave a protective efficacy of 59% against malaria and 50% against severe anaemia (Schellenberg *et al.*, 2001). This approach to malaria control is currently being examined by WHO but, again, it is important to recognise that the parasite may be moving more rapidly than those who determine antimalarial drug policy, hence resistance to SP threatens this strategy.

3.3. Case Management of Uncomplicated Malaria

3.3.1. Background

Numerically, this is the principal way in which antimalarial drugs are employed (there are perhaps 120 million cases treated annually in

Africa), and it has a large impact on morbidity and mortality. Efficient case management of uncomplicated malaria relies heavily on the availability of effective, affordable and accessible drugs. In the past, chloroquine was widely used, inexpensive and safe, but its efficacy is now so low—almost everywhere—that it is no longer an acceptable treatment. As recounted above, many countries changed first-line treatment to SP, but found that resistance developed (very quickly in the case of SE Asia, perhaps more slowly in the case of east Africa). Public health structures and budgets in many tropical countries (especially in Africa) are not robust enough to sustain frequent changes in malaria drug policy, and there has been an intense search for a strategy that might lengthen the 'useful therapeutic life' of drugs.

Based initially on observations made in Thailand, ACT is now the strategy that is being recommended. The logic underpinning combination therapy has been set out by White (2004). The artemisinin derivatives reduce the parasite biomass by around 4-logs for each asexual cycle and this makes them the most rapidly efficacious antimalarial drugs in use. But using artemisinins on their own is dogged by high rates of recrudescence (almost certainly because all the drugs in this class are very rapidly eliminated, and long courses of treatment are impractical). In combination with a second drug, ACT, the rapid reduction of the parasite biomass produced by the artemisinin component reduces the rate at which parasite populations develop mutations to the second drug.

Drugs can, of course, be co-administered with artemisinins (e.g. AQ is often co-administered with artesunate) but, to be practicable for outpatient use, an ACT regimen needs to be co-formulated: that is the various drugs must all be formulated in the same tablet. Lumefantrine–artemether (Coartem) is the only co-formulated ACT that has been approved by rigorous regulatory scrutiny (and therefore, the only ACT that could be purchased by the International Public Purse) but others are under development. As outlined above, there are concerns regarding the safety of the artemisinin drug group in the first trimester of pregnancy. So far, these concerns are largely theoretically based on data from animal models: work continues to define the degree of risk, if any, to people.

3.3.2. Lumefantrine–artemether (Coartem)

Lumefantrine is incompletely bioavailable from the gut and is eliminated with a half-life of 1–6 days; the disposition of artemether is briefly reviewed above (Ezzet *et al.*, 2000). Coartem is used for the treatment of uncomplicated multi-resistant *P. falciparum* malaria. It must be given twice daily for 3 days, and achieves impressive efficacy in clinical trial. The manufacturer is to be congratulated on the effort that has been made to get packaging right in an effort to optimise adherence (and thereby optimise operational effectiveness). Concerns linger that such a six-dose treatment might prove too complicated to achieve high operational effectiveness. Recent work has shown that adherence to the six-dose regimen can be high (Fogg *et al.*, 2004), but this has not been rigorously tested when patients pay for the drug. Coartem is quite an expensive drug but, once again, the manufacturer is to be congratulated for its 'deal' with the WHO, in which drug costs in poor countries can be minimised. Recent disturbing data suggest the selection of resistance by the lumefantrine component of Coartem (Sisowath *et al.*, 2005).

3.3.3. Chlorproguanil–Dapsone–Artesunate (CDA)

CD (Lapdap^{TM}) was licenced by the UK regulatory authorities in July 2003 and, since then, has been approved by 21 African regulatory authorities. Some current ACT regimens use co-administered drugs (sometimes these are co-packaged), and CD may be co-administered with artemisinins (several studies of this are ongoing) but co-formulation is probably an essential pre-requisite for optimal adherence. With this in mind, the manufacturer of CD is developing CDA (with public funding mainly from MMV (see above)) (www.mmv.org). Phase-III clinical trials are planned for 2005.

3.3.4. Dihydroartemisinin–Piperaquine (DHA–PQ)

Piperaquine (PQ) is a member of the 4-aminoquinoline group that includes chloroquine. PQ proved to be effective and well tolerated when used alone, and no cross-resistance with chloroquine was observed. The initial ACT regimen that included PQ comprised DHA, PQ, primaquine and trimethoprim (referred to as CV8). This has fortunately been rationalised more recently to a dual combination of PQ with DHA (as 'Artekin'; Holleykin Pharmaceuticals). Like CDA, this drug combination is now being developed for submission to regulatory authorities, funded by MMV, and Phase-III trials are planned for 2005 (www.mmv.org).

3.3.5. Other Management

Uncomplicated malaria requires little supportive care and, in high-transmission areas, patients are usually managed without admission to hospital. Rehydration (by mouth) is important because febrile patients may become dehydrated rapidly: oral rehydration solutions are appropriate for outpatient care. Acetaminofen (paracetamol) is probably the safest antipyretic drug, and can be given orally or rectally (although suppositories are expensive).

3.4. Case Management of Severe *P. falciparum* Malaria

It is estimated that there are about 12 million cases of severe malaria treated annually in Africa, with a mortality rate exceeding 10% (assuming competent management). Effective management of severe malaria syndromes is expensive, and relies heavily on hospital and human resources (which are often not equal to the task in tropical countries). It may strike the reader as odd, but whereas the management of uncomplicated malaria has been heavily hit by drug resistance; this is not the case for severe *P. falciparum* malaria in Africa where quinine and the artemisinin drugs remain effective (some resistance to quinine is seen in SE Asia). The principal clinical challenges are initial resuscitation, and then keeping the patient alive long enough to permit the antiparasitic drugs to work.

- The objective of treatment is to save life: secondary considerations, such as parasite clearance and fever clearance, are relegated until the patient has been resuscitated.

- Treatment should be started immediately after the diagnosis is proved (in some cases it is appropriate to start as soon as the diagnosis is *suspected*).
- A drug regimen should be chosen appropriate for the known local pattern of drug resistance. Thus, although quinine remains appropriate in Africa, the artemisinins may be preferred in SE Asia (SEAQUAMAT group, 2005).
- Drug dosage should be calculated by body weight, rather than estimated. This is especially important with quinine which has small therapeutic indices.
- The antimalarial drug should be given parenterally. Oral (or nasogastric dosing) is best avoided: aspiration is a constant risk and drug absorption may be unreliable because of ileus.
- Loading doses of quinine should be given unless the patient has received parenteral quinine or oral halofantrine within the previous 24 hours.
- Therapeutic response should be monitored frequently.
- Drugs should be given orally as soon as patients are able to swallow and retain tablets. This may be quinine but more convenient drugs are usually chosen at this stage, following local guidelines.
  - (a) *Quinine (see drug monographs above)*. The only contraindication to the use of quinine is reliable evidence of serious quinine allergy. Haemolysis, pregnancy, jaundice and renal failure are not contraindications (Warrell, 1999). Quinine has a narrow therapeutic range, and doses should always be adjusted for body weight. A loading dose should be given to achieve therapeutic concentrations more rapidly: there is some evidence from clinical trials of the clinical benefit of a loading dose, but the practice is based largely upon sound pharmacokinetic data and empirical considerations. Contraindications to the use of a loading dose are: (a) treatment with quinine or quinidine in the previous 24 hours and (b) treatment with halofantrine in the previous 24 hours. If patients develop severe malaria following mefloquine treatment, a full dose of quinine should be given. Quinine must never be given as a bolus intravenous injection: the risk of serious adverse reactions is high. The preferred means of administration is by

slow, constant-rate infusion of the drug diluted in crystalloid solution. If intravenous administration is impossible, quinine may be given intramuscularly. Maintenance quinine doses are usually given every 8 hours, but in African children 12-hourly maintenance is effective. In SE Asia, quinine is given for 7 days. Courses are generally shorter in semi-immune African patients (5 days being standard in many countries). To prevent accumulation of quinine, the maintenance dose should be reduced to one-half after 48 hours of parenteral treatment. If possible, blood slides should be examined during treatment: after 24 hours of treatment, counts usually fall in a log-normal manner and asexual parasitaemia should disappear within 5 days (gametocytes may persist, but they are non-pathogenic and of no clinical, although of some public health, relevance). A rising, or unchanging, parasite count after 24 hours of quinine treatment may indicate drug resistance: this is particularly likely in infections acquired in SE Asia.

(b) *Artemisinins (see drug monographs above)*. Intravenous artesunate is superior to intravenous quinine in non-immune patients in SE Asia (SEAQUAMAT group, 2005), where sensitivity to quinine is declining (Roper *et al.*, 2003). An initial loading dose is recommended followed by maintenance doses at 12 hours and, thereafter, daily for up to 7 days or until an oral antimalarial drug can be taken. Suppositories of artemisinin and artesunate (Cao *et al.*, 1997) have proved effective in adults and children with cerebral and other forms of severe malaria in China and SE Asian countries. This is a particularly promising route of administration for use at the most peripheral level of the health service particularly for Africa (Barnes *et al.*, 2004). If malaria is suspected or confirmed in a patient with an acute fever who is unable to swallow tablets, these suppositories may prevent the evolution to severe disease.

(c) Supportive care. A description of the various syndromes of severe malaria, and their management, is outside the scope of the present chapter, and the reader is referred to specific reviews of the subject (Anon, 2000).

3.5. Management of Malaria Outside the Formal Sector

The previous sections stressed the use of drugs in the formal health sector. However, throughout much of the tropics, certainly throughout Africa, a large proportion of antimalarial drug use involves no contact with healthcare professionals. This is a very large topic, and beyond the scope of the present chapter: the reader is referred to Guyatt and Snow (2004).

Communities tend to have a poly pharmacy approach to treating fever, with combinations of traditional remedies, purchased drugs and formal clinic consultation. Sometimes the initial 'choice' of drug is inappropriate: for example, multiple exposures to diversely named proprietary antipyretics/analgesics can delay the start of effective antimalarial drugs. But, assuming that the drug bought over-the-counter is an appropriate choice, it is empirically obvious that adherence with dose and regimen recommendations will be major determinants of outcome. Low adherence is, of course, a common problem in industrialised nations, but poses a particular threat to effective self-medication for malaria, especially in the case of young children and pregnant women. Explanations for this include early resolution of symptoms, limited budgets and poor awareness of correct doses (on the part of both purchaser and vendor). Overdosing is probably less frequent than under dosing but is not uncommon. This 'informal' use of antimalarial drugs has not generally received much research attention in the past but much effort is now being made to study and exploit this area.

4. CONCLUSIONS

We have barely held our own against the burden of mortality and morbidity from malaria in recent years despite a great deal of progress in our understanding of the parasite and the pathophysiology that it initiates. We already possess many of the necessary tools to improve malaria control, but their implementation is currently sub-optimal. This is mainly for reasons of economics and logistics (exacerbated by lack of human resources for complex interventions). So, while it is true that new tools will always be needed, the most immediate concern is obtaining the wherewithal to implement existing control measures.

It seems that we shall be reliant on antimalarial drugs for many decades to come. Africa will certainly need access to novel antimalarial drugs in due course, and drug discovery efforts are happening. But replacements for first-line drugs are needed immediately, and the discovery/development of novel compounds takes many years. So, for some time to come, we shall be reliant on the intelligent deployment of existing drugs and drug combinations. Thanks to the efforts of academia, international organisations (such as WHO, MMV and the Wellcome Trust) and a few pharmaceutical companies, a variety of drugs and drug combinations will become available in the next 2 or 3 years. But we need to keep costs and practicality in the forefront of our minds. Chloroquine and SP are the principal drugs for malaria management in Africa right now, and they cost a few US cents per treatment. Resistance is making us think of using drugs that cost multiples of a dollar: this in a setting where many Ministries of Health are faced with declining drug budgets, and escalating problems in other areas (not least HIV). New approaches to case definitions/diagnosis and case management may be needed in this setting.

It is important to be aware that the data underpinning development of antimalarial drugs need to pass Regulatory scrutiny—the stage that the next wave of drugs is approaching—are insufficient to decide the role of a new drug for the Public Health. Decision makers need data on operational effectiveness (efficacy data from randomised trials are simply too 'artificial'), safety (with data sets in the tens of thousands) and impact on the evolution of drug resistance. There is an urgent need to use behavioural and epidemiological data on fever and drug exposure risks to better estimate the likely adverse drug reaction profiles under different endemicity and drug management scenarios. And even when such operational data are available, experience shows us that the business of splicing new drugs into the public health is extremely complicated—often taking us beyond science and into national politics. Any attempt to understand the vast complexities of human malaria requires an ability to think 'from molecule to policy' and this will require continued multi-disciplinary communication and effort.

REFERENCES

Anon. (2000). Severe falciparum malaria. World Health Organization. *Transactions of the Royal Society of Tropical Medicine and Hygiene* **94**, supplement 1.

Bakyaita, N., Dorsey, G., Yeka, A., Banek, K., Staedke, S.G., Kamya, M.R., Talisuna, A., Kironde, F., Nsobya, S., Kilian, A., Reingold, A., Rosenthal, P.J. and Wabwire-Mangen, F. (2005). Sulfadoxine-pyrimethamine plus chloroquine or amodiaquine for uncomplicated falciparum malaria: a randomized, multisite trial to guide national policy in Uganda. *American Journal of Tropical Medicine and Hygiene* **72**(5), 573–580.

Barnes, K.I., Mwenechanya, J., Tembo, M., McIlleron, H., Folb, P.I., Ribeiro, I., Little, F., Gomes, M. and Molyneux, M.E. (2004). Efficacy of rectal artesunate compared with parenteral quinine in initial treatment of moderately severe malaria in African children and adults: a randomised study. *Lancet* **363**, 1598–1605.

Borrmann, S., Issifou, S., Esser, G., Adegnika, A.A., Ramharter, M., Matsiegui, P.B., Oyakhirome, S., Mawili-Mboumba, D.P., Missinou, M.A., Kun, J.F., Jomaa, H. and Kremsner, P.G. (2004). Fosmidomycin–clindamycin for the treatment of *Plasmodium falciparum* malaria. *Journal of Infectious Diseases* **190**(9), 1534–1540.

Bray, P.G., Hawley, S.R., Mungthin, M. and Ward, S.A. (1996). Physicochemical properties correlated with drug resistance and the reversal of drug resistance in *Plasmodium falciparum*. *Molecular Pharmacology* **50**, 1559–1566.

Bray, P.G., Janneh, O., Raynes, K.J., Mungthin, M., Ginsburg, H. and Ward, S.A. (1999). Cellular uptake of chloroquine is dependent on binding to ferriprotoporphyrin IX and is independent of NHE activity in *Plasmodium falciparum*. *Journal of Cell Biology* **145**, 363–376.

Bray, P.G., Mungthin, M., Ridley, R.G. and Ward, S.A. (1998). Access to hematin: the basis of chloroquine resistance. *Molecular Pharmacology* **54**, 170–179.

Canfield, C.J., Pudney, M. and Gutteridge, W.E. (1995). Interactions of atovaquone with other antimalarial drugs against *Plasmodium falciparum* in vitro. *Experimental Parasitology* **80**, 373–381.

Cao, X.T., Bethell, D.B., Pham, T.P., Ta, T.T., Tran, T.N., Nguyen, T.T., Pham, T.T., Nguyen, T.T., Day, N.P. and White, N.J. (1997). Comparison of artemisinin suppositories, intramuscular artesunate and intravenous quinine for the treatment of severe childhood malaria. *Transactions of the Royal Society of Tropical Medicine and Hygiene* **91**, 335–342.

Centers for Disease Control. (1985). Adverse reactions to Fansidar and updated recommendations for its use in the prevention of malaria. *Morbidity and Mortality Weekly Report* **8**, 713–714.

Clark, R.L., White, T.E., Clode, S., Gaunt, I., Winstanley, P. and Ward, S.A. (2004). Developmental toxicity of artesunate and an artesunate combination in the rat and rabbit. *Birth Defects Research B Developmental and Reproductive Toxicology* **71**(6), 380–394.

Day, K.P. and Marsh, K. (1991). Naturally acquired immunity to *Plasmodium falciparum*. *Parasitology Today* **7**(3), 68–71.

Dollery, C. (1999a). In: *Therapeutic Drugs*, pp. A208–A213. Edinburgh: Churchill Livingstone.

Dollery, C. (1999b). In: *Therapeutic Drugs*, pp. C177–C182. Edinburgh: Churchill Livingstone.

Dollery, C. (1999c). In: *Therapeutic Drugs*, pp. D13–D18. Edinburgh: Churchill Livingstone.

Dollery, C. (1999d). In: *Therapeutic Drugs*, pp. P296–P300. Edinburgh: Churchill Livingstone.

Dollery, C. (1999e). In: *Therapeutic Drugs*, pp. Q16–Q21. Edinburgh: Churchill Livingstone.

Eckstein-Ludwig, U., Webb, R.J., Van Goethem, I.D., East, J.M., Lee, A.G., Kimura, M., O'Neill, P.M., Bray, P.G., Ward, S.A. and Krishna, S. (2003). Artemisinins target the SERCA of *Plasmodium falciparum*. *Nature* **424**(6951), 957–961.

Ezzet, F., van Vugt, M., Nosten, F., Looareesuwan, S. and White, N.J. (2000). Pharmacokinetics and pharmacodynamics of lumefantrine (benflumetol) in acute falciparum malaria. *Antimicrobial Agents and Chemotherapy* **44**, 697–704.

Fogg, C., Bajunirwe, F., Piola, P., Biraro, S., Checchi, F., Kiguli, J., Namiiro, P., Musabe, J., Kyomugisha, A. and Guthmann, J.P. (2004). Adherence to a six-dose regimen of artemether–lumefantrine for treatment of uncomplicated Plasmodium falciparum malaria in Uganda. *American Journal of Tropical Medicine and Hygiene* **71**(5), 525–530.

Guyatt, H.L. and Snow, R.W. (2004). The management of fevers in Kenyan children and adults in an area of seasonal malaria transmission. *Transactions of the Royal Society of Tropical Medicine and Hygiene* **98**(2), 111–115.

Hatton, C., Peto, T., Bunch, C., Pasvol, G., Russel, S., Singer, C., Edwards, G. and Winstanley, P.A. (1986). Frequency of severe neutropaenia associated with amodiaquine prophylaxis against malaria. *Lancet* **1**, 411–413.

Kublin, J.G., Cortese, J.F., Njunju, E.M., Mukadama, R.A., Wirima, J.J., Kazembe, P.N., Djimde, A.A., Kouriba, B. and Plowe, C.V. (2003). Re-emergence of chloroquine-sensitive *Plasmodium falciparum* malaria after cessation of chloroquine use in Malawi. *JID* **187**, 1870–1875.

McGready, R., Cho, T., Keo, N.K., Thwai, K.L., Villegas, L., Looareesuwan, S., White, N.J. and Nosten, F. (2001). Artemisinin antimalarials in pregnancy: a prospective treatment study of 539 episodes of multidrug-resistant *Plasmodium falciparum*. *Clinical Infectious Diseases* **33**, 2009–2016.

Murphy, S., Watkins, W.M., Bray, P.G., Lowe, B., Winstanley, P.A., Peshu, N. and Marsh, K. (1995). Parasite viability during treatment of severe falciparum malaria: differential effects of artemether and quinine. *American Journal of Tropical Medicine and Hygiene* **53**(3), 303–305.

Nosten, F., Rogerson, S.J., Beeson, J.G., McGready, R., Mutabingwa, T.K. and Brabin, B. (2004). Malaria in pregnancy and the endemicity spectrum: what can we learn? *Trends in Parasitology* **20**(9), 425–432.

Nosten, F., ter Kuile, F.O., Luxemburger, C., Woodrow, C., Kyle, D.E., Chongsuphajaisiddhi, T. and White, N.J. (1993). Cardiac effects of antimalarial treatment with halofantrine. *Lancet* **341**, 1054–1056.

Nosten, F., van Vugt, M., Price, R., Luxemburger, C., Thway, K.L., Brockman, A., McGready, R., ter Kuile, F., Looareesuwan, S. and White, N.J. (2000). Effects of artesunate–mefloquine combination on the incidence of *Plasmodium falciparum* malaria and mefloquine resistance in Western Thailand: a prospective study. *Lancet* **356**, 297–302.

Olliaro, P. and Mussano, P. (2003). Amodiaquine for treating malaria. *Cochrane Database Systems Reviews* (2), CD000016. Update of: (2000). *Cochrane Database Systems Reviews* (2), CD000016.

Plowe, C.V., Cortese, J.F., Djimde, A., Nwanyanwu, O.C., Watkins, W.M., Winstanley, P.A., Estrada-Franco, J.G., Mollinedo, R.E., Avila, J.C., Cespedes, J.L., Carter, D. and Doumbo, O.K. (1997). Mutations in *Plasmodium falciparum* dihydrofolate reductase and dihydropteroate synthase and epidemiologic patterns of pyrimethamine-sulfadoxine use and resistance. *Journal of Infectious Diseases* **176**, 1590–1596.

Riou, B., Barriot, P., Rimailho, A. and Baud, F.J. (1988). Treatment of severe chloroquine poisoning. *New England Journal of Medicine* **318**, 1–6.

Roper, C., Pearce, R., Bredenkamp, B., Gumede, J., Drakeley, C., Mosha, F., Chandramohan, D. and Sharp, B. (2003). Antifolate antimalarial resistance in southeast Africa: a population-based analysis. *Lancet* **361**(9364), 1174–1181.

Schellenberg, D., Menendez, C., Kahigwa, E., Aponte, J., Vidal, J., Tanner, M., Mshinda, H. and Alonso, P. (2001). Intermittent treatment for malaria and anaemia control at time of routine vaccinations in Tanzanian infants: a randomised, placebo-controlled trial. *Lancet* **357**(9267), 1471–1477.

Sisowath, C., Stromberg, J., Martensson, A., Msellem, M., Obondo, C., Bjorkman, A. and Gil, J.P. (2005). In vivo selection of *Plasmodium falciparum* pfmdr1 86N coding alleles by artemether–lumefantrine (Coartem). *Journal of Infectious Diseases* **191**(6), 1014–1017.

South East Asian Quinine Artesunate Malaria Trial (SEAQUAMAT) group. (2005). Artesunate versus quinine for treatment of severe falciparum malaria: a randomised trial. *Lancet* **366**, 717–725.

Senior, K. (2005). Shortfall in front-line antimalarial drug likely in 2005. *Lancet Infectious Diseases* **5**(2), 75.

Shulman, C.E., Dorman, E.K., Cutts, F., Kawuondo, K., Bulmer, J.N., Peshu, N. and Marsh, K. (1999). Intermittent sulphadoxine–pyrimethamine to prevent severe anaemia secondary to malaria in pregnancy: a randomised placebo-controlled trial. *Lancet* **353**(9153), 632–636.

Sisowath, C., Stromberg, J., Martensson, A., Msellem, M., Obondo, C., Bjorkman, A. and Gil, J.P. (2005). In vivo selection of Plasmodium falciparum pfmdr1 86N coding alleles by artemether–lumefantrine (Coartem). *Journal of Infectious Diseases* **191**(6), 1014–1017.

Warrell, D.A. (1999). Management of severe malaria. *Parasitologia* **41**, 287–294.

Watkins, W.M. and Mosobo, M. (1993). Treatment of *Plasmodium falciparum* malaria with pyrimethamine–sulfadoxine: selective pressure for resistance is a function of long elimination half-life. *Transactions of the Royal Society of Tropical Medicine and Hygiene* **87**, 75–78.

Wellems, T.E., Panton, L.J., Gluzman, I.Y., do Rosario, V.E., Gwadz, R.W., Walker-Jonah, A. and Krogstad, D. (1990). Chloroquine resistance not linked to mdr-like genes in a *Plasmodium falciparum* cross. *Nature* **345**, 253–255.

Wellems, T.E. and Plowe, C.V. (2001). Chloroquine-resistant malaria. *Journal of Infectious Diseases* **184**, 770–776.

White, N.J. (1994). Clinical pharmacokinetics and pharmacodynamics of artemisinin and derivatives. *Transactions of the Royal Society of Tropical Medicine and Hygiene* **88**(supplement 1), S41–S43.

White, N.J. (2004). Antimalarial drug resistance. *Journal of Clinical Investigation* **113**(8), 1084–1092.

White, N.J., Miller, K.D. and Churchill, F.C. (1988). Chloroquine treatment of severe malaria in children. Pharmacokinetics, toxicity and new dosage recommendations. *New England Journal of Medicine* **319**, 1493–1500.

Winstanley, P.A., Coleman, J.W., Maggs, J.M., Breckenridge, A.M. and Park, B.K. (1990). The toxicity of amodiaquine and its principal metabolites towards mononuclear leukocytes and granulocyte–monocyte colony forming units. *British Journal of Clinical Pharmacology* **29**, 479–485.

Winstanley, P.A., Edwards, G., Orme, M.L.E. and Breckenridge, A.M. (1987). The disposition of amodiaquine in man after oral administration. *British Journal of Clinical Pharmacology* **23**, 1–7.

Winstanley, P.A., Newton, C.R., Watkins, W.M., Mberu, E., Ward, S.A., Warn, P.A., Mwangi, I., Waruiru, C., Pasvol, G., Warrell, D.A. and Marsh, K. (1993). Towards optimal parenteral quinine regimens for young children with cerebral malaria: importance of unbound quinine concentration. *Transactions of the Royal Society of Tropical Medicine and Hygiene* **87**, 201–206.

Useful Websites:

http://www.mmv.org/FilesUpld/208.pdf.
http://www.rocheuk.com/ProductDB/Documents/rx/pil/Lariam_PIL.pdf.

Insecticide-Treated Nets

Jenny Hill[1], Jo Lines[2] and Mark Rowland[3]

[1]*Child and Reproductive Health Group, Liverpool School of Tropical Medicine, Pembroke Place, Liverpool L3 5QA, UK*
[2]*Malaria Knowledge Programme, London School of Hygiene and Tropical Medicine, Keppel Street, London WC1E 7HT, UK*
[3]*Gates Malaria Partnership, London School of Hygiene and Tropical Medicine, Keppel Street, London WC1E 7HT, UK*

ADVANCES IN PARASITOLOGY VOL 61
ISSN: 0065-308X
DOI: 10.1016/S0065-308X(05)61003-2

ABSTRACT

Insecticide-treated nets (ITNs) are the most powerful malaria control tool to be developed since the advent of indoor residual spraying (IRS) and chloroquine in the 1940s, and as such they have been an important component of global and national malaria control policies since the mid-1990s. Yet a decade later, coverage is still unacceptably low: only 3% of African children are currently sleeping under an ITN, and only about 20% are sleeping under any kind of net. This review charts the scientific, policy and programmatic progress of ITNs over the last 10 years. Available evidence for the range of programmatic delivery mechanisms used at country level is presented alongside the key policy debates that together have contributed to the evolution of ITN delivery strategies over the past decade. There is now global consensus around a strategic framework for scaling up ITN usage in Africa, which recognizes a role for both the public sector (targeting vulnerable groups to promote equity) and the private sector (sustainable supply). So, while progress with increasing coverage to date has been slow, there is now global support for the rapid scale-up of ITNs among vulnerable groups by integrating ITN delivery with maternal and child health programmes (and immunization in particular), at the same time working with the private sector in a complementary and supportive manner to ensure that coverage can be maintained for future generations of African children.

1. INTRODUCTION

Insecticide-treated nets (ITNs) first came to the attention of public health experts over 20 years ago, when the first studies to evaluate the impact of the novel application of pyrethroid insecticides to the traditional mosquito net on reducing malaria vector exposure were undertaken in Africa and Asia (Darriet *et al.*, 1984; Ranque *et al.*, 1984; Charlwood and Graves, 1987; Lines *et al.*, 1987). These studies confirmed the safety of pyrethroid insecticides used to treat the nets and demonstrated substantial effects on various entomological measures such as human biting rates, feeding behaviour and survival. The success of these initial studies led quickly to Phase II and III clinical field trials, which provided the crucial evidence that ITNs were successful in reducing both malaria morbidity and, importantly, all-cause child mortality.

The mortality trials showed that ITNs are the most powerful malaria control tool to be developed since the advent of indoor residual spraying (IRS) and chloroquine, more than four decades earlier. As a result, they have been an important component of global and many national malaria control policies since the mid-1990s. Yet a decade later, coverage is still unacceptably low. Why is this?

This review charts the progress of ITNs over the last ten years, from efficacy and effectiveness studies to more recent technological advances, and from incorporation of ITNs into global and national malaria control policies to their deployment using a range of programmatic delivery mechanisms.

2. EFFICACY STUDIES

2.1. The Impact of ITNs on Malaria Morbidity

2.1.1. Children and Adults

There is a large body of evidence from over 81 trials conducted in a range of malaria transmission settings worldwide showing that use of ITNs substantially reduces the frequency and severity of malaria. A recent systematic review of 22 of these trials (those which constituted randomized controlled trials) conducted in children and adults in sub-Saharan Africa (13), Latin America (5), Thailand (2), Pakistan (1) and Iran (1) showed that ITNs reduced clinical episodes by around 50% in both stable and unstable malarious areas and for both *Plasmodium falciparum* and *P. vivax* infections (Lengeler, 2004). The protective efficacy tended to be higher when the control group had no nets as compared to untreated nets, and in areas of unstable malaria the impact of ITNs against *P. falciparum* infections was greater than against *P. vivax*. One trial demonstrated a 45% reduction in the number of cases of severe malarial disease presenting to health facilities (Nevill *et al.*, 1996). Studies variously included parasite prevalence, high parasitaemia, anaemia, splenomegaly and anthropometric measures as outcomes, with the majority of trials using 2–5 different outcomes (see Table 1). Five studies which assessed high parasitaemia as an outcome showed a protective efficacy range from 20% (3 trials with untreated nets in the control group) (Snow *et al.*, 1988; Lindsay *et al.*, 1989a; D'Alessandro *et al.*, 1995a) to 29% (2 trials with controls with no nets) (Habluetzel *et al.*, 1997; ter Kuile *et al.*, 2003a). ITNs also had a beneficial impact on both anaemia (9 trials) and anthropometric outcomes (3 trials).

However, efficacy is expected to depend on vector behaviour. Although the trial evidence is remarkably consistent, there are still some important gaps. For example, until recent studies (Magris, 2004), there was no convincing evidence that ITNs are effective against forest malaria transmitted by *Anopheles darlingi* in the Amazon basin (Zimmerman and Voorham 1997). In the case of the south-east Asian forest malaria vectors, especially *An. dirus*, ITNs are believed to have been highly effective in routine programmes, but there is surprisingly little evidence from rigorous formal randomized trials. A recent study in a forested area of Cambodia with *An. dirus* indicates a protective efficacy of 35% in children under five (Sochantha *et al.*, 2006). In particular, it is widely believed that ITNs are not and cannot be efficacious against vectors that bite early in the evening. This is indeed a sensible expectation, but in fact ITNs have been shown to be surprisingly effective against *An. sinensis* in China (IDRC and WHO, 1996), *An. albimanus* in South America (Richards *et al.*, 1994; Kroeger *et al.*, 1995), *An. culicifacies* in India (Curtis *et al.*, 1999) and Pakistan (Rowland *et al.*, 1996), and *An. stephensi* in Afghanistan (Rowland *et al.*, 2004), despite the fact that these four species are early evening biters.

2.1.2. Pregnant Women

Six randomized controlled trials to determine the impact of ITNs in pregnant women (Dolan *et al.*, 1993; D'Alessandro *et al.*, 1996; Shulman *et al.*, 1998; Browne *et al.*, 2001; Njagi *et al.*, 2003; ter Kuile *et al.*, 2003b) and one non-randomized trial of the impact of socially marketed ITNs (Marchant *et al.*, 2002) have been conducted across a range of malaria

Table 1 Insecticide-treated nets and curtains for preventing malaria: randomization and outcomes

Study	Types of controls	Unit of allocation[a]	Child mortality[b]	Uncomplicated episodes[c]	Parasite prevalence[c]	High parasitaemia	Anaemia	Splenomegaly	Anthropometry
Burkina Faso (Habluetzel)	No nets	Groups of villages	X		X	X	X		
Cameroon (Moyou-Somo)	No nets	Household			X			X	
Colombia (Kroeger)	Untreated nets	Village		X Pf/Pv					
Ecuador (Kroeger)	Untreated nets	Village		X Pf/Pv					
Gambia (D'Alessandro)	Untreated nets	Village	X (X)		X	X	X	X	X
Ghana (Binka)	No nets	Village	X (X)		X	X	X		
Gambia (Snow I)	Untreated nets	Household		X	X	X	X		
Gambia (Snow II)	Untreated nets	Village		X	X	X	X	X	
Iran (Zaim I)	Untreated nets	Village		X Pf/Pv					
Ivory Coast (Henry)	No nets	Village		X	X		X		
Kenya (Nevill)	No nets	Village	X[d]		X				X
Kenya (Phillips-Howard)	No nets	Village	X	X	X	X	X		X
Kenya (Sexton)	No nets	Household		X					
Madagascar (Rabarison)	Untreated nets	Household		X					
Nicaragua (Kroeger)	No nets	Village		X Pv					
Pakistan (Rowland)	No nets	Household		X Pf/Pv	X Pf/Pv				
Peru Amazon (Kroeger)	Untreated nets	Village		X Pv					
		Village		X Pv					

Table 1 (*continued*)

Study	Types of controls	Unit of allocation[a]	Child mortality[b]	Uncomplicated episodes[c]	Parasite prevalence[c]	High parasitaemia	Anaemia	Splenomegaly	Anthropometry
Peru Coast (Kroeger)	Untreated nets								
Sierra-Leone (Marbiah)	No nets	Village		X			X	X	
Tanzania (Fraser-Hurt)	No nets	Individual			X		X		
Thailand (Kamol-Ratanakul)	Untreated nets	Household		X Pf/Pv					
Thailand (Luxemburger)	Untreated nets	Individual		X Pf/Pv	X Pf/Pv			X	

Source: Lengeler (2004). Copyright © Cochrane Library. Reproduced with permission.
[a]Randomization by village considered by cluster.
[b]Studies marked X also measured malaria-specific child mortality.
[c]Pf/Pv indicates *P. falciparum* and *P. vivax*; all other studies included *P. falciparum* only.
[d]Also included severe disease.

transmission settings in sub-Saharan Africa. Among the earlier studies, two studies in areas with low, seasonal transmission (Thailand and The Gambia) showed ITNs significantly reduced parasitaemia and maternal anaemia and increased birth weight (D'Alessandro *et al.*, 1996; Dolan *et al.*, 1993), but studies in higher transmission settings (coastal Kenya and Ghana) showed no impact on these outcomes (Shulman *et al.*, 1998; Browne *et al.*, 2001). However, three more recent trials in high transmission areas observed improvements in anaemia, severe anaemia, maternal and placental malaria and birth weight outcomes (Marchant *et al.*, 2002; Njagi *et al.*, 2003; ter Kuile *et al.*, 2003b). The results of these studies are summarized in Table 2.

In addition to variations in impact in different transmission settings, the timing of ITN use during pregnancy is significant. The risk of peripheral malaria parasitaemia is greatest in the first 20 weeks of gestation and ITNs are therefore likely to have their greatest impact during this period. Four of the six randomised controlled trials to determine the impact of ITNs during pregnancy gave ITNs to all members of the community, regardless of pregnancy status, so the majority of pregnant women became pregnant after the intervention was introduced—i.e. they were protected from the start of their pregnancy. We do not have sufficient evidence of the impact ITNs when used from the second or even third trimesters of pregnancy, as is the case in a programmatic setting when most women first access ANC.

2.1.3. *ITNs in Combination with Other Malaria Control Interventions*

While ITN efficacy studies have mainly focused on single interventions, the programmatic reality is that several malaria control interventions, such as ITNs and intermittent preventative treatment (IPT) or case management and ITNs, are delivered alongside each other as part of integrated maternal and child health programmes. It is therefore important to understand the effectiveness and cost-effectiveness of combined interventions. However, only one study has assessed the combined effect of IPT with ITNs on malaria in pregnancy using a factorial design with four intervention groups—IPT + ITNs, IPT alone, ITNs alone, and no intervention (Njagi *et al.*, 2003). The study,

Table 2 Studies of use of insecticide-treated nets during pregnancy

Country (reference)	Transmission (entomological inoculation rate)	Control group	No. (ITN/control)	Comments		Anaemia[a]	Severe anaemia[b]	Maternal malaria	Placental malaria	Low birth weight (difference from mean birth weight)
Thailand (Dolan *et al.*, 1993)	Low (<1)	No net	103/204	All gravidae, ANC-based randomization	control (*N* = 30 no net)	**PR: 0.5**	NA	RR: 0.51	NA	PR: 0.64
					Control no net + untreated net (N = 204)	PR: 0.73	NA	**RR: 0.81**	NA	PR: 1.01
The Gambia (D'Alessandro *et al.*, 1996)	Low seasonal (1–10)	No net or untreated	305/341	Primigravidae	Rainy season	NA	PR: 1.18	**PR: 0.61**	NA	**+ 130 g**
					Dry season	NA	**PR: 0.32**	PR: 1.11	NA	–135 g
Kenya (Shulman *et al.*, 1998)	Intermediate seasonal (10–30)	No net	263/228	Primigravidae, village-based randomization; hospital ANC attendees		PR: 0.99	OR: 0.71	OR: 0.75	OR: 0.75	0 g
Ghana (Browne *et al.*, 2001)	High seasonal (300)	No net	1033/928	All gravidae, household children <5 years		OR: 0.88	OR: 0.80	OR: 0.89	NA	OR: 0.87
Kenya (ter Kuile *et al.*, 2003)	High perennial (100–300)	No net	1377/1377	All gravidae	Gravidae 1 to 4	**HR: 0.79**[c]	HR: 0.70[c]	**PR: 0.62**	**PR: 0.77**	**PR: 0.72 + 78 g**
					Gravidae 5 +	HR: 1.00[c]	HR: 1.24[c]	PR: 0.80	**PR: 0.72**	PR: 1.12 – 27 g
Kenya (Njagi, 2002)	High perennial (100–300)	No net	480/483	Primi + secundigravidae ANC-based randomization		**PR: 0.59**[d]	NA	**PR: 0.70**	**PR: 0.61**	PR: 0.68 + 67 g
Tanzania (Marchant *et al.*, 2002)	High perennial (100–300)	No net	239/266	All gravidae, non-randomized, social marketing		**PR: 0.88**	**RR: 0.62**	RR: 0.77[e]	NA	NA

Source: ter Kuile (2003). Reproduced with permission.
Bold type indicates statistically significant differences. ANC, antenatal clinics; HR, hazard ratio; N, number; NA, not applicable; OR, odds ratio; PR, prevalence ratio; RR, risk ratio.
[a]Any anaemia (haemoglobin <11 or <10 g/dL, or haematocrit <30%).
[b]Severe anaemia (haemoglobin <8 or <7 g/dL).
[c]Gravidae 1–4: *N* = 451, gravidae 5 +: *N* = 313.
[d]Primigravidae only; 16% [–35 to –48] in secundigravidae.
[e]Significant reduction in high-density parasitaemia (RR 0.62 [0.41–0.95]).

which assessed the impact of ITNs distributed to women during their second trimester as part of routine antenatal care services, showed that both ITNs and IPT are effective in reducing maternal and placental malaria and maternal anaemia (see Table 2), but IPT alone had a greater impact on maternal anaemia than ITNs alone. A small additional benefit of combining IPT with ITNs was observed.

It would be expected that a combined intervention of repellent plus ITN would be more effective than ITN alone against malaria transmitted by vector species that bite both in the early evening and at night, although no randomized trial has yet been undertaken. However a case–control study carried out on a population that had been the subject of a social marketing (SM) project of ITN and skin repellents indicated that regular users of ITN and DEET repellent acquired 69% protection against *P. vivax* malaria episodes, compared to 46% protection with ITN alone (Rowland *et al.*, 2004).

2.1.4. Untreated Nets

As one might expect, untreated nets do give partial protection against malaria. The evidence for this is not extensive, and has mostly been collected since the advent of ITNs, but it is nevertheless consistent in implying that the protection against malaria by untreated net use is about half that given by ITN use (Clarke *et al.*, 2001; Schellenberg *et al.*, 2001; Guyatt and Snow, 2002). If this is true, it casts an interesting light on the observation that over 80% of nets in Africa are untreated (WHO, 2005a). It means that, at the time of these surveys, these untreated nets, which were presumably mostly supplied by unsubsidized commercial sources, were preventing more child mortality in Africa than the treated nets supplied by projects.

There is evidence that untreated nets divert mosquitoes from the occupant to unprotected people nearby. However, this probably acts to the benefit of children, since they are the most likely members if the family to be actually sleeping under a net in net-owning households (http://www.NetMarkAfrica.org). There is also evidence that high levels of untreated net use can confer some protection against malaria on individuals with no nets in the same community (Clarke *et al.*, 2001; Hii *et al.*, 2001; Smith *et al.*, 2002).

2.2. The Impact of ITNs on Childhood Mortality

2.2.1. Protective Efficacy and Lives Saved

Child mortality (children aged 1–59 months) from all causes is the main outcome of public health interest. Five randomized controlled trials in areas of stable malaria transmission in sub-Saharan Africa (Burkina Faso, The Gambia, Ghana, western Kenya and coastal Kenya) examined the impact of ITNs on childhood mortality. In four of these, the intervention was distribution of ITNs to everyone in the community, and background levels of net use in the control group were low (Binka *et al.*, 1996; Nevill *et al.*, 1996; Habluetzel *et al.*, 1997; Phillips-Howard *et al.*, 2003). In one trial, pre-existing background levels of untreated net use were high, and the intervention consisted of treating these nets with insecticide (D'Alessandro *et al.*, 1995b). The protective efficacy for the four trials with no-net controls was 17%, compared to 23% for the trial with controls with untreated nets (see Figure 1) and the summary rate differences were almost identical, 5.5 versus 5.6 lives saved per year for every 1000 under five children protected (Lengeler, 2004).

Measured as a ratio, the protective efficacy provided by ITN use appears to be lower in areas with high malaria transmission (entomological inoculation rate >1000) than in areas with lower transmission, but the magnitude of the risk difference was remarkably constant over a wide range of transmission intensities. Hence, we can say with some confidence that, in most endemic rural areas of sub-Saharan Africa, maintaining ITN coverage for just 200 under five children will prevent one death per year (Lengeler, 2004). It is estimated that approximately 370 000 deaths could be avoided annually if every child in sub-Saharan Africa was protected by ITNs (14% of a population at risk of 480 million, or 67 million children).

2.2.2. Mass Effect versus Individual Barrier Protection

The coverage levels of ITNs achieved in clinical trials is high, usually in excess of 80–90%, and there have been relatively few trials with lower levels of coverage. However, little is known about how impact

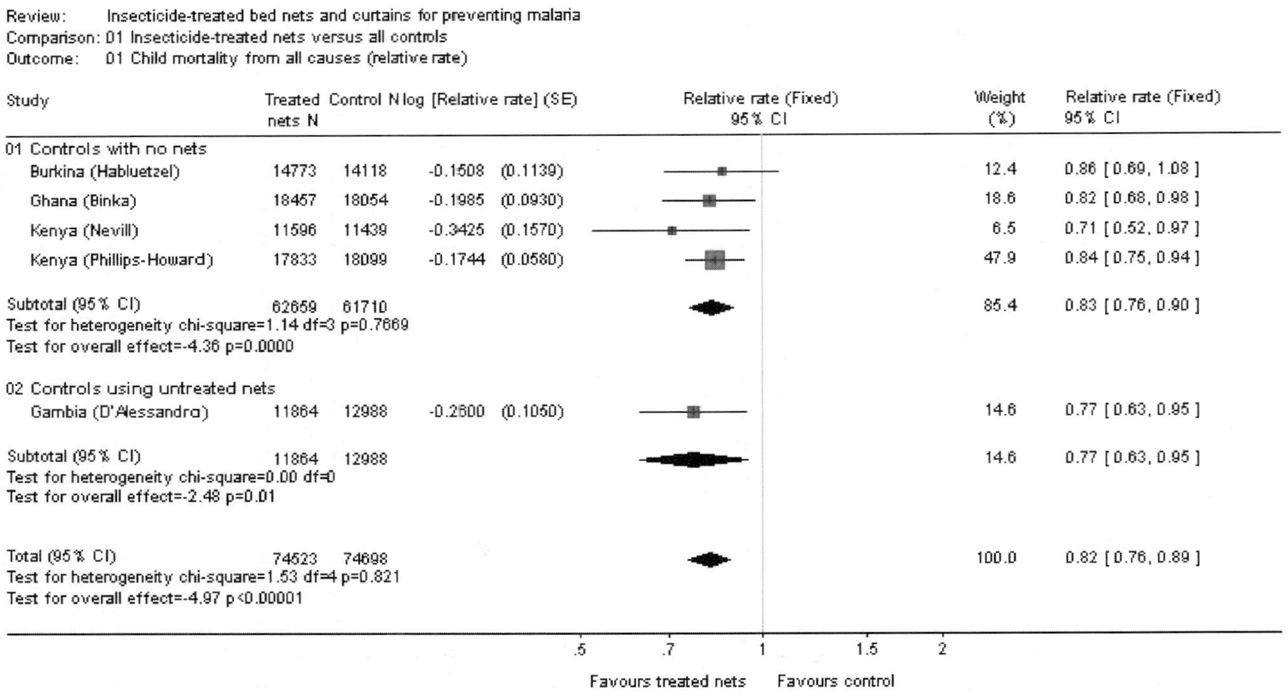

Figure 1 Comparison of insecticide-treated nets versus all controls: child mortality from all causes (relative rate). *Source*: Lengeler, 2004. Copyright © Cochrane Library. Reproduced with permission.

varies with coverage level. It is known that ITNs kill some of the mosquitoes that come to bite (Lines *et al.*, 1987). High levels of ITN coverage can result in mass killing of the mosquito population, which tends to reduce the mean lifespan of vector females and can produce substantial reductions in the local sporozoite rate of the vector population (Magesa *et al.*, 1991). This kind of 'mass effect' on vectors produces an epidemiological 'community effect', by which the presence of large number of ITNs in a community gives health benefits even to non-users (IDRC and WHO, 1996). Studies in Ghana (Binka *et al.*, 1998) and western Kenya (Hawley *et al.*, 2003) showed that children in control areas but living within a few hundred metres of an intervention area experienced similar reductions in mortality to children in the intervention areas. Similar benefits of a mass effect on malaria morbidity have been detected in a study on the Kenyan coast (Howard *et al.*, 2000). On the other hand, no such effect was observed in trials in The Gambia, perhaps because of a higher level of mosquito movement between intervention and non-intervention villages (D'Alessandro *et al.*, 1995b; Quinones *et al.*, 1998).

Two of the six randomized controlled trials of the impact of ITNs during pregnancy described above assessed the impact of ITNs distributed through antenatal clinics and randomized individual women, rather than villages, to the different interventions. The mass-killing effect on mosquito populations in the other four trials, which were group-randomized, may therefore have resulted in an underestimation of impact of ITNs during pregnancy, as pregnant women in the control groups may have received some protection from the mass effect (D'Alessandro *et al.*, 1996; Shulman *et al.*, 1998; Browne *et al.*, 2001; ter Kuile *et al.*, 2003b).

An important factor to consider in the interpretation of the mass effect is that it is a positive externality, i.e. it depends on ITN coverage at the community level, not on individual behaviour, and requires that these ITNs retain good insecticidal activity. Thus the degree of mass effect observed in clinical trials is unlikely to be matched under operational conditions, where ITN retreatment rates are notoriously low. The development of long-lasting insecticidal nets (LLINs) (see Section 6) may help to extend the effective duration of the mass effect, but this is not yet clear.

More studies are needed to determine how the intensity of the mass effect varies with coverage levels and over time. Strong mass effects are unlikely to be seen with highly zoophilic vectors (such as *An. culicifacies*). In terms of coverage, it would be helpful for planning purposes to define a target threshold level of coverage for the mass effect, just as 80% coverage is conventionally regarded as a target for house-spraying. In reality, it is unlikely that this kind of threshold exists for ITNs. Rather, the strength of the mass effect probably varies continuously across all levels of coverage. This is consistent with theoretical expectation, and with the observation that even full ITN coverage does not interrupt transmission completely.

2.3. The Impact of ITNs on Other Diseases and Nuisance Insects

While ITNs have the potential to provide personal protection or transmission control against a number of vector-borne diseases in which the vector bites at night such as leishmaniasis and Chagas disease (Kroeger *et al.*, 2002; Kroeger *et al.*, 2003), few studies have actually been carried out. A household-randomized trial of ITN versus IRS was carried out in the city of Kabul, Afghanistan, against anthroponotic cutaneous leishmaniasis (ACL) transmitted by sand flies (Reyburn *et al.*, 2000). Over the course of a year the incidence of new cases was reduced by 67% among households with ITNs, compared to 48% among households with IRS, relative to the control group. ITNs were the more popular intervention and there was a high demand for ITNs in the urban population. Because of the scale of the problem, the size of the population at risk in Kabul, and the non-fatal nature of the disease, no donor was able or willing to address the problem with the number of nets that would be required, and the largest epidemic of ACL in the world continues unabated. Earlier Taych *et al.* (1997) had used bednets impregnated with pyrethroids in Aleppo, Syria to control ACL transmitted by *Phlebotomus sergenti*.

ITNs provide protection against a number of nuisance insects and this is sometimes cited as a reason for their popularity (Alaii *et al.*, 2003). The nuisance mosquito *Culex quinquefasciatus* is often more abundant than anophelines and were it not for the protection given against culicines the popularity and effectiveness of ITN would be hampered (Magesa *et al.*, 1991; Hewitt *et al.*, 1997; Asidi *et al.*, 2005). ITNs are very effective against susceptible *C. quinquefasciatus* in Asia but owing to pyrethroid resistance they are not very effective in killing *C. quinquefasciatus* in E. or W. Africa (Hewitt *et al.*, 1997; Asidi *et al.*, 2005; Graham *et al.*, 2005). Despite this, ITN remain popular in Africa because of a barrier effect even when holed (Asidi *et al.*, 2005). *C. quinquefasciatus* is, of course, an important urban vector of filariasis in E. Africa and Asia but no concerted studies have been carried out on whether ITNs might provide any protection against infection rates or morbidity due to filariasis. ITNs have also been shown to reduce risk of Japanese encephalitis infection in children < 10 years old combined with vaccination (Dapeng *et al.*, 1994).

ITNs also provide protection against head lice and bedbugs (Lindsay *et al.*, 1989b), and reduction in infestations has been used as an indirect indicator of ITN use during trials of ITN in naïve populations (Rowland *et al.*, 1996). Bedbugs have recently become resistant to pyrethroids in foci of E. Tanzania where ITN have been in use for several years, and are no longer being controlled (whereas the anophelines remain susceptible), and it is greatly feared that this will undermine the current popularity of ITN (Myamba *et al.*, 2002). Alternative insecticides need to be sought for use on nets.

2.4. Acquisition of Malarial Immunity

Both theory and the available observational evidence suggest that children protected by ITNs do have reduced levels of immunity compared to unprotected children. They nevertheless suffer less disease on balance, because the substantial decrease in exposure more than compensates for this slight increase in vulnerability. This straightforward and reassuring conclusion requires qualification of two kinds.

The first concerns the question of what happens if the protection is withdrawn. If a child has been using an ITN but is suddenly deprived of it, then, in theory, we expect disease incidence and severity to be increased, during the period while the child's levels of immunity re-adjust to the new and higher levels of exposure. There is nevertheless every reason to expect that the previous health benefits, gained from earlier use of the ITN, will greatly exceed and outweigh the health costs during this post-withdrawal period of 'rebound' disease. More-over, in practice, it is much more likely that the protection will decline slowly, as the insecticide wears off and as the net develops holes and, because this happens gradually, no noticeable rebound effect is likely. This lack of a rebound effect on all-cause childhood mortality has been documented in two six-year follow-up studies in Burkina Faso and western Kenya (Diallo *et al.*, 2004; Eisele *et al.*, 2005).

The second and more serious issue is whether there might be cir-cumstances in which reducing exposure to malaria is actually unde-sirable and potentially harmful. The best way to understand how this could be is to think of the examples of mumps (for men) and rubella (for women). These are viral infections which cause generally mild and non-severe disease in children, and one infection gives complete immunity. However, if a person does not get infected as a child, and does get infected as an adult, he or she is at high risk of severe disease: mumps often infects and destroys the testes of adult men, and rubella causes severe damage to the foetus in pregnant women. In the absence of a vaccine, and assuming that one cannot avoid exposure com-pletely, where would the best place to live in be in order to avoid these problems? The answer is: somewhere with very intense transmission, so that everyone is exposed and infected in childhood, and more or less all adults are already immune. In an area of less intense trans-mission, on the other hand, there is a greater chance of being infected not as a child but as an adult. In this scenario, the lifetime risk of being harmed by the infection is actually higher. So reducing trans-mission from very high to moderate intensity will actually increase the population burden of disease. This can be the case if (and only if) the pathogenic effects of infection at a young age are less severe than at some older age (Coleman *et al.*, 2001).

That malaria might be like this was first suggested by data from five hospitals in two different parts of Africa, each with markedly differ-ent transmission patterns, in which severe malaria incidence was es-timated by dividing the number of severe malaria admissions by the nominal catchment population of the facility (Snow *et al.*, 1994). These data seemed to show the highest disease rates in intermediate transmission intensities. It was hypothesized that children aged 1–5 years might be more vulnerable than infants to cerebral malaria, and that children born into the most intense transmission conditions might be relatively protected from this vulnerability by the partial immunity developed in their first year of life. Reducing their exposure in infancy might leave them more vulnerable to life-threatening cerebral disease than slightly older children. This suggestion caused a good deal of controversy (Molineaux, 1997) because of its implication that there might be circumstances in which transmission reduction through vector control (including ITNs) could actually be harmful.

Fortunately, this hypothesis was not borne out by further examination. First, the suggestion that mortality rates might peak at intermediate intensities was not confirmed by a more extensive collation of data from epidemiological studies (Lengeler *et al.*, 1997). More detailed analysis and modelling of age-specific disease rates (Coleman *et al.*, 1999) showed that this kind of phenomenon, if it occurs at all in malaria, cannot be strong enough to make ITNs not cost-effective as an intervention. Finally, long-term follow-up of vector control in Burkina Faso and Kenya confirmed that the benefits of this control were sustained even among five-year-old children who had been born in the reduced transmission conditions (Diallo *et al.*, 2004; Eisele *et al.*, 2005).

3. EFFECTIVENESS AND COST-EFFECTIVENESS STUDIES

3.1. Effectiveness of ITNs

3.1.1. ITNs Alone

Studies to determine whether the high efficacy of ITNs found in highly controlled clinical trials can be replicated when ITNs are deployed under programme conditions (Phase IV trials) have been limited. The few studies that have been conducted have however documented good impact in both small- and large-scale programme settings (see Table 3). There are many inherent difficulties in measuring impact under programme conditions, the major one being that programmes deliver interventions to specific target groups within the whole population, so that there are no contemporaneous control populations for those target groups for impact assessment (Lengeler and Snow, 1996). Nevertheless, measurement of effectiveness is necessary to determine the cost-effectiveness of different programme approaches in order to inform resource allocation. Potential options for measuring the impact of ITNs in programmatic settings include population-based prospective surveillance, health facility-based passive surveillance, repeated cross-sectional surveys, and case–control studies, but further research is needed to find optimal methodologies.

Results from the first of the effectiveness studies in The Gambia (D'Alessandro *et al.*, 1995b) sounded a note of caution. The study assessed the impact on mortality of the government's programme of delivering free insecticide for the treatment of privately owned nets, using prospective surveillance in sentinel sites, and found a 25% reduction in all-cause mortality. While this result in itself was impressive, it was in stark contrast to the earlier Phase III trial, which had shown a 42% mortality reduction (Alonso *et al.*, 1991). The substantial difference observed between efficacy and effectiveness of ITNs is unlike many other medical interventions, such as vaccinations, and has major implications for the widescale deployment of ITNs. The reduction in the efficacy of ITNs seen in programmatic settings is due to limitations in access, ineffective application of insecticides, poor public awareness, user behaviour and adherence in the home, and weaknesses in the health systems and other models currently used to deliver ITNs. In the case of the Gambian studies, the key factors identified as contributing to the reduction in efficacy between Phase III and Phase IV trials were low ITN use among children in some areas and sub-optimal insecticide residues on nets.

Two further studies to measure effectiveness of ITNs in The Gambia programme's second year, one to measure mortality and the other to measure morbidity, explored the feasibility of using a case–control design (D'Alessandro *et al.*, 1997). For the mortality study, children aged 1–9 years who died were matched by age and sex with two

Table 3 Impact of using ITNs on overall mortality, mild malaria disease, parasitaemia and anaemia, measured under operational conditions

Country	Study	Impact (Protective efficiency)[a]				Source
		Overall mortality	Mild disease (fever and parasitaemia)	Parasitaemia	Anaemia	
The Gambia	Longitudinal surveillance	25–40%				D'Alessandro *et al.* (1995b)
The Gambia	Case–control Study	0%	59%[b]			D'Alessandro *et al.* (1997)
Pakistan	Case–control study		0%[c] 78%[d] 69%[e]			Rowland *et al.* (1997)
Tanzania	Cross-sectional survey			62%	63%	Abdulla *et al.* (2001)
Tanzania	Case–control study	27%[f]				Schellenberg *et al.* (2001)

Source: WHO (2002b). Copyright © WHO. Reproduced with permission.
[a]Impact under operational conditions.
[b]Matched with health centre controls.
[c]Matched with village controls.
[d]*Plasmodium falciparum.*
[e]*Plasmodium vivax.*
[f]Reduction in post-neonatal child death (combined with coverage data this suggests that ITNs prevented 1 in 20 post-neonatal child deaths; if the effect of untreated nets is taken into account, this increases to 1 in 10 post-neonatal child deaths prevented).

healthy controls from the same village. The study showed no impact on mortality. For the morbidity study, children aged 1–9 years attending specific health centres who had fever and parasitaemia were matched by age with a child attending the same health facility without fever or parasitaemia and with an additional healthy control from the case's village. A protective effect was detected when cases were compared with controls recruited at health centres but not when compared with the controls from the villages.

A case–control study design was also used to measure the effectiveness of ITNs in Afghan refugee communities in two villages in Pakistan, which had only partial coverage of ITNs. The study, which compared the slide-positivity rates obtained at health centres for ITN users and non-users, showed a protective effect of 78% against *P. falciparum* and of 69% against *P. vivax* (see Rowland *et al.*, 1997). This provided a relatively cheap method for measuring effectiveness in remote programme settings. The level of protection shown by the case–control method was slightly higher than that shown by a prospective household randomized trial of ITNs carried out in the same villages three years earlier (Rowland *et al.*, 1996) probably because the case–control method identified ITN users more accurately than the household trial. A similar case–control study of the impact of the sale of ITNs in a remote rural Zambian village documented reduction in malarial parasitaemia and improved haemoglobin levels in children (McClean and Senthilselvan, 2002).

The more recent evaluation of a large SM programme in Tanzania, covering a population of 480 000, has shown compelling evidence of the effectiveness of an alternative delivery strategy for ITNs. Annual community-based cross-sectional surveys over 3 years measuring parasitaemia and anaemia among ITN users and non-users revealed a substantial reduction in anaemia (protective efficacy of 63%) and parasitaemia (protective efficacy of 62%) in children aged under 2 years (Abdulla *et al.*, 2001). Demographic surveillance in an area of 60 000 people within the same SM programme was used to determine impact on child survival (children aged 1 month to 4 years) using a case–control approach. An ITN coverage rate for infants of 50% was associated with a 27% increase in child survival among ITN users compared to non-users (Schellenberg *et al.*, 2001). The study design, comparing users and non-users, meant that these results measured the effectiveness of personal protection rather than a mass effect as described above.

Large-scale SM of ITNs has been carried out in Afghanistan by non-governmental organizations (NGOs) over the last decade (covering about 2 million people), and to assess its impact, repeated cross-sectional surveys were compared with a clinic-based case–control approach. Findings with the two approaches were comparable against *P. falciparum* malaria (odds ratios of 0.31 and 0.41, respectively) but both showed a lower impact against *P. vivax* malaria, owing to an inability to distinguish new infections from relapses of old infections acquired before the ITN sales programme began (Rowland *et al.*, 2002).

3.1.2. ITNS as Part of National Malaria Control Programmes

The impact of widescale deployment of ITNs as part of national malaria control programmes in China and Vietnam (Ettling, 2002) has been impressive. In China, the number of malaria cases has dropped by 99% over the past 50 years as a result of a combination of malaria control interventions including ITNs (Tang, 2000). Governmental spraying of over 2.4 million privately owned nets with deltamethrin in Sichuan Province, China, resulted in marked reductions in the number of malaria cases (Cheng *et al.*, 1995).

It will be important to continue to measure the effectiveness of ITN delivery strategies as they evolve and as new strategies are tested. For example, there is an urgent need to evaluate the effectiveness of the ITN delivery strategies targeting vulnerable groups that have been promoted recently, such as mass distribution of ITNs through expanded programme on immunization (EPI) campaigns and distribution through routine antenatal clinics and EPI services (see Section 8.1).

3.2. Cost-Effectiveness of ITNs

The most comprehensive study, taking account of data across a range of settings, is that of Goodman *et al.* (1999). As well as reviewing the studies that had estimated ITN cost-effectiveness up to that time, these authors used Monte Carlo modelling to generate cost-effectiveness estimates using published data on costs, effectiveness and some important co-factors. For the intervention of distributing ITNs free of charge to the whole population, as was done in most of the large epidemiological field trials, they estimated the cost per disability-adjusted life-year (DALY) averted to be in the range US$19 to US$85. This was interpreted as either 'attractive' or 'highly attractive' by conventional standards. They also considered the situation where there is already a moderately high level of pre-existing net coverage, and an alternative mode of intervention was to treat these existing nets with insecticide. This was found to be even better value for money: US$4 to US$10 per DALY averted, and highly attractive by conventional standards.

These results were consistent with the conclusions of previous studies. Since then, there have been a few further reports in the same range. One of the most careful studies came from a major trial in Kisumu, Kenya, which estimated a cost-effectiveness of US$34 per life-year gained (Wiseman *et al.*, 2003).

Although this body of evidence is consistent, its usefulness is limited by the fact that the intervention tested in most of these trials—provision of free ITNs for everyone in the community—is not the intervention that has been implemented in most large-scale programmes. Unlike most trials, routine implementation programmes have generally resulted in partial coverage, either through SM of ITNs, or by targeting ITN distribution to the most vulnerable groups, children under five years of age and/or pregnant women. This is important because of the evidence that full ITN coverage can reduce the density and sporozoite rate of local vector populations, which in turn can have a community effect, giving additional epidemiological protection to everyone in the area (see Section 2.2).

The Kilombero Valley Insecticide-Treated Net (KINET) SM trial in Tanzania therefore provides a critical link between the efficacy evidence and these routine programmes. The trial sold ITNs, and compared mortality rates between individual children who did and did not sleep under one of these ITNs, excluding the community effect and allowing for socioeconomic and other confounding factors. The cost-effectiveness estimates were reassuringly similar to those from the previous community-randomized trials: the estimated protective efficacy of individual ITN use against all-cause mortality was 27%, the estimated cost per death averted was US$1559 and the cost per DALY averted was US$57 (Hanson *et al.*, 2003). These figures fell to US$1018 and US$37, respectively, when the protection given by untreated nets (bought from unsubsidized commercial sources) was included.

ITNs also have important economic benefits (as well as health benefits) at the household level. For example, a study in Ahero, Kenya, estimated that households with ITNs saved US$0.25 in health care expenditure over a two-week period (Meltzer *et al.*, 2003).

If it is accepted that ITN coverage can reliably be assumed to have good health impact, then the relative efficiency of alternative delivery systems, measured as the cost-per-net-delivered or the cost-per-ITN-year, becomes a key issue. Two notable reports came from Malawi (Stevens *et al.*, 2005) and Kenya (Guyatt *et al.*, 2002). Unfortunately, many more data are hidden in unpublished project reports, and a thorough review of this question is beyond the scope of this paper.

4. RISK ASSESSMENT

Synthetic pyrethroids were first developed in the early 1970s, and rapidly entered widespread use in agriculture. Since then, they have gained and kept a reputation of being one of the safest classes of insecticide, in terms of hazards to both human health and the environment.

Pyrethroids are formally classified as 'moderately toxic', which is lower than most other commonly used classes of insecticide. They break down quickly in tissue, soil and water, and therefore do not accumulate through prolonged exposure or through concentration in food chains. Pyrethroids are not carcinogenic, genotoxic or toxic to reproduction in experimental animals.

A brief review of the safety of pyrethroid-treated nets was published by Zaim *et al.* (2000). The first formal toxicological risk assessment of the use of pyrethroids on nets was published by Barlow *et al.* (2001), and a similar generic approach has since been endorsed and recommended by the World Health Organization (WHO) (Barlow and Sullivan, 2004). All these studies concluded that exposure in practical conditions from net treatment and use of treated nets is unlikely to be hazardous.

Perhaps the most important issue about which there is still room for doubt is neuro-developmental toxicity: the possibility that exposure *in utero* or in infancy might influence the development of the nervous system. In Europe there has been some public concern and debate as to whether pyrethroids might have endocrine and neuro-developmental effects, and precautionary regulations now forbid the sale of pyrethroid-treated nets in some European Union countries. The evidence in this debate has been reviewed by Kolaczinski and Curtis (2004). It should also be emphasized that the balance of likely risks and benefits looks very different in Europe from what it does in malaria-endemic countries, where some remaining uncertainties about safety must be set against the much more substantial and certain benefits of protection against malaria. Recently, the WHO commissioned a further external and independent review of its current recommendations concerning the safety aspects of pyrethroids in public health (WHO, 2005d). This reported that further evidence is necessary before firm conclusions can be reached about neuro-developmental effects. However, it did conclude that pyrethroids 'do not pose any significant health risk when they are used in compliance with their directions for use, which are intended to limit human exposure within the levels recommended for their specific applications', and did not recommend any changes to WHO's current recommendations.

5. MONITORING AND IMPACT OF INSECTICIDE RESISTANCE

In the long term, resistance is probably the most important threat to the effectiveness of ITNs. Pyrethroid resistance mechanisms of two kinds have been reported.

'Knockdown resistance' (kdr) is caused by one or more substitution mutations in the target molecule on the surface of the nerve. Two kdr mutations have been reported in *An. gambiae*. One, which was first discovered in Kenya, is confined to permethrin (Ranson *et al.*, 2000). The other, which confers cross resistance to a variety of pyrethroids, was probably first selected in response to the use of agricultural pyrethroids (Chandre *et al.*, 2000; Diabate *et al.*, 2002). It is now widespread in West Africa. Some experimental hut studies have confirmed that resistant insects are more likely to survive exposure to ITNs (Kolaczinski *et al.*, 2000), while others indicate that resistance offers little or no protection (Hougard *et al.*, 2003). There is some evidence that the presence of this resistance at high gene frequencies does not prevent ITNs from being epidemiologically effective (Darriet *et al.*, 1998; Henry *et al.*, 2005). It is thought that this might be because resistant insects are less irritated by the pyrethroid and persist for longer in seeking entry to a treated net, and hence pick up a higher dosage so there is no differential survival between resistant and susceptible genotypes (Corbel *et al.*, 2004).

The other type of resistance is an oxidase-based detoxification mechanism, which breaks down the pyrethroid before it can reach the nerves. This is found in *An. funestus* in southern Africa and resulted in failure of the IRS campaigns with pyrethroids and necessitated a switch back to DDT (Hargreaves *et al.*, 2000). It is not known whether this mechanism would be protective against ITNs in southern Africa. Oxidase mechanisms have also been found in *An. gambiae* from West Africa, but so far less is known about its importance (Etang *et al.*, 2004).

Recent evidence indicates that the situation for pyrethroids is changing for the worse. A comparative experimental hut trial against *An. gambiae* carried out simultaneously in areas of pyrethroid resistance and susceptibility in southern and northern Benin produced only 19% mortality and no reduction of blood-feeding in deliberately holed nets in the pyrethroid-resistant south but 95% mortality and 95% reduction in blood-feeding in the susceptible north (R. N'Guessan and M. Rowland, unpublished observations). This is the first unequivocal demonstration of resistance in *An. gambiae* undermining the effectiveness of ITNs under field conditions.

Further work to measure the epidemiological impact of resistance is urgently needed. This can be done as part of village-randomized trials of ITNs, ideally in two areas—one with a high frequency and one with a low frequency of resistance. In areas where both are present the impact of resistance might be measured quite simply by comparing the sporozoite rates in resistant and susceptible insects in the same area.

The prospects for finding alternative compounds for use on nets are daunting. Compared to other classes of insecticide, pyrethroids are extremely safe for people and do very little damage to the environment, but they are highly toxic to insects. Their rapid mode of action and excito-repellent effects are especially important for the personal protective effect of mosquito nets. Other insecticides that might be effective in similarly small quantities as pyrethroids exist, but may not be safe enough for use on nets (Guillet *et al.*, 2001). Other alternatives are safe but have a very slow action, and so might be good at killing blood-seeking mosquitoes and hence transmission control but not at preventing them from biting the occupant of the net. Use of a slow-acting alternative in combination with a pyrethroid may provide the ideal 'cocktail' and might even reduce the rate of selection of pyrethoid resistance (Asidi *et al.*, 2005). Exploring alternative insecticides has been neglected, but it is now an active area of research, and it is likely that one or more non-pyrethroid compounds will be shown to be useful and effective on nets in the next few years.

6. TECHNOLOGICAL ADVANCES

To remain effective, ITNs need to be re-treated with insecticide about once a year or after two or three washes. This is a major constraint to the effective use of ITNs in rural Africa since systems for providing re-treatment are either absent or inadequate. To address this problem some manufacturers have sought to develop LLINs in which insecticide remains present on the net at toxic concentrations even after several washes. This is an active and competitive area of research. There is growing evidence that a number of products, based on differing technologies, are fulfilling the criteria and proving more wash-resistant than conventional ITNs. These products are taking an increasing share of the market, particularly among international donors and implementing agencies.

Long-lasting insecticidal nets are defined by WHO as nets treated with insecticide either incorporated into or coated around the fibres, which resist multiple washes and whose biological activity lasts as long as the net itself (WHO, 2005b).

The first LLIN to become commercially available and obtain WHO approval was Olyset® (WHOPES [WHO Pesticides Evaluation Scheme], 2001). This is a polyethylene net in which permethrin is incorporated within the fibres during net manufacture and over time migrates to the surface of the yarn to replace residues removed by washing. After seven years of continuous use in rural villages in Tanzania, the permethrin content of Olyset nets was still 35% of the initial loading dose and 90% of the nets were still fully active against *An. gambiae* in terms of knockdown in 3-minute exposure bioassay tests, although mortality rates after 24 hours were rather low (Tami *et al.*, 2004). Experimental hut trials of Olyset nets tested after 3 years' field use in Côte d'Ivoire produced a level of mortality among *An. gambiae* and *C. quinquefasciatus* no different from that of new, unused Olyset nets (N'Guessan *et al.*, 2001). Migration and replenishment of permethrin to the surface of the net after washing (regeneration) is temperature-dependent and can be accelerated by heating (WHOPES, 2001). Heating nets under field conditions may be impractical and in any event does not appear to be necessary to maintain the personal protective effect of Olyset. It is unclear whether Olyset can produce consistently high mortality of mosquitoes throughout the lifespan of the net.

PermaNet® is a more recent LLIN in which polyester nets are treated with a deltamethrin-containing wash-resistant resin which is coated on to the fibres during manufacture of the nets. The first-generation PermaNets produced variable field results owing to quality control problems during manufacture (WHOPES, 2004); efficacy persisted after washing in a South American study (Ordonez Gonzalez *et al.*, 2002) but showed a decline with successive washes in some African and Asian studies (Müller *et al.*, 2002; Graham *et al.*, 2005). With the launch of PermaNet 2.0 in 2002, this problem has been solved. Tests by independent agencies in laboratory and experimental huts have shown that effectiveness of PermaNet 2.0 persists for at least 20 WHO-standardized washes (WHOPES, 2004; Graham *et al.*,

2005). After obtaining interim approval from WHOPES in 2004, sales of PermaNet 2.0 have soared and this LLIN is presently dominating the market.

It is unclear whether PermaNet 2.0 or any other resin-based LLIN will remain effective throughout the 4–5 year lifespan presumed for polyester nets. Attrition of insecticide during normal use may accrue from a combination of washing, friction and general wear and tear, and the standardized washing procedure used in WHO Phase 1 and 2 trials applies only the first of these factors. The acid test of any LLIN is persistence of effectiveness over several years of normal use in village conditions, and for PermaNet 2.0 these studies have only recently been initiated.

The vast majority of nets in current use are not LLINs and have either never been treated or were treated only on issue (WHO, 2005b). An important technical development is the treatment kit (KO Tab 1-2-3) which combines a conventional insecticide tablet with a binding agent which can be applied to ordinary nets in the field through simple dipping and provides a genuinely wash-resistant treatment. Chemical assay using high-performance liquid chromatography showed that insecticide was removed by washing at a rate only slightly greater than that of Perma-Net, and after 30 washes the treated nets were still fully effective in mosquito bioassays (Yates *et al.*, 2005). This recent development raises the prospect of conventional nets being made long-lasting through simple dipping in the home. If widely taken up, this could have a major impact on malaria in Africa. The effect of netting material on persistence and wash-resistance of long-lasting formulations has still to be determined and it is presently unclear whether such formulations would perform equally well on nets made of cotton, nylon or polyethylene.

In 2004, the WHO (2004) guide prices were $2.18 for a medium size conventional untreated polyester net, and $4.80 for an LLIN. However, in recent enquiries the prices appear to have increased which presumably reflects the fact that demand greatly exceeds supply. The present production capacity of PermaNet is 25 million per year and will increase to 60 million by end of 2006 (M. Vestergaard, personal communication). Olyset production stands at 5 million per annum and will grow to 20 million per annum by 2006 (Sumitomo press release, 10 March 2005). Based on the combined statements from these manufacturers, overall production of LLIN is projected to grow to 60–80 million annually. However, announcing bold and ambitious plans for investment in new capacity is one way in which these manufacturers can defend their current positions on the LLIN market. It is therefore possible that capacity will in fact expand rather more slowly than the more optimistic projections would suggest. Nevertheless, if these projections hold and an LLIN will last on average of 5 years before needing replacement, global coverage of these LLIN will eventually stabilize at around 300–400 million.

Several other major agrochemical and textile manufacturers are developing their own LLINs, and it is anticipated that in the not too distant future all commercial nets will be LLINs. It is hoped that competition will help to lower prices of LLINs. Some of their manufacturers are the producers of alternative insecticides that may ultimately supplement or replace the pyrethroids on nets, and it will be necessary to subject these too to LLIN technology.

7. EVOLUTION OF ITN POLICY

The evolution of ITN policy over the past 10 years has been driven by key milestones in the evidence provided by the research on ITNs described above in terms of target groups (from efficacy studies) and delivery strategies (from cost-effectiveness studies). The main policy debate has been on how best to achieve a balance between equity on the one hand and sustainability on the other. Central, and closely linked, themes within this debate have been 'who should pay? (and how much can they afford for how long?)' and 'mass versus targeted deployment of ITNs'. Another key policy debate has been on the relative roles of ITNs versus IRS for malaria vector control.

7.1. Equity versus Sustainability

The debate on how to increase ITN coverage has much in common with food aid and agricultural development. The basic strategic choice is between providing commodities completely free to poor communities to achieve equity and more developmental approaches where subsidies are used to build and promote more sustainable systems, which can thrive after donor support wanes. The dilemma is therefore how to achieve rapid impact while encouraging growth of more sustainable solutions.

Efficacy studies have provided powerful evidence for ITNs as a cost-effective public health tool (see Section 3) to reduce mortality and morbidity in vulnerable groups, namely young children and pregnant women. While ITNs also afford health benefits to other population groups, it is generally acknowledged that free ITNs for everyone at risk from malaria globally would require levels of funding and health systems capacity not currently available. As long as this remains the case, some form of prioritization will be necessary, thereby according public sector priority to the most vulnerable.

Vulnerable groups therefore became the focus of global policy (WHO, 2002a) and targets for increased ITN coverage (WHO, 2000). It has however been argued that by targeting only pregnant women and children with ITNs, the 'mass effect' detected in some (but not all) trials would not be seen and that this would compromise the level of protection. However, the evidence is inconsistent (see Section 2.2.2).

Even with prioritization of vulnerable groups, it is recognized that public sector capacity will be stretched and that the commercial sector has an important role to play both in supporting the public sector in achieving its goals in the immediate term and also in sustaining high coverage levels in the longer term.

7.2. Role of the Commercial Sector

The World Malaria Report (WHO, 2005a) showed that coverage with any net is generally much higher (up to 10-fold) than coverage with ITNs, with ITNs constituting a median of just 18% of nets owned by households. In other words, about five out of every six nets found in African households have been supplied by the commercial sector and only one out of six by the public sector, demonstrating that the commercial sector plays a significant role in providing nets.

There are, however, important differences between nets and insecticide. While nets are widely available, insecticide markets are almost non-existent. Secondly, untreated nets are a 'private good', meaning that the benefits are confined to those sleeping nets, whereas insecticide treatment provides a positive externality through the 'mass effect' (see Section 2.2.2). In the presence of an externality, demand is likely to fall short of the optimal level of demand required for impact, providing a rationale for public intervention in the provision of insecticide, such as public financing or provision of public information. This is the approach used in China and Viet Nam, which have the largest and longest-sustained ITN programmes in the world.

These differences between nets and insecticide have two important implications for ITN programmes: (i) the commercial sector already plays an important role in the distribution of nets, and should be supported by the public sector through the so-called 'enabling environment', the success of which has been demonstrated in Tanzania (Magesa *et al.*, 2005); (ii) provision of insecticide treatment kits and/ or services should constitute an important component of all ITN programmes, except where LLINs are used.

7.3. Who Should Pay?

There has been much debate about the relative roles of the public sector, the commercial private sector, and the community in terms of who should pay for ITNs (Curtis *et al.*, 2003; Lines *et al.*, 2003). One school of thought is that the public sector (governments of malaria-endemic countries and development partners) should provide (and sustain) free nets for everyone to maximize the mass effect and hence the health and development benefits. The alternative view is that the public sector in resource-poor settings should focus on the most vulnerable and at the same time support the public health contribution made by the commercial sector. A recent estimate of the international investment required to provide 80% coverage of those at risk from malaria with available malaria interventions by 2010 of US$1900 million per year is far beyond current levels of investment for malaria control, and malaria-endemic countries are concerned as to whether investments will grow to cover needs and be sustained (WHO, 2005b). The World Health Assembly's most recent resolution on malaria control upholds the alternative view, that member states should pursue the rapid scale-up of targeted free, or highly subsidized, ITNs and IPT to vulnerable groups (WHO, 2005c).

The precise balance to be achieved between subsidized approaches to delivering ITNs to vulnerable groups and commercial market development for ITN distribution will vary from place to place and over time, as coverage levels increase and as markets develop (Figure 2).

7.4. Role of ITNs Relative to IRS

The relative role and effectiveness of ITNs versus IRS for the control of malaria is a major policy consideration for governments of malaria-endemic countries. In a direct effort to address questions on this issue by policy makers, the Roll Back Malaria (RBM) initiative released a consensus statement regarding personal protection and vector control options for prevention of malaria (RBM, 2004).* The statement affirms that, in Africa, ITNs and IRS are both very effective for malaria vector control but that the evidence concerning the relative cost-effectiveness of these two interventions is mixed. It also raises an important programmatic consideration that the choice between these two interventions depends not only on short-term epidemiological impact but also on considerations of feasibility and sustainability in the long term and at the scale required, and on the availability of appropriate delivery systems. There is therefore no generalized recommendation for the region as a whole, and choices need to be made on the basis of local context.

IRS has some important advantages in areas of unstable or epidemic malaria in that it has rapid and reliable short-term impact, and can be targeted at the communities at highest risk, on an annual basis and in response to changing transmission patterns. IRS is, however, relatively demanding in terms of the logistics, infrastructure, skills, planning systems and coverage levels that are needed for its successful and effective operation. Nevertheless, such systems have been

---

*http://rbm.who.int/partnership/wg/wg_itn/docs/RBMWINStatementVector.pdf

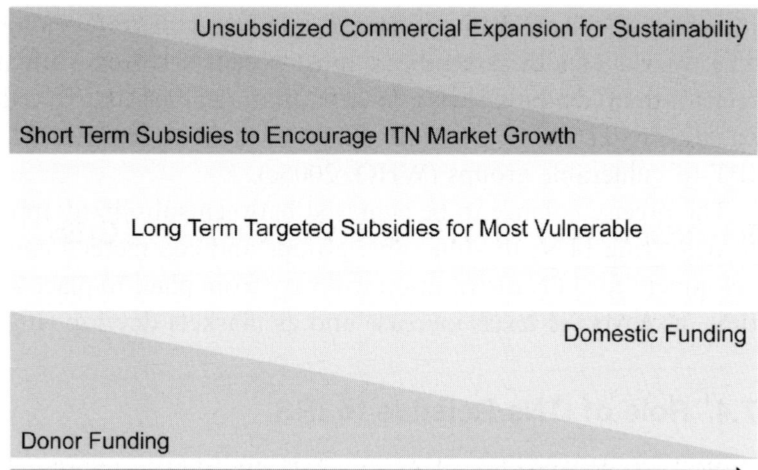

Figure 2   Striking a balance between subsidized and commercial strategies for the supply of insecticide-treated nets. *Source:* WHO, 2005e. Copyright © WHO. Reproduced with permission.

successfully and effectively maintained for many years in some African countries, and every effort should be made to sustain these systems in the future.

In most countries of Africa south of the Sahara, however, the vast majority of the rural population is exposed to stable malaria and the infrastructure, capacity and systems needed for large-scale IRS do not exist. In these circumstances, ITNs have important advantages. As well as being less demanding than IRS in terms of infrastructure and organization, ITNs allow vector control resources to be targeted towards those most at risk in stable endemic settings, i.e. pregnant women and young children, and hence best use can be made of initial resources. In addition to personal protection, ITNs provide community-level benefits, which are thought to increase proportionally with coverage across all coverage levels, and will contribute to early gains in equity as programs scale up.

The RBM statement concludes: 'In high transmission and stable endemic malaria settings of Africa south of the Sahara facing a choice of methods to implement and scale up, RBM strongly recommends that countries and RBM partners focus preventive vector control efforts on increasing coverage of insecticide-treated nets (ITNs) rather than investing in the creation of new large-scale IRS programs'.

8. EVOLUTION OF ITN DELIVERY STRATEGIES

8.1. National Level

8.1.1. Projects

Projects to deliver ITNs began in Asia and the Pacific region in the late 1980s and in Africa slightly later, in the early 1990s. With the exception of China, Viet Nam, Solomon Islands and The Gambia, all of which have national programmes, ITN distribution was, until a few years ago, limited to discrete, relatively small-scale projects run by a combination of government agencies, NGOs and development partners, but with limited inter-agency collaboration between partners. There are now essentially four models for delivering ITNs: (i) subsidized sales (community-based and SM); (ii) free goods; (iii) total market approach (TMA); and (iv) unsubsidized commercial sales. The earlier projects were based on subsidized sales and free goods, with limited targeting. The importance of the role of the commercial sector has been recognized relatively recently in the evolution of ITN delivery strategies, and has brought with it support for TMA.

8.1.1.1. Subsidized Sales. Earlier models for delivering ITNs focused on community-based approaches where community volunteers, with support from Ministries of Health, were involved in the promotion, treatment and sale of ITNs, which generated revolving funds intended for continuation of activities. An example of this approach was the UNICEF-supported Bamako Initiative in Kenya in the early 1990s, but problems with inefficient community management of funds and lack of a viable re-supply system for ITN commodities left the project unsustainable without continued external support

(McPake *et al.*, 1993). Many other community-based initiatives to deliver ITNs have run into similar problems (Chavasse *et al.*, 1999) and emphasis soon broadened to include SM models.

SM approaches to the delivery of ITNs were attempted in the Central African Republic in 1994, where the approach was successful in creating very high demand for heavily subsidized ITNs but the project was terminated prematurely due to civil unrest (Chavasse *et al.*, 1999). At first the project sold pre-treated nets through retail outlets and pharmacies but retailers started to resell nets at higher prices elsewhere, so that the SM agency had to resort to selling the products directly to consumers themselves, thereby undermining the potential efficiency of the SM approach in which the commercial sector is used for ITN distribution, alleviating the burden on public health systems. SM of ITNs in Afghanistan through rural clinics and mobile teams in more remote areas has led to a steady increase in coverage since 1992 (Rowland *et al.*, 2002; Kolaczinski *et al.*, 2004). In such war-torn countries, commercial networks are unstable or slow to develop and this results in a longer dependence on development programmes to meet the continuing demand.

SM approaches to delivering ITNs in politically stable countries have evolved to include a variety of distribution mechanisms, including use of existing commercial channels, subsidized commercial channels (PSI, 2005a)[†] and public health facilities (PSI, 2005b),[‡] and subsidized promotion campaigns, e.g. in the absence of supply inputs (see Section 8.1.1.3.).

Malawi has one of the largest ITN distribution programmes in Africa, delivering over 3 million ITNs by the end of 2004 (PSI, 2005b). SM has been used to deliver ITNs through a combination of channels, to pregnant women (at heavily subsidized prices) through antenatal clinics and to the general population through a combination of community-based and private sector distribution, the latter mainly in urban centres. Coverage of households owning at least one net has increased from 5% in 2000 to 43% in 2003, with 35% of children under five years of age and 31% of pregnant women now

---

[†]http://www.psi.org/malaria/malaria-resources/Tanzania%20ITN%20Program.pdf
[‡]http://www.psi.org/malaria/malaria-resources/Malawi%20ITN%20Program.pdf

sleeping under an ITN (WHO, 2005a). The cost of this approach was estimated to be US$1.92 per ITN delivered (Stevens *et al.*, 2005).

8.1.1.2. Free Goods, Including Vouchers.   The provision of free goods can apply to ITNs and/or insecticides. The provision of free insecticide to treat privately owned nets bought through commercial channels in China and Viet Nam has already been described. This approach is now being tested in parts of Africa (Cameroon and Uganda). In Cameroon, this operation was successful and there is evidence that the prospect of free insecticide also stimulated purchase of new nets from the local market (Manga *et al.*, 2004).[§]

The distribution of free ITNs is usually targeted, such as the distribution of free ITNs to pregnant women through antenatal clinics in Kenya, to children through immunization campaigns in Togo, Zambia and Ghana, to populations living in malaria transmission zones in Eritrea, and to flood victims in Mozambique. While there is some documentation of the costs and successes of this approach when used on a limited scale for targeting pregnant women through antenatal clinics in Kenya (Guyatt *et al.*, 2002; Guyatt and Ochola, 2003) and children through measles campaigns in Ghana (Grabowsky *et al.*, 2005), and more recently on a national scale in Togo (WHO, 2005a), there are insufficient data to assess its costs on a larger scale or its sustainability in the longer term. Similarly, there is little evidence on the cost-effectiveness of delivering ITNs through routine immunization (as opposed to campaigns), though this approach has the potential for targeting groups missed by immunization campaigns and for routine follow-up of ITNs distributed during campaigns (J. Webster and J. Hill, unpublished observations).

One of the most attractive methods of delivering ITN subsidies is the delivery of vouchers which can be exchanged for goods at commercial retail outlets either free or at a discount, since this supports local trade and at the same time alleviates the burden on the public health system of the distribution costs, logistics and management functions associated with ITNs. While there have been several pilot schemes, Tanzania is the only country to have adopted this approach

---

[§]http://www.afro.who.int/ddc/bulletins/2004-03.pdf

on a national scale to target pregnant women attending antenatal clinics (Worrall *et al.*, 2005). Preliminary anecdotal evidence suggests that the voucher programme is working well, but there are as yet no data on its cost-effectiveness and viability on a large scale.

8.1.1.3. Total Market Approach.   SM using a TMA has been used more recently with significant success in both Tanzania and Nigeria, and is currently favoured by some donors over traditional SM. TMA differs from traditional SM in that rather than selling an SM branded product at prices just below those of the unsubsidized commercial sector, SM approaches are applied to local net brands through demand creation, in addition to which local net manufacturers are encouraged to package nets with insecticide kits before sale.

A major challenge for programme design using TMA is the great diversity across Africa in the structure and size of net markets (see Section 8.2), and the challenges of engaging with the more disseminated markets found in West and Central Africa.

8.1.1.4. Unsubsidized Commercial Sales.   The importance of local net markets, which sell locally stitched nets in West and Central Africa and manufactured nets in East Africa, have been consistently underestimated but recent evidence has now confirmed that most nets currently in use in Africa have been bought from these markets (WHO, 2005a) and that coverage is surprisingly equitable (Webster, *et al.*, 2005).

Each of these approaches (Sections 8.1.1.1. to 8.1.1.4.) has been successful to varying degrees in increasing ITN coverage, but these successes need to be understood in the context of national programmes which take into account the challenges of going to full scale and sustaining high levels of coverage.

8.1.2. Moving from Projects to Programmes: Going to Full Scale

The launch of the RBM initiative by the Director General of the WHO in 1998 provided new impetus for partners to come together to agree strategies to scale up key malaria control interventions, including

ITNs. The RBM strategic framework for 'scaling-up insecticide-treated netting programmes in Africa' summarizes the evidence and captures the consensus approach for scaling up ITNs by a broad range of national and international partners, including ministries of health, development partners, United Nations agencies, NGOs and research institutions (WHO, 2002a), and a second edition has recently been produced following still broader consultation among governments and their partners in Africa (WHO, 2005e).[¶] The strategic framework builds on the work already being undertaken to develop national consensus strategies to deploy ITNs in several sub-Saharan African countries. Crucially, the framework recognizes that the public sector alone does not have the capacity or the resources to deliver ITNs to everyone at risk and needs to prioritize vulnerable groups, and that the commercial sector has an important role to play. It provides a conceptual framework in which both public and private sector partners can work in a complementary and supportive manner (see Figure 3).

The key consideration for countries embarking on nationwide strategies for increasing ITN coverage is therefore not 'which model?' but which 'combination of approaches?' and how best to manage implementation of the range of approaches adopted in order to promote positive and supportive interactions. The combination of approaches adopted by any one country will very much depend on the local country context, and the approaches are expected to evolve over time as coverage increases and as commercial markets develop (Figure 2).

8.1.3. Current ITN Coverage

The 2005 World Malaria Report stated that, 'with the exception of the most recent survey that covered all areas at risk of malaria in Eritrea—the population-weighted coverage of ITN usage in African children under five years of age is 3%' (WHO, 2005a). This figure was based on 34 surveys conducted in the median year 2001, and therefore excluded more recent efforts to deploy large numbers of ITNs

---

[¶]http://www.rollbackmalaria.org/partnership/wg/wg_itn/docs/WINITN_Strategic Framework.pdf

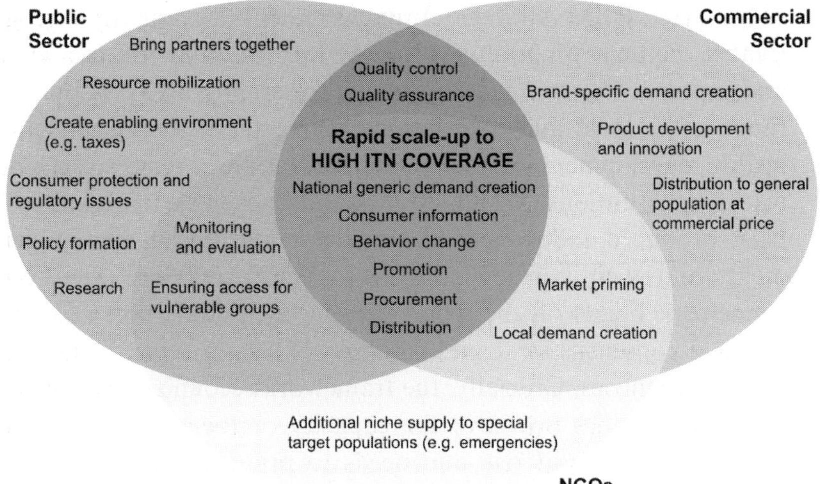

Figure 3   National scaling-up of ITN usage: a conceptual framework for partners. *Source*: WHO, 2005e. Copyright © WHO. Reproduced with permission.

through campaigns and subsidized delivery mechanisms. Nevertheless, with the exception of Eritrea (endemic regions only), Malawi, Togo (children aged 9–59 months only), São Tomé and Principé, and possibly Tanzania, few countries have achieved the Abuja target of 60% coverage of vulnerable groups with ITNs by the end of 2005. This inability to deploy ITNs to groups at particular risk from malaria throughout malaria-endemic Africa more than 20 years after their invention is especially depressing to those who have fought hard to promote ITNs, but there is a strong sense globally that the corner has finally been turned given recent policy statements and the push for the Millennium Development Goals (UNDP, 2005).[#]

8.2. Regional Level

According to the most recent survey data (WHO, 2005a), some four out of five nets in use in Africa are untreated. This means that the great majority of nets used in African households were bought by their owners

---

[#]http://www.millenniumproject.org/reports/tf_malaria.htm

from unsubsidized commercial markets. Yet there are major geographical contrasts, both between Africa and other continents and within Africa, in the state of commercial net supplies and in ITN policies.

In many parts of West Africa, for example, net use is a long-standing tradition. Nets are made by local tailors from a wide variety of materials and fabrics, according to the buyer's specified preferences. These nets are mostly large and rectangular, and are often stronger and heavier than the knitted polyester nets favoured elsewhere. Coverage rates vary widely, but can be high: household net ownership rates exceed 50% in Mali as a whole, and reach 90% in the famously remote locality of Tombouctou (http://www.NetMarkAfrica.org). Net ownership is also surprisingly equitable in this region, and in some countries, poor and rural households are more likely to have an untreated commercial net than rich urban households (Webster *et al.*, 2005).

In East Africa, there is also a pervasive local market in nets, but in this case it is dominated by factory-made nets, mostly of light-knitted polyester fabric, including a high proportion of conical nets. In this region, net use is more strongly concentrated in urban areas and in less-poor socioeconomic groups (Webster *et al.*, 2005).

The importance and potential of local net supplies and informal textile markets tend to be underestimated by ITN projects, but they can be very responsive to changes in demand. Within weeks of an ITN advertising campaign on Nigerian television, wholesale net traders in local markets had started to sell insecticide treatment kits packaged with their own nets, at prices that competed well with the nets imported by the project. But the big success story is that of Tanzania, which has been transformed over the last ten years. Nets used to be very rare and expensive and untreated, and they are now very common and cheap and treated; national ITN coverage is close to Abuja target levels and shows every sign of being sustainable (Lines and Addington, 2001).

In south-east Asia, net ownership is even more common and widespread, and it is not unusual for most people to be using nets. The malaria programme in Cambodia has for years reported net coverage rates based on the numbers of ITNs distributed by the government and NGO projects, assuming that communities in forested malarious areas were too poor to buy nets for themselves. A recent survey has now shown that coverage rates everywhere are high, and project nets represent less than one-third of the total number of nets in households.

9. CONCLUSIONS AND NEEDS

While there is currently unprecedented political and financial support for increasing access to ITNs as a key strategy to controlling malaria, with consequent benefits to poverty reduction, there are still many questions concerning the effectiveness of different, as well as combined, approaches to scaling up ITN interventions, including those listed below.

- What is the effectiveness of different approaches to increasing coverage of ITNs (with and without IPT) in programme settings, by combining ITN delivery with maternal and child health programmes? (This will require new methodologies for measuring effectiveness as it is no longer ethical to deny the intervention to control groups.)
- What is the cost effectiveness of use of single interventions such as ITNs versus use of combined interventions, or use of ITNs and IPT to prevent malaria in children and pregnant women, use of repellents and ITN in regions with early and late biting vectors, and ITN versus artemisin-based combination therapy for long-term transmission control?

Similarly, there remain substantial gaps in knowledge on the efficacy of ITNs in different programmatic scenarios as well as on the epidemiological impact of ITNs in certain geographical zones and of long-term use, as follows:

- What is the impact of ITNs at different levels of coverage to determine better the relationship between individual and mass protection, in order to guide delivery strategies?
- What is the impact of ITNs targeting pregnant women through antenatal clinics (the current policy recommended by WHO), where women may not benefit from the mass effect seen in group-randomized trials? (There has been only one study to date.)
- What is the impact of ITNs in a programme setting where the

majority of women attend antenatal clinics in the second trimester? (To date only two trials have assessed the impact of ITNs delivered through these clinics.)

- What is the impact of long-term use of ITNs on malaria transmission intensity and on the development of immunity?
- What is the efficacy of ITNs in Latin America? (This requires the design and execution of well-conceived large-scale trials that take into account the low incidence of malaria, high prevalence of *P. vivax* and relapsing cases, and the relationship between human activity and crepuscular biting patterns of some malaria vectors in the Americas.)
- What is the potential role of ITNs against other vector-borne diseases such as visceral leishmaniasis (kala-azar) or lymphatic filariasis in India or Africa, or Chagas disease in South America?

And finally, while the last five years have brought us what is arguably the most important technical development (that of LLINs), a fundamental technical challenge remains—the development of insecticide resistance. Knockdown resistance has already become widespread in West Africa but it is unclear whether this or other resistance mechanisms will become an obstacle to control, or whether the barrier effect will mean that ITNs remain effective when IRS is compromised by resistance. Nevertheless, the search to develop alternative insecticides and mixtures to replace pyrethroids needs to begin now. A related issue is measurement of the duration of effectiveness of an ITN (or an LLIN), which currently relies on purely entomological measures. Conventional definitions of 'adequate insecticidal activity', as measured in entomological bioassays, are arbitrary and have never been calibrated in epidemiological terms.

REFERENCES

Abdulla, S., Schellenberg, J.A., Nathan, R., Mukasa, O., Marchant, T., Smith, T., Tanner, M. and Lengeler, C. (2001). Impact on malaria morbidity of a programme supplying insecticide treated nets in children aged under 2 years in Tanzania: community cross sectional study. *British Medical Journal* **322**, 270–273.

Alaii, J.A., Van Den Brone, H.W., Kachur, S.P., Mwenesi, H., Vulule, J.M., Hawley, W.A., Meltzer, M.I., Nahlen, B.L. and Phillips-Howard, P.A. (2003). Perceptions of bed nets and malaria prevention before and after a randomized-controlled trial of permethrin treated bed nets in western Kenya. *American Journal of Tropical Medicine and Hygiene* **68**(Suppl. 4), 142–148.

Alonso, P.L., Lindsay, S.W., Armstrong, J.R., Conteh, M., Hill, A.G., David, P.H., Fegan, G., De Francisco, A., Hall, A.J. and Shenton, F.C. (1991). The effect of insecticide-treated bed nets on mortality of Gambian children. *Lancet* **337**, 1499–1502.

Asidi, A.N., N'Guessan, R., Koffi, A.A., Curtis, C.F., Hougard, J.M., Chandre, F., Corbel, V., Darriet, F., Zaim, M. and Rowland, M.W. (2005). Experimental hut evaluation of bed nets treated with an organophosphate (chlorpyrifos methyl) or a pyrethroid (lambdacyhalothrin) alone and in combination against insecticide resistant *A. gambiae* and *C. quinquefasciatus* mosquitoes. *Malaria Journal* **4**, 25.

Barlow, S.M. and Sullivan, F.M. (2004) *A Generic Risk Assessment Model for Insecticide Treatment and Subsequent Use of Mosquito Nets.* WHO/CDS/WHOPES/GCDPP/2004.6, WHO/PCS/04.1

Barlow, S.M., Sullivan, F.M. and Lines, J. (2001). Risk assessment of the use of deltamethrin on bednets for the prevention of malaria. *Food and Chemical Toxicology* **39**, 407–422.

Binka, F.N., Indome, F. and Smith, T. (1998). Impact of spatial distribution of permethrin-impregnated bed nets on child mortality in rural northern Ghana. *American Journal of Tropical Medicine and Hygiene* **59**, 80–85.

Binka, F.N., Kubaje, A., Adjuik, M., Williams, L.A., Lengeler, C., Maude, G.H., Armah, G.E., Kajihara, B., Adiamah, J.H. and Smith, P.G. (1996). Impact of permethrin impregnated bednets on child mortality in Kassena-Nankana district, Ghana: a randomized controlled trial. *Tropical Medicine and International Health* **1**, 147–154.

Browne, E.N., Maude, G.H. and Binka, F.N. (2001). The impact of insecticide-treated bednets on malaria and anaemia in pregnancy in Kassena-Nankana district, Ghana: a randomized controlled trial. *Tropical Medicine and International Health* **6**, 667–676.

Chandre, F., Darriet, F., Duchon, S., Finot, L., Manguin, S., Carnevale, P. and Guillet, P. (2000). Modifications of pyrethroid effects associated with kdr mutation in *Anopheles gambiae*. *Medical and Veterinary Entomology* **14**, 81–88.

Charlwood, J.D. and Graves, P.M. (1987). The effect of permethrin-impregnated bednets on a population of *Anopheles farauti* in coastal Papua New Guinea. *Medical and Veterinary Entomology* **1**, 319–327.

Chavasse, D., Reed, C. and Attawell, K. (1999). *Insecticide Treated Nets: A Handbook for Managers*. Malaria Consortium.

Cheng, H., Yang, W., Kang, W. and Liu, C. (1995). Large-scale spraying of bednets to control mosquito vectors and malaria in Sichuan, China. *Bulletin of the World Health Organization* **73**, 321–328.

Clarke, S.E., Bough, C., Brown, R.C., Pinder, M., Walraven, G.E. and Lindsay, S.W. (2001). Do untreated bed nets protect against malaria? *Transactions of the Royal Society of Tropical Medicine and Hygiene* **95**, 457–462.

Coleman, P.G., Goodman, C.A. and Mills, A. (1999). Rebound mortality and the cost-effectiveness of malaria control: potential impact of increased mortality in late childhood following the introduction of insecticide treated nets. *Tropical Medicine and International Health* **4**, 175–186.

Coleman, P.G., Perry, B.D. and Woolhouse, M.E. (2001). Endemic stability—a veterinary idea applied to human public health. *Lancet* **357**, 1284–1286.

Corbel, V., Chandre, F., Brengues, C., Akogbeto, M., Lardeux, F., Hougard, J.M. and Guillet, P. (2004). Dosage-dependent effects of permethrin-treated nets on the behaviour of *Anopheles gambiae* and the selection of pyrethroid resistance. *Malaria Journal* **3**, 22.

Curtis, C., Maxwell, C., Lemnge, M., Kilama, W.L., Steketee, R.W., Hawley, W.A., Bergevin, Y., Campbell, C.C., Sachs, J., Teklehaimanot, A., Ochola, S., Guyatt, H. and Snow, R.W. (2003). Scaling-up coverage with insecticide-treated nets against malaria in Africa: who should pay? *Lancet Infectious Diseases* **3**, 304–307.

Curtis, C.F., Mnzava, A.E., Misra, S. and Rowland, M. (1999). Malaria control: bednets or spraying? Summary of the presentations and the discussion. *Transactions of the Royal Society of Tropical Medicine and Hygiene* **93**, 460.

D'Alessandro, U., Langerock, P., Bennett, S., Francis, N., Cham, K. and Greenwood, B.M. (1996). The impact of a national impregnated bed net programme on the outcome of pregnancy in primigravidae in The Gambia. *Transactions of the Royal Society of Tropical Medicine and Hygiene* **90**, 487–492.

D'Alessandro, U., Olaleye, B., Langerock, P., Bennett, S., Cham, K., Cham, B. and Greenwood, B.M. (1997). The Gambian National Impregnated Bed Net Programme: evaluation of effectiveness by means of case–control studies. *Transactions of the Royal Society of Tropical Medicine and Hygiene* **91**, 638–642.

D'Alessandro, U., Olaleye, B.O., Mcguire, W., Langerock, P., Bennett, S., Aikins, M.K., Thomson, M.C., Cham, M.K., Cham, B.A. and Greenwood, B.M. (1995b). Mortality and morbidity from malaria in Gambian children after introduction of an impregnated bednet programme. *Lancet* **345**, 479–483.

D'Alessandro, U., Olaleye, B.O., Mcguire, W., Thomson, M.C., Langerock, P., Bennett, S. and Greenwood, B.M. (1995a). A comparison of the efficacy of insecticide-treated and untreated bed nets in preventing malaria in Gambian children. *Transactions of the Royal Society of Tropical Medicine and Hygiene* **89**, 596–598.

Dapeng, L., Konghuma, Z., Jinduo, S., Renguo, Y., Hongru, H., Baoxin, L., Yong, L. and Wang (1994). The protective efficacy of bednets impregnated with pyrethroid insecticide and vaccination against Japanese encephalitis. *Transactions of the Royal Society of Tropical Medicine and Hygiene* **88**, 632–634.

Darriet, F., Guillet, P., N'Guessan, R., Doannio, J.M., Koffi, A., Konan, L.Y. and Carnevale, P. (1998). Impact of resistance of *Anopheles gambiae* s.s. to permethrin and deltamethrin on the efficacy of impregnated mosquito nets. *Med Trop (Mars)* **58**, 349–354.

Darriet, F., Robert, V., Tho Vien, N. and Carnevale, P., eds (1984). *Evaluation of the Efficacy of Permethrin Impregnated Intact and Perforated Mosquito Nets Against Vectors of Malaria.* World Health Organization, WHO/VBC/84.899.

Diabate, A., Baldet, T., Chandre, F., Akogbeto, M., Guiguemde, R.T., Darriet, F., Brengues, C., Guillet, P., Hemingway, J., Small, G.J. and Hougard, J.M. (2002). The role of agricultural use of insecticides in resistance to pyrethroids in *Anopholes gambiae* s.l. in Burkina Faso. *American Journal of Tropical Medicine and Hygiene* **67**, 617–622.

Diallo, D.A., Cousens, S.N., Cuzin-Ouattara, N., Nebie, I., Ilboudo-Sanogo, E. and Esposito, F. (2004). Child mortality in a West African population protected with insecticide-treated curtains for a period of up to 6 years. *Bulletin of the World Health Organization* **82**, 85–91.

Dolan, G., ter Kuile, F.O., Jacoutot, V., White, N.J., Luxemburger, C., Malankirii, L., Chongsuphajaisiddhi, T. and Nosten, F. (1993). Bed nets for the prevention of malaria and anaemia in pregnancy. *Transactions of the Royal Society of Tropical Medicine and Hygiene* **87**, 620–626.

Eisele, T.P., Lindblade, K.A., Wannemuehler, K.A., Gimnig, J.E., Odhiambo, F., Hawley, W.A., ter Kuile, F.O., Phillips-Howard, P., Rosen, D.H., Nahlen, B.L., Vulule, J.M. and Slutsker, L. (2005). Effect of sustained insecticide-treated bed net use on all-cause child mortality in an area of intense perennial malaria transmission in western Kenya. *American Journal of Tropical Medicine and Hygiene* **73**, 149–156.

Etang, J., Chandre, F., Guillet, P. and Manga, L. (2004). Reduced bio-efficacy of permethrin EC impregnated bednets against an *Anopheles gambiae* strain with oxidase-based pyrethroid tolerance. *Malaria Journal* **3**, 46.

Ettling, M.B. (2002). *The Control of Malaria in Viet Nam from 1980 to 2000: What Went Right?* Manila: World Health Organization Regional Office for the Western Pacific.

Goodman, C.A., Coleman, P.G. and Mills, A.J. (1999). Cost-effectiveness of malaria control in sub-Saharan Africa. *Lancet* **354**, 378–385.

Grabowsky, M., Nobiya, T., Ahun, M., Donna, R., Lengor, M., Zimmerman, D., Ladd, H., Hoekstra, E., Bello, A., Baffoe-Wilmot, A. and Amofah, G. (2005). Distributing insecticide-treated bednets during measles vaccination: a low-cost means of achieving high and equitable coverage. *Bulletin of the World Health Organization* **83**, 195–201.

Graham, K., Kayedi, M.H., Maxwell, C., Kaur, H., Rehman, H., Malima, R., Curtis, C.F., Lines, J.D. and Rowland, M.W. (2005). Multi-country field trials comparing wash-resistance of PermaNet and conventional insecticide-treated nets against anopheline and culicine mosquitoes. *Medical and Veterinary Entomology* **19**, 72–83.

Guillet, P., N'Guessan, R., Darriet, F., Traore-Lamizana, M., Chandre, F. and Carnevale, P. (2001). Combined pyrethroid and carbamate 'two-in-one' treated mosquito nets: field efficacy against pyrethroid-resistant *Anopheles* and *Culex*. *Medical and Veterinary Entomology* **15**, 105–112.

Guyatt, H.L., Gotink, M.H., Ochola, S.A. and Snow, R.W. (2002). Free bednets to pregnant women through antenatal clinics in Kenya: a cheap, simple and equitable approach to delivery. *Tropical Medicine and International Health* **7**, 409–420.

Guyatt, H. and Ochola, S. (2003). Use of bednets given free to pregnant women in Kenya. *Lancet* **362**, 1549–1550.

Guyatt, H.L. and Snow, R.W. (2002). The cost of not treating bednets. *Trends in Parasitology* **18**(1), 12–16.

Habluetzel, A., Diallo, D.A., Esposito, F., Lamizana, L., Pagnoni, F., Lengeler, C., Traore, C. and Cousens, S.N. (1997). Do insecticide-treated curtains reduce all-cause child mortality in Burkina Faso? *Tropical Medicine and International Health* **2**, 855–862.

Hanson, K., Kikumbih, N., Armstrong, S.J., Mponda, H., Nathan, R., Lake, S., Mills, A., Tanner, M. and Lengeler, C. (2003). Cost-effectiveness of social marketing of insecticide-treated nets for malaria control in the United Republic of Tanzania. *Bulletin of the World Health Organization* **81**, 269–276.

Hargreaves, K., Koekemoer, L.L., Brooke, B.D., Hunt, R.H., Mthembu, J. and Coetzee, M. (2000). *Anopheles funestus* resistant to pyrethroid insecticides in South Africa. *Medical and Veterinary Entomology* **14**, 181–189.

Hawley, W.A., Phillips-Howard, P.A., ter Kuile, F.O., Terlouw, D.J., Vulule, J.M., Ombok, M., Nahlen, B.L., Gimnig, J.E., Kariuki, S.K., Kolczak, M.S. and Hightower, A.W. (2003). Community-wide effects of permethrin-treated bed nets on child mortality and malaria morbidity in western Kenya. *American Journal of Tropical Medicine and Hygiene* **68**, 121–127.

Henry, M.C., Assi, S.B., Rogier, C., Dossou-Yovo, J., Chandre, F., Guillet, P. and Carnevale, P. (2005). Protective efficacy of lambdacyhalothrin treated nets in *A. gambiae* pyrethroid resistance areas of Cote d'Ivoire. *American Journal of Tropical Medicine and Hygiene* **75**, 859–864.

Hewitt, S., Ford, E., Urhaman, H., Mohammad, N. and Rowland, M. (1997). The effect of bed nets on unprotected people: open-air studies in an Afghan refugee village. *Bulletin of Entomological Research* **87**, 455–459.

Hii, J.L.K., Smith, T., Alexander, N., Mai, A., Ibam, E. and Alpers, M.P. (2001). Area effects of bed net use in a malaria endemic area in Papua New Guinea. *Transactions of the Royal Society of Tropical Medicine and Hygiene* **95**, 7–13.

Hougard, J.M., Corbel, V., N'Guessan, R., Darriet, F., Chandre, F., Akogbeto, M., Baldet, T., Guillet, P., Carnevale, P. and Traore-Lamizana, M. (2003). Efficacy of mosquito nets treated with insecticide mixtures or mosaics against insecticide resistant *A. gambiae* and *C. quinquefasciatus* in Cote d'Ivoire. *Bulletin of Entomological Research* **93**, 491–498.

Howard, S.C., Omumbo, J., Nevill, C., Some, E.S., Donnelly, C.A. and Snow, R.W. (2000). Evidence for a mass community effect of insecticide-treated bednets on the incidence of malaria on the Kenyan coast. *Transactions of the Royal Society of Tropical Medicine and Hygiene* **94**, 357–360.

IDRC and WHO (1996). *NetGain: A New Method for Preventing Malaria Deaths.* IDRC, WHO.

Kolaczinski, J.H. and Curtis, C.F. (2004). Chronic illness as a result of low-level exposure to synthetic pyrethroid insecticides: a review of the debate. *Food and Chemical Toxicology* **42**(5), 697–706.

Kolaczinski, J.H., Fanello, C., Herve, J.P., Conway, D.J., Carnevale, P. and Curtis, C.F. (2000). Experimental and molecular genetic analysis of the impact of pyrethroid and non-pyrethroid insecticide impregnated bednets for mosquito control in an area of pyrethroid resistance. *Bulletin of Entomological Research* **90**, 125–132.

Kolaczinski, J.H., Mohammed, N., Khan, Q.S., Jan, Z., Rehman, N., Leslie, T.J. and Rowland, M. (2004). Subsidized sales of insecticide-treated nets in Afghan refugee camps demonstrate the feasibility of a transition from humanitarian aid towards sustainability. *Malaria Journal* **3**, 15.

Kroeger, A., Mancheno, M., Alarcon, J. and Pesse, K. (1995). Insecticide-impregnated bed nets for malaria control: varying experiences from Ecuador, Colombia, and Peru concerning acceptability and effectiveness. *American Journal of Tropical Medicine and Hygiene* **3**(4), 313–323.

Kroeger, A., Avila, E.V. and Morison, L. (2002). Insecticide impregnated curtains to control domestic transmission of cutaneous leishmaniasis in Venezuala: cluster randomised trial. *British Medical Journal* **325**, 810–813.

Kroeger, A., Villegas, E., Ordonez-Gonzalez, J., Pabon, E. and Scorza, J.V. (2003). Prevention of the transmission of Chagas' disease with pyrethroid-impregnated materials. *American Journal of Tropical Medicine and Hygiene* **68**, 307–311.

Lengeler, C. (2004). Insecticide-treated bed nets and curtains for preventing malaria. *Cochrane Database Systematic Reviews*. CD000363.

Lengeler, C., Smith, T.A. Armstrong Schellenberg, J. (1997). Focus on the effect of bednets on malaria morbidity and mortality. *Parasitology Today* 13, 123–124; author reply 125–126

Lengeler, C. and Snow, R.W. (1996). From efficacy to effectiveness: insecticide-treated bednets in Africa. *Bulletin of the World Health Organization* **74**, 325–332.

Lindsay, S.W., Snow, R.W., Armstrong, J.R. and Greenwood, B.M. (1989b). Permethrin-impregnated bednets reduce nuisance arthropods in Gambian houses. *Medical and Veterinary Entomology* **3**, 377–383.

Lindsay, S.W., Snow, R.W., Broomfield, G.L., Janneh, M.S., Wirtz, R.A. and Greenwood, B.M. (1989a). Impact of permethrin-treated bednets on malaria transmission by the *Anopheles gambiae* complex in The Gambia. *Medical and Veterinary Entomology* **3**, 263–271.

Lines, J. and Addington, W. (2001). Insecticide-treated nets in Tanzania. Correspondence. *Lancet* **358**, 671.

Lines, J., Lengeler, C., Cham, K., De Savigny, D., Chimumbwa, J., Langi, P., Carroll, D., Mills, A., Hanson, K., Webster, J., Lynch, M., Addington, W., Hill, J., Rowland, M., Worrall, E., Macdonald, M., Kilian, A. (2003). Scaling-up and sustaining insecticide-treated net coverage. *Lancet Infectious Diseases* 3, 465–466; discussion 467–468.

Lines, J.D., Myamba, J. and Curtis, C.F. (1987). Experimental hut trials of permethrin-impregnated mosquito nets and eave curtains against malaria vectors in Tanzania. *Medical and Veterinary Entomology* **1**, 37–51.

Magesa, S., Lengeler, C., De Savigny, D., Miller, J., Njau, R., Kramer, K., Kitua, A. and Mwita, A. (2005). Creating an enabling environment for taking insecticide treated nets to national scale: The Tanzanian experience. *Malaria Journal* **4**, 34.

Magesa, S.M., Wilkes, T.J., Mnzava, A.E., Njunwa, K.J., Myamba, J., Kivuyo, M.D., Hill, N., Lines, J.D. and Curtis, C.F. (1991). Trial of pyrethroid impregnated bednets in an area of Tanzania holoendemic for malaria. Part 2. Effects on the malaria vector population. *Acta Tropica* **49**, 97–108.

Magris, M.C. (2004). *Malaria control using lambda-cyhalothrin treated nets in Yanomami communities in Amazonas state, Venezuala.* Ph.D. thesis, University of London.

Manga, L., Bagayoko, M., Ameneshewa, B., Faye, O., Lyimo, E.O., Govere, J., Fondjo, E., Masimike, M., Sillah, J. and Tewolde, G. (2004).

Mass mosquito net impregnation campaigns: an effective way to increase net re-impregnation rates. *WHO AFRO: Communicable Diseases Bulletin for the African Region* **2.1**, 1–3.

Marchant, T., Schellenberg, J.A., Edgar, T., Nathan, R., Abdulla, S., Mukasa, O., Mponda, H. and Lengeler, C. (2002). Socially marketed insecticide-treated nets improve malaria and anaemia in pregnancy in southern Tanzania. *Tropical Medicine and International Health* **7**, 149–158.

McClean, K.L. and Senthilselvan, A. (2002). Mosquito bed nets: implementation in rural villages in Zambia and the effect on subclinical parasitaemia and haemoglobin. *Tropical Doctor* **32**, 139–142.

McPake, B., Hanson, K. and Mills, A. (1993). Community financing of health care in Africa: an evaluation of the Bamako initiative. *Social Science and Medicine* **36**, 1383–1395.

Meltzer, M.I., Terlouw, D.J., Kolczak, M.S., Odhacha, A., ter Kuile, F.O., Vulule, J.M., Alaii, J.A., Nahlen, B.L., Hawley, W.A. and Phillips-Howard, P.A. (2003). The household-level economics of using permethrin-treated bednets to prevent malaria in children less than five years of age. *American Journal of Tropical Medicine and Hygiene* **68**(Suppl. 4), 149–160.

Molineaux, L. (1997). Malaria and mortality: some epidemiological considerations. *Annals of Tropical Medicine and Parasitology* **91**(7), 811–825.

Müller, O., Ido, K. and Traoré, C. (2002). Evaluation of a prototype long-lasting insecticide-treated mosquito net under field conditions in rural Burkina Faso. *Transactions of the Royal Society of Tropical Medicine and Hygiene* **96**, 483–484.

Myamba, J., Maxwell, C.A., Asidi, A. and Curtis, C.F. (2002). Pyrethroid resistance in tropical bedbugs, *Cimex lectularis*, associated with use of treated bednets. *Medical and Veterinary Entomology* **16**, 448–451.

Nevill, C.G., Some, E.S., Mung'ala, V.O., Mutemi, W., New, L., Marsh, K., Lengeler, C. and Snow, R.W. (1996). Insecticide-treated bednets reduce mortality and severe morbidity from malaria among children on the Kenyan coast. *Tropical Medicine and International Health* **1**, 139–146.

N'Guessan, R., Darriet, F., Doannio, J.M., Chandre, F. and Carnevale, P. (2001). Olyset net efficacy against pyrethroid-resistant *Anopheles gambiae* and *Culex quinquefasciatus* after 3 years' field use in Cote te d'Ivoire. *Medical and Veterinary Entomology* **15**, 97–104.

Njagi, J.K. (2002). *The effects of sulfadoxine-pyrimethamine intermittent treatment and pyrethroid impregnated bed nets on malaria morbidity and birth weight in Bondo district, Kenya.* Department of Microbiology, Faculty of Medicine, University of Nairobi, and Danish Bilharzia Laboratory. Nairobi and Copenhagen.

Njagi, J.K., Magnussen, P., Estambale, B., Ouma, J. and Mugo, B. (2003). Prevention of anaemia in pregnancy using insecticide-treated bednets and sulfadoxine-pyrimethamine in a highly malarious area of Kenya: a randomized controlled trial. *Transactions of the Royal Society of Tropical Medicine and Hygiene* **97**, 277–282.

Ordonez Gonzalez, J., Kroeger, A., Avina, Ai. and Pabon, E. (2002). Wash resistance of insecticide-treated materials. *Transactions of the Royal Society of Tropical Medicine and Hygiene* **96**, 370–375.

Phillips-Howard, P.A., ter Kuile, F.O., Nahlen, B.L., Alaii, J.A., Gimnig, J.E., Kolczak, M.S., Terlouw, D.J., Kariuki, S.K., Shi, Y.P., Kachur, S.P., Hightower, A.W., Vulule, J.M., Hawley, W.A. (2003). The efficacy of permethrin-treated bed nets on child mortality and morbidity in western Kenya II. Study design and methods. *American Journal of Tropical Medicine and Hygiene*, 68, 10–15.

PSI (2005a). *SMARTNET: A Tanzanian Public /Private Partnership to Prevent Malaria*. Unpublished report.

PSI (2005b). *The Malawi ITN Delivery Model*. Unpublished report.

Quinones, M.L., Lines, J., Thomson, M.C., Jawara, M. and Greenwood, B.M. (1998). Permethrin-treated bed nets do not have a 'mass-killing effect' on village populations of *Anopheles gambiae* s.l. in The Gambia. *Transactions of the Royal Society of Tropical Medicine and Hygiene* **92**, 373–378.

Ranque, P., Toure, Y.T., Soula, G., Du, L., Diallo, Y., Traore, O., Duflo, B. and Balique, H. (1984). [Utilization of mosquitoes impregnated with deltamethrin in the battle against malaria]. *Parasitologia* **26**, 261–268.

Ranson, H., Jensen, B., Vulule, J.M., Wang, X., Hemingway, J. and Collins, F.H. (2000). Identification of a point mutation in the voltage-gated sodium channel gene of Kenyan *Anopheles gambiae* associated with resistance to DDT and pyrethroids. *Insect Molecular Biology* **9**, 491–497.

RBM (2004) *RBM Consensus Statement on Insecticide Treated Netting: Personal Protection and Vector Control Options for Prevention of Malaria.*

Reyburn, H., Ashford, R., Mohsen, M., Hewitt, S. and Rowland, M. (2000). A randomized controlled trial of insecticide treated bednets and chaddars or top-sheets, and residual spraying or interior rooms for the prevention of cutaneous leishmaniasis in Kabul, Afghanistan. *Transactions of the Royal Society of Tropical Medicine & Hygiene* **94**, 361–366.

Richards, F.O., Jr., Flores, R.Z., Sexton, J.D., Beach, R.F., Mount, D.L., Cordon-Rosales, C., Gatica, M. and Klein, R.E. (1994). Effects of permethrin-impregnated bed nets on malaria vectors of northern Guatemala. *Bulletin of the Pan American Health Organization* **28**, 112–121.

Rowland, M., Bouma, M., Ducornez, D., Durrani, N., Rozendaal, J., Schapira, A. and Sondorp, E. (1996). Pyrethroid impregnated bed nets for self protection from malaria for Afghan refugees. *Transactions of the Royal Society of Tropical Medicine & Hygiene* **90**, 357–361.

Rowland, M., Freeman, T., Downey, G., Hadi, A. and Saeed, M. (2004). Deet mosquito repellent sold through social marketing provides protection against malaria in an area of all-night mosquito biting and partial coverage of insecticide treated nets: a case control study of effectiveness. *Tropical Medicine and International Health* **9**, 343–350.

Rowland, M., Hewitt, S., Durrani, N., Saleh, P., Bouma, M. and Sondorp, E. (1997). Sustainability of pyrethroid-impregnated bednets for malaria control in Afghan communities. *Bulletin of the World Health Organization* **75**, 23–29.

Rowland, M., Webster, J., Saleh, P., Chandramohan, D., Freeman, T., Pearcy, B., Durrani, N., Rab, A. and Mohammed, N. (2002). Prevention of malaria in Afghanistan through social marketing of insecticide treated nets: evaluation of coverage and effectiveness by cross-sectional surveys and passive surveillance. *Tropical Medicine and International Health* **7**, 813–822.

Schellenberg, J.R., Abdulla, S., Nathan, R., Mukasa, O., Marchant, T.J., Kikumbih, N., Mushi, A.K., Mponda, H., Minja, H., Mshinda, H., Tanner, M. and Lengeler, C. (2001). Effect of large-scale social marketing of insecticide-treated nets on child survival in rural Tanzania. *Lancet* **357**, 1241–1247.

Shulman, C.E., Dorman, E.K., Talisuna, A.O., Lowe, B.S., Nevill, C., Snow, R.W., Jilo, H., Peshu, N., Bulmer, J.N., Graham, S. and Marsh, K. (1998). A community randomized controlled trial of insecticide-treated bednets for the prevention of malaria and anaemia among primigravid women on the Kenyan coast. *Tropical Medicine and International Health* **3**, 197–204.

Smith, T., Genton, B., Betuela, I., Rare, L. and Alpers, M.P. (2002). Mosquito nets for the elderly? *Transactions of the Royal Society of Tropical Medicine and Hygiene* **96**, 37–38.

Snow, R.W., Bastos De Azevedo, I., Lowe, B.S., Kabiru, E.W., Nevill, C.G., Mwankusye, S., Kassiga, G., Marsh, K. and Teuscher, T. (1994). Severe childhood malaria in two areas of markedly different falciparum transmission in east Africa. *Acta Tropica* **57**, 289–300.

Sochantha, T., Hewitt, S., Nguon, C., Okell, L., Alexander, N., Rowland, M. and Socheat, D. (2006). Insecticide-treated bed nets for the prevention of *Plasmodium falciparum* malaria in Cambodia: a cluster-randomised trial. Unpublished observations.

Snow, R.W., Rowan, K.M., Lindsay, S.W. and Greenwood, B.M. (1988). A trial of bed nets (mosquito nets) as a malaria control strategy in a rural area of The Gambia, West Africa. *Transactions of the Royal Society of Tropical Medicine and Hygiene* **82**, 212–215.

Stevens, W., Wiseman, V., Ortiz, J. and Chavasse, D. (2005). The costs and effects of a nationwide insecticide-treated net programme: the case of Malawi. *Malaria Journal* **4**, 22.

Tami, A., Mubyazi, G., Talbert, A., Mshinda, H., Duchon, S. and Lengeler, C. (2004). Evaluation of Olyset insecticide-treated nets distributed seven years previously in Tanzania. *Malaria Journal* **3**, 19.

Tang, L. (2000). Progress in malaria control in China. *Chinese Medical Journal (England)* **113**, 89–92.

Taych, A., Jalouk, J. and Al-Khiami, A.M. (1997). *A cutaneous leishmaniasis control trial using pyrethroid impregnated bednets in villages near Aleppo Syria*. World Health Organistion, Geneva. WHO/LEISH/97.41.

ter Kuile, F.O., Terlouw, D.J., Phillips-Howard, P.A., Hawley, W.A., Friedman, J.F., Kolczak, M.S., Kariuki, S.K., Shi, Y.P., Kwena, A.M., Vulule, J.M. and Nahlen, B.L. (2003a). Impact of permethrin-treated bed nets on malaria and all-cause morbidity in young children in an area of intense perennial malaria transmission in western Kenya: cross-sectional survey. *American Journal of Tropical Medicine and Hygiene* **68**, 100–107.

ter Kuile, F.O., Terlouw, D.J., Phillips-Howard, P.A., Hawley, W.A., Friedman, J.F., Kariuki, S.K., Shi, Y.P., Kolczak, M.S., Lal, A.A., Vulule, J.M. and Nahlen, B.L. (2003b). Reduction of malaria during pregnancy by permethrin-treated bed nets in an area of intense perennial malaria transmission in western Kenya. *American Journal of Tropical Medicine and Hygiene* **68**, 50–60.

ter Kuile, T. (2003c). Insecticide treated nets for the control of malaria in pregnancy: a summary of seven controlled studies. *PREMA Newsletter* **3**.

UNDP (2005). *Coming to Grips with Malaria in the New Millennium*. Task Force on HIV/AIDS, Malaria, TB, and Access to Essential Medicines, Working Group on Malaria.

Webster, J., Lines, J., Bruce, J., Armstrong-Schellenberg, J.R. and Hanson, K. (2005). Which delivery systems reach the poor? A review of equity of coverage of ever-treated nets, never-treated nets and immunization to reduce child mortality in Africa. *Lancet Infectious Diseases* **5**(11), 709–717.

WHO (2000). *The African Summit on Roll Back Malaria, Abuja, Nigeria*, World Health Organization, WHO/CDS/RBM/2000.17.

WHO (2002a). *Scaling-Up Insecticide Treated Netting Programmes in Africa: A Strategic Framework for Coordinated National Action*, World Health Organization, WHO/CDS/RBM/2002.43.

WHO (2002b). *Insecticide-Treated Mosquito Net Interventions: A Manual for Malaria Control Programme Managers by Webster, J., Lines, J. and Hill, J.*, World Health Organization. WHO/CDS/RBM/2002.45.

WHO (2004). *Sources and Prices of Selected Products for the Prevention, Diagnosis and Treatment of Malaria*. 66 pp. A joint WHO RBM UNICEF UNAIDS PSI MSH project. WHO/HTM/RBM/2004.

WHO (2005a). *World Malaria Report*, World Health Organization.

WHO (2005b). *58th World Health Assembly: Malaria report by the Secretariat*. WHO58.8.

WHO (2005c). *58th World Health Assembly: Resolution on malaria control.* WHA58.2.

WHO (2005d). *Safety of Pyrethroids for Public Health Use.* WHO/CDS/ WHOPES/GCDPP/2005.10, WHO/PCS/RA/2005.1

WHO (2005e). *Scaling-Up Insecticide treated Netting Programmes in Africa: A Strategic Framework for Coordinated National Action.* World Health Organization. 2nd edition.

WHOPES [WHO Pesticide Evaluation Scheme]. (2001). *Report of the 5th WHOPES Working Group Meeting, WHO/HQ 30–31 October 2001.* WHO/CDS/WHOPES/2001.4.

WHOPES [WHO Pesticide Evaluation Scheme] (2004). *Report of the 7th WHOPES Working Group Meeting, WHO/HQ 2–4 December 2003.* WHO/CDS/WHOPES/2004.8.

Wiseman, V., Hawley, W.A., ter Kuile, F.O., Phillips-Howard, P.A., Vulule, J.M., Nahlen, B.L. and Mills, A.J. (2003). The cost-effectiveness of permethrin-treated bed nets in an area of intense malaria transmission in western Kenya. *American Journal of Tropical Medicine and Hygiene* **68**(Suppl. 4), 161–167.

Worrall, E., Hill, J., Webster, J. and Mortimer, J. (2005). Experience of targeting subsidies on insecticide-treated nets: what do we know and what are the knowledge gaps? *Tropical Medicine and International Health* **10**, 19–31.

Yates, A., N'Guessan, R., Kaur, H. and Rowland, M. (2005). Evaluation of KO Tab 1-2-3: a dip-it-yourself long-lasting insecticide formulation for use on mosquito nets. *Malaria Journal* **4**, 52.

Zaim, M., Aitio, A. and Nakashima, N. (2000). Safety of pyrethroid-treated mosquito nets. *Medical and Veterinary Entomology* **14**, 1–5.

Zimmerman, R.H. and Voorham, J. (1997). Use of insecticide-impregnated mosquito nets and other impregnated materials for malaria control in the Americas. *Rev Panam Salud Publica* **2**, 18–25.

Control of Chagas Disease

Yoichi Yamagata[1] and Jun Nakagawa[2]

[1]*Institute for International Cooperation, Japan International Cooperation Agency, 10-5, Ichigaya Honmura-cho, Shinjuku-ku, Tokyo 162-8433, Japan*
[2]*Japan International Cooperation Agency, Apdo. postal 1752, Tegucigalpa, M.D.C., Honduras*

ADVANCES IN PARASITOLOGY VOL 61
ISSN: 0065-308X
DOI: 10.1016/S0065-308X(05)61004-4

ABSTRACT

The Southern Cone Initiative (Iniciativa de Salud del Cono Sur, INCOSUR) to control domestic transmission of *Trypanosoma cruzi* is a substantial achievement based on the enthusiasm of the scientific community, effective strategies, leadership, and cost-effectiveness. INCOSUR triggered the launch of other regional initiatives in Central America and in the Andean and Amazon regions, which have all made progress. The Central American Initiative targeted the elimination of an imported triatomine bug (*Rhodnius prolixus*) and the control of a widespread native species (*Triatoma dimidiata*), and faced constraints such as a small scientific community, the difficulty in controlling a native species, and a vector control programme that had fragmented under a decentralized health system. International organizations such as the Japan International Cooperation Agency (JICA) have played an important role in bridging the gaps between fragmented organizational resources. Guatemala achieved virtual elimination of *R. prolixus* and 'reduction of *Tri. Dimidiata* and El Salvador and Honduras revitalized their national programmes. The programme also revealed new challenges. *Tri. dimidiata* control needs to cover a large geographic area efficiently with stratification, quality control, community mobilization, and information management. Stakeholders such as the National Chagas Program, the local health system and their communities, as well as local government must share responsibilities to continue comprehensive vector control.

1. INTRODUCTION

Control of Chagas disease caused by the parasite *Trypanosoma cruzi* in Latin America over the last two decades has been a substantial public health achievement. The incidence of Chagas disease was reduced by over 65% between 1990 and 2000, from an estimated 700 000 cases per year to fewer than 200 000 (Schmunis *et al.*, 1996; WHO, 2002). The Southern Cone Initiative (Iniciativa de Salud del Cono Sur, INCOSUR) was launched in 1991, aimed at elimination of the main vector, the reduviid bug *Triatoma infestans,* and elimination of transfusional transmission of *T. cruzi* in Argentina, Bolivia, Brazil, Chile, Paraguay, and Uruguay (PAHO, 1993). Since transmission by triatomine bugs accounts for over 80% of Chagas disease transmission, and the initiative successfully eliminated domestic *Tri. infestans* over large areas, this large-scale regional cooperation has significantly reduced disease transmission (Table 1) (WHO, 2002). The interruption of domiciliary transmission of *T. cruzi* by *Tri. infestans* has already been certified in Uruguay, Chile, four provinces in Argentina, 10 states in Brazil, and one state in Paraguay (PAHO, 1998, 1999a, 2000a, 2002a, 2003a). This success suggested that Chagas disease control is no longer a technical issue, but a political, economic, and organizational problem (Dias and Schofield, 1999; Schofield and Dias, 1999; Dias *et al.,* 2002).

Based on the success of INCOSUR, the concept of region-wide control of Chagas disease has expanded to other regions such as Central America, where the endemic countries are facing new challenges in vector control. The World Health Organization (WHO) adopted the common goal of the elimination of Chagas disease in Latin America by the year 2010. In 1997, Belize, Costa Rica, El Salvador, Guatemala, Honduras, Nicaragua, and Panama launched the Central American Initiative (Iniciativa de los países de Centroamérica, IPCA) and Colombia, Ecuador, Peru, and Venezuela launched the Andean Initiative (1997) to control vectorial and transfusional transmission of the disease. Mexico has begun a dialogue

Table 1 Change of seroprevalence (%) of *T. cruzi* infection in five Southern Cone countries, 1981–1999

Country	1981–1991		1995–1999		Age group (years)
	Seroprevalence	Year	Seroprevalence	Year	
Argentina	4.8	1983	1.0	1995	18
Brazil	5.0	1981	0.3	1999	0–7
Chile	5.4	1990	0.2	1999	0–4
Paraguay	9.7	1991	3.9	1996	18
Uruguay	2.4	1985	0.1	1996	0–12

Source: WHO (2002).

with IPCA, seeking to join in the control activities. In addition, the Amazon region has discussed launching a regional initiative for surveillance and control of sylvatic vector species. IPCA has made the most significant progress to date, especially in vector control. IPCA, however, must deal with an entomological, social, and political situation, which is different from that of the Southern Cone countries. The aims of this paper are to review the lessons of the Southern Cone Initiative and their application in Central America, and to discuss strategies to tackle the new challenges of sustainable triatomine control.

2. THE SOUTHERN CONE INITIATIVE

INCOSUR (the Southern Cone Initiative) provided valuable lessons for implementing Chagas disease control in the Americas. Recent reviews have evaluated the achievements of INCOSUR (e.g. Dias and Schofield, 1999; Morel, 1999; Schofield and Dias, 1999; Silveira and Vinhaes, 1999; Dias *et al.*, 2002; WHO, 2002; Moncayo, 2003). These reviews summarize the following points:

(i)   INCOSUR established the appropriate technology and strategy to interrupt the transmission of Chagas disease.
(ii) A control programme with strong leadership at the central level was a vital factor.
(iii) The regional initiative was feasible, valuable, and cost-effective.
(iv) The scientific community played an important role in providing expertise and continuity for the initiative.

2.1. Technology and Strategy Development

INCOSUR established a three-phase control strategy: preparation, attack, and maintenance (Dias, 1991; Schofield and Dias, 1999). (i) The preparatory phase identified infested villages and surveyed seroprevalence in children, using established indices.* (ii) The attack phase involved large-scale residual spraying of pyrethroid insecticides in the domestic and peridomestic structures in the infested villages. (iii) The maintenance phase consisted of vector surveillance by vector control personnel and the local community, and additional spraying of insecticides in any reinfested houses.

Tri. infestans is the most important and most widely distributed vector of Chagas disease in South America, and has the following characteristics that make it vulnerable to this strategy: (i) relatively slow rate of repopulation; (ii) limited range of habitats (domestic and peri-domestic areas, except for some sylvatic populations in parts of central Bolivia); (iii) limited capacity for active dispersal; (iv) complete suscep-tibility to modern pyrethroid insecticides; and (v) low genetic vari-ability, suggesting a low tendency to develop insecticidal resistance (Dias and Schofield, 1999; WHO, 2002). The massive triatomine con-trol campaign in Brazil between 1983 and 1986 demonstrated the ef-fectiveness of the triatomine control strategy, reducing the number of *Tri. infestans*-infested municipalities from 711 to 83, and seroprevalence in the 0–7 year age group from 5% to 0.3% (WHO, 1997b). Based on this success and various technical guidelines developed in member countries, the WHO Expert Committee on the Control of Chagas Dis-ease provided the technical guidelines (WHO, 1991) for implementing national programmes in other countries in South and Central America.

2.2. Cost-Effectiveness

Cost-effectiveness of any large-scale vector control campaign is the crucial basis for the political decision to launch the regional initia-tives. Chagas disease was ranked as the fourth most serious parasitic

---

*Principal entomological indices were: house infestation index = percentage of houses infested by triatomines among number of houses examined; dispersion index = percentage of villages infested with triatomines among number of villages examined; density index = number of triatomines captured per house examined; crowding index = number of triatomines captured per house infested with triato-mines; colonization index = percentage of houses infested with triatomine nymphs among number of houses infested with triatomines. Among these indices, the house infestation index is the most commonly used (Schofield, 2001).

disease globally (after malaria, schistosomiasis, and intestinal worms) in terms of annual loss of disability adjusted life years (DALYs), which is equivalent to over US$ 6.5×10^6 per year (World Bank, 1993). In Latin America, Chagas disease is the most important of the parasitic diseases. Schofield and Dias (1991) projected that the internal rate of return on investment on triatomine control was estimated to be 14% per year by savings in medical costs. Subsequently, the Chagas disease control programme in Brazil was shown to have prevented an estimated 89% of potential disease transmission (Akhavan, 2000), and the internal rate of return of Chagas disease vector control was estimated to be over 60% in Argentina (Basombrío et al., 1998).

This economic benefit, however, would be lost quickly without continued vector-surveillance activity. Analysis showed that the absence of surveillance after the attack phase would reduce the benefit of the initiative to zero after 11 years (Schofield and Dias, 1991; Akhavan, 2000; Dias et al., 2002). Vector surveillance by community participation detected infestation more precisely than active surveillance by health personnel when the infestation level was low (Dias, 1988, 1991; Wanderley, 1991). The risk of reinfestation from the peridomestic to the domestic habitat always persists; thus a combination of community-based surveillance and selective application of insecticides would be cost-beneficial (Schofield and Dias, 1991; Akhavan, 2000; Dias et al., 2002).

2.3. Organization

INCOSUR successfully strengthened national programmes for Chagas disease control. At the beginning of the initiative, only Argentina and Brazil had established national programmes. Their triatomine control campaign started with a "vertical" structure with its own human and financial resources (Dias, 1991; Schmunis and Dias, 2000; Liese et al., 1991). During the decentralization of the health system that started in the mid-1980s, the vector control organizations were progressively dismantled, and the personnel were allocated to the newly established local health systems (Dias and Schofield, 1999). However, most of the Southern Cone countries managed to establish a continuous vector control programme in accordance with their health system needs, by maintaining a strong national-level perspective of the role of vector control. While Paraguay maintained a vertical programme, Chile and Uruguay carried out vector control activity at the regional and departmental levels to which the national level provided human and financial resources, technical guidance and logistics (Schmunis and Dias, 2000).

2.4. Regional Coordination

The regional initiative made it possible to tackle issues such as accomplishing wide geographic coverage, control of boundary areas, and regional quality control of the vector programme. Under the common objectives, progress in each country was monitored and evaluated cooperatively through regional meetings and Pan American Health Organization (PAHO) evaluation missions to each country. The use of evaluation teams from neighbouring countries afforded excellent opportunities for shared experience and, in some cases, resource-sharing. Setting attainable goals and certifying the progress created healthy competition, and motivated member countries. The certification of interruption of Chagas disease transmission by PAHO was particularly important politically as well as technically. The decision to certify five countries as free of domiciliary transmission was publicized widely by WHO. International organizations facilitated these regional activities. PAHO provided a political framework for the initiative, and facilitated the regional exchange of knowledge and personnel. ECLAT (Latin America Triatomine Research Network), supported by the European Union, promoted regional networking among scientists, and helped to link scientific effort with the vector control operation.

The recent focus of the initiative is in the maintenance phase of the elimination of *Tri. infestans* and the control of secondary species of vectors in Argentina, Chile, Brazil, and Uruguay. Currently, Bolivia has the most active vector control programme in South America, backed by a substantial loan from the Inter-American Development Bank (IDB). Bolivia launched a national programme in 1991, but was unable to achieve its operational targets until the IDB loan was implemented in 1998; Bolivia has now sprayed more than 600 000 houses, 80% of the target (PAHO, 2003a). Paraguay continues to focus on vector control and surveillance activities. Peru participated in the initiative meeting for the first time in 1996, and has launched control activities against *Tri. infestans* in the southern part of the country.

INCOSUR demonstrated that multicountry initiatives are feasible and valuable in strengthening the vector control programmes of the member countries. The scientific community played an important role in maintaining political continuity for Chagas disease control, by convincing policy makers with scientific evidence. Organizing and promoting the scientific community was a vital factor in providing expertise and continuity for the vector control programmes. INCOSUR is now seen as a model for regional cooperation in disease control, and its control strategy is effective throughout the Americas (Schofield and Dias, 1999). The success of the initiative has become a motivating factor for the other countries in the Americas to tackle Chagas disease. Molyneux and Morel (1998) have discussed the similarities between the successful programme of onchocerciasis control and with that for Chagas disease, where, despite significant biological differences, process and programmatic comparisons are valid.

3. THE CENTRAL AMERICAN INITIATIVE

IPCA was created to duplicate the success of the Southern Cone countries. IPCA, however, differs from INCOSUR in the following ways: (i) its creation was concurrent with decentralization of the health system; (ii) a smaller number of scientists with limited influence on political decisions are present in the region; and (iii) a widely distributed species of vector with domestic, peridomestic, and sylvatic populations is the main vector (*Tri. dimidiata*). The initiative had limited success during the first few years, but was revitalized with international cooperation. In 1999 in the department of Yoro, the Honduran government and Médecins sans Frontières (MSF) launched a project for prevention and treatment of Chagas disease. Guatemala and the JICA jointly launched a triatomine control project in 2000, which expanded to El Salvador and Honduras in 2003.

3.1. History and Political Framework

Chagas disease has long been known to be a serious endemic disease in Central America. The earliest recorded cases of human infection of *T. cruzi* in Central America were reported in El Salvador (Segovia, 1913), Panama (Miller, 1931), Guatemala (Reichenow, 1933), and Costa Rica (von Bullow, 1941). The percentage of infected people was determined, at the village level, to be 11.7% in Costa Rica (Zeledón *et al.*, 1975), 18.4% in El Salvador (Cedillos, 1975), and 8.8% in Panama (Sousa and Johnson, 1971). In addition, the seroprevalence among blood donors was between 19.8% and 28% in Honduras (Ponce and Zeledón, 1973; Ponce, 1999).

The first advance in Chagas disease control was made by eliminating blood transfusional transmission of *T. cruzi.* In 1987, with support from PAHO, Honduras started a national programme to control the transmission of *T. cruzi* by blood transfusion, and achieved 100% coverage of blood screening by 1991. A similar programme was launched in El Salvador in 1992 with assistance from Honduras and PAHO, reaching 100% coverage by 1997 (Ponce, 1999). The coverage increased gradually in other countries, reaching 99% in Guatemala, 81% in Nicaragua, and 95% in Panama by 2002 (PAHO, 2005b).

The success in vector control of the INCOSUR programme inspired Central American countries such as Belize, Costa Rica, El Salvador, Guatemala, Honduras, Nicaragua, and Panama to launch IPCA in 1997. The first discussions on the initiative took place during the ECLAT workshop in Ecuador in 1995, when a series of resolutions formed the basis for approaching the national authorities of Central America to begin the initiative (Schofield *et al.*, 1996). The Honduran Vice-Minister of Health indicated his support for the Southern Cone Initiative by participating in its annual meeting in 1997. Following this, the 13th Health Sector Meeting in Central America (RESSCA) declared that the control of Chagas disease was a priority. At a follow-up Central American meeting in Honduras,

Table 2   Chagas disease in Central America

	Seroprevalence[a]	Incidence[b]	Main vectors
Belize	675	26	*Tri. dimidiata*
Guatemala	730 000	28 387	*R. prolixius, Tri. dimidiata*
Honduras	300 000	11 490	*R. prolixius, Tri. dimidiata*
El Salvador	322 000	10 594	*Tri. dimidiata*
Nicaragua	67 000	2660	*R. prolixius, Tri. dimidiata*
Costa Rica	130 000	3320	*Tri. dimidiata*
Panama	220 000	5346	*R. pallescens*
Total	1 769 675	61 823	

[a]WHO estimates, based on reports from Ministries of Health.
[b]Incidence calculated using the model of Hayes and Schofield (1990).

during which IPCA was launched (WHO, 1998a), the population at risk in the region was estimated to be more than 9 million, of whom 1.7 million were currently infected (Table 2). In 1998, the 51st World Health Assembly acknowledged IPCA, and resolved to eliminate Chagas disease transmission in the Americas by the end of 2010 (WHO, 1998b).

IPCA set three objectives: (i) elimination of *Rhodnius prolixus*; (ii) decreased house infestation by *Tri. dimidiata*; and (iii) elimination of transfusional transmission of *T. cruzi* (PAHO, 1999b). The elimination of *R. prolixus* was set as the primary objective. The first meeting of IPCA in 1998 recommended that all participating countries should determine the distribution of triatomines by species, and implement the attack phase of vector control with internal and external funding (PAHO, 1999b). Annual meetings of the initiative have been held since 1998, and PAHO began to dispatch evaluation missions to member countries in 2002. Technical guidelines for vector control were provided by local and international experts (e.g. Schofield, 2000, 2001; WHO, 2002), and species-specific guidelines were also developed in thematic workshops (PAHO, 2002b, 2003a, b).

IPCA attracted several non-governmental organizations (NGOs) and international cooperation agencies to work for the control of Chagas disease. Among them, JICA, which has so far made the largest external contribution in Central America. The JICA project was launched in Guatemala in 2000, and provided Japanese long- and short-term consultants and volunteers as well as materials (insecticide, spray pumps, and vehicles). Guatemala contributed salaries for the vector control personnel, transportation costs, and insecticide. PAHO, the secretariat of IPCA, provided technical support for the project via regional meetings, seminars, and support of evaluation missions. PAHO evaluation missions have since visited Guatemala in 2002 and Honduras and El Salvador in 2003. JICA is currently providing collaborative support to these three countries.

3.2. Chagas Disease Vectors

R. prolixus and *Tri. dimidiata* are the main vectors of *T. cruzi* in Central America (Figure 1). In this region, 15 species of vectors have been reported, but these two have the widest dispersion with domiciliary populations (Schofield, 2000). *R. pallescens* is an important vector in Panama, and other species such as *Tri. nitida* have also been occasionally found infected in domestic areas.

R. prolixus is the most efficient vector transmitting *T. cruzi* in Central America. The vectorial capacity of *R. prolixus* was found to be three times that of *Tri. dimidiata* (Ponce *et al.*, 1993; Ponce, 1995). Paz-Bailey *et al.* (2002) showed that the prevalence of human infection with *T. cruzi* is four times higher in villages infested with *R. prolixus* (38.8%) than in areas infested with *Tri. dimidiata* (8.9%). The efficiency of *R. prolixus* as a vector is partially attributable to its ability to reach high population densities. Over 11 000 *R. prolixus* individuals have been found in a single house, while the density of *Tri. dimidiata* is usually much less than 100 per house (Schofield, 2000). The seroprevalence of schoolchildren (7–14 years old) in the *R. prolixus*-infested departments was 7.9% in Guatemala and 10.8% in Nicaragua (Rizzo *et al.*, 2003; MINSA, 2003). In Honduras, the highest seroprevalence recorded was 17.8% at the municipality (subdivision of department) level (PAHO, 2003c).

R. prolixus was considered a feasible target for elimination from Central America. The population of *R. prolixus* in Central America is confined to domestic areas (mainly thatched-roof houses), and its genetic variation is much less than that among South American populations in Colombia and Venezuela. This suggests that *R. prolixus* was imported from South America (Dujardin *et al.*, 1998; Schofield

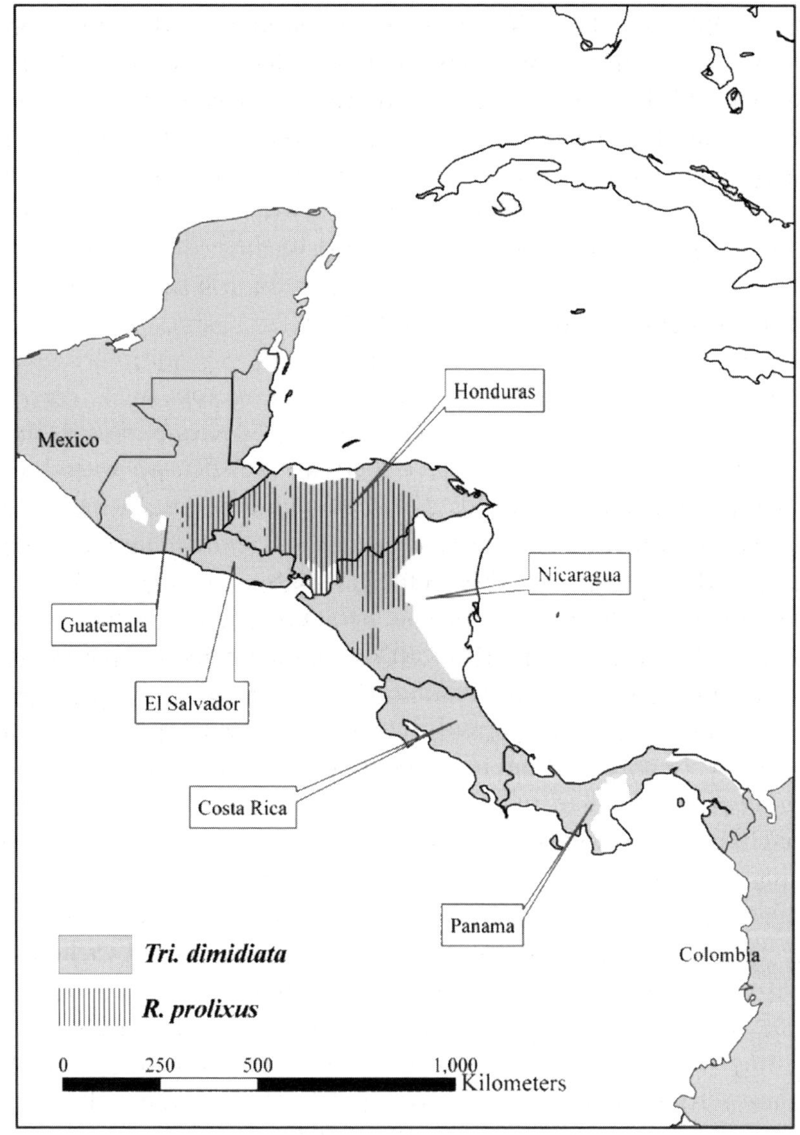

Figure 1 Geographic distribution of *R. prolixus* and *Tri. dimidiata* in Central America. (Data from PAHO, 2002c, 2003b, c, 2004; WHO, 2002.)

and Dujardin, 1997). At the beginning of the 20th century, *R. prolixus* was reported in El Salvador but by the early 1950s it was widely distributed from northern Costa Rica to the south of Mexico

(Dias, 1952). By the 1990s, however, *R. prolixus* had almost completely disappeared from Mexico, Costa Rica, and El Salvador (Zeledón, 1981; PAHO, 2003c). This reduction is attributed to the decrease in thatched-roof houses during the last 40 years and to widespread insecticide spraying by the malaria eradication campaigns that started in the mid-1950s. Preliminary entomological surveys, which studied vector infestation at the department level, also demonstrated an apparent reduction in the distribution of *R. prolixus* in Central America (Tabaru *et al.*, 1999; PAHO, 2003c).

Rapid entomological assessments for identifying infested villages, by community members and trained ministry personnel, demonstrated that the distribution of *R. prolixus* in Central America was concentrated around the borders of Honduras. During 2000–2002, Guatemala identified a total of 296 infested villages, the majority of them concentrated in the eastern region of the country on the border with Honduras (PAHO, 2003c, 2005b). Honduras had the widest distribution, from the western border with Guatemala to the eastern border with Nicaragua (PAHO, 2003c), and identified 65 infested villages during 2003–2004, most of them located in western departments such as Copán and Ocotepeque (PAHO, 2005b; Secretaría de Salud de Honduras, unpublished information). Nicaragua also identified 50 infested villages on the borders with Honduras (MINSA, 2003; PAHO, 2005b). At the same time, a small number of dispersed villages were found to be infested in distant Guatemalan departments such as El Quiché (one infested village), Huehuetenango (two), and Baja Verapaz (one), which probably indicates either accidental dispersal by travellers or surviving colonies from a declining distribution of *R. prolixus*.

Tri. dimidiata is a major threat in Central America, despite its relatively low efficiency as a vector of *T. cruzi*. The distribution of *Tri. dimidiata* is much wider than that of *R. prolixus*, from Mexico to northern South America (Carcavallo *et al.*, 1999). Despite the low population density, human transmission of *T. cruzi* has been confirmed in *Tri. dimidiata*-infested areas (Ponce and Zeledón, 1973; Zeledón *et al.*, 1975; Ponce *et al.*, 1993). The seroprevalence of schoolchildren in the *Tri. dimidiata*-infested departments was 5.2% in Honduras and 4.7% in Guatemala (PAHO, 2003a; Rizzo *et al.*, 2003). *Tri. dimidiata* appears to be responsible for the acute cases in El Salvador (PAHO, 2004).

Unlike *R. prolixus*, the elimination of *Tri. dimidiata* is not a feasible goal because of the existence of peridomestic and sylvatic populations. *Tri. dimidiata* mainly infests crevices in the mud walls of houses and peridomestic structures such as chicken pens. Sylvatic populations have been reported in Belize, Costa Rica, and Guatemala (Zeledón, 1981). The vector colonizes not only rural areas, but also parts of major cities such as San Salvador and Tegucigalpa (Ponce and Zeledón, 1973; Cedillos, 1975). Thus reduction of its domestic population is the only feasible control strategy (WHO, 2002).

The preliminary entomological surveys confirmed vector infestation in most of the departments in Guatemala (21 of 22 departments), El Salvador (14 of 14), and Nicaragua (15 of 17) (Tabaru *et al.*, 1999; PAHO, 2000b, 2002c). Rapid entomological assessments in Guatemala identified over 1700 infested villages, and demonstrated that the dispersion index at the department level was 15–85%, while the house infestation index was 2.4–36% (MSPAS, 2002; Nakagawa *et al.*, 2005). The dispersion index in Honduras was 65–78%, and the infestation index was 17–25% (PAHO, 2005b). In El Salvador, the dispersion index was 8–82% and the infestation index was 12–33% (Ministerio de Salud de El Salvador, unpublished information). Domestic as well as peridomestic infestation was observed in most areas. In El Salvador, no specimen of *R. prolixus* has been recorded since 1999, in spite of active searches (PAHO, 2003c).

Populations of *Tri. dimidiata* are difficult to detect. The existing survey methods cannot detect all infestations, which makes targeted control activity impractical. Monroy *et al.* (1998a, b) demonstrated that less than 10% of *Tri. dimidiata* can be collected by the most commonly used method (man–hour survey), and that other survey methods (white-paper and flush-out methods) were less effective in detecting infestation. It was also found that the effectiveness of the man–hour survey can be improved by focusing on the areas close to beds, where more than 30% of the vectors were found (Monroy *et al.*, 1998b).

The efficacy of residual spraying of pyrethroids was verified in Central America. Third-generation pyrethroids were shown to be highly effective in South America for triatomine control, such as β-cyfluthrin (12.5% suspension concentrate (SC) at target dose of 25 mg of active ingredient (a.i.)/m^2), cyfluthrin (10% wettable powder (WP) at 50 mg a.i./m^2), deltamethrin (10% SC or 5% WP at 25 mg a.i./m^2), and λ-cyhalothrin (10% WP at 30 mg a.i./m^2) (Zerba, 1999). Control trials against *R. prolixus* and *Tri. dimidiata* in Central America demonstrated the effectiveness of these pyrethroids (Oliveira Filho, 1997; Tabaru *et al.*, 1998; Acevedo *et al.*, 2000), and the domestic infestation rate was reduced to zero with a single application during 12 months evaluation (Tabaru *et al.*, 1998; Acevedo *et al.*, 2000).

3.3. Control of *Rhodnius prolixus*

The population of *R. prolixus* has been reduced drastically by the control campaign, suggesting that elimination is feasible in the near future. Based on the entomological findings of Tabaru *et al.* (1999), Guatemala and Japan launched a vector control project in five eastern departments of Guatemala (Zacapa, Chiquimula, Jalapa, Jutiapa, and Santa Rosa) in 2000, and in an additional four (Alta Verapaz, Baja Verapaz, El Progreso, and Quiche) in 2002. Residual spraying of pyrethroids targeted all the houses in the 296 infested villages (the so-called "eradication strategy"), as recommended by Schofield (2000) and PAHO (2003c). The first round of the spraying covered 33 000 houses, and the post-spraying evaluation (4–18 months after the first spraying) showed that the number of infested villages had declined to nine (Figure 2) (Nakagawa *et al.*, 2003a, b). After the second spraying, only one village was found to be infested, and it was subsequently retreated (MSPAS, unpublished information).

Honduras and Nicaragua, in 2000, also launched vector control against *R. prolixus* with external funding. In Honduras, infested villages in two departments (Intibuca and Yoro) were sprayed, with assistance from NGOs such as MSF and World Vision. Geographic coverage of the vector control was expanded significantly in 2000, when the Honduran government and international organizations such as JICA, the Canadian International Development Agency (CIDA) and World Vision jointly launched vector control projects in six *R. prolixus*-infested departments. These stakeholders, together with PAHO, co-developed a national strategic plan that became a foundation for strong donor harmonization of Chagas disease

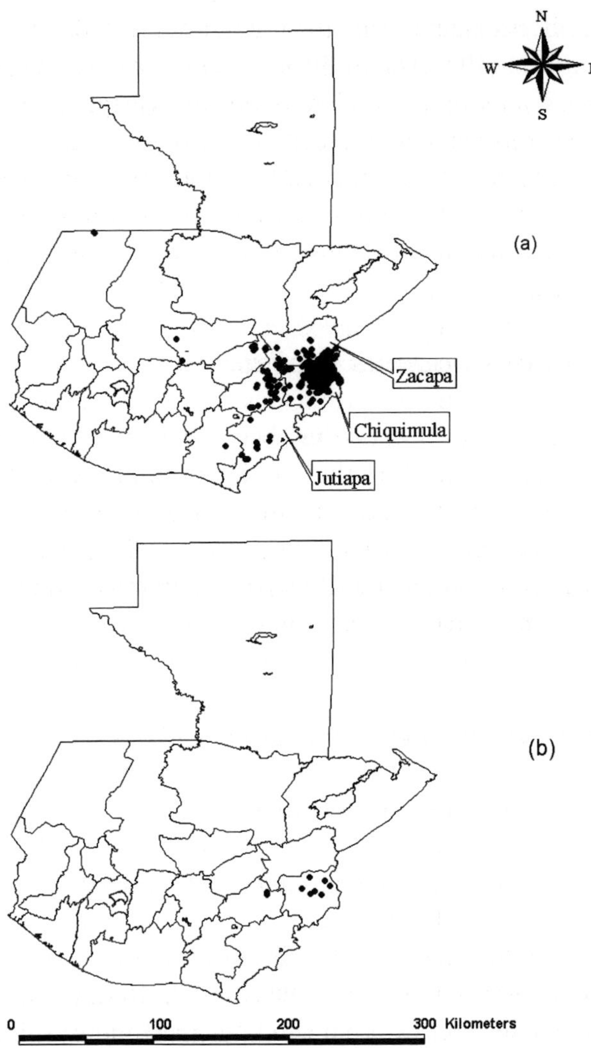

Figure 2 Change in distribution of villages infested with *R. prolixus* in Guatemala, before (a) and after (b) the first round of insecticide spraying. Black dots indicate villages in which at least one bug was found. (Data from Ministerio de Salud Publica y Asistencia Técnica, courtesy of H. Alvarez and K. Hashimoto.)

control. Nicaragua sprayed all the 50 infested villages in eight departments, with financial assistance from the government of Taiwan (PAHO, 2003a–c). The second round of the spraying is in the planning stage, and the impact of the spraying has not yet been evaluated.

Because of a shortage of vector control personnel, due to the decentralization of the health system, the Honduran projects implemented a "school-based exploration" to identify infested villages by interviewing schoolchildren. Environmental Health Technicians (Técnicos de Salud Ambiental, TSAs) visited primary schools and asked pupils of 4th–6th grades whether they had seen *R. prolixus*, shown in colour pictures with which they were presented. A total of 65 villages in eight departments were identified as infested with *R. prolixus* (PAHO, 2005b). Community members were trained and involved in the spraying activities, to overcome the shortage of vector control personnel.

Community-based surveillance has been established in selected villages in Guatemala, to evaluate progress towards the elimination of *R. prolixus*. The Health Areas (HAs) have trained volunteers in 61 villages in four departments (Jalapa, Jutiapa, Santa Rosa, and Zacapa) to detect and report reinfestation by *R. prolixus*. No reinfestation by *R. prolixus* has been reported in these villages since 2004 (Hashimoto *et al.*, personal communication).

3.4. Control of *Triatoma dimidiata*

Insecticide spraying against *Tri. dimidiata* was effective in reducing domestic populations, though repeated spraying together with surveillance was necessary to assure the minimum level of infestation. Villages with infestation levels higher than 5% were targeted for spraying. This strategy was based on the finding that in Brazil transmission of *T. cruzi* was rare below that level of infestation (Dias, 1987). Residual spraying targeted all houses constructed with mud walls, and peridomestic structures such as chicken pens in the relevant villages. Second and third rounds of spraying were applied in villages with persistent infestation (i.e. infestation rates higher than 5%) to maximize the impact of the spraying.

The vector control project has reduced the house infestation rate of *Tri. dimidiata* in Guatemala. More than 1700 villages were identified as targets for intervention, and the first round of spraying covered more than 1300 villages, followed by a second round in over 300 villages. Postspraying monitoring demonstrated a reduction in the infestation level (Figure 3). The infestation rate in the department of Zacapa decreased

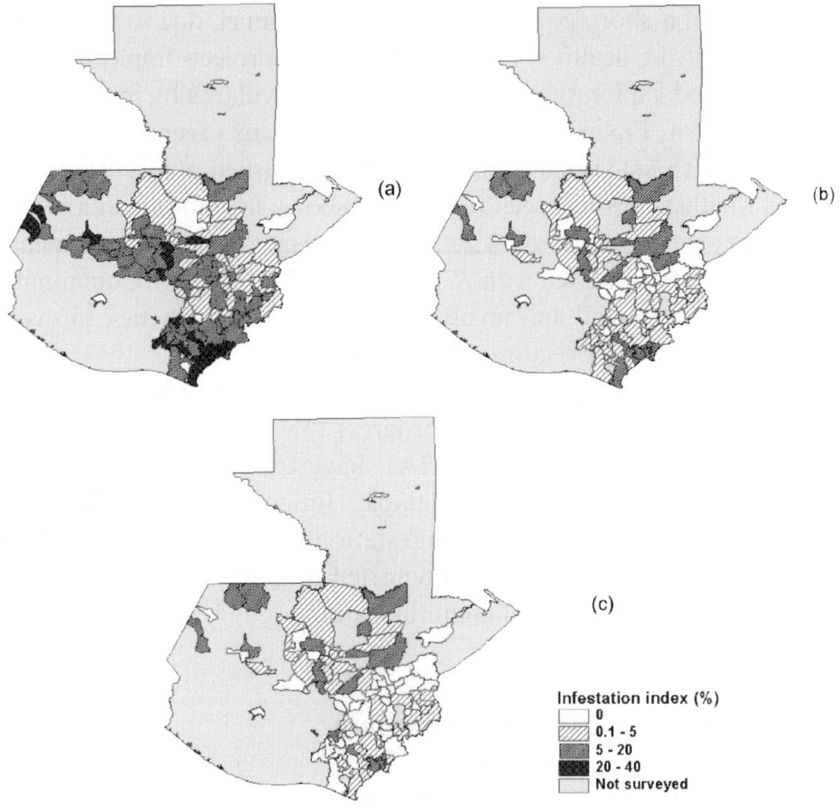

Figure 3 Difference in the house infestation rate (%) of *Tri. dimidiata* before (a) and after two rounds (b and c) of insecticide spraying in Guatemala. The figure shows the house infestation at the municipality level. (Data from Ministerio de Salud Publica y Asistencia Técnica, courtesy of H. Alvarez and K. Hashimoto.)

by 97% (from 5.3% to 0.5%), and by 75% (from 36% to 8.9%) in Jutiapa after the first round of spraying (Nakagawa *et al.*, 2003a, b). The second round of the spraying reduced the infestation rate to zero in Zacapa and 4.1% in Jutiapa (MSPAS, unpublished information).

Post-intervention surveillance together with additional spraying in Jutiapa demonstrated a general reduction of *Tri. dimidiata* infestation, as well as highlighting areas with persistent post-spraying infestation (Figure 4). In Jutiapa, where the initial infestation level was the highest in Guatemala, villages with initially high infestation rates were

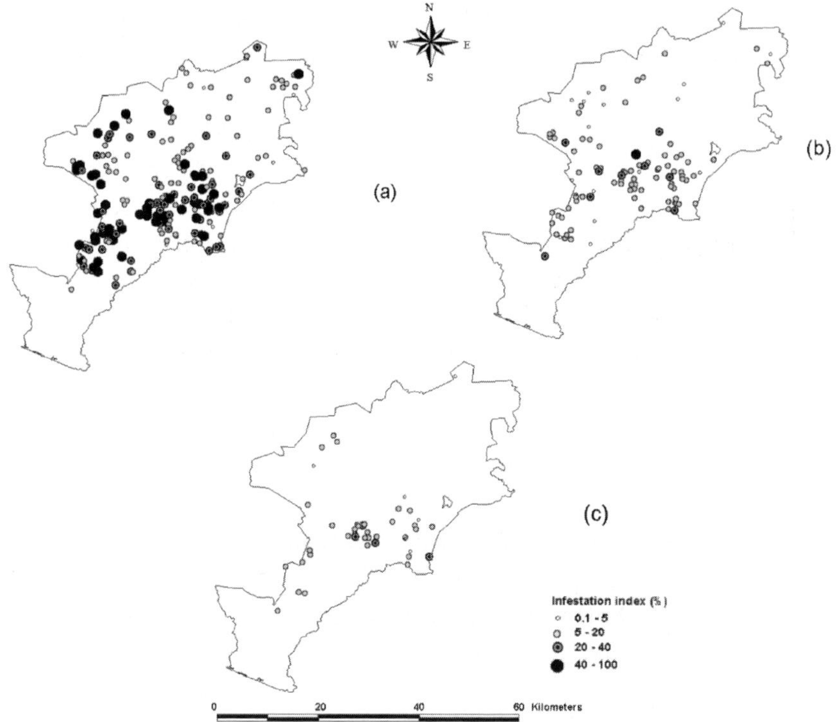

Figure 4 Change in the house infestation rate (%) of *Tri. dimidiata* in the department of Jutiapa in Guatemala before (a) and after two rounds (b and c) of insecticide spraying. Black circles indicate villages with infestation rates of 40–100%; dark gray, 20–40%; light gray, 5–12%; and open circles, 0.1–5%. (Data from Ministerio de Salud Publica y Asistencia Técnica, courtesy of R. Trampe and K. Hashimoto.)

more persistent than other villages, requiring three rounds of spraying. Infestation rates in the villages sprayed three times was reduced by 90%, reaching an average infestation of 4.1% (range 0–25%). The infestation rates in the villages receiving a single spraying remained less than 5% between 12 and 33 months, except for 26 villages with rates as high as 55%. These villages were those adjacent to the villages with the highest pre-intervention levels of infestation, suggesting the need for geographical clustering of the number of spray rounds. More than 70% of the positive houses were colonized by nymphs, which were more often observed in domestic than peridomestic sites, indicating that some indoor bugs survived the spray round (MSPAS, unpublished information; Nakagawa *et al.*, 2003b). Although the check-and-spray method was effective in reducing the infestation to the initial target of less than 5%, the operational cost was high.

Implementation of community-based surveillance was crucial to detect infestation of *Tri. dimidiata*. In agreement with the experience of INCOSUR, community-detection of infestation was better than that by vector control personnel when the infestation level was low (Wanderley, 1991). Schoolchildren in Guatemala demonstrated their capacity to detect and kill the bugs, or to report them to their school (Hashimoto *et al.*, 2005a). The trial of community-based surveillance in Guatemala and Honduras involved the local health systems, community leaders, NGOs, and schools. The communities were encouraged to report infestations, to improve houses, and to clean peridomestic areas. However, the number of reports of infestation from infested communities dropped quickly in the absence of a proper response by the local health unit (Suzuki, personal communication).

Other Central American countries started control activities against *Tri. dimidiata*, though their geographic coverage was limited. Western departments in El Salvador (Santa Ana, Ahuachapán, and Sonsonate) and Honduras (Copán and Choluteca) started residual spraying activities against *Tri. dimidiata* in 2004. Nicaragua's current focus is the elimination of *R. prolixus*, and the control of *Tri. dimidiata* is in the planning stages.

3.5. Organization and Management

Organization and management of the vector control campaigns are complicated in a decentralized health system, despite chemical control of triatomine bugs being technically straightforward. The current challenge of INCOSUR is the maintenance of integrity and quality of the national programmes during the irreversible trend of decentralization (Schofield and Dias, 1999), which also applies to IPCA. When IPCA was launched in 1997, the vertical organization and skilled personnel for vector control had almost disappeared from Central America. The process of this fragmentation of the vector control programme had been most advanced in Honduras, followed by El Salvador and, to a lesser degree, by Guatemala. In all three cases, no single organization was ready to undertake, by itself, large-scale vector control.

JICA's technical cooperation programme aimed at bridging the fragmented organizational resources in each country (Figure 5).

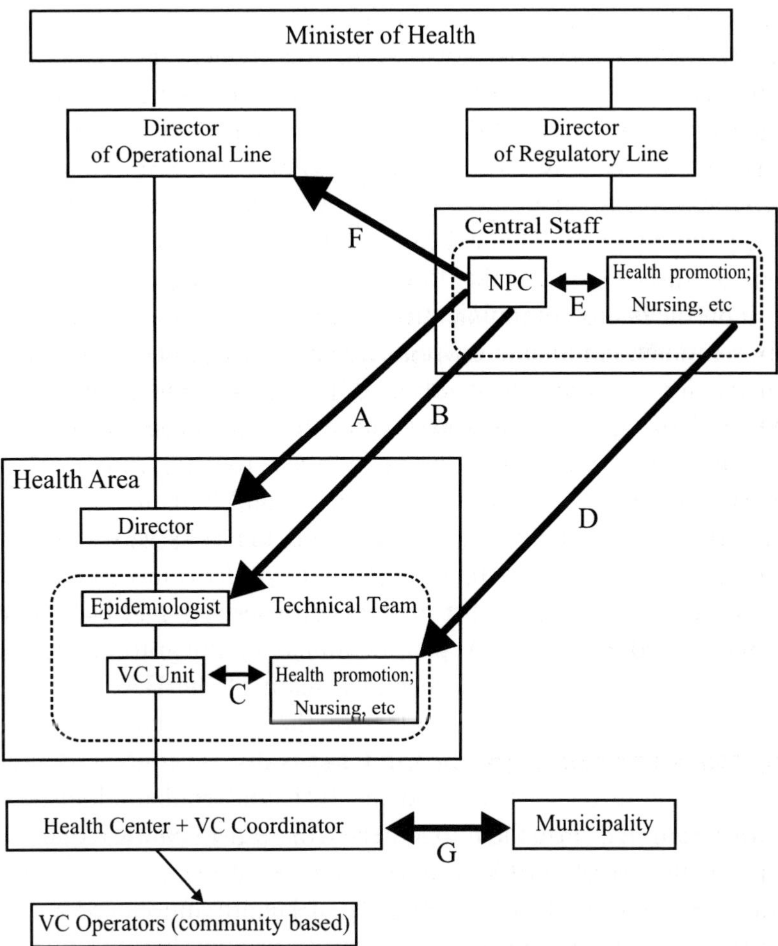

Figure 5 Organizational chart showing collaboration for the attack phase of the control of Chagas disease in Central America. Arrow A shows policy advice; B and D, technical guidance; C and E, technical collaboration within the health sector; and F, reporting from the central staff of the regulatory line to the operational line. The alphabetical order roughly follows the history of the projects supported by JICA: Guatemala 2000 (A, B); El Salvador 2004 (C); Guatemala 2004 (D, E, F); and Honduras 2004 (G).

Although this strategy was consistent with all the JICA-supported projects, the tactics varied by country in response to different processes and stages of decentralization. In Guatemala in 2000, local vector control units had not been fully integrated into HAs (normally equivalent to departments). Direct contact between the National Program of Chagas disease control (NPC) and the HAs was difficult because the latter differed not only by hierarchical level (central vs. local) but also by line of command (regulatory vs. operational). JICA sent from Japan a long-term consultant to the NPC and four volunteers to the HAs to facilitate technical and political dialogue between them (diagonal arrows A and B of Figure 5, respectively). As a part of the NPC, the Medical Entomology Section reinforced its traditional authority over the local vector control personnel. Some common means of communication included supervisory visits, quarterly seminars, comments on reports, and daily phone calls and fax transmissions (Yamagata *et al.*, 2003). A Geographic Information System (GIS) approach was introduced for the purpose of monitoring, but also proved to be a useful political tool for convincing the Ministry of Health to invest in insecticides and human resources for spraying. Bridging between the NPC and the HAs was crucial for acceleration of the attack phase against *R. prolixus* in Guatemala.

In El Salvador, where most of the health services had been decentralized by 2003, the JICA project aimed at integrating the local vector control units into the technical team of the HA. The epidemiologist and the health promoters of the HA, in particular, were expected to play important roles in Chagas disease control. A vector control training course was held in 2004, and epidemiologists and health promoters attended together with vector control operators (horizontal arrow C of Figure 5).

In Guatemala in 2004, the Ministry of Health announced a policy of rapid decentralization. By that time, *R. prolixus* had virtually disappeared from the country except for the department of Chiquimula, and the local vector control units had been integrated into HAs. However, involvement of different health specialists at the local level into Chagas disease control was possible only with central authorization of each speciality (diagonal arrow D, Figure 5). In order to do so, the NPC had to brief the relevant central staff (horizontal arrow

E, Figure 5) as well as the director responsible for operations (upward diagonal arrow F, Figure 5).

In Honduras, Environmental Health Technicians (TSAs), the former vector control operators, had been overloaded with additional tasks such as safe water supply, sanitation, and rabies control. In addition, they were inadequately staffed to conduct operations themselves. A variety of stakeholders, such as municipalities and communities, had been involved to fill the shortage of health personnel and finance (horizontal arrow G, Figure 5). Community-based operators conducted insecticide spraying with technical and logistic support from the HA and NGOs such as MSF and World Vision. NPC played a larger role in coordination and resource management than in operations. GIS was utilized for bridging between endemic municipalities and external partners, particularly international NGOs and donor countries such as Canada. Some local government authorities started to take responsibility for vector control operations. NPC paid special attention to avoiding the fragmentation of areas to be treated.

4. CHALLENGES IN CENTRAL AMERICA

The collaboration between IPCA and the decentralized health system has revealed new challenges. While the elimination of *R. prolixus* in Central America will be attainable in the near future, the control of *Tri. dimidiata* remains a difficult task. The key challenges lie in efficient geographic coverage and sustainability. Central American countries require control activity that will produce maximum results with minimum investment. In addition, attaining sustainability is important to permit long-term maintenance.

4.1. Efficient Geographic Coverage of *Triatoma dimidiata* Control

Stratification of high-risk areas, according to the precontrol infestation level, is crucial to cover extensive geographic areas efficiently. *Tri. dimidiata* appears to form several foci with high infestation rates in south-eastern Guatemala (departments of Santa Rosa and Jutiapa), western El Salvador (departments of Santa Ana, Ahuachapán, Sonsonate, and La Libertad) and south-western Honduras (departments of Copán and Ocotepeque). These foci should be sprayed two to three times in the attack phase, followed by an intensive maintenance phase, which includes housing improvement. Cross-border assessment of the distribution of *Tri. dimidiata* foci is necessary, together with analysis of the relationship between the initial infestation rates and the number of spray rounds required. In departments where the precontrol level of infestation and colonization were particularly low, such as Alta Verapaz in north-central Guatemala, the focus needs to be on surveillance rather than control (Nakagawa *et al.*, 2005). Ecological niche modelling, which demonstrated high predictive accuracy in defining the geographic distribution of *Tri. brasiliensis* and *Tri. barberi* (Townsend Peterson *et al.*, 2002; Costa *et al.*, 2002), would also be useful in limiting and stratifying target areas for the control of *Tri. dimidiata*.

Determination of the minimum resource requirement is vital for the efficient control of *Tri. dimidiata*. Unlike the elimination strategy, the control strategy has no clear endpoint. Elimination of vectorial transmission of *T. cruzi* may be a possible goal; however, the level of infestation corresponding to that goal is not yet known. The tentative operational target, an infestation rate lower than 5%, may be too expensive for countries with decentralized health systems, such as Honduras. Where the vector is *Tri. dimidiata*, which has a low vectorial capacity, an infestation higher than 5% may be acceptable, as was the case with *Tri. brasiliensis* in north-east Brazil, where the critical infestation rate was 20% (C.J. Schofield, personal communication). In order to establish the acceptable level of domestic infestation, a combination of vector control, chemotherapy, and subsequent serological survey could be applied to the *Tri. dimidiata*-infested areas, as has been done in *R. prolixus*-infested areas of Honduras.

Efficient geographic coverage also requires affordable vector-surveillance methods with active participation by municipalities and communities, in order to cover the infested area. Development of alternative indices can lessen the financial burden for a decentralized health administration. Existing entomological indices require trained vector personnel to conduct standard survey methods (person–hour survey) and data analysis, which is difficult in a subnational decentralized health administration with poor resources. Community-based surveillance is an alternative method, although the data may not be as quantitative or reliable as the person–hour survey. Organizing periodic "National triatomine-hunting campaigns" to encourage residents to capture triatomines can create fairly uniform hunting pressure over a large geographic area, and can provide quantitative data such as the number of bugs captured per community, municipality, and department. Such data can be useful in making operational decisions and monitoring the level of infestation.

Improvement of the effectiveness of residual spraying must complement efficient geographic coverage for the best results. Combined quality control and community mobilization can assure the effectiveness of residual spraying against *Tri. dimidiata*. Three annual spraying rounds in Jutiapa resulted in fair, but not complete, reduction of *Tri. dimidiata*. Quality control of the spraying is valuable in order to improve the penetration of triatomine habitats such as deep crevices in the walls, particularly when community-based operators are involved. This quality control alone, however, does not guarantee adequate spraying coverage in all the target houses which have abundant habitats for the vector. Community mobilization in improving housing conditions can complement residual spraying by reducing hiding places for the vector, such as piles of clothing, stacks of mud bricks, and firewood.

Information management and networking is strategically vital to tackle these challenges. For efficient and effective control of *Tri. dimidiata*, information such as GIS analysis of entomological and epidemiological data, cross-border studies of vector distribution, cost-effectiveness analysis of the control activity, and effectiveness of community-based surveillance, should be accumulated and properly managed at national as well as regional (Central American) levels. This information should also be shared with all the stakeholders. Regional networks of scientists such as ECLAT, Chagas Disease Intervention Activities (CDIA-EU), and research-funding programmes such as the Special Program for Research and Training in Tropical Diseases (TDR) should play an increasing role in identifying operational research needs, linking the needs and research institutions with expertise, and accumulating a knowledge base. International organizations can also facilitate information management and technical standardization by networking stakeholders and providing funding. Information management at different administrative levels is discussed further in the following section.

4.2. Sustainable Vector Control via Integration of the Maintenance Phase

The control of *Tri. dimidiata* needs further integration into the general local administration, because it will be a long-term process involving most departments and municipalities in Central America. NPC and HAs have to lead such integration via technology transfer, information sharing, and mobilization of financial resources.

Figure 6 shows a hypothetical model of decentralization and integration of the maintenance phase of Chagas disease vector control. Technology (T) for vector survey and control, including planning, monitoring, and housing improvement, is transferred gradually from central NPC (top left) to municipal administration or the community (bottom right). Reciprocally, the data (D) on the vector distribution and on the control performance are reported from bottom right to top left. The diagonal flows of T and D replace the classical lines of command and reporting in the vertical programme.

Some municipalities need financial support in addition to technology. Despite their limited financial capacity, NPC and HA can stimulate potential funding resources by providing the municipalities with the relevant information. As shown in Figure 6, the raw data (D) from the implementation level are processed by the NPC or the HA, and translated into information (I) relevant and attractive to the funding agencies. This information may include epidemiological data, an estimate of number of target houses for spraying, unit cost, and the benefit of successful operations. The funding agencies would eventually support the municipalities with funds for implementation (F). Possible financial resources include the development budget of the union of municipalities, the Poverty Reduction Fund, the National Fund for Social Investment, bank loans, and other development funds.

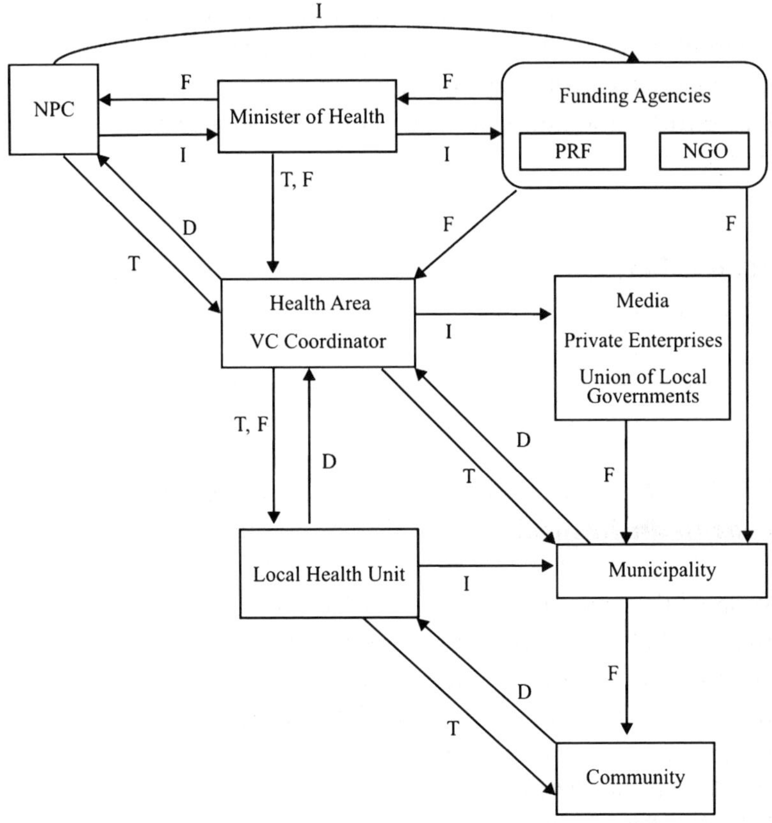

Figure 6   A hypothetical organizational chart for the maintenance phase of Chagas disease vector control. The figure comprises two basic movements: technology transfer (T) and triangular trade between data (D), information (I) and finance (F). (T) is decentralized to the local level (downward), and integrated to a more general organization (to the right). Data (D) are analysed at the more central and specific organization, and processed into information (I), which is essential for the mobilization of financial resources (F). NGO, Non-Governmental Organization; NPC, National Program of Chagas Disease Control; PRF, Poverty Reduction Fund.

In this context, the function of the NPC and the HA in the maintenance of vector control is more coordination rather than operation. The new functions of NPC and HA include: (i) transfer of appropriate vector control technologies to the local administration; (ii) translation of the data into relevant information; (iii) brokering of the information for fund raising; (iv) assurance of the quality of vector control; and (v) monitoring of the vector situation. GIS is useful for compilation of locally collected data as well as for negotiation with development partners to attract investment in vector control or housing improvement.

5. CHAGAS DISEASE CONTROL INITIATIVES IN OTHER REGIONS

Beside the Southern Cone and Central American regions, crucial areas in the control of Chagas disease are the Andean and Amazon regions and Mexico.

5.1. Andean Region

Colombia, Ecuador, Peru, and Venezuela launched the Andean Initiative in 1997, aiming at interrupting vectorial and transfusional transmission of *T. cruzi* (WHO, 1997a). The main triatomine species are *R. prolixus, R. ecuadoriensis, Tri. dimidiata,* and *Tri. infestans.* It is estimated that 25 million people are at risk and 5 million are infected (Moncayo, 2003).

Before this initiative, since the 1950s, Venezuela executed an impressive Chagas disease vector control programme combined with a strong rural housing project (Aché and Matos, 2001). The achievement of the programme was significant, reducing the house infestation rate in rural areas from 60–80% to 1.6–4.0% and seroprevalence from 44.5% to 9.2%, between 1958 and 1998 (Aché and Matos, 2001). However, the programme has been reduced since the 1980s due to financial constraints and decentralization of the health system (Dias and Schofield, 1999). The impact of the reduced level of activity has become evident in the recent reported increase in infestation rate and seroprevalence (Feliciangeli *et al.*, 2003). Apart from Venezuela, no Andean countries had previous experience in triatomine control; nevertheless the initiative made some progress. Ecuador launched a triatomine control campaign in 2004, targeting the elimination of *Tri. dimidiata* in western provinces (Guayas and Manabí) where the vector is exclusively domestic (Guhl, 2005). Baseline surveys have been implemented in Colombia and Ecuador, and Peru has made progress in the control of *Tri. infestans* (Schofield, 2003). Meetings of those taking part in the initiative are held annually to review progress and to plan future actions.

5.2. Amazon Region

The Amazon basin has more than 10 sylvatic triatomine species, but has been considered free from human Chagas disease. However, human cases of Chagas disease have been reported in the area recently, possibly as a result of increasing human migration and domestic invasion by sylvatic triatomines (Coura *et al.*, 2002). In order to prevent further spread of the disease, accurate detection of acute cases by microscopical examination of blood films (Coura *et al.*, 2002) and ecological surveillance combining epidemiological studies and remote sensing are necessary (Guhl and Schofield, 2004; Schofield, 2003).

Based on the increased need to control Chagas disease in this region, eight countries (Brazil, Colombia, Ecuador, French Guyana, Guyana, Peru, Surinam, and Venezuela) launched a regional initiative (Iniciativa de los países Amazónicos para la Vigilancia y Control de la Enfermedad de Chagas, AMCHA) in 2005. This initiative aims at establishing epidemiological surveillance systems as well as effective control methods that are suitable for this region (PAHO, 2005a). Regional meetings have been held since 2004, and delegates from these countries have developed strategic plans to implement this initiative.

5.3. Mexico

Despite the size of the population at risk and the widespread distribution of triatomines, the Mexican government has been reluctant to recognize Chagas disease as a serious health issue. In Mexico, 30 triatomine species have been reported, and over 1 million people are estimated to be infected with *T. cruzi* (Guzman-Bracho, 2001). A small population of *R. prolixus* has also been reported (Ramsey *et al.*, 2000). Mexican researchers have been active in the field, but few disease control measures have been taken until recently. In 2002, Mexico became a part of the regional effort to control Chagas disease by participating in the annual meetings of IPCA, and a large-scale campaign against Chagas disease is in the planning stages (Ramsey *et al.*, 2003).

6. CONCLUSION

Interruption of Chagas disease transmission in Central America by 2010, as proposed by IPCA, seems achievable, although the process of maintenance, especially with *Tri. dimidiata,* needs to be accelerated. The vector control technologies and strategy developed by INCOSUR were largely applicable to Central American conditions. There are, however, some Central American situations that challenge this vector control strategy: the rapid decentralization of the health system and residual and reinfesting populations of *Tri. dimidiata.* Regional and international cooperation is managing the challenge of decentralization by promoting integration of vector control into the local health system (attack phase) and into the local administration (maintenance phase). International organizations and bilateral donor agencies have worked to develop the capacity of NPC to include the new techniques of technology transfer, information management, and advocacy for financial resource mobilization.

The Central American experience of triatomine control could be useful for strengthening other regional initiatives. The Andean initiative needs to control indigenous species with limited resources, and INCOSUR is facing challenges to continue the maintenance phase against *Tri. infestans* with a decentralized health system and declining investment in Chagas disease control. Other national and regional programmes to control vector-borne disease, such as malaria and dengue fever, also have to maintain vector control in similar situations. Despite the differences in control technology and strategy, the experience with common challenges such as management of a vector-control programme in a decentralized health system can be shared among different programmes, which can help to improve effectiveness, efficiency, and sustainability.

ACKNOWLEDGEMENTS

This review was written as part of the regional effort to combat Chagas disease in the Americas in collaboration with stakeholders in Central and South American countries as well as with international organizations such as PAHO, JICA, ECLAT, CIDA, MSF, and World Vision. We thank the vector control teams of the Ministry of Health of Guatemala, El Salvador, Honduras, and other Central and South American countries for their pursuit of Chagas disease vector control. We also thank C. Cordon-Rosales, E. Gil, G. de Margerie, M. Kojima, K. Hashimoto, K. Mizuno, C. Monroy, C. Nakagawa, K. Ota, C. Ponce, E. Ponce, B. Singer, and C. Schofield for advice.

REFERENCES

Acevedo, F., Godoy, E. and Schofield, C.J. (2000). Comparison of intervention strategies for control of *Triatoma dimidiata* in Nicaragua. *Memorias do Instituto Oswaldo Cruz* **95**, 867–871.

Aché, A. and Matos, A.J. (2001). Interrupting Chagas disease transmission in Venezuela. *Revista do Instituto de Medicina Tropical de São Paulo* **1**, 37–43.

Akhavan, D. (2000). *Analise de Custo-efetividade do Programa de Controle da Doença de Chagas no Brasil*. Brasilia: Pan American Health Organization.

Basombrío, M A , Schofield, C.J., Rojas, C.L. and Del Rey, E.C. (1998). A cost-benefit analysis of Chagas disease control in north-western Argentina. *Transactions of the Royal Society of Tropical Medicine and Hygiene* **92**, 137–143.

Carcavallo, R., Curto de Casas, S.I., Sherlock, I.A., Giron, I.G., Jurberg, J., Galvao, C., Mena Segura, C.A. and Noireau, F. (1999). Geographical distribution and Alti-latitudinal dispersion. In: *Atlas of Chagas' Disease Vectors in the Americas* (R. Carcavallo, I.G. Giron, J. Jursberg and H.E. Lent, eds), Vol. III, pp. 747–792. Rio de Janeiro: Editora Fiocruz.

Cedillos, R.A. (1975). Chagas' disease in El Salvador. *Bulletin of Pan American Health Organization* **9**, 135–141.

Costa, J., Townsend Peterson, A. and Ben Beard, G. (2002). Ecologic niche modeling and differentiation of populations of *Triatoma brasiliensis* Neiva, 1991, the most important Chagas' disease vector in northeastern Brazil (Hemiptera, Reduviidae, Triatominae). *American Journal of Tropical Medicine and Hygiene* **67**, 516–520.

Coura, J.R., Junqueira, A.C., Fernandes, O., Valente, S.A. and Miles, M.A. (2002). Emerging Chagas disease in Amazonian Brazil. *Trends in Parasitology* **18**, 171–176.

Dias, E. (1952). Doenças de Chagas nas Américas III. Américas Central. *Revista Brasileira de Malariologia e Doenças Tropicais* **4**, 75–84.

Dias, J.C. (1987). Control of Chagas disease in Brazil. *Parasitology Today* **3**, 336–341.

Dias, J.C. (1988). Controle de vetores de doença de Chagas no Brasil e riscos de reinfestação domiciliária por vetores secundários. *Memoria do Instituto Oswaldo Cruz* **83**(supplement 1), 387–391.

Dias, J.C. (1991). Chagas disease control in Brazil: which strategy after the attack phase? *Annales de Societe Belge de Medicine Tropicale* **71**(supplement 1), 75–86.

Dias, J.C. and Schofield, C.J. (1999). The evolution of Chagas disease (American trypanosomiasis) control after 90 years since Carlos Chagas discovery. *Memoria do Instituto Oswaldo Cruz* **94**(supplement 1), 103–121.

Dias, J.C., Silveira, A.C. and Schofield, C.J. (2002). The impact of Chagas disease control in Latin America: a review. *Memoria do Instituto Oswaldo Cruz* **97**, 603–612.

Dujardin, J.P., Munoz, M., Chavez, T., Ponce, C., Moreno, J. and Schofield, C.J. (1998). The origin of *Rhodnius prolixus* in Central America. *Medical and Veterinary Entomology* **12**, 113–115.

Feliciangeli, M.D., Campbell-Lendrum, D., Martinez, C., Gonzalez, D., Coleman, P. and Davies, C. (2003). Chagas disease control in Venezuela: lessons for the Andean region and beyond. *Trends in Parasitology* **19**, 44–49.

Guhl, F. (2005). *Memoria del Primer Taller Internacional sobre Control de la Enfermedad de Chagas*. Bogota: Universidad de Los Andes.

Guhl, F. and Schofield, D.J. (2004). *Proceedings of the ECLAT-AMCHA International Workshop on Chagas Disease Surveillance in the Amazon Region, Palmari, Brazil*. Bogota: Universidad de Los Andes.

Guzman-Bracho, C. (2001). Epidemiology of Chagas disease in Mexico: an update. *Trends in Parasitology* **17**, 372–376.

Hashimoto, K., Kojima, M., Nakagawa, J. and Yamagata, Y. (2005). Effectiveness of health education through primary school teachers. *Technology and Development* **18**, 71–76.

Hayes, R.J. and Schofield, C.J. (1990). Estimación de las tasas de incidencia de infecciones y parasitosis crónicas a partir de la prevalecía: la enfermedad de Chagas en América Latina. *Boletín de la Oficina Sanitaria Panamericana* **108**, 308–316.

Liese, B., Sachdeva, P.S. and Glynn Cochrane, D. (1991). *Organizing and Managing Tropical Disease Control Programs. Lessons of Success*. Washington, DC: World Bank.

Miller, J. (1931). Chagas disease in Panama: report of three cases. *Southern Medical Journal* **24**, 645–647.

MINSA. (2003). *Informe para la Misión de Evaluación OPS/OMS*. Managua: Ministerio de Salúd, Republica de Nicaragua.

Molyneux, D.H. and Morel, C. (1998). Oncocerciasis and Chagas' disease control: the evolution of control via applied research through changing development scenarios. *British Medical Bulletin* **54**, 327–339.

Moncayo, A. (2003). Chagas disease: current epidemiological trends after the interruption of vectorial and transfusional transmission in the Southern Cone countries. *Memoria do Instituto Oswaldo Cruz* **98**, 577–591.

Monroy, C., Mejia, M., Rodas, A., Hashimoto, T. and Tabaru, Y. (1998a). Assessing methods for the density of *Triatoma dimidiata*, the principal vector of Chagas' disease in Guatemala. *Medical Entomology and Zoology* **49**, 301–307.

Monroy, C., Mejia, M., Rodas, A., Rosales, R., Horio, M. and Tabaru, Y. (1998b). Comparison of indoor searches with whole house demolition collections of the vectors of Chagas disease and their indoor distribution. *Medical Entomology and Zoology* **49**, 195–200.

Morel, C.M. (1999). Chagas disease, from discovery to control – and beyond: history, myths and lessons to take home. *Memoria do Instituto Oswaldo Cruz* **94**(supplement 1), 3–16.

MSPAS. (2002). *Programa de Prevención y Control de la Enfermedad de Chagas: Informe para Misión de Evaluación OPS/OMS*. Guatemala City: Ministerio de Salud Publica y Asistencia Social de Guatemala.

Nakagawa, J., Cordon-Rosales, C., Juarez, J., Itzep, C. and Nonami, T. (2003a). Impact of residual spraying on *Rhodnius prolixus* and *Triatoma dimidiata* in the department of Zacapa in Guatemala. *Memoria do Instituto Oswaldo Cruz* **98**, 277–281.

Nakagawa, J., Hashimoto, K., Cordon-Rosales, C., Abraham Juarez, J., Trampe, R. and Marroquin, L.M. (2003b). The impact of vector control on *Triatoma dimidiata* in the Guatemalan department of Jutiapa. *Annals of Tropical Medicine and Parasitology* **97**, 288–297.

Nakagawa, J., Juárez, J., Nakatsuji, K., Akiyama, T., Hernández, G., Macal, R., Flores, C., Ortiz, M., Marroquín, L., Banba, T. and Wakai, S. (2005). Geographic characterization of triatomine infestation in north-central Guatemala. *Annals of Tropical Medicine and Parasitology* **99**, 1–9.

Oliveira Filho, A. (1997). Uso de nuevas herramientas para el control de triatominos en diferentes situaciones entomológicas en el continente americano. *Revista da Sociedade Brasileira de Medicina Tropical* **30**, 41–46.

PAHO. (1993). *Iniciativa del Cono Sur*. Washington, DC: Pan American Health Organization document no. PNSP/92-18. rev.1.

PAHO. (1998). *Iniciativa de Salud del Cono Sur. VIIa. Reunión de la Comisión Intergubernamental para la Eliminación de Triatoma infestans y la Interrupción de la Tripanosomiasis americana por Transfusión.* Washington, DC: Pan American Health Organization document no. OPS/HCP/HCT/114.98.

PAHO. (1999a). *Iniciativa de Salud del Cono Sur. VIIIa. Reunión de la Comisión Intergubernamental para la Eliminación de Triatoma infestans y la Interrupción de la Tripanosomiasis americana por Transfusión.* Washington, DC: Pan American Health Organization document no. OPS/HCP/HCT/151.99.

PAHO. (1999b). *Primera Reunión de la Comisión Intergubernamental de la Iniciativa de Centroamérica y Belice para la interrupción de la Transmisión Vectorial de la Enfermedad de Chagas por Rhodnius prolixus, Disminución de la Ingestación Domiciliar por Triatoma dimidiata.* Washington, DC: Pan American Health Organization document no. OPS/HCP/HCT/145/99.

PAHO. (2000a). *Iniciativa de Salud del Cono Sur. IXa. Reunión de la Comisión Intergubernamental para la Eliminación de Triatoma infestans y la Interrupción de la Tripanosomiasis americana por Transfusión.* Washington, DC: Pan American Health Organization document no. OPS/HCP/HCT/175.00.

PAHO. (2000b). *Segunda Reunión de la Comisión Intergubernamental de la Iniciativa de Centroamérica y Belice para la Interrupción de la Transmisión Vectorial de la Enfermedad de Chagas por Rhodnius prolixus, Disminución de la Infestación Domiciliar por Triatoma dimidiata.* Washington, DC: Pan American Health Organization document no. OPS/HCP/HCT/164/00.

PAHO (2002a). *El Control de la Enfermedad de Chagas en los Países el CONOSUR de América: Historia de Una Iniciativa Internacional 1991/2001* (online). Available at: http://www.paho.org/Spanish/AD/DPC/CD/dch-historia-incosur.pdf.

PAHO. (2002b). *Iniciativa de Salud del Cono Sur. XIa. Reunión de la Comisión Intergubernamental para la Eliminación de Triatoma infestans y la Interrupción de la Tripanosomiasis americana por Transfusión.* Washington, DC: Pan American Health Organization document no. OPS/HCP/HCT/216/02.

PAHO. (2002c). *Taller para el Establecimiento de Pautas Técnicas en el Control de Triatoma dimidiata.* Washington, DC: Pan American Health Organization document no. OPS/HCP/HCT/214/02.

PAHO. (2003a). *Iniciativa de Salud del Cono Sur. XIIa. Reunión de la Comisión Intergubernamental para la Eliminación de Triatoma infestans y la Interrupción de la Tripanosomiasis americana por Transfusión.* Washington, DC: Pan American Health Organization document no. OPS/DPC/CD/270/03.

PAHO. (2003b). *Quinta Reunión de la Comisión Intergubernamental de la Iniciativa de los Países de Centro América, para la Interrupción de la Transmisión Vectorial y Transfusión de la Enfermedad del Chagas.* Washington, DC: Pan American Health Organization document no. OPS/HCP/HCT/235/03.

PAHO. (2003c). *Reunión Internacional para el Establecimiento de Criterios de Certificación de la Eliminación de Rhodius prolixus (Stahl, 1859).* Washington, DC: Pan American Health Organization document no. OPS/DPC/CD/245/03.

PAHO. (2004). *Sexta Reunión de la Comisión Intergubernamental de la Iniciativa de los Países de Centro América, para la Interrupción de la Transmisión Vectorial y Transfusional de la Enfermedad de Chagas.* Washington, DC: Pan American Health Organization document no. OPS/DPC/CD/282/04.

PAHO. (2005a). *International Meeting on Surveillance and Prevention of Chagas Disease in the Amazon Region.* Washington, DC: Pan American Health Organization document no. OPS/DPC/CD/321/05.

PAHO. (2005b). *Septima reunión de la comisión intergubernamental de la iniciativa de los países de Centro América, para la interrupción de la transmisión vectorial y transfusional de la enfermedad de Chagas.* Washington, D.C.: Pan American Health Organization document no. OPS/DPC/CD/345/05.

Paz-Bailey, G., Monroy, C., Rodas, A., Rosales, R., Tabaru, R., Davies, C. and Lines, J. (2002). Incidence of *Trypanosoma cruzi* infection in two Guatemalan communities. *Transactions of the Royal Society of Tropical Medicine and Hygiene* **96**, 48–52.

Ponce, C. (1995). La Enfermedad de Chagas en Centroamérica. *The International Workshop on Population Genetics and Control of Triatominae, Santo Domingo de los Colorados – 40.* Mexico City: INDRE.

Ponce, C. (1999). La enfermedad de Chagas transfusional en Honduras y otros países de américa central. *Medicina (Buenos Aires)* **59**(supplement II), 135–137.

Ponce, C., Ponce, E., Flores, M. and Avila, G. (1993). Intervention trials of new tools to control transmission of Chagas disease in Honduras. *Memoria do Instituto Oswaldo Cruz* **12**(supplement), 57.

Ponce, C. and Zeledón, R. (1973). Chagas disease in Honduras. *Bulletin of the Pan American Health Organization* **75**, 239–248.

Ramsey, J., Lopez, A.T. and Pohls, J.L., eds. (2003). *Iniciativa para la Vigilancia y el Control de la Enfermedad de Chagas en la Republica Mexicana.* Cuernavaca: Instituto Nacional de Salud Publica.

Ramsey, J., Ordóñez, R., Cruz-Celis, A., Alvear, A.L., Chávez, V., López, R., Pintor, J.R., Gama, F. and Carrillo, S. (2000). Distribution of domestic triatominae and stratification of Chagas disease transmission in Oaxaca, Mexico. *Medical and Veterinary Entomology* **14**, 19–30.

Reichenow, E. (1933). *Sobre la Existencia de la Enfermedad de Chagas en Guatemala*. Guatemala City: Dirección de Sanidad Publica.

Rizzo, N.R., Arana, B.A., Diaz, A., Cordon-Rosales, C., Klein, R.E. and Powell, M.R. (2003). Seroprevalence of *Trypanosoma cruzi* infection among school-age children in the endemic area of Guatemala. *American Journal of Tropical Medicine and Hygiene* **68**, 678–682.

Schmunis, G.A. and Dias, J.C. (2000). Health care reform, decentralization, prevention and control of vector-borne diseases. *Cadernos de Saude Publica* **16**(supplement 2), 117–123.

Schmunis, G.A., Zicker, F. and Moncayo, A. (1996). Interruption of Chagas' disease transmission through vector elimination. *Lancet* **348**, 1171.

Schofield, C. J. (2000). *Challenge of Chagas Disease Vector Control in Central America*. World Health Organization, document no. WHO/CDS/WHOPES/GCDPP/2000.1.

Schofield, C. J. (2001). *Field Testing and Evaluation of Insecticides for Indoor Residual Spraying against Domestic Vectors of Chagas Disease*. World Health Organization, document no. WHO/CDS/WHOPES/GCDPP/2000.1.

Schofield, C.J. (2003). Regional initiatives against Chagas disease vectors in Latin America. In: *Iniciativa para la Vigilancia y el Control de la Enfermedad de Chagas* (J. Ramsey, A.T. Lopez and J.L. Phols, eds), pp. 67–75. Cuernavaca: Instituto Nacional de Salud Publica.

Schofield, C.J. and Dias, J.C. (1991). A cost-benefit analysis of Chagas disease control. *Memoria do Instituto Oswaldo Cruz* **86**, 285–295.

Schofield, C.J. and Dias, J.C. (1999). The Southern Cone Initiative against Chagas disease. *Advances in Parasitology* **42**, 1–27.

Schofield, C.J. and Dujardin, J.P. (1997). Chagas disease vector control in Central America. *Parasitology Today* **13**, 141–144.

Schofield, C.J., Dujardin, J.P. and Jurberg, J. (1996). *Proceedings of the International Workshop on Population Genetics and Control of Triatominae, Santo Domingo de los Colorados, Ecuador*. Mexico City: INDRE.

Segovia, J. (1913). Un caso de tripanosomiasis. *Archivo de Hospital Rosales (San Salvador)* **8**, 249–254, quoted by Cedillos, R.A. (1975). Chagas disease in El Salvador. *Bulletin of Pan American Health Organization* **9**, 135–141.

Silveira, A. and Vinhaes, M. (1999). Elimination of vector-borne transmission of Chagas disease. *Memorias do Instituto Ostwaldo Cruz* **94**(Suppl.), 405–411.

Sousa, O. and Johnson, M. (1971). Frequency and distribution of *Trypanosoma cruzi* and *Trypanosoma rangeli* in the republic of Panama. *American Journal of Tropical Medicine and Hygiene* **20**, 405–410.

Tabaru, Y., Monroy, C., Rodas, A., Mejia, M. and Rosales, R. (1998). Chemical control of *Triatoma dimidiata* and *Rhodnius prolixus*

(Reduviidae: Triatominae), the principal vector of Chagas' disease in Guatemala. *Medical Entomology and Zoology* **49**, 87–92.

Tabaru, Y., Monroy, C., Rodas, A., Mejia, M. and Rosales, R. (1999). The geographical distribution of vectors of Chagas' disease and population at risk of infection in Guatemala. *Medical Entomology and Zoology* **50**, 9–17.

Townsend Peterson, A., Sánchez-Cordero, V., Ben Beard, C. and Ramsey, J. (2002). Ecologic niche modeling and potential reservoirs for Chagas disease, Mexico. *Emerging Infectious Disease* **8**, 662–667.

Von Bullow, T. (1941). *Tripanosomiasis americana. Revista Medicina de Costa Rica* 4, 497–520, quoted by Zeledón, R., Solano, G., Burstin, L. and Swartzwelder, J.C. (1975). Epidemiological pattern of Chagas' disease in an endemic area of Costa Rica. *American Journal of Tropical Medicine and Hygiene* **24**, 214–225.

Wanderley, D.M. (1991). Vigilância entomológica da doença de Chagas no Estado de São Paulo. *Revista de Saúde Publica* **25**, 28–32.

WHO. (1991). *Control of Chagas Disease. First Report of the WHO Expert Committee*. Geneva: World Health Organization.

WHO. (1997a). Andean countries initiative launched in Colombia. *TDR News* **53**, 3.

WHO. (1997b). Chagas disease. Interruption of transmission. *Weekly Epidemiological Record* **72**, 1–5.

WHO. (1998a). Chagas disease: Central American initiative launched. *TDR News* **55**, 6.

WHO (1998b). *51st World Health Assembly*, Resolution WHA 51.14.

WHO. (2002). *Control of Chagas Disease. Second Report of the WHO Expert Committee*. Geneva: World Health Organization.

World Bank. (1993). *World Development Report 1993*. New York: Oxford University Press.

Yamagata, Y., Nakagawa, J., Shimoda, M. and Tabaru, Y. (2003). Management of infectious disease control in a decentralized organization: the case of the Japan-Guatemala Project for Chagas' disease control in Guatemala. *Technology and Development* **16**, 47–54.

Zeledón, R. (1981). *El Triatoma dimidiata (Latreille, 1811) y su Relación con la Enfermedad de Chagas*. San Jose, Costa Rica: Editora Universidad Estatal a Distancia.

Zeledón, R., Solano, G., Burstin, L. and Swartzwelder, J.C. (1975). Epidemiological pattern of Chagas' disease in an endemic area of Costa Rica. *American Journal of Tropical Medicine and Hygiene* **24**, 214–225.

Zerba, E. (1999). *Past and Present of Chagas Vector Control and Future Needs*. World Health Organization, document no. WHO/CDS/WHOPES/GCDPP/99.1.

Human African Trypanosomiasis: Epidemiology and Control

E.M. Fèvre[1], K. Picozzi[1], J. Jannin[2], S.C. Welburn[1] and I. Maudlin[1]

[1]*Centre for Infectious Diseases, Royal (Dick) School of Veterinary Studies, University of Edinburgh, Easter Bush, Roslin, Midlothian, EH25 9RG, UK*
[2]*World Health Organization, 20 Avenue Appia, CH-1211 Geneva 27, Switzerland*

ADVANCES IN PARASITOLOGY VOL 61
ISSN: 0065-308X
DOI: 10.1016/S0065-308X(05)61005-6

ABSTRACT

Human African trypanosomiasis (HAT), or sleeping sickness, describes not one but two discrete diseases: that caused by *Trypanosoma brucei rhodesiense* and that caused by *T. b. gambiense*. The Gambian form is currently a major public health problem over vast areas of central and western Africa, while the zoonotic, Rhodesian form continues to present a serious health risk in eastern and southern Africa. The two parasites cause distinct clinical manifestations, and there are significant differences in the epidemiology of the diseases caused. We discuss the differences between the diseases caused by the two parasites, with an emphasis on disease burden, reservoir hosts, transmission, diagnosis, treatment and control. We analyse how these differences impacted on historical disease control trends and how they can inform contemporary treatment and control options. We consider the optimal ways in which to devise HAT control policies in light of the differing biology and epidemiology of the parasites, and emphasise, in particular, the wider aspects of control policy, outlining the responsibilities of individuals, governments and international organisations in control programmes.

1. INTRODUCTION

Human African trypanosomiasis (HAT), or sleeping sickness, is a parasitic disease transmitted by tsetse flies of the genus *Glossina*, and caused by a group of parasites called trypanosomes. There are three sub-species of *Trypanosoma brucei*, the protozoan causative organism of HAT: *T. b. brucei*, *T. b. gambiense* and *T. b. rhodesiense*. All of these species infect mammals, but only *T. b. gambiense* and *T. b. rhodesiense* infect and cause clinical disease in humans. While infection with either *T. b. rhodesiense* or *T. b. gambiense* is termed HAT or sleeping sickness, the clinical features of the infections, the treatment protocols used, the geographical range of the parasites, and the epidemiology and transmission and the control options that are available, differ. Thus, each form of HAT is, in effect, a separate disease entity. In this review, these differences will be highlighted, and the clinical and epidemiological characteristics of infection with both parasites will be discussed. Policy options for HAT control depend for their success on a sound understanding of basic disease characteristics, and policy should thus be formulated with disease-specific conditions in mind. Recently, Pépin and Méda (2001) reviewed the epidemiology of gambiense HAT. While we will, of necessity, cover some of the basic aspects of the epidemiology of the gambiense disease here, we refer the reader to that excellent review for full coverage of the gambiense form of the disease. We will, however, cover important policy issues for both rhodesiense and gambiense HAT.

T. b. rhodesiense causes an acute infection in humans, the condition of the patient deteriorating rapidly as the parasite moves from the blood and lymphatic systems (early stage infection) through to the central nervous system (CNS). When parasites cross the blood–brain barrier and enter the CNS, the patient is said to be in the meningo-encephalitic, or late stage of infection. The pathology resulting from infection with the parasite is described in detail by Kristensson and Bentivoglio (1999). Briefly, initial infection results in a chancre at the site of inoculation by the tsetse fly; the chancre, well illustrated by Moore *et al.* (2002), is a localised immune response resulting in inflammation. Parasites then move to the lymph nodes and are disseminated in the circulatory system, multiplying in both the blood and lymph. Following invasion of the CNS, inflammation of the brain tissue occurs (meningo-encephalitis), as well as cellular infiltration of spinal nerve tissue and inflammation of visceral organs. In the absence of treatment, death usually occurs within 6–8 months (Apted, 1970; Odiit *et al.*, 1997), though there is evidence of geographic variation in the speed at which *T. b. rhodesiense* infections progress to the late stage (MacLean *et al.*, 2004)—differences that may be due to either variation in parasite genotypes or host responses to infection. *T. b. gambiense*, by contrast, is usually described as causing a chronic infection, often with a long pauci-symptomatic stage of some years, and a chronic meningo-encephalitic condition during the late stage (Apted, 1970; Taelman *et al.*, 1987). The important epidemiological distinction between these clinical conditions is the length of the clinical course and the degree of disability resulting from infection. The impact of these most basic differences on disease transmission and control polices is profound.

2. DISEASE BURDEN AND DISTRIBUTION

A continent-wide prevalence of both forms of HAT of 300 000 cases has been estimated by the World Health Organization (WHO); over the last 10 years, an average of 30 000 new cases (incidence) of both forms of the disease have been reported annually (World Health Organization, 2003), although this is generally thought to be an under-estimate resulting from low detection rates—60 million people live in risk areas, and as many of these have poor access to diagnostic and health care facilities, under-reporting rates are high. Over the past three years, the number of reported cases has been decreasing, but it is uncertain whether this is a reflection of successful control or some other, possibly stochastic, factor. *T. b. rhodesiense* is by far, less significant than *T. b. gambiense* in terms of the number of cases of the disease across the African continent. It remains a significant issue at regional and local levels however; Odiit (2003) found that at a local level in a *T. b. rhodesiense* epidemic area, the ratio of malaria to HAT cases was 178, while the ratio in terms of Disability-Adjusted Life Years (DALYs), an equitable measure of disease burden (Murray, 1994), was 2.

Foci of gambiense HAT cover west and central Africa, and are particularly active in areas with civil disturbances. Rhodesiense HAT, on the other hand, occurs in well-documented foci in Uganda, Tanzania and Kenya, but for other countries in eastern and southern Africa, such as Zambia (Wurapa *et al.*, 1984), Malawi and Mozambique (Perez-Martin *et al.*, 1991), the burden imposed by the disease is not clear, and the epidemiological characteristics are not as well understood, as elsewhere; HAT occurs amongst the poorest and most marginalised communities with poor access to health care facilities (Odiit *et al.*, 2004a). Even in Uganda, where reporting might be considered of higher quality than in many other countries, patients may visit health facilities between two and seven times before an accurate HAT diagnosis is made and, among 119 patients studied (Odiit *et al.*, 2004b), inappropriate diagnosis, referrals, lack of diagnostic facilities and patient delays accounted for a mean of 60 days of delay before commencement of treatment for *T. b. rhodesiense*. This increases the risk of late stage disease development with the consequent risk of death from the infection and, in *T. b. gambiense* areas, the risk of transmission. In countries less likely than Uganda to recognize HAT at local health centre levels, it is certain that there are many misdiagnoses and that many patients die unaccounted for. Molyneux (2001a) noted that the Ebola virus kills around 70% of patients quickly, while HAT kills 100% slowly, in the absence of treatment. Thus, in the marginalised and often war-torn areas in which HAT occurs, failure to reach a hospital implies death of the patient. Both *T. b. rhodesiense* and *T. b. gambiense* are resurging in affected countries as a result of a lack of infrastructure, funding and political priority given to HAT (Barrett, 1999).

T. b. gambiense was first described by Forde (1902) and named *T. gambiense* by Dutton (1902). *T. b. rhodesiense*, originally called *T. rhodesiense*, was first identified by Stephens and Fantham (1910) in Zambia, and was first incriminated explicitly as the cause of HAT in Uganda by MacKichan (1944) in an outbreak in the Busoga region. However, it had certainly existed there previously and been confused with *T. b. gambiense* (Fèvre *et al.*, 2004)—the parasite responsible for early outbreaks in various parts of East Africa has been confused by the fact that only one species of human-infective trypanosome had been identified at that time. HAT has a focal distribution, and established foci are generally stable through time, persisting with few or no cases during endemic periods but expanding outwards during epidemics, and sometimes spreading to new areas where disease transmission then becomes autochthonous (Fèvre *et al.*, 2001). Although there are concerns that the geographical distribution of the two diseases might soon overlap (Enyaru *et al.*, 1999), there is no evidence that this has yet happened. In addition, endemic foci of the two diseases have remained stable through time, and there is no clear evidence to show that areas where *T. b. gambiense* was once endemic are now affected by *T. b. rhodesiense*, or vice versa (Fèvre *et al.*, 2004). The life cycle and morphology of the human-infective trypanosomes, including the obligate developmental stages in the tsetse fly, are well understood (Vickerman, 1985); the details of the developmental stages of the parasite are less important in the context of this discussion than the transmission cycle (Baker, 1974); that for *T. b. rhodesiense* is shown in Figure 1. The vectors of human and animal trypanosomes on the African continent are tsetse flies of the genus

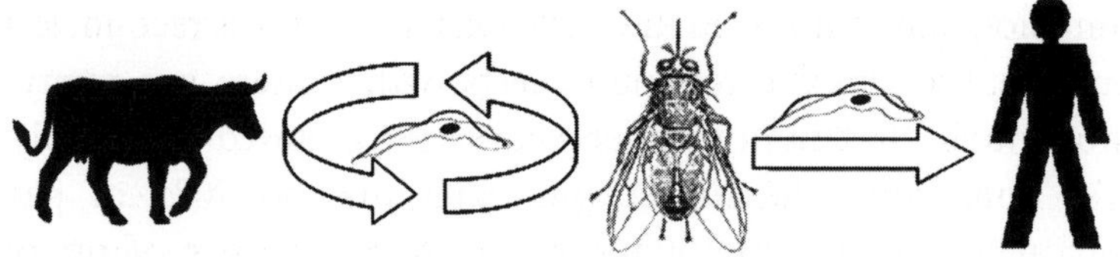

Figure 1   The transmission cycle of *T.b. rhodesiense* (after Baker, 1974). The full life cycle of HAT is given by Vickerman (1985); in the context of this review, it is the transmission cycle that is of importance. *T.b. rhodesiense* and *T. b. brucei* occur in a tsetse–bovid–tsetse cycle. The occasional infection of humans with *T.b. rhodesiense* results in HAT. The nature of human-fly contact and the acute nature of the disease make it unlikely that humans act as a reservoir of infection. By contrast, in *T.b. gambiense*, which is chronic, and for which the role of an animal reservoir is uncertain, humans are the main reservoir (Welburn *et al.*, 2001a). See text for discussion.

Glossina. Trypanosomes take approximately 20–40 days to develop in the tsetse host (Dale *et al.*, 1995) depending on the susceptibility of the fly, which remains infectious until the end of its life, which lasts approximately 5–6 weeks in the field (Welburn and Maudlin, 1999).

3. THE VECTOR—TSETSE FLIES

Tsetse are distributed across most of sub-Saharan Africa only—their range does not extend beyond the African continent. Ford and Katondo (1977) published the most authoritative printed maps available of tsetse distributions as well as details of the datasets used to construct them; these maps represent agglomerated country data and information from specific surveys. While such maps are of value in helping to define, broadly, which areas are affected or at risk, continent-scale tsetse distribution data are deceiving; these flies in general, and certain species of *Glossina* in particular, have highly focal distributions bounded by very specific habitat requirements, such that even within areas considered part of the 'tsetse belt' they occur in pockets determined by environmental variables. For example, *G. tachinoides*, a riverine species of tsetse, is sensitive to desiccation and generally prefers the shaded areas afforded by riverine forest habitats (Nash, 1936; Laveissière and Boreham, 1976), and thus remains relatively close to the shelter of its preferred environment, particularly in the dry season. The rivers and streams along which such habitat is found can be very small; thus, continental maps of the distribution of the species show, at best, the general geographical area across which it might occur, and not where it actually occurs. In Figure 2 (Figure 2, which is Plate 5.2 in the separate colour plate section), the country-level and focus-specific distributions can be compared. Recently, given known associations of different tsetse species with particular eco-climatic zones and types of vegetation, large-scale, low-resolution satellite imagery has been used to predict the geographical extent of tsetse (Rogers and Robinson, 2004). The use of such technologies is a significant advance, allowing continental mapping at an affordable cost. Mapping tsetse habitat and changes in the extent of this habitat on a regional or even local scale can also be carried out with higher resolution imagery (Kitron *et al.*, 1996; de la Rocque *et al.*, 2001), although ground truthing of data becomes more of an issue at this scale (Table 1).

Tsetse are K-strategists (Leak, 1999), females producing a few, regularly spaced offspring that are deposited in soil at the larval stage—a more mature form than the offspring of many other insects, resulting in a higher chance of survival (Hargrove, 2004). Tsetse of both sexes feed exclusively on blood, and both sexes are therefore potential vectors of trypanosomes. Some species of tsetse are thought to be more efficient vectors than others, either for behavioural (habitat preferences, host preferences) or genetic (resistance to infection with trypanosomes) reasons (Welburn *et al.*, 1989; Snow *et al.*, 1991; Welburn and Maudlin, 1999; Sane *et al.*, 2000). Broadly speaking, however, all

Table 1 General divisions of tsetse species by habitat type, with some examples of each group. There are 33 species and sub-species of tsetse recognised (Gooding and Krafsur, 2004)

General habitat type	Morsitans group	Palpalis group	Fusca group
	Savannah	Riverine	Forest
Species (example)	*G. morsitans sub-morsitans*	*G. palpalis palpalis*	*G. fusca fusca*
	G. pallidipes	*G. fuscipes fuscipes*	*G. brevipalpis*
	G. swynnertoni	*G. tachinoides*	*G. longipennis*
	G. austeni	*G. palpalis gambiensis*	*G. medicorum*

tsetse are potential vectors, and their presence thus presents a risk for parasite transmission.

4. TRYPANOSOMIASIS IN ANIMALS

4.1. Species Other than *Trypanosoma brucei*

Although it is not the purpose of this review to examine the biology of all trypanosomes, this discussion would not be complete without mention of the livestock trypanosomes and their impact. In sub-Saharan Africa, *Trypanosoma congolense* and *T. vivax* are also transmitted by tsetse. Production losses as a result of these infections have a considerable impact on the livelihoods of livestock keepers, and thus on the rural economy more generally (Kristjanson *et al.*, 1999; Shaw, 2004). Although *T. brucei* and its sub-species also infect livestock, it is not highly pathogenic to many breeds of African indigenous cattle (Wilde and French, 1945; Wellde *et al.*, 1989a, b) or pigs. Full descriptions of the clinical and pathological aspects of trypanosomiasis in various domestic animal species can be found elsewhere (Stephen, 1986; Taylor and Authié, 2004). The lack of pathogenicity of *T. brucei* infections in animals has profound implications for the epidemiology of this parasite and, in particular, its human-infective sub-species (Coleman and Welburn, 2004). *T. b. rhodesiense* is a zoonotic parasite, and wild and domestic animals serve as reservoirs. The nature of animal reservoirs of *T. b. gambiense* is somewhat less certain; certainly, this parasite can infect animals, but they may not play an important role in disease transmission (and hence be of epidemiological importance). For *T. b. rhodesiense*, however, the importance of the reservoir has implications for the control of transmission to humans.

4.2. Hosts and Reservoirs of *Trypanosoma brucei*

4.2.1. Wild Hosts

Traditionally, the bushbuck (*Tragelaphus scriptus*) has been considered the archetypal animal reservoir host for *T. b. rhodesiense*, a perception resulting from the fact that a human-infective trypanosome was first isolated from this species by Heisch *et al.* (1958). Other wild animals, especially bovids, may also be hosts (Ashcroft *et al.*, 1959; Geigy *et al.*, 1971; Mwambu and Woodford, 1972); even lions (*Panthera leo*) have been found to become infected (Sachs *et al.*, 1967), though these infections were probably through feeding on other infected animals (Bertram, 1973; Moloo *et al.*, 1973). The Blood Incubation Infectivity Test (BIIT) (Rickman and Robson, 1970a) has been used extensively to test trypanosomes isolated from wild species and determine their human infectivity status; for example, Robson *et al.* (1972) assessed the possible reservoir status of wild carnivore, bovine and porcine hosts in the Lambwe Valley, Kenya, and Geigy *et al.* (1975) conducted similar studies in the Serengeti region of Tanzania. Herder *et al.* (2002) recently used PCR to detect *T. brucei s.l.* in apes, ungulates, carnivores and rodents in Cameroon. In many African countries, there has been a drastic change in land use as pressure to grow more food and more cash crops has increased. While MacKichan (1944) observed that wild game animals were plentiful in the mid-1940s in Uganda, most of the country currently supports very little wild game and correspondingly few wild species of bovids (Eltringham and Malpas, 1993). Work in southwestern Ethiopia also suggests that anthropogenic changes are having an effect on the tsetse population and consequently on HAT. Some *Glossina* species that occurred there are no longer present, and game animals are being hunted out to make room for raising domestic stock (Nigatu *et al.*, 1992). In areas where wild animals are no longer abundant, domestic hosts (see below) are usually the principal reservoirs. Fairbairn (1948) suggested that *T. b. rhodesiense* in humans during epidemics of the disease in Tanzania probably represented spill-over infections from wild animal reservoirs, and in areas of Tanzania and elsewhere with abundant wildlife, this is likely to still be the case—recently highlighted by the occurrence of *T. b. rhodesiense* in tourists returning from safari holidays in East Africa (Sinha *et al.*, 1999; Nieman and Kelly, 2000; Moore *et al.*, 2002; Stich *et al.*, 2002; Jelinek *et al.*, 2003). Bloodmeal analysis of tsetse in the Serengeti National Park in Tanzania (Rogers and Boreham, 1973) found that warthogs (*Phacochoerus africanus*), for example, were a preferred source of food for the flies; like pigs (Waiswa *et al.*, 2003), they are good maintenance hosts of *T. brucei s.l.* Warthogs have also been found infected in other ecosystems, such as the Luangwa Valley, Zambia (Awan, 1979; Rickman *et al.*, 1991). Land-use pressures are resulting in an increasing overlap of wildlife and domestic animal grazing areas (Bourn and Blench, 1999); transmission of human-infective trypanosomes from wildlife to humans or to their livestock thus continues to be a public health issue.

4.2.2. Domestic hosts

A number of domestic animal species, including pigs, dogs, goats, sheep and cattle may carry human-infective trypanosome species (Stephen, 1970). Bruce and co-workers (1910, 1911) were the first to suggest that domestic animals might be important in the epidemiology of trypanosomiasis, and attached particular importance to cattle as a potential reservoir. Parasites isolated from domestic bovids were able to produce patent infections in monkeys; Bruce *et al.* (1910) commented:

> no branch of sleeping sickness investigation is of greater practical importance than the identification of animals which can serve as reservoirs of the sleeping sickness parasite (p. 236).

While Heisch *et al.* (1958) were the first to demonstrate the zoonotic potential of *T. brucei s.l.* isolated from wildlife, Onyango *et al.* (1966) were the first to isolate *T. brucei s.l.* parasites from domestic cattle and successfully infect a human. Their study was conducted on the Kenyan shores of Lake Victoria, where a prevalence of *T. brucei s.l.* of 21.2% was found in cattle (Onyango *et al.*, 1966). Large numbers of cattle are kept in East Africa, in intimate contact with humans. Both humans and cattle may also have close contact with tsetse fly habitat making cattle a potentially important reservoir of parasites. Maudlin *et al.* (1990) found that 4.9% of cattle tested in Iyolwa county, southeast Uganda during 1988 were carrying *T. brucei s.l.* infections, and 25% of these were human serum resistant, indicating that they were probably *T. b. rhodesiense.* Welburn *et al.* (2001b) found that in a *T. b. rhodesiense* epidemic area, 18% of cattle were carrying human-infective parasites. Resistance to lysis when incubated in human serum *in vitro* has been an important tool in identifying the human-infective phenotype (Rickman and Robson, 1970b), in the absence (until recently) of genetic tools to identify this trait.

In contrast to the above emphasis on the role of domestic animals as *T. b. rhodesiense* reservoirs, Okia *et al.* (1994) insisted that cattle do not play an important role in the epidemiology of HAT. They questioned HAT patients and controls in southeast Uganda on their behaviour, and observed that cases of HAT had fewer animals grazing near areas of human–tsetse contact than controls. It is important to note, however, that it is the combination of contacts of both livestock and humans with tsetse in their habitats that is of significance in terms of transmission, and not contact between humans and the livestock themselves. These interactions have been successfully studied in the context of assessing the risk to animals of infection with the livestock trypanosomes in West Africa (Wacher *et al.*, 1994; de la Rocque *et al.*, 1999).

Recently, it has been noted that pigs are of increasing importance as a source of income for livestock farmers in many parts of East Africa, and that this presents new challenges for the control of zoonotic diseases including cysticercosis and trypanosomiasis (Phiri *et al.*, 2003; Waiswa *et al.*, 2003). In areas of Uganda where pigs are abundant, Waiswa *et al.* (2003) found them carrying a high prevalence of human serum-resistant isolates. A number of studies have identified pigs as important sources of tsetse bloodmeals (Okoth and Kapaata, 1988; Clausen *et al.*, 1998, Spath, 2000). Together, these studies indicate that it is necessary to improve our understanding of the role of suids in HAT epidemiology in areas where they are abundant, and particularly where pigs and cattle exist together. Pigs are also thought to act as a reservoir of *T. b. gambiense* in West and Central Africa and numerous studies have found pigs infected with this trypanosome (Gibson *et al.*, 1978; Mehlitz *et al.*, 1982; Schares and Mehlitz, 1996). *T. b. gambiense* can, therefore, survive in pigs, as well as other animal species. However, it has been possible to locally eliminate *T. b. gambiense* transmission by treatment of the human reservoir alone, without recourse to animal targeted interventions (Pépin and Méda, 2001), and the strains of *T. brucei s.l.* found in pigs in HAT-affected areas may not match those found in humans

(Jamonneau *et al.*, 2004). Thus, while animals can sustain *T. b. gambiense*, these animals are unlikely to have a fundamental role in the epidemiology and transmission of this parasite to humans (Welburn *et al.*, 2001a). Further studies would be necessary to identify the risk posed by animal hosts in the persistence of *T. b. gambiense* in foci where large-scale human treatments have been carried out.

5. DIAGNOSIS

While it is not our intention to provide a full review of diagnostic methods available for trypanosome identification, we summarise below the current most significant available technologies. Serological tests, while not specific enough to be used for clinical decision making for individual cases, are used to screen large portions of the population rapidly; the direct detection of parasites remains essential for clinical decisions (e.g. whether or not to treat a patient). Diagnostic methods for *T. b. gambiense* have been recently reviewed by Chappuis *et al.* (2005).

5.1. Microscopy

The direct detection of parasites by microscopy is the 'gold standard' diagnostic technique for trypanosomes; microscopy based on wet blood films is, however, accurate only at or above concentrations of 10^4 parasites per mL, a parasite concentration that is well above those often seen in human patients, particularly in *T. b. gambiense* infections. Concentration techniques such as the mini-haematocrit centrifugation technique (Woo, 1970)—originally developed for avian trypanosomes (Bennett, 1962)—or the miniature anion exchange centrifugation (m-AECT; Lumsden *et al.*, 1979), improve detection levels to 500 and 100 parasites per mL by microscopy, respectively (World Health Organization, 1998). Stage determination of HAT (a therapeutic decision tool—see Section 6) has traditionally also relied on the direct observation of trypanosomes within the cerebrospinal fluid (CSF), either directly or after concentration by centrifugation (Cattand *et al.*, 1988). WHO criteria for the indirect determination of CNS invasion are an elevated leukocyte count of more than 5 cells/µL or increased protein concentrations $>37\,\text{mg}/100\,\text{mL}$ (World Health Organization, 1998). It has been suggested that the cut-off cell count for second stage determination be raised to 20 cells/µL (Bisser *et al.*, 1997), although recent work has shown that there is an increased risk of pentamidine treatment failure when patients with cell counts between 11 and 20 cells/µL are assumed to be in the early stage of infection (Lejon *et al.*, 2003).

5.2. CATT

The detection of *T. b. gambiense* has relied heavily on the Card Agglutination Test for Trypanosomiasis (CATT/*T. b. gambiense*) since its development in 1978 (Magnus *et al.*, 1978). Based on detecting the presence of antibodies directed against a dominant variant antigen type (VAT) of *T. b. gambiense*, LiTat 1.3, CATT has a specificity of 90–95% and a sensitivity of 92–100% (Noireau *et al.*, 1987; Jamonneau *et al.*, 2000; Truc *et al.*, 2002). Whole, fixed and stained trypanosomes expressing this VAT are combined with human serum on a simple card, resulting in a visually detectable level of agglutination in patients with previous exposure to *T. b. gambiense*; confirmatory positive diagnosis relies on subsequent parasitological confirmation (Simarro *et al.*, 1999). Each CATT costs approximately US$ 0.40 (Pépin and Méda, 2001), so that this test remains fundamental to large-scale screening for *T. b. gambiense*, although Robays *et al.* (2004) emphasise that it needs to be integrated into a well-managed screening programme to be truly effective; Chappuis *et al.* (2005) describe a field algorithm for *T. b. gambiense* diagnosis involving the CATT test. CATT cannot differentiate between past and current infections and therefore cannot be used to assess treatment efficacy. There are also a small number of *T. b. gambiense* variants that do not express the specific test antigen (Dukes *et al.*, 1992; Kanmogne *et al.*, 1996; Enyaru *et al.*, 1998). The CATT test does not work on *T. b. rhodesiense* (Enyaru *et al.*, 1999), although some preliminary work has shown promise on field-adapted antigen detection tests for *T. b. rhodesiense* (Akol *et al.*, 1999). Diagnosis for *T. b. rhodesiense* must therefore be made either clinically, or through parasitological or molecular methods.

5.3. Other Field Serological Tests for *T. b. gambiense*

There are other serological tests for *T. b. gambiense* infection. One is the Latex/*T. b. gambiense* (Büscher *et al.*, 1999), which is a variant of the CATT/*T. b. gambiense* test but directed against three VAT (LiTat 1.3, 1.5 and 1.6), and which has a specificity of up to 99% and a sensitivity between 84% and 100%. Another is the Latex/IgM (Lejon *et al.*, 1998b, 2002), used to detect elevated IgM in the CNS of second stage patients: when *T. b. gambiense* trypanosomes invade the CNS, the inflammatory response results in elevated levels of IgM, up to 16x greater than normal (Bisser *et al.*, 2002). The specificity and sensitivity of this test are 89% and 93%, respectively. Latex/IgM agglutination may also be applicable to stage determination in *T. b. rhodesiense* infection where similar changes in antibody levels have been demonstrated—although this remains to be evaluated (Itazi, 1981; Lejon *et al.*, 2002). Chappuis *et al.* (2005) provide an in-depth review of these tests.

5.4. ELISA

The enzyme-linked immunosorbent assay (ELISA) is a more complicated method of antibody detection than those previously mentioned. The principle remains the same, in that the test relies on the detection of antigens or antibodies relating to the parasite presence within human serum. Most targets originally identified for ELISA-based diagnosis such as immunodominant surface glycoproteins (Lejon *et al.*, 1998a) or whole purified trypanosome preparations (Olaho-Mukani *et al.*, 1994) have since been transferred to a simplified agglutination test.

5.5. PCR

The Polymerase Chain Reaction (PCR) is a diagnostic method that multiplies specific fragments of DNA. PCR has been used to assess the presence of *T. b. gambiense* infection in both blood and CSF of patients from the Ivory Coast, Cameroon and Uganda (Kanmogne *et al.*, 1996; Enyaru *et al.*, 1998; Truc *et al.*, 1999; Kyambadde *et al.*, 2000) with a sensitivity of 100% in parasitologically positive samples

(Truc *et al.*, 1999; Kyambadde *et al.*, 2000; Jamonneau *et al.*, 2003). PCR is recognised as being the most sensitive diagnostic method for HAT when compared with parasitological means, but due to the very low parasitaemia in chronic *T. b. gambiense* infections, there have been difficulties in calculating the sensitivity of this test. Currently the detection limit of PCR is thought to be 1 trypanosome/10 mL of cattle blood (Masake *et al.*, 2002) or 25 trypanosomes/mL of human blood (Kanmogne *et al.*, 1996). Inhibitory factors present in human blood result in the discrepancy between bovine and human studies (Contamin *et al.*, 1995). While much effort has focused on the detection of genetic material from *T. brucei s.l.* (Sloof *et al.*, 1983; Kabiri *et al.*, 1999), diagnostic markers are now available to differentiate the two human pathogenic sub-species.

5.5.1. *T. b. rhodesiense*

In 2001, Welburn *et al.* demonstrated the potential of the serum resistance associated (SRA) gene as a specific molecular marker for *T. b. rhodesiense* (Welburn *et al.*, 2001b). The protein encoded by the SRA gene had been identified as responsible for human serum resistance in *T. b. rhodesiense* (de Greef *et al.*, 1989; de Greef and Hamers, 1994). This target has since been identified as a ubiquitous marker for *T. b. rhodesiense* throughout eastern Africa, and a further sub-division of these parasites is possible through selective markers for southern and northern isolates (Gibson *et al.*, 2002; Gibson and Ferris, 2003).

5.5.2. *T. b. gambiense*

The specific detection of *T. b. gambiense* by PCR has focused predominantly on identification of variant specific glycoprotein (VSG) genes, such as LiTat 1.3 and AnTat 11.17 (Magnus *et al.*, 1978; Thi *et al.*, 1991; Bromidge *et al.*, 1993). Due to the sequence variation that exists within the VSG repertoire, there are occasionally foci detected where established molecular targets are not present within the parasite genomes (Enyaru *et al.*, 1993). An alternative diagnostic target is the receptor-like flagellar pocket glycoprotein TgsGP (Berberof *et al.*,

2001); this region has been shown to provide a specific marker for *T. b. gambiense* (Radwanska *et al.*, 2002a).

5.6. New Technology in Diagnostics

Jannin and Cattand (2004) have recently reviewed novel diagnostics. The continued development of technologies involved in the diagnosis of HAT appears to be diverging; from the highly advanced computer-based analysis of protein signatures (Papadopoulos *et al.*, 2004) to the modification and combination of existing methods to provide greater sensitivity to field-based diagnosis. One such development of the latter is PNA-FISH, a method that relies on the detection of *T. brucei s.l.* parasites on a microscope slide by fluorescein-labelled peptide nucleic acid (PNA) probes (Radwanska *et al.*, 2002a, b), the detection limits of which are five parasites per mL, five times the sensitivity of PCR. Advances in the simplification of DNA-based analysis by loop-mediated isothermal amplification (LAMP) (Kuboki *et al.*, 2003), with a single heating step and visual colorimetric identification of amplicons (Notomi *et al.*, 2000), have also successfully detected human-infective parasites.

5.7. Field Diagnostics: Realistic and Appropriate Technologies

The development of novel diagnostic tests, particularly those based on DNA technologies, is to be applauded, and certainly contributes greatly to our understanding of epidemiological systems—for example, assessing the extent of the animal reservoir of *T. b. rhodesiense* (Kyambadde *et al.*, 2000; Welburn *et al.*, 2001b). Such information provides a basis from which appropriately targeted control interventions can be designed and, with time, highly sensitive and specific DNA detection methods are becoming increasingly miniaturised and portable (Callahan *et al.*, 2002). However, for African rural health centres with small budgets dealing with a multitude of diseases, it is the most basic, cost-effective diagnostic techniques that will remain the mainstay of the diagnostic toolbox for the foreseeable future. These tools include, first and foremost, clinical diagnosis, and then microscopy and the CATT (Abel *et al.*, 2004). The direct observation of parasites through microscopy in blood or other tissues is particularly important, even when CATT is used. To prevent unnecessary treatment for *T. b. gambiense* of CATT false-positive patients with toxic drugs, a parasitological diagnosis based on CSF or lymph gland exudate usually follows (World Health Organization, 1998). There have been some exceptions to this (Simarro *et al.*, 2001), but it holds as a general rule. Screening of peripheral blood and/or CSF are, equally, key for *T. b. rhodesiense* diagnosis and staging (and thus deciding on the drug regimen to follow). It cannot be over-emphasised that, particularly for *T. b. rhodesiense* affected areas, the provision of a microscope and trained microscopist at a health centre is probably the best method for improving the level of detection of HAT (Odiit *et al.*, 2004b) and reducing the burden suffered by patients. The historical achievements with HAT control were entirely based on routine microscopy and regular surveillance of at risk populations when microscopy was the only, albeit insensitive, available tool. This approach reduced the problem of HAT as a public health problem over large areas.

6. TREATMENT

The epidemiological characteristics and clinical course of *T. b. rhodesiense* and *T. b. gambiense* are different. Similarly, the drugs used to treat them differ (Fairlamb, 2003). The choice of treatment is dependent on the parasite species involved and on the stage of the disease; drugs for the treatment of late stage disease are able to cross the blood–brain barrier in order to clear trypanosomes in the CSF. Various reviews have recently been published on issues relating to treatment of HAT (Legros *et al.*, 2002; Bouteille *et al.*, 2003), and the biochemical properties of the different drugs (Docampo and Moreno, 2003). A historical review of the development of drugs that have been used against trypanosomiasis is given by Ollivier and Legros (2001). Hospitalisation is required during adminiistration of all the drugs currently used, particularly for the late stage (World Health Organization, 1995); this may be for a period of longer than one month, adding an extra burden on families of patients and on the health system—though Burri *et al.* (2000) recently described a shorter (10-day) treatment course for late stage *T. b. gambiense* using melarsoprol, which has been shown to be as effective as the standard course on long-term follow-up (Schmid *et al.*, 2004), and has been adopted as the recommended course by WHO.

T. b. rhodesiense is preferably treated with suramin or melarsoprol (an arsenical compound) in the early and late stages respectively, whereas *T. b. gambiense* is treated with pentamidine—the drug of choice (Pépin and Milord, 1994)—or suramin, in the early stage and melarsoprol in the late stage (World Health Organization, 1995; Van Nieuwenhove, 1999). Pentamidine is less effective against early stage *T. b. rhodesiense* (Apted, 1980). Although there are an increasing number of clinical failures with melarsoprol in the treatment of *T. b. gambiense* (Pépin *et al.*, 1994; Burri and Keiser, 2001; Matovu *et al.*, 2001a), no significant reduction in efficacy has yet been demonstrated for *T. b. rhodesiense*. The alternative, registered drug for melarsoprol-refractory-late-stage *T. b. gambiense* treatment is eflornithine (Van Nieuwenhove, 1999), but it cannot be used for *T. b. rhodesiense* (Iten *et al.*, 1995). Nifurtimox, used mainly for the treatment of Chagas disease (caused by *Trypanosoma cruzi*) in South America (Rodriques Coura and de Castro, 2002), is being studied in combination with eflornithine. Eflornithine, also called difluoromethyl-ornithine (DFMO), is an effective anti-trypanocidal drug (Burri and Brun, 2003) which was originally developed as an anti-cancer agent (Wickware, 2002), and is also used as a topical treatment for excess facial hair (Hickman *et al.*, 2001); despite its efficacy, however, it is difficult to administer for HAT treatment, as it is very expensive (Van Nieuwenhove, 2000) and is recommended only for relapsing—melarsoprol refractory—cases of *T. b. gambiense* (Pépin *et al.*, 2000). The total cost of treating a patient with eflornithine has been estimated as US\$ 675, against US\$ 253 for melarsoprol, US\$ 114 for suramin and US\$ 107 for pentamidine, when drugs are purchased commercially (World Health Organization, 1998). For comparison, anti-retroviral therapy for HIV/AIDS costs approximately US\$ 300 per person per year (Reid *et al.*, 2004).

Though pentamidine is not as toxic as other HAT drugs, there have been some reports of drug failure due to resistance; these early stage cases of *T. b. gambiense* are then treated with suramin. Suramin is a relatively toxic drug, which can result in severe adverse reactions such as anaphylactic shock (particularly if used to treat HAT during co-infections with onchocerciasis), cutaneous reactions such as exfoliate dermatitis (May and Allolio, 1991; World Health Organization, 1995), and neurotoxic side effects. In late stage treatments, melarsoprol results in an encephalopathic reaction in approximately 5% of cases (Haller *et al.*, 1986; Pépin *et al.*, 1995; Blum *et al.*, 2001). There is a growing number of reports of drug failures with melarsoprol (Pépin *et al.*, 1994; Brun *et al.*, 2001), which could be due to parasite resistance or lack of bioavailability—though this latter point has been recently challenged (Burri and Keiser, 2001). The mode of uptake of melarsoprol may be similar to that of pentamidine and also diminazine aceturate (Barrett and Fairlamb, 1999); thus, there is a possibility of cross resistance not only with early stage HAT drugs, but also with curative treatments of trypanosomiasis in animals (Barrett, 2001), for which diminazine would be the drug of choice in most instances (Geerts *et al.*, 2001).

The prospects for new drugs to combat HAT are bleak (Legros *et al.*, 2002). HAT is one of the group of so-called neglected diseases (Banerji, 2003; Jannin *et al.*, 2003; Molyneux, 2004), which have recently seen a number of programmes (such as the 'Drugs for Neglected Diseases Initiative'—DNDi) to promote drug discovery and drug availability. Jannin and Cattand (2004) review some of the new compounds that are under investigation for trypanosomiasis therapy.

7. CONTROL

7.1. Historical Paradigms for Control: Biology and Necessity

Welburn *et al.* (2004) discuss the socio-historical context of the study of HAT in Africa, and emphasise that, until recently, our understanding of the historical disease trends was limited to conjecture from scant sociological studies (Lyons, 1992). A lack of scientific data has been the cause of some important historical misunderstandings about the epidemiology of HAT (Köerner *et al.*, 1995; Fèvre *et al.*, 2004).

Historically, the effects of the bipartite geographical distribution of HAT have been both technically and politically profound. The colonial authorities did not recognise the essential differences between the two diseases (caused by *T. b. rhodesiense* and *T. b. gambiense*) as being important in control terms. The problems facing the colonial regimes were apparently mutually exclusive, either HAT in humans or nagana in animals. In addition, in tackling HAT in the east and west of the continent, different technologies evolved with progressive scientific advances; yet authorities stopped short of acknowledging that these differences were firmly rooted in the differing biologies of the diseases and not, as was perceived, in vague political agendas. Thus, francophone Africa pursued technologies suited for the control of Gambian HAT, while anglophone Africa pursued technologies suited primarily to nagana and secondarily to Rhodesian HAT. In each case, the rationale was entirely logical; most of francophone Africa was heavily forested (e.g. the Congo River Basin) and inhabited by riverine tsetse species with low population densities. Anglophone Africa, by contrast, was concerned with vast areas of savanna suitable for rearing cattle, the economic importance of which was of far more concern to the colonial authorities. Apart from large epidemics (Langlands, 1967), which were rare, the occasional Rhodesian HAT outbreak, which tended to be self limiting, was of little concern.

The post colonial period saw, at first, a lively debate between francophone and anglophone technologists who came from different, and one has to say competing, backgrounds. In tsetse control, this led to a plethora of trapping technologies which worked in one setting but, when tested in another setting, were apparently ineffective. Similarly, when insecticide 'pour-ons' were refined, they worked well in settings where there were high densities of cattle but not in settings where cattle were at low densities—this would include most of the forested parts of Africa (Hargrove, 2003b). In human-targeted HAT control, active case finding worked well in *T. b. gambiense* areas but not in *T. b. rhodesiense* areas. Areas with *T. b. rhodesiense* often had high densities of flies and high rates of transmission, where flies were dealt with as a priority concurrently with human-targeted interventions. In *T. b. gambiense* areas, flies need not be dealt with as a high priority but rather as a longer term objective (Gouteux and Artzrouni, 1996). Time, communication systems and technology have resolved these differences and science is now in a position to offer appropriate technologies for appropriate settings, irrespective of cultural barriers.

Thus, historical differences in approaches, which became intertwined with politics, were, in fact, grounded in the realities of parasite biology from an early stage. The details of these disease-driven differences are given below; with the technological toolbox now available for the study of the epidemiology of HAT, we need to return to these biological differences in the effective design of control programmes, and note that there is unlikely to be one effective, trans-continental control paradigm (Molyneux, 2001b).

7.1.1. Approaches Adopted in West Africa

In the early years of HAT control through drugs, effective treatments were simply not available and mortality rates were high; thus, patients themselves were used as the testing ground for optimising treatment regimens, often with dubious results (Eckart, 2002). Eventually, chemotherapy was deployed on a large scale—sometimes prophylactically (Van Hoof *et al.*, 1946), and for the control of gambian HAT, combining active case-detection and drug treatment of positive cases is now the cornerstone of disease prevention and control (Ekwanzala *et al.*, 1996). Lapeyssonnie (1992) outlines the historical context in which tens of millions of people were screened during colonial times for *T. b. gambiense*, and treated (if positive) with arsenical-based therapies, then tryparsamide (Ollivier and Legros, 2001); the approach he outlines, which was undertaken in particular by French and Belgian colonial authorities, was to screen everyone, everywhere, in affected foci. This was the method originally devised by Eugène Jamot in Cameroon in 1917 (Ducloux, 1988; Louis *et al.*, 2002): as a result of Jamot's successful screening campaigns, the number of cases in Cameroon was reduced by 300-fold (Lapeyssonnie, 1992), and similarly dramatic reductions were achieved in other *T. b. gambiense* affected areas. In order to reduce transmission of a disease, it is necessary to reduce the size of the reservoir of that disease (the early stage of *T. b. gambiense* is long, and the relative lack of clinical signs means that patients may continue to serve as sources of infections for tsetse as they go about their daily activities). Reducing the size of the human reservoir will reduce the chances of further generations of tsetse becoming infected and passing on the infection, so that transmission will eventually be interrupted (Welburn *et al.*, 2001a). During the late 1990s, over 8000 cases of *T. b. gambiense* HAT were detected annually in Angola, mainly through active case detection (Stanghellini and Josenando, 2001), with a high proportion of late stage cases. Active case detection continues, therefore, to be key in controlling *T. b. gambiense*. There is evidence of transplacental transmission of *T. b. gambiense* (Lingam *et al.*, 1985; Triolo *et al.*, 1985; Rocha *et al.*, 2004) and some evidence that this may also occur in *T. b. rhodesiense* (Traub *et al.*, 1978), and isolated reports of possible sexual transmission of *T. b. gambiense* (Rocha *et al.*, 2004). This passing of parasites from mother to foetus or through sexual transmission is mainly of clinical interest, however, and is unlikely to drive the epidemiology of these diseases.

7.1.2. *Approaches Adopted in East Africa*

Dealing with outbreaks or epidemics of *T. b. rhodesiense* requires a different approach from that of *T. b. gambiense* control. While finding and treating infected patients is of course a necessary ethical duty and medical task, such activities will not stem the actual transmission of parasites. Humans are unlikely to serve as reservoirs of *T. b. rhodesiense*; the high burden imposed on the individual infected with *T. b. rhodesiense* at an early stage ensures their removal from transmission zones. Rather, we have seen that livestock and other animal hosts of this zoonotic sub-species need to be the focus of control activities.

Around the Lake Victoria Basin, affected by a major HAT epidemic that killed hundreds of thousands of people (Langlands, 1967) and that we now know was due to the rapid spread of *T. b. rhodesiense* (Köerner *et al.*, 1995; Fèvre *et al.*, 2004), active case finding was not considered. Rather, affected populations were isolated in what were effectively concentration camps (Hodges, 1910; Eckart, 2002), and tsetse infested areas were forcibly evacuated (Anon, 1909). Uptake of parasites by the flies was thus limited, and opportunities for further transmission were reduced. In eastern Africa generally, tsetse habitat was cleared, both indiscriminately on a large scale and more selectively, targeting certain vegetation types (Swynnerton, 1925; Ford *et al.*, 1970). Later, when it became clear that animals served as a parasite reservoir, contact between these animals and tsetse was also prevented; at the time, game animals served as the most important reservoir (Heisch *et al.*, 1958), and these were culled in large numbers where they occurred close to human habitations (Bruce *et al.*, 1911; Potts and Jackson, 1952; Ford, 1970).

7.2. Overlap of *T. b. gambiense* and *T. b. rhodesiense*: Policy Implications

Uganda is the only country in Africa known to be affected by both *T. b. rhodesiense* and *T. b. gambiense*. Up to the present, however, within the country the distribution of these parasites has been quite separate; *T. b. gambiense* affects populations in the West Nile region in the north-west, close to the Sudanese and Congo borders, and has been dealt with mainly by non-governmental organisations (NGOs) in the recent past (Paquet *et al.*, 1995). *T. b. rhodesiense* traditionally occurs, with far fewer cases per annum in the south-east's Busoga region, in the Lake Victoria Basin (Odiit *et al.*, 2004a). This geographical separation is a major factor in both the differential diagnosis of HAT in the country, which is mainly through microscopy, and in the treatment of the disease, as the drugs required differ (see above). Recently, however, *T. b. rhodesiense* has spread beyond its traditional range— an epidemic is underway as a result of the movement of infected livestock (Fèvre *et al.*, 2001) to the previously unaffected Teso region, and the possible occurrence of rhodesiense has been noted in other previously unaffected regions (Enyaru *et al.*, 1999) in the west. Field evidence shows that the expansion has not been curtailed despite control efforts (Fèvre *et al.*, in press), and *T. b. rhodesiense* is now present very close to areas that were once foci of *T. b. gambiense* (Morris, 1959). Additionally, there were no reported cases of *T. brucei s.l.* in the livestock reservoir in studies in Teso before recent events; since then, a prevalence of up to 40% has been reported (Welburn *et al.*, 2001b). These important changes, coupled with the knowledge that restocking of cattle herds was taking place extensively across the country, has led to the fear that HAT might spread to other areas from which it had previously been absent. Furthermore, as the treatments and diagnostic protocols for *T. b. rhodesiense* and *T. b. gambiense* HAT are different, the potential for the overlap of the two human disease-causing species would have serious implications for control activities and patient management. A CATT negative result, for example, could, in this scenario, be due to either problems with test sensitivity or the fact that the parasite is *T. b. rhodesiense* and thus undetectable using CATT. This would raise questions as to the grounds for treatment of such cases, or indeed the necessary treatment for parasitologically positive cases (given the identical morphologies of the causative organisms).

7.3. Modern Paradigms for Control: Options for Policy

The control of trypanosomiasis is concerned with reducing parasite transmission from host to vector and on to further hosts. An important concept in the study of infectious disease epidemiology is R_0, the basic reproduction number (Anderson and May, 1992), which describes the number of new infections that arise as a result of one infected case in a susceptible population. If R_0 is less than 1 ($R_0 < 1$), then each infected individual gives rise, on average, to less than one new infection, and in a given population over a period of time, an outbreak would not sustain itself. For values of R_0 greater than 1 ($R_0 > 1$), the opposite is true as each infected individual gives rise to more than one new infection; the higher the value of R_0, the more difficult it is to control the spread of a disease (Rogers, 1988). The choices for the optimal control strategy depend on whether it is the vector or the mammalian host that is the target and, if the mammal, whether it is the human, livestock or wildlife species. The one-size-fits-all approach certainly does not fit with a disease like HAT, in which each of the 200 distinct foci (see Figure 1) may present quite different transmission scenarios.

7.3.1. Choice 1: Human Treatments

Treatment of patients for HAT will be an ethical necessity as long as patients are acquiring infections, despite the problems with drug resistance and toxicity. For *T. b. rhodesiense*, this is a 'fire-fighting' exercise; we have seen that curing humans does not prevent transmission and disease spread because of the existence of an animal reservoir. *T. b. rhodesiense* control has to go beyond treatment of humans, and deal with transmission from the reservoir, which is domestic livestock in most areas, and wildlife species where they exist (see below). For *T. b. gambiense*, treating human patients has the dual effect of preventing individual suffering and preventing further infections: transmission control programmes reduce the size of the main reservoir of parasites, humans. In West and Central Africa, therefore, human-targeted interventions will be cost-effective when there are many cases of disease, though as cases become rarer as control progresses, the cost-effectiveness per case diagnosed will decrease. Human case finding therefore needs sustained commitment and central organisation to make it efficient.

At an international level, the neglected status of HAT (both *T. b. gambiense* and *T. b. rhodesiense* infection) has resulted in an increasingly poor likelihood of new drugs being developed and questions over the availability of existing ones. Inputs are required from international organisations and governments, who need to be convinced to support HAT drug design and delivery—various initiatives have already been designed to do this (Zumla, 2002; Banerji, 2003; Jannin *et al.*, 2003).

7.3.2. Choice 2: Vector Control

There are a range of possible tsetse-targeted interventions that can be used to prevent trypanosomiasis transmission. These include the use of baits or traps, the use of insecticides either on their own (through various methods of deployment such as aerial spraying or ground spraying) or in combination with traps (Allsopp and Hursey, 2004).

(a) *Use of baits and/or traps.* A wide range of traps and targets has been developed to attract and trap tsetse (Leak, 1999). These exploit the attraction of these insects to certain colours, particularly blue and black (Steverding and Troscianko, 2004), and to certain shapes (Vale, 1982). Traps can be supplemented with chemical attractants; for example, cow urine and its constituents are particularly attractive to certain species of tsetse (Bursell *et al.*, 1988; Vale *et al.*, 1988). Traps cost between US$5 and 15 (Laveissière and Grebaut, 1990; Brightwell *et al.*, 1991; Okoth, 1991) each. While the deployment of traps has certain benefits in terms of the control programme, being visible to the population, their use as effective tsetse control tools requires enough traps per unit area to significantly reduce the density of the tsetse population. For example, Lancien (1991) reported using 10 unbaited traps per square km in Uganda for *G. f. fuscipes* control, and Hargrove (2003a) estimated that four baited targets per square km would be necessary for *Glossina pallidipes* in a closed area (not susceptible to the immigration of flies). Centralised organisation is likely to be needed for a deployment on this scale—a $5\,km^2$ village would need 50 traps, the deployment of which would ideally be co-ordinated with neighbouring villages. Fifty traps would cost up to US\$ 500; where the average income is perhaps US\$ 1 per day per individual, even for the village as a whole this might be prohibitive without external support. There have been some studies showing that communities can take charge of trapping under the right circumstances (Gouteux and Sinda, 1990; Okoth *et al.*, 1991), but the financial and time constraints make this unrealistic over a large area. Although the use of insecticide-treated bed nets has more immediate and tangible benefit in controlling malaria than do tsetse traps in preventing trypanosomiasis—by reducing malaria incidence by up to 50% (Lengeler, 2004), there are many problems with convincing communities in malarious areas to use bed nets, mainly relating to cost (Guyatt *et al.*, 2002). This is likely to be even more the case in areas affected by HAT. For longer-term effectiveness, Dransfield and Brightwell (2004) have emphasised the importance of real, rather than nominal, participation of local communities in tsetse control operations; without such participation they suggest that the disease will simply increase in prevalence. However, we must ask whether it is plausible to do more to prevent a neglected disease without some serious centralised effort.

(b) *Use of insecticides.* Insecticidal control, through distribution of insecticides over wide areas from aircraft and ground spraying of residual compounds, as well as the constraints to such techniques, has been recently reviewed (Allsopp, 2001; Allsopp and Hursey, 2004). Such methods are expensive, but have been successful in reducing tsetse densities over treated areas. This success, however, is dependent on a serious and sustained investment in infrastructure and therefore on a centralised and 'top-down' disease management system. Agencies providing funding for such control may also be concerned about the environmental impact of insecticide distribution in the environment.

(c) *Integrated control.* Where trypanosomiasis is endemic, other diseases, in particular tick-borne diseases (TBD), often occur concurrently (Bauer *et al.*, 1992; Mattioli *et al.*, 1998). From a disease control perspective, the integrated control of both groups of diseases presents logistical and economic advantages (Holmes, 1997; Eisler *et al.*, 2003), although such integration must be based on a sound understanding of disease transmission systems in specific areas to have the desired effect (Coleman *et al.*, 2001). Pour-on and spray formulations of pyrethroid insecticides are particularly suitable for integrated control as they can be applied by farmers themselves with minimal inputs, and often in low volume (Vale *et al.*, 1999). Individual animals are protected from acquiring new infections if vectors are killed before they feed, and the animal itself becomes a living, impregnated, tsetse target. The challenge is optimising the delivery of the insecticidal compounds to the livestock (different frequency of spraying, different application methods). Such control is particularly suitable in decentralised systems as, once the demand for such services is established, market forces will deal with delivery. Integrated control of tsetse and ticks thus becomes self-sufficient. Dip tanks serve a similar disease-control purpose, but their effective use requires more inputs and organisation.

(d) *Sterile insect technique.* Early in the last century, almost complete elimination of tsetse was achieved on Principe Island over a 4-year period, through the combined efforts of bush clearing, the killing of wildlife and tsetse trapping using the Maldonado process of wearing sticky cloth that attracts flies (Bruto da Costa *et al.*, 1916). Currently, it is proposed that elimination or eradication of tsetse from wide areas might involve the use of the sterile insect technique (SIT) (Kabayo, 2002); this effectively involves the replacement of the wild male tsetse population with males that have been sterilised, either chemically or through exposure to ionizing radiation (Vreysen *et al.*, 2000). Although female tsetse can be experimentally mated more than once, their first mating with a single male is sufficient to produce a lifetime of off-spring, and in the wild, females are unlikely to mate again. If the probability that a female will mate with a sterile male fly can be kept high across several generations, by keeping the so-called over-flooding ratio of males high (generally accepted to be 1:10 for tsetse) the fertility of the tsetse population will decrease. In order to achieve this ratio, the population of flies needs to be brought down by the use of insecticides or intensive trapping prior to the release of sterile males.

SIT has been effective for the elimination of the New World Screwworm fly, *Cochliomyia hominivorax*, from the southern USA and Mexico (Krafsur *et al.*, 1987), and was also used after the fly was introduced to Libya in 1988 (Lindquist *et al.*, 1992). Before 1997, a single species of tsetse (*Glossina austeni*) existed on Zanzibar island, Tanzania (Vreysen *et al.*, 2000); in that year, an SIT programme eliminated this fly. While such a programme has thus been shown to be effective, it was achieved at a huge cost (Molyneux, 2001b), as large 'factories' are required for rearing and sterilizing millions of flies, which are then distributed from aircraft. In future, SIT may be useful, if funds allow, for confined areas with a low risk of inward migration from untreated areas; the prohibitive logistics and costs required to deal with multiple tsetse species across many countries, however, makes wholescale eradication of tsetse using SIT a hypothetical solution. Reichard (1999) points out that SIT is designed to cover large geographic areas and 'consequently, requires active and continuous international participation.' Smaller scale, farmer-oriented control activities are more likely to be successful in the short and medium terms.

7.3.3. *Choice 3: Animal Treatments for Human Health Benefit*

Animal-targeted interventions include chemotherapy of reservoir species with either curative or prophylactic trypanocides. The drugs available currently include the salts of only three compounds: diminazene aceturate, homidium bromide/homidium chloride and isometamidium chloride. Diminazine is used for curative rather than prophylactic treatment, while the latter two drugs have a prophylactic effect. Trypanosomiasis control in animals might be undermined by the development of resistance to these veterinary drugs (Geerts *et al.*, 2001). Resistance of *T. congolense* to isometamidium chloride has been reported in Kenya (Gray *et al.*, 1993) and resistance to all available trypanocides has been recorded in different parts of Ethiopia (Codjia *et al.*, 1993; Afewerk *et al.*, 2000) and Burkina Faso (Clausen *et al.*, 1992); resistance of *T. vivax* to all trypanocides other than diminazine has been reported in Kenya and Somalia (Schonefeld *et al.*, 1987). Drug resistance is thus a potentially serious issue which would undermine control activities. Although not yet a problem at the clinical level, recent studies *in vitro* (Matovu *et al.*, 1997) have shown reduced sensitivity to diminazine and isometamidium of human serum resistant (i.e. *T. b. rhodesiense*) stocks isolated in the Busoga focus in Uganda. In that study, which set out specifically to test the potential usefulness of animal treatments for public health purposes, parasites were found to have reduced sensitivity to both drugs simultaneously (multi-drug resistance). Combination therapy may therefore be necessary for animal treatment, especially in areas where animals are a reservoir of human-infective trypanosomes (see White and Olliaro (1996) for a discussion of the rationale of combination therapies).

Geerts *et al.* (2001) argue that preventing drug resistance in animal trypanosomes may in fact depend on limiting treatments to clinical cases, as mass treatment of herds may impose a strong selection pressure on the trypanosome population to develop resistance (Matovu *et al.*, 2001b). Drug resistance mechanisms of trypanosomes are poorly understood (Barrett, 2001); there is evidence in laboratory strains, however, to suggest that there may be cross-resistance between diminazene and melarsoprol, as the mode of uptake of both compounds by trypanosomes is similar (Barrett and Fairlamb, 1999). In both cases, uptake of the drugs is mediated in part by an amino-purine transporter across the trypanosome membrane (termed the P2 transporter), first described by Carter and Fairlamb (1993). If trypanocidal drugs are used appropriately and in a controlled manner during mass drug administration, the impact on the development of drug resistance would be limited while reducing the risk of spreading human-infective parasites. This requires collaboration between medical and veterinary sectors in the formulation of policy.

In eastern Uganda, during the start of an epidemic of HAT in the late 1990s, up to 18% of domestic cattle were harbouring human-infective *T. b. rhodesiense* (Welburn *et al.*, 2001b); cattle are a significant reservoir of human-infective trypanosomes, and treating them in the context of a bovine trypanosomiasis control programme could theoretically prevent human disease. Welburn *et al.* (2001a) quantified the impacts of this control technique, and found that it would have a significant public health impact, in an established HAT focus. The model was based on a previous model of trypanosome transmission (Rogers, 1988), which is a one-vector (tsetse) and two-host model (humans and cattle); Welburn *et al.* (*op. cit.*) added an extra component, that of the effects of drug treatment on both mammalian components of the life cycle. Given the knowledge that humans are not a significant reservoir of the parasite, and a situation in which at least 60% of *T. b. rhodesiense*-infected cattle are promptly treated with a trypanocidal drug, an outbreak of *T. b. rhodesiense* HAT will die out because the number of flies acquiring infections and further infecting humans and other animals will not be high enough. Reducing the size of the animal reservoir in order to minimise the chances of human hosts becoming infected with trypanosomes, is an application of the R_0 concept for *T. b. rhodesiense*—keeping the number of infective reservoirs low enough to interrupt, or at least reduce, transmission of the parasite.

Treating cattle would have the added effect of improving animal health by clearing other, non-human-infective trypanosomes of livestock. Cost-effective prevention strategies are a necessity in countries where human and animal health services are increasingly decentralised and where few funds are available generally for health improvement activities (Jeppsson and Okuonzi, 2000; Jeppsson, 2001; Bossert and Beauvais, 2002). Interventions aimed at domestic livestock, which ultimately improve human health are also relevant in other contexts. Rowland *et al.* (2001) treated cattle with deltamethrin pour-on insecticides to prevent transmission of malaria by zoophilic mosquitoes in peridomestic habitats in Pakistan, and the effective control of schistosomiasis caused by *Schistosoma japonicum* may depend, in some areas, on control of the parasite in the cattle reservoir (Guo *et al.*, 2001). Habtewold *et al.* (2004) have adopted a similar approach in Ethiopia in an attempt to reduce the incidence of malaria in households using pour-ons primarily to control tsetse. The perceived benefits to human health would, it is hoped, provide the impetus to promote and sustain the tsetse control strategy. Combining targeted chemotherapy with pour-ons or other methods of reducing transmission might present a user-friendly system applicable in areas with poor professional veterinary coverage. Understanding the biology and epidemiology of zoonotic diseases in their reservoir hosts (Cleaveland *et al.*, 2001; Woolhouse *et al.*, 2001) is essential to the appropriate design of public health interventions and disease control programmes.

7.4. Responsibility for Control

As we have seen, the control of epidemic HAT was historically the remit of governments, while endemic HAT received little attention. However, governments are increasingly unable to provide sufficient funds for such activities, and international organisations and NGOs are filling up this gap (Paquet *et al.*, 1995; Moore *et al.*, 1999; Abel *et al.*, 2004). NGOs are able to address specific issues in a targeted manner; however, it should be a long-term aim of such projects to devolve the activities to either national or local governments eventually. The following questions then arise: Where do the responsibilities for disease control lie? With government? With communities? With third parties such as NGOs? What role should international organisations play? The answers to these questions lie in the long-term goals of control programmes, in the availability of funding and economic development generally, and in the public health priority given to HAT over other disease by the players at different institutional levels. Molyneux (2001c) highlighted the conflict between the trend towards decentralisation and the need for a vertical approach to HAT control.

7.4.1. Government

Traditionally, as discussed above, trypanosomiasis control has been centralised at the government level; tsetse control, for example, has often been the remit of specialised sections of the government veterinary services. Rogers *et al.* (1994) reviewed a range of tsetse control activities across Africa, and concluded that governments there have effectively privatised tsetse control, moving towards a situation where the local population is responsible for control, albeit with some outside assistance in terms of expertise or funding. The degree of support provided for communities determines whether the programme can be termed community driven (Dransfield and Brightwell, 2004), and governments are likely to continue, at the very least, to set priority areas and facilitate interaction of communities with outside organisations.

Medical supervision of HAT treatment is necessarily hospital based, and HAT drug distribution is likely always to remain centralised and be the responsibility of Ministries of Health or specialised organisations—particularly given the poor availability of drugs at an international level. States, therefore, will always have a key role to play, though the degree to which they choose to devolve tsetse and livestock trypanosomiasis control will vary, usually as a function of the financial situation.

If the SIT does become a key component in governments' policies for trypanosomiasis control through the PATTEC initiative—(the Pan African Tsetse and Trypanosomiasis Eradication Campaign)— (Kabayo, 2002), a hitherto unseen level of international government commitment and co-ordination to trypanosomiasis control will be necessary, pooling resources for the re-establishment of a centralised system. Recently, the African Development Fund has agreed the finance to create sustainable tsetse and trypanosomiasis free areas in East and West Africa involving SIT and other technologies (African Development Fund, 2004). This project, which covers Burkina Faso, Mali, Ghana, Ethiopia, Uganda and Kenya, is being coordinated by PATTEC. Uganda is the only country seriously affected by HAT in this group and we must hope that this ambitious scheme proves successful in reducing the incidence of disease.

7.4.2. Community Control

As mentioned above, it is not practical (unlike with malaria) for individuals to treat themselves for HAT. Control undertaken by the community thus involves controlling transmission. In *T. b. gambiense* areas, where treatment of humans is a key component of overall prevention strategies, community control will supplement the necessarily centralised strategies, and will assist in the longer term prevention of new outbreaks. Laveissière *et al.* (1998) found that community health workers are more cost-effective than mobile teams for *T. b. gambiense* control in Côte d'Ivoire, and also found that community workers could be effective in deploying targets against tsetse (Laveissière *et al.*, 1994). Similarly, Okoth *et al.* (1991) have shown that communities can be encouraged to produce their own tsetse traps. These examples, while involving the community, are still dependent on a high degree of outside support.

Farmer-based tsetse control has been recently reviewed (Brightwell *et al.*, 2001; Dransfield and Brightwell, 2004), and it has been stressed that this needs to be driven by demand rather than supply. That is, a successful farmer-based programme to reduce tsetse density and control trypanosome transmission must be developed in conjunction with the community, and answer the specific needs of that community (White, 1996), rather than employ members of the community simply to undertake technical roles for an overall purpose which was not developed with their consultation and input. In reality, a combination of approaches is likely to be adopted, depending on the urgency with which control needs to be undertaken (epidemic vs. endemic situations).

7.4.3. Third Parties

NGOs have been very effective at HAT control (Paquet *et al.*, 1995). Their efforts are a form of disaster relief in war-torn or socially disrupted areas (Nathan *et al.*, 2004), and the withdrawal of such organisations needs to be planned with local health authorities to enable local partners to continue efforts once these authorities become re-established.

While health concerns have become global, it often remains the remit of national bodies to deal with specific disease issues. The international community, however, does have a role in ensuring that priorities are maintained even for the most neglected diseases (Dentico and Ford, 2005)—in particular, such diseases which affect poor, marginalised populations with few external linkages (Smith *et al.*, 2004).

International organisations and NGOs have a key long-term role in lobbying for increased drug production and supply (Wickware, 2002), and there have, to date, been sterling efforts involving HAT (Banerji, 2003; Pécoul, 2004), which have undoubtedly saved many thousands of lives. Only time will show how sustainable these efforts can be.

8. CONCLUSIONS

HAT, or sleeping sickness, describes not one but two discrete diseases; the Gambian and Rhodesian forms of the disease which present very different clinical pictures, the former chronic and the latter acute. The Gambian form is currently a major public health problem over vast areas of Africa from Sudan in the north through north-west Uganda, the Democratic Republic of the Congo to Angola in the south. The Rhodesian form continues to present a serious health risk in the Lake Victoria Basin, particularly in eastern Uganda, and there are small pockets of disease endemic in other countries of east and central Africa, which occasionally give rise to epidemics. A line drawn from north to south through sub-Saharan Africa, roughly following the Rift Valley, neatly differentiates the distribution of the two diseases with the Gambian form to the west and the Rhodesian to the east of this notional line.

Apart from these clinical and geographical differences, there are significant differences between the two diseases in their epidemiology, and any attempt to control them must take account of these differences. Outbreaks of the Gambian form of the disease, which have at times been on a massive scale both in terms of distribution and incidence, can be and have been brought under control by the simple expedient of case finding and effective treatment at a local level. The proven effectiveness of this approach reflects the fact that while domestic and wild animals may harbour *T. b. gambiense* trypanosomes, the major reservoir of Gambian disease lies in the human population. In the case of an epidemic of Rhodesian HAT, simple case finding and treatment will never be sufficient to achieve control as the major reservoir of *T. b. rhodesiense* trypanosomes lies not in the human population, but in animals; in the past the reservoir resided in game animals which in many parts of modern Africa have been replaced by domestic livestock as the major reservoir of disease. Any attempt to control the incidence and spread of Rhodesian HAT must now also address the question of controlling infections in the livestock reservoir. In practice, at the community level, this will involve both treatment of human cases and chemotherapy and/or insecticidal treatment of livestock to reduce local transmission by tsetse in the area at risk. To prevent the spread of disease, livestock from affected areas should be suitably screened and treated before being traded into adjacent unaffected zones.

For the most part, we have been describing tactics designed to contain outbreaks of human disease at a local level. It has, however, been the long-held desire of many African countries to free themselves from the threat of HAT on a permanent basis. In eastern Africa, in particular, this aim was prompted largely by the economic benefits which could accrue from simultaneously removing nagana in livestock (Shaw, 2004). Such longer term aims can be achieved only by removal of the tsetse fly on a permanent basis—i.e. elimination. In considering elimination rather than disease control, we immediately enter controversial waters: modellers do not agree on whether elimination on a permanent basis is achievable (Rogers and Randolph, 2002; Hargrove, 2003b); ecologists do not agree whether this aim is desirable or even environmentally abusive (Bourn *et al.*, 2001); economists argue about cost/benefit ratios (Shaw, 2004); technologists do not agree on the most appropriate technology to adopt (Vale *et al.*, 1999; Vreysen *et al.*, 2000; Allsopp, 2001); sociologists suggest that failures in the past reflect our inability properly to involve local communities at the correct level (Barrett and Okali, 1998; Brightwell *et al.*, 2001; Dransfield and Brightwell, 2004); politicians and donor agencies worry about the cost of large-scale tsetse control projects which, if they fail to achieve elimination, may become on-going burdens on their budgets which, in the case of human health, have many pressing demands in sub-Saharan Africa (Molyneux, 2001c). It has not been the purpose of this review to recommend one course of action over another—the choices made must be tailored to the needs and circumstances of individual African nations who must make their own assessments of the specific risks involved. Suffice to say that the history of tsetse control is littered with expensive projects with a few limited success stories—success may be more likely in a scenario where a range of approaches is combined. The failures may not always be laid at the door of technology, but often lie at the human level, whether that of the local community, state or international community.

ACKNOWLEDGEMENTS

This work was supported by the Animal Health Programme of the UK Department for International Development, though the views expressed do not necessarily represent those of DFID.

REFERENCES

Abel, P.M., Kiala, G., Loa, V., Behrend, M., Musolf, J., Fleishmann, H., Theophile, J., Krishna, S. and Stich, A. (2004). Retaking sleeping sickness control in Angola. *Tropical Medicine and International Health* **9**, 141–148.

Afewerk, Y., Clausen, P.H., Abebe, G., Tilahun, G. and Mehlitz, D. (2000). Multiple-drug resistant *Trypanosoma congolense* populations in village cattle of Metekel district, north-west Ethiopia. *Acta Tropica* **76**, 231–238.

African Development Fund. (2004). *Creation of sustainable tsetse and trypanosomiasis free areas in East and West Africa: appraisal report*. Available at: http://www.afdb.org. Tunis: African Development Fund.

Akol, M.N., Olaho-Mukani, W., Odiit, M., Enyaru, J.C.K., Matovu, E., Magona, J. and Okitoi, N.D. (1999). Trypanosomosis agglutination card test for *Trypanosoma brucei rhodesiense* sleeping sickness. *East African Medical Journal* **76**, 38–41.

Allsopp, R. (2001). Options for vector control against trypanosomiasis in Africa. *Trends in Parasitology* **17**, 15–19.

Allsopp, R. and Hursey, B.H. (2004). Insecticidal control of tsetse. In: *The Trypanosomiases* (I. Maudlin, P.H. Holmes and M.A. Miles, eds), pp. 491–507. Wallingford: CABI.

Anderson, R.M. and May, R.M. (1992). *Infectious Diseases of Humans: Dynamics and Control*. Oxford: University Press Oxord.

Anonymous (1909). Sleeping sickness news: preventative measures in Uganda. *Sleeping Sickness Bureau Bulletin* **1**, 118–119.

Apted, F.I. (1980). Present status of chemotherapy and chemopropylaxis of human trypanosomiasis in the Eastern Hemisphere. *Pharmacology and Therapeutics* **11**, 391–413.

Apted, F.I.C. (1970). Clinical manifestations and diagnosis of sleeping sickness. In: *The African Trypanosomiases* (W.E. Kershaw, ed.), pp. 661–683. London: George Allen and Unwin.

Ashcroft, M.T., Burtt, E. and Fairbairn, H. (1959). The experimental infection of some African wild animals with *Trypanosoma rhodesiense, T. brucei* and *T. congolense. Annals of Tropical Medicine and Parasitology* **53**, 147–161.

Awan, M.A. (1979). Identification by the blood incubation infectivity test of *Trypanosoma brucei* subspecies isolated from game animals in the Luangwa Valley, Zambia. *Acta Tropica* **36**, 343–347.

Baker, J.R., 1974. Epidemiology of African sleeping sickness. In: *Trypanosomiasis and Leishmaniasis with Special Reference to Chagas Disease* (Ciba Foundation, ed.), pp. 29–50. Amsterdam: Elsevier.

Banerji, J. (2003). New initiative to develop drugs for neglected diseases. *Essential Drugs Monitor* **33**, 28.

Barrett, K. and Okali, C., 1998. *Partnerships for Tsetse Control: Community Participation and Other Options.* Working Document No 6. Harare, Zimbabwe: PAAT Advisory Group Co-ordinators.

Barrett, M.P. (1999). The fall and rise of sleeping sickness. *Lancet* **353**, 1113–1114.

Barrett, M.P. (2001). Veterinary link to drug resistance in human African trypanosomiasis? *Lancet* **358**, 603–604.

Barrett, M.P. and Fairlamb, A.H. (1999). The biochemical basis of arsenical-diamidine cross-resistance in African trypanosomes. *Parasitology Today* **15**, 136–140.

Bauer, B., Kabore, I., Liebisch, A., Meyer, F. and Petrichbauer, J. (1992). Simultaneous control of ticks and tsetse flies in Satiri, Burkina-Faso, by the use of flumethrin pour on for cattle. *Tropical Medicine and Parasitology* **43**, 41–46.

Bennett, G.F. (1962). The haematocrit centrifuge for laboratory diagnosis of hematozoa. *Canadian Journal of Zoology* **40**, 124–125.

Berberof, M., Perez-Morga, D. and Pays, E. (2001). A receptor-like flagellar pocket glycoprotein specific to *Trypanosoma brucei gambiense. Molecular and Biochemical Parasitology* **113**, 127–138.

Bertram, B.C. (1973). Sleeping sickness survey in the Serengeti area (Tanzania) 1971. 3. Discussion of the relevance of the *Trypanosoma* survey to the biology of large mammals in the Serengeti. *Acta Tropica* **30**, 36–48.

Bisser, S., Bouteille, B., Sarda, J., Stanghellini, A., Ricard, D., Jauberteau, M.O., Marchan, F., Dumas, M. and Breton, J.C. (1997). Apport des examens biochimiques dans le diagnostic de la phase nerveuse de la trypanosomose humaine africaine. *Bulletin de la Société de Pathologie Exotique* **90**, 321–326.

Bisser, S., Lejon, V., Preux, P.M., Bouteille, B., Stanghellini, A., Jauberteau, M.O., Büscher, P. and Dumas, M. (2002). Blood–cerebrospinal fluid barrier and intrathecal immunoglobulins compared to field diagnosis of central nervous system involvement in sleeping sickness. *Journal of the Neurological Sciences* **193**, 127–135.

Blum, J., Nkunku, S. and Burri, C. (2001). Clinical description of encephalopathic syndromes and risk factors for their occurrence and outcome during melarsoprol treatment of human African trypanosomiasis. *Tropical Medicine and International Health* **6**, 390–400.

Bossert, T.J. and Beauvais, J.C. (2002). Decentralization of health systems in Ghana, Zambia, Uganda and the Philippines: a comparative analysis of decision space. *Health Policy and Planning* **17**, 14–31.

Bourn, D. and Blench, R. (1999). *Can Livestock and Wildlife Co-exist? An Interdisciplinary Approach*. London: ODI.

Bourn, D., Reid, R., Rogers, D., Snow, W. and Wint, W. (2001). *Environmental Change and the Autonomous Control of Tsetse and Trypanosomiasis in sub-Saharan Africa*. Oxford: Environmental Research Group.

Bouteille, B., Oukem, O., Bisser, S. and Dumas, M. (2003). Treatment perspectives for human African trypanosomiasis. *Fundamental & Clinical Pharmacology* **17**, 171–181.

Brightwell, B., Dransfield, B., Maudlin, I., Stevenson, P. and Shaw, A. (2001). Reality vs. rhetoric—a survey and evaluation of tsetse control in East Africa. *Agriculture and Human Values* **18**, 219–233.

Brightwell, R., Dransfield, R.D. and Kyorku, C. (1991). Development of a low-cost tsetse trap and odour baits for *Glossina pallidipes* and *G. longipennis* in Kenya. *Medical and Veterinary Entomology* **5**, 153–164.

Bromidge, T., Gibson, W., Hudson, K. and Dukes, P. (1993). Identification of *Trypanosoma brucei gambiense* by PCR amplification of variant surface glycoprotein genes. *Acta Tropica* **53**, 107–119.

Bruce, D., Hamerton, A.E., Bateman, H.R. and Mackie, F.P. (1910). Cattle as a sleeping sickness reservoir. *Sleeping Sickness Bureau Bulletin* **2**, 235–236.

Bruce, D., Hamerton, A.E., Bateman, H.R., Mackie, F.P. and Bruce, L. (1911). Experiments designed to discover the source of the infection of sleeping sickness. *Reports of the Sleeping Sickness Commission of the Royal Society* **11**, 71–111.

Brun, R., Schumacher, R., Schmid, C., Kunz, C. and Burri, C. (2001). The phenomenon of treatment failures in Human African Trypanosomiasis. *Tropical Medicine and International Health* **6**, 906–914.

Bruto da Costa, B.F., Firminto Sant'Anna, J., Correia dos Santos, A. and de Araujo Alvares, M.G. (1916). *Sleeping Sickness: a Record of Four Years' War Against it in Principe, Portugese West Africa*. London: Baillière, Tindall and Cox.

Burri, C. and Brun, R. (2003). Eflornithine for the treatment of human African trypanosomiasis. *Parasitology Research* **90**, S49–S52.

Burri, C. and Keiser, J. (2001). Pharmacokinetic investigations in patients from northern Angola refractory to melarsoprol treatment. *Tropical Medicine & International Health* **6**, 412–420.

Burri, C., Nkunku, S., Merolle, A., Smith, T., Blum, J. and Brun, R. (2000). Efficacy of new, concise schedule for melarsoprol in treatment of sleeping sickness caused by *Trypanosoma brucei gambiense*: a randomised trial. *Lancet* **355**, 1419–1425.

Bursell, E., Gough, A.J.E., Beevor, P.S., Cork, A., Hall, D.R. and Vale, G.A. (1988). Identification of components of cattle urine attractive to tsetse flies, *Glossina* spp (Diptera, Glossinidae). *Bulletin of Entomological Research* **78**, 281–291.

Büscher, P., Lejon, V., Magnus, E. and Van Meirvenne, N. (1999). Improved latex agglutination test for detection of antibodies in serum and cerebrospinal fluid of *Trypanosoma brucei gambiense* infected patients. *Acta Tropica* **73**, 11–20.

Callahan, J.D., Brown, F., Osorio, F.A., Sur, J.H., Kramer, E., Long, G.W., Lubroth, J., Ellis, S.J., Shoulars, K.S., Gaffney, K.L., Rock, D.L. and Nelson, W.M. (2002). Use of a portable real-time reverse transcriptase-polymerase chain reaction assay for rapid detection of foot-and-mouth disease virus. *Journal of the American Veterinary Medical Association* **220**, 1636–1642.

Carter, N.S. and Fairlamb, A.H. (1993). Arsenical-resistant trypanosomes lack an unusual adenosine transporter. *Nature* **361**, 173–176.

Cattand, P., Miezan, B.T. and de Raadt, P. (1988). Human African trypanosomiasis: use of double centrifugation of cerebrospinal fluid to detect trypanosomes. *Bulletin of the World Health Organization* **66**, 83–86.

Chappuis, F., Loutan, L., Simarro, P., Lejon, V. and Büscher, P. (2005). Options for field diagnosis of human African trypanosomiasis. *Clinical Microbiology Reviews* **18**, 133–146.

Clausen, P.H., Adeyemi, I., Bauer, B., Breloeer, M., Salchow, F. and Staak, C. (1998). Host preferences of tsetse (Diptera: Glossinidae) based on bloodmeal identifications. *Medical and Veterinary Entomology* **12**, 169–180.

Clausen, P.H., Sidibe, I., Kabore, I. and Bauer, B. (1992). Development of multiple drug resistance of *Trypanosoma congolense* in Zebu cattle under high natural tsetse fly challenge in the pastoral zone of Samorogouan, Burkina Faso. *Acta Tropica* **51**, 229–236.

Cleaveland, S., Laurenson, M.K. and Taylor, L.H. (2001). Diseases of humans and their domestic mammals: pathogen characteristics, host range and the risk of emergence. *Philosophical Transactions of the Royal Society of London Series B—Biological Sciences* **356**, 991–999.

Codjia, V., Mulatu, W., Majiwa, P.A., Leak, S.G., Rowlands, G.J., Authie, E., d'Ieteren, G.D. and Peregrine, A.S. (1993). Epidemiology of bovine trypanosomiasis in the Ghibe valley, southwest Ethiopia. 3. Occurrence of populations of *Trypanosoma congolense* resistant to diminazene, isometamidium and homidium. *Acta Tropica* **53**, 151–163.

Coleman, P.G., Perry, B.D. and Woolhouse, M.E.J. (2001). Endemic stability—a veterinary idea applied to human public health. *Lancet* **357**, 1284–1286.

Coleman, P.G. and Welburn, S.C. (2004). Are fitness costs associated with resistance to human serum in *Trypanosoma brucei rhodesiense*? *Trends in Parasitology* **20**, 311–315.

Contamin, H., Fandeur, T., Bonnefoy, S., Skouri, F., Ntoumi, F. and Mercereau-Puijalon, O. (1995). PCR typing of field isolates of *Plasmodium falciparum*. *Journal of Clinical Microbiology* **33**, 944–951.

Dale, C., Welburn, S.C., Maudlin, I. and Milligan, P.J.M. (1995). The kinetics of maturation of trypanosome infections in tsetse. *Parasitology* **111**, 187–191.

de Greef, C. and Hamers, R. (1994). The serum resistance-associated (*SRA*) gene of *Trypanosoma brucei rhodesiense* encodes a variant surface glycoprotein-like protein. *Molecular and Biochemical Parasitology* **68**, 277–284.

de Greef, C., Imberechts, H., Matthyssens, G., Van Meirvenne, N. and Hamers, R. (1989). A gene expressed only in serum resistant variants of *Trypanosoma brucei rhodesiense*. *Molecular and Biochemical Parasitology* **36**, 169–176.

de la Rocque, S., Augusseau, X., Guillobez, S., Michel, V., De Wispelaere, G., Bauer, B. and Cuisance, D. (2001). The changing distribution of two riverine tsetse flies over 15 years in an increasingly cultivated area of Burkina Faso. *Bulletin of Entomological Research* **91**, 157–166.

de la Rocque, S., Bengaly, Z., Michel, J.F., Solano, P., Sidibé, I. and Cuisance, D. (1999). Importance des interfaces spatiales et temporelles entre les bovins et les glossines dans la transmission de la trypanosomose animale en Afrique de l'Ouest. *Revue d'Elevage et de Médecine Vétérinaire des Pays Tropicaux* **52**, 215–222.

Dentico, N. and Ford, N. (2005). The courage to change the rules: a proposal for an essential Health R&D treaty. *Public Library of Science Medicine* **2**, 96–99.

Docampo, R. and Moreno, S.N. (2003). Current chemotherapy of human African trypanosomiasis. *Parasitology Research* **90**, S10–S13.

Dransfield, R.D. and Brightwell, R. (2004). Community participation in tsetse control. In: *The Trypanosomiases* (I. Maudlin, P.H. Holmes and M.A. Miles, eds), pp. 533–546. Wallingford: CABI.

Ducloux, M. (1988). Eugène Jamot (1879–1937): un fils du Limousin. *Bulletin de la Société de Pathologie Exotique* **81**, 419–426.

Dukes, P., Gibson, W.C., Gashumba, J.K., Hudson, K.M., Bromidge, T.J., Kaukus, A., Asonganyi, T. and Magnus, E. (1992). Absence of the LiTat 1.3 (CATT antigen) gene in *Trypanosoma brucei gambiense* stocks from Cameroon. *Acta Tropica* **51**, 123–134.

Dutton, J.E. (1902). Note on a *Trypanosoma* occurring in the blood of man. *British Medical Journal* **2**, 881–884.

Eckart, W.U. (2002). The colony as laboratory: German sleeping sickness campaigns in German East Africa and in Togo, 1900–1914. *History and Philosophy of the Life Sciences* **24**, 69–89.

Eisler, M.C., Torr, S.J., Coleman, P.G., Machila, N. and Morton, J.F. (2003). Integrated control of vector-borne diseases of livestock—pyrethroids: panacea or poison? *Trends in Parasitology* **19**, 341–345.

Ekwanzala, M., Pépin, J., Khonde, N., Molisho, S., Bruneel, H. and De Wals, P. (1996). In the heart of darkness: sleeping sickness in Zaire. *Lancet* **348**, 1427–1430.

Eltringham, S.K. and Malpas, R.C. (1993). The conservation status of Uganda game and forest reserves in 1982 and 1983. *African Journal of Ecology* **31**, 91–105.

Enyaru, J.C., Matovu, E., Akol, M., Sebikali, C., Kyambadde, J., Schmidt, C., Brun, R., Kaminsky, R., Ogwal, L.M. and Kansiime, F. (1998). Parasitological detection of *Trypanosoma brucei gambiense* in serologically negative sleeping-sickness suspects from north-western Uganda. *Annals of Tropical Medicine and Parasitology* **92**, 845–850.

Enyaru, J.C.K., Allingham, R., Bromidge, T., Kanmogne, G.D. and Carasco, J.F. (1993). The isolation and genetic heterogeneity of *Trypanosoma brucei gambiense* from north-west Uganda. *Acta Tropica* **54**, 31–39.

Enyaru, J.C.K., Odiit, M., Winyi-Kaboyo, R., Sebikali, C.G., Matovu, E., Okitoi, D. and Olaho-Mukani, W. (1999). Evidence for the occurrence of *Trypanosoma brucei rhodesiense* sleeping sickness outside the traditional focus in south-eastern Uganda. *Annals of Tropical Medicine and Parasitology* **93**, 817–822.

Fairbairn, H. (1948). Sleeping sickness in Tanganyika Territory, 1922–1946. *Tropical Medicine Bulletin* **45**, 1–17.

Fairlamb, A.H. (2003). Chemotherapy of human African trypanosomiasis: current and future prospects. *Trends in Parasitology* **19**, 488–494.

Fèvre, E.M., Coleman, P.G., Odiit, M., Magona, J.W., Welburn, S.C. and Woolhouse, M.E.J. (2001). The origins of a new *Trypanosoma brucei rhodesiense* sleeping sickness outbreak in eastern Uganda. *Lancet* **358**, 625–628.

Fèvre, E.M., Coleman, P.G., Welburn, S.C. and Maudlin, I. (2004). Re-analyzing the 1900–1920 sleeping sickness epidemic in Uganda. *Emerging Infectious Diseases* **10**, 567–573.

Fèvre, E.M., Picozzi, K., Fyfe, J., Waiswa, C., Odiit, M., Coleman, P.G. and Welburn, S.C. (2005). A burgeoning epidemic of sleeping sickness in Uganda. *Lancet* **366**, 745–747.

Ford, J. (1970). Control by destruction of the larger fauna. In: *The African Trypanosomiases* (H.W. Mulligan, W.H. Potts and W.E. Kershaw, eds), pp. 557–571. London: George Allen and Unwin.

Ford, J. and Katondo, K.M. (1977). Maps of tsetse fly (*Glossina*) distribution in Africa, 1973 according to sub-generic groups on scale of 1:5,000,000. *Bulletin of Animal Production in Africa* **25**, 188–194.

Ford, J., Nash, T.A.M. and Welch, J.R. (1970). Control by clearing of vegetation. In: *The African Trypanosomiases* (H.W. Mulligan, W.H. Potts and W.E. Kershaw, eds), pp. 543–556. London: George Allen and Unwin.

Forde, R.M. (1902). The discovery of the human *Trypanosoma*. *British Medical Journal* **2**, 1741.

Geerts, S., Holmes, P.H., Diall, O. and Eisler, M.C. (2001). African bovine trypanosomiasis: the problem of drug resistance. *Trends in Parasitology* **17**, 25–28.

Geigy, R., Jenni, L., Kauffmann, M., Onyango, R.J. and Weiss, N. (1975). Identification of *T. brucei* subgroup strains isolated from game. *Acta Tropica* **32**, 190–205.

Geigy, R., Mwambu, P.M. and Kauffmann, M. (1971). Sleeping sickness survey in Musoma District, Tanzania. IV. Examination of wild mammals as a potential reservoir for *T. rhodesiense*. *Acta Tropica* **18**, 221–230.

Gibson, W., Backhouse, T. and Griffiths, A. (2002). The human serum resistance associated gene is ubiquitous and conserved in *Trypanosoma brucei rhodesiense* throughout East Africa. *Infection, Genetics and Evolution* **25**, 1–8.

Gibson, W. and Ferris, V. (2003). Conservation of the genomic location of the human serum resistance associated gene in *Trypanosoma brucei rhodesiense*. *Molecular and Biochemical Parasitology* **130**, 159–162.

Gibson, W., Mehlitz, D., Lanham, S.M. and Godfrey, D.G. (1978). The identification of *Trypanosoma brucei gambiense* in Liberian pigs and dogs by isoenzymes and by resistance to human plasma. *Tropenmedizin und Parasitologie* **29**, 335–345.

Gooding, R.H. and Krafsur, E.S. (2004). Tsetse genetics: applications to biology and systematics. In: *The Trypanosomiases* (I. Maudlin, P.H. Holmes and M.A. Miles, eds), pp. 95–111. Wallingford: CABI.

Gouteux, J.P. and Artzrouni, M. (1996). Faut-il ou non un contrôle des vecteurs dans la lutte contre la maladie du sommeil? Une approche biomathématique du problème. *Bulletin de la Société de Pathologie Exotique* **89**, 299–305.

Gouteux, J.P. and Sinda, D. (1990). Community participation in the control of tsetse flies—large-scale trials using the pyramid trap in the Congo. *Tropical Medicine and Parasitology* **41**, 49–55.

Gray, M.A., Kimarua, R.W., Peregrine, A.S. and Stevenson, P. (1993). Drug sensitivity screening in vitro of populations of *Trypanosoma congolense* originating from cattle and tsetse flies at Nguruman, Kenya. *Acta Tropica* **55**, 1–9.

Guo, J.G., Ross, A.G., Lin, D.D., Williams, G.M., Chen, H.G., Li, Y., Davis, G.M., Feng, Z., McManus, D.P. and Sleigh, A.C. (2001). A baseline study on the importance of bovines for human *Schistosoma japonicum* infection around Poyang Lake, China. *American Journal of Tropical Medicine and Hygiene* **65**, 272–278.

Guyatt, H.L., Ochola, S.A. and Snow, R.W. (2002). Too poor to pay: charging for insecticide-treated bednets in highland Kenya. *Tropical Medicine and International Health* **7**, 846–850.

Habtewold, T., Prior, A., Torr, S.J. and Gibson, G. (2004). Could insecticide-treated cattle reduce Afrotropical malaria transmission? Effects of deltamethrin-treated Zebu on *Anopheles arabiensis* behaviour and survival in Ethiopia. *Medical and Veterinary Entomology* **18**, 408–417.

Haller, L., Adams, H., Merouze, F. and Dago, A. (1986). Clinical and pathological aspects of human African trypanosomiasis (*T. b. gambiense*). with particular reference to reactive arsenical encephalopathy. *American Journal of Tropical Medicine and Hygiene* **35**, 94–99.

Hargrove, J.W. (2003a). Optimized simulation of the control of tsetse flies *Glossina pallidipes* and *G. m. morsitans* (Diptera: Glossinidae) using odour-baited targets in Zimbabwe. *Bulletin of Entomological Research* **93**, 19–29.

Hargrove, J.W. (2003b). *Tsetse Eradication: Sufficiency, Necessity and Desirability*. Research report. Edinburgh: DFID Animal Health Programme, Centre for Tropical Veterinary Medicine, University of Edinburgh, UK.

Hargrove, J.W. (2004). Tsetse population dynamics. In: *The Trypanosomiases* (I. Maudlin, P.H. Holmes and M.A. Miles, eds), pp. 113–137. Wallingford: CABI.

Heisch, R.B., McMahon, J.P. and Manson-Bahr, P.E.C. (1958). The isolation of *Trypanosoma rhodesiense* from a bushbuck. *British Medical Journal* **2**, 1203–1204.

Herder, S., Simo, G., Nkinin, S. and Njiokou, F. (2002). Identification of trypanosomes in wild animals from southern Cameroon using the polymerase chain reaction (PCR). *Parasite* **9**, 345–349.

Hickman, J.G., Huber, F. and Palmisano, M. (2001). Human dermal safety studies with eflornithine HCl 13.9% cream (Vaniqa), a novel treatment for excessive facial hair. *Current Medical Research and Opinion* **16**, 235–244.

Hodges, A.D.P. (1910). Progress report on the Uganda sleeping sickness camps from December, 1906, to November, 1909. *Sleeping Sickness Bureau Bulletin* **2**, 260–271.

Holmes, P.H. (1997). New approaches to the integrated control of trypanosomosis. *Veterinary Parasitology* **71**, 121–135.

Itazi, O.K. (1981). *Radial Immunodiffusion as a Diagnostic Test for African Human Trypanosomiasis in Cases with Neurological Involvement.* Report of the 17th meeting. Arusha: International Scientific Council for Trypanosomiasis Research and Control.

Iten, M., Matovu, E., Brun, R. and Kaminsky, R. (1995). Innate lack of susceptibility of Ugandan *Trypanosoma brucei rhodesiense* to DL-alpha-difluoromethylornithine (DFMO). *Tropical Medicine and Parasitology* **46**, 190–194.

Jamonneau, V., Ravel, S., Koffi, M., Kaba, D., Zeze, D.G., Ndri, L., Sane, B., Coulibaly, B., Cuny, G. and Solano, P. (2004). Mixed infections of trypanosomes in tsetse and pigs and their epidemiological significance in a sleeping sickness focus of Cote d'Ivoire. *Parasitology* **129**, 693–702.

Jamonneau, V., Solano, P., Garcia, A., Lejon, V., Dje, N., Miezan, T.W., N'Guessan, P., Cuny, G. and Büscher, P. (2003). Stage determination and therapeutic decision in human African trypanosomiasis: value of polymerase chain reaction and immunoglobulin M quantification on the cerebrospinal fluid of sleeping sickness patients in Cote d'lvoire. *Tropical Medicine & International Health* **8**, 589–594.

Jamonneau, V., Truc, P., Garcia, A., Magnus, E. and Büscher, P. (2000). Preliminary evaluation of LATEX/*T.b.gambiense* and alternative versions of CATT/*T.b.gambiense* for the serodiagnosis of human african trypanosomiasis of a population at risk in Cote d'Ivoire: considerations for mass-screening. *Acta Tropica* **76**, 175–183.

Jannin, J. and Cattand, P. (2004). Treatment and control of human African trypanosomiasis. *Current Opinion in Infectious Diseases* **17**, 565–571.

Jannin, J., Simarro, P.P. and Louis, F.J. (2003). Le concept de maladie negligée. *Médecine Tropicale* **63**, 219–221.

Jelinek, T., Bisoffi, Z., Bonazzi, L., van Thiel, P., Bronner, U., de Frey, A., Gundersen, S.G., McWhinney, P., Ripamonti, D. and European Network on Imported Infectious Disease Surveillance. (2003). Cluster of African trypanosomiasis in travelers to Tanzanian national parks. *Emerging Infectious Diseases* **8**, 634–635.

Jeppsson, A. (2001). Financial priorities under decentralization in Uganda. *Health Policy and Planning* **16**, 187–192.

Jeppsson, A. and Okuonzi, S.A. (2000). Vertical or holistic decentralization of the health sector? Experiences from Zambia and Uganda. *International Journal of Health Planning and Management* **15**, 273–289.

Kabayo, J.P. (2002). Aiming to eliminate tsetse from Africa. *Trends in Parasitology* **18**, 473–475.

Kabiri, M., Franco, J.R., Simarro, P.P., Ruiz, J.A., Sarsa, M. and Steverding, D. (1999). Detection of *Trypanosoma brucei gambiense* in sleeping sickness suspects by PCR amplification of expression-site-associated genes 6 and 7. *Tropical Medicine and International Health* **4**, 658–661.

Kanmogne, G.D., Asonganyi, T. and Gibson, W.C. (1996). Detection of *Trypanosoma brucei gambiense*, in serologically positive but aparasitaemic sleeping-sickness suspects in Cameroon, by PCR. *Annals of Tropical Medicine and Parasitology* **90**, 475–483.

Kitron, U., Otieno, L.H., Hungerford, L.L., Odulaja, A., Brigham, W.U., Okello, O.O., Joselyn, M., MohamedAhmed, M.M. and Cook, E. (1996). Spatial analysis of the distribution of tsetse flies in the Lambwe Valley, Kenya, using Landsat TM satellite imagery and GIS. *Journal of Animal Ecology* **65**, 371–380.

Köerner, T., de Raadt, P. and Maudlin, I. (1995). The 1901 Uganda sleeping sickness epidemic revisited: a case of mistaken identity? *Parasitology Today* **11**, 303–305.

Krafsur, E.S., Whitten, C.J. and Novy, J.E. (1987). Screwworm eradication in North and Central America. *Parasitology Today* **3**, 131–137.

Kristensson, K. and Bentivoglio, M. (1999). Pathology of African trypanosomiasis. In: *Progress in Human African Trypanosomiasis, Sleeping Sickness* (M. Dumas, B. Bouteille and A. Buguet, eds), pp. 157–181. Paris: Springer.

Kristjanson, P.M., Swallow, B.M., Rowlands, G.J., Kruska, R.L. and de Leeuw, P.N. (1999). Measuring the costs of African animal trypanosomosis, the potential benefits of control and returns to research. *Agricultural Systems* **59**, 79–98.

Kuboki, N., Inoue, N., Sakurai, T., Di Cello, F., Grab, D.J., Suzuki, H., Sugimoto, C. and Igarashi, I. (2003). Loop-mediated isothermal amplification for detection of African trypanosomes. *Journal of Clinical Microbiology* **41**, 5517–5524.

Kyambadde, J.W., Enyaru, J.C.K., Matovu, E., Odiit, M. and Carasco, J.F. (2000). Detection of trypanosomes in suspected sleeping sickness patients in Uganda using the polymerase chain reaction. *Bulletin of the World Health Organization* **78**, 119–124.

Lancien, J. (1991). Lutte contre la maladie du sommeil dans le sud-est Ouganda par piégeage des Glossines. *Annales de la Société Belge de Médecine Tropicale* **71**, 35–47.

Langlands, B.W. (1967). *The Sleeping Sickness Epidemic of Uganda, 1900–1920: A Study in Historical Geography.* Occasional Paper No. 1. Kampala: Makerere University College.

Lapeyssonnie, L. (1992). Geometrie et passion. La lutte contre la maladie du sommeil. *Annales de la Société Belge de Médecine Tropicale* **72**, 7–12.

Laveissière, C. and Boreham, P.F.L. (1976). Ecologie de *Glossina tachinoides* Westwood, 1850, en savane humide d'Afrique de l'Ouest. I. Préférences trophiques. *Cahiers ORSTOM, série Entomologie Médicale et Parasitologie* **14**, 187–200.

Laveissière, C. and Grebaut, P. (1990). Recherches sur les pièges à glossines (Diptera: Glossinidae). Mise au point d'un modèle économique: le piège "Vavoua". *Tropical Medicine and Parasitology* **41**, 185–192.

Laveissière, C., Grebaut, P., Lemasson, J.-J., Méda, H.A., Couret, D., Doua, F., Brou, N. and Cattand, P. (1994). *Les Communautés Rurales et la Lutte Contre la Maladie du Sommeil en Fôret de Côte d'Ivoire.* WHO/TRY/94.1. Geneva: World Health Organization.

Laveissière, C., Meda, A.H., Doua, F. and Sane, B. (1998). Detecting sleeping sickness: a comparison between the efficacy of mobile teams and community health workers. *Bulletin of the World Health Organization* **76**, 559–564.

Leak, S.G.A. (1999). *Tsetse Biology and Ecology: Their Role in the Epidemiology and Control of Trypanosomosis.* Wallingford: CABI International.

Legros, D., Ollivier, G., Gastellu-Etchegorry, M., Paquet, C., Burri, C., Jannin, J. and Büscher, P. (2002). Treatment of human African trypanosomiasis—present situation and needs for research and development. *Lancet Infectious Diseases* **2**, 437–440.

Lejon, V., Büscher, P., Magnus, E., Moons, A., Wouters, I. and Van Meirvenne, N. (1998a). A semi-quantitative ELISA for detection of *Trypanosoma brucei gambiense* specific antibodies in serum and cerebrospinal fluid of sleeping sickness patients. *Acta Tropica* **69**, 151–164.

Lejon, V., Büscher, P., Sema, N.H., Magnus, E. and Van Meirvenne, N. (1998b). Human African trypanosomiasis: a latex agglutination field test for quantifying IgM in cerebrospinal fluid. *Bulletin of the World Health Organization* **76**, 553–558.

Lejon, V., Kwete, J. and Büscher, P. (2003). Towards saliva-based screening for sleeping sickness? *Tropical Medicine and International Health* **8**, 585–588.

Lejon, V., Legros, D., Richer, M., Ruiz, J.A., Jamonneau, V., Truc, P., Doua, F., Dje, N., N'Siesi, F.X., Bisser, S., Magnus, E., Wouters, I., Konings, J., Vervoort, T., Sultan, F. and Büscher, P. (2002). IgM quantification in the cerebrospinal fluid of sleeping sickness patients by a latex card agglutination test. *Tropical Medicine and International Health* **7**, 685–692.

Lengeler, C. (2004). Insecticide-treated bed nets and curtains for preventing malaria. *Cochrane Database of Systematic Reviews* **2**, CD000363.

Lindquist, D.A., Abusowa, M. and Hall, M.J.R. (1992). The New-World screwworm fly in Libya—a review of its introduction and eradication. *Medical and Veterinary Entomology* **6**, 2–8.

Lingam, S., Marshall, W.C., Wilson, J., Gould, J.M., Reinhardt, M.C. and Evans, D.A. (1985). Congenital trypanosomiasis in a child born in London. *Developmental Medicine and Child Neurology* **27**, 670–674.

Louis, F.J., Simarro, P.P. and Lucas, P. (2002). Maladie du sommeil: cent ans d'évolution des strategies de lutte. *Bulletin de la Société de Pathologie Exotique* **95**, 331–336.

Lumsden, W.H., Kimber, C.D., Evans, D.A. and Doig, S.J. (1979). *Trypanosoma brucei*: miniature anion-exchange centrifugation technique for detection of low parasitaemias: adaptation for field use. *Transactions of the Royal Society of Tropical Medicine and Hygiene* **73**, 312–317.

Lyons, M. (1992). *The Colonial Disease: A Social History of Sleeping Sickness in Northern Zaire, 1900–1940.* Cambridge: Cambridge University Press.

MacKichan, I.W. (1944). Rhodesian sleeping sickness in eastern Uganda. *Transactions of the Royal Society of Tropical Medicine and Hygiene* **38**, 49–60.

MacLean, L., Chisi, J.E., Odiit, M., Gibson, W.C., Ferris, V., Picozzi, K. and Sternberg, J.M. (2004). Severity of human African trypanosomiasis in East Africa is associated with geographic location, parasite genotype, and host inflammatory cytokine response profile. *Infection and Immunity* **72**, 7040–7044.

Magnus, E., Vervoort, T. and Van Meirvenne, N. (1978). A card agglutination test with stained trypanosomes (CATT) for the serological diagnosis of *T.b. gambiense* trypanosomiasis. *Annales de la Société Belge de Médecine Tropicale* **58**, 169–176.

Masake, R.A., Njuguna, J.T., Brown, C.C. and Majiwa, P.A. (2002). The application of PCR–ELISA to the detection of *Trypanosoma brucei* and *T. vivax* infections in livestock. *Veterinary Parasitology* **105**, 179–189.

Matovu, E., Enyaru, J.C.K., Legros, D., Schmid, C., Seebeck, T. and Kaminsky, R. (2001a). Melarsoprol refractory *T.b. gambiense* from Omugo, north-western Uganda. *Tropical Medicine & International Health* **6**, 407–411.

Matovu, E., Iten, M., Enyaru, J.C.K., Schmid, C., Lubega, G.W., Brun, R. and Kaminsky, R. (1997). Susceptibility of Ugandan *Trypanosoma brucei rhodesiense* isolated from man and animal reservoirs to diminazene, isometamidium and melarsoprol. *Tropical Medicine & International Health* **2**, 13–18.

Matovu, E., Seebeck, T., Enyaru, J.C.K. and Kaminsky, R. (2001b). Drug resistance in *Trypanosoma brucei* spp., the causative agents of sleeping sickness in man and nagana in cattle. *Microbes and Infection* **3**, 763–770.

Mattioli, R.C., Jaitner, J., Clifford, D.J., Pandey, V.S. and Verhulst, A. (1998). Trypanosome infections and tick infestations: susceptibility in N'Dama, Gobra zebu and Gobra × N'Dama crossbred cattle exposed to natural challenge and maintained under high and low surveillance of trypanosome infections. *Acta Tropica* **71**, 57–71.

Maudlin, I., Welburn, S.C., Gashumba, J.K., Okuna, N. and Kalunda, M. (1990). The role of cattle in the epidemiology of sleeping sickness. *Bulletin de la Société Française de Parasitologie* **8**, 788.

May, E. and Allolio, B. (1991). Fatal toxic epidermal necrolysis during suramin therapy. *European Journal of Cancer* **27**, 1338.

Mehlitz, D., Zillmann, U., Scott, C.M. and Godfrey, D.G. (1982). Epidemiological studies in the animal reservoir of gambiense sleeping sickness. Part III. Characterization of *Trypanozoon* stocks by isoenzymes and sensitivity to human serum. *Tropenmedizin und Parasitologie* **33**, 113–118.

Moloo, S.K., Losos, G.J. and Kutuza, S.B. (1973). Transmission of *Trypanosoma brucei* to cats and dogs by feeding of infected goats. *Annals of Tropical Medicine and Parasitology* **67**, 331–334.

Molyneux, D.H. (2001a). African trypanosomiasis. Failure of science and public health. In: *World Class Parasites: The African Trypanosomes* (S.J. Black and J.R. Seed, eds), Vol 1, pp. 1–10. Boston: Kluwer Academic.

Molyneux, D.H. (2001b). Sterile insect release and trypanosomiasis control: a plea for realism. *Trends in Parasitology* **17**, 413–414.

Molyneux, D.H. (2001c). Vector-borne infections in the tropics and health policy issues in the twenty-first century. *Transactions of the Royal Society of Tropical Medicine and Hygiene* **95**, 233–238.

Molyneux, D.H. (2004). "Neglected" diseases but unrecognised successes—challenges and opportunities for infectious disease control. *Lancet* **364**, 380–383.

Moore, A., Richer, M., Enrile, M., Losio, E., Roberts, J. and Levy, D. (1999). Resurgence of sleeping sickness in Tambura County, Sudan. *American Journal of Tropical Medicine and Hygiene* **61**, 315–318.

Moore, D.A.J., Edwards, M., Escombe, R., Agranoff, D., Bailey, J.W., S.B., S. and Chiodini, P.L. (2002). African trypanosomiasis in travelers returning to the United Kingdom. *Emerging Infectious Diseases* **8**, 74–76.

Morris, K.R.S. (1959). The epidemiology of sleeping sickness in East Africa. I. A sleeping sickness outbreak in Uganda in 1957. *Transactions of the Royal Society of Tropical Medicine and Hygiene* **53**, 384–393.

Murray, C.J.L. (1994). Quantifying the burden of disease: the technical basis for disability-adjusted life years. *Bulletin of the World Health Organization* **72**, 429–445.

Mwambu, P.M. and Woodford, M.H. (1972). Trypanosomes from game animals of the Queen Elizabeth National Park, western Uganda. *Tropical Animal Health and Production* **4**, 152–155.

Nash, T.A.M. (1936). The relationship between maximum temperature and seasonal longevity of *Glossina submorsitans* Westw. and *G. tachinoides* in Northern Nigeria. *Bulletin of Entomological Research* **27**, 273–279.

Nathan, N., Tatay, M., Piola, P., Lake, S. and Brown, V. (2004). High mortality in displaced populations of northern Uganda. *Lancet* **363**, 1402.

Nieman, R.E. and Kelly, J.J. (2000). African trypanosomiasis. *Clinical Infectious Diseases* **30**, 985.

Nigatu, W., Abebe, M., Hadis, M. and Lulu, M. (1992). The effect of re-settlement and agricultural activities on tsetse populations in Gambella, south-western Ethiopia. *Insect Science and Its Application* **13**, 763–770.

Noireau, F., Gouteux, J.P. and Duteurtre, J.P. (1987). Valeur diagnostique du test d'agglutination sur carte (Testryp CATT) dans le dépistage de masse de la trypanosomiase humaine au Congo. *Bulletin de la Société de Pathologie Exotique* **80**, 797–803.

Notomi, T., Okayama, H., Masubuchi, H., Yonekawa, T., Watanabe, K., Amino, N. and Hase, T. (2000). Loop-mediated isothermal amplification of DNA. *Nucleic Acids Research* **28**, E63.

Odiit, M. (2003). *Epidemiology of* Trypanosoma brucei rhodesiense *sleeping sickness in Eastern Uganda.* Ph.D. thesis. University of Edinburgh, Edinburgh, UK.

Odiit, M., Amulen, D., Kansiime, F., Enyaru, J.C.K. and Okitoi, D. (1997). *Comparison of the Epidemiology of Sleeping Sickness and the Environment Profile in Tororo District.* Paper presented at the Proceedings of the 24th Meeting of the International Scientific Council for Trypanosomiasis Research and Control (ISCTRC), publication 119, Maputo, Mozambique.

Odiit, M., McDermott, J.J., Coleman, P.G., Fèvre, E.M., Welburn, S.C. and Woolhouse, M.E.J. (2004a). Spatial and temporal risk factors for the early detection of *T. b. rhodesiense* sleeping sickness patients in Tororo and Busia districts, Uganda. *Transactions of the Royal Society of Tropical Medicine and Hygiene* **98**, 569–576.

Odiit, M., Shaw, A., Welburn, S.C., Fèvre, E.M., Coleman, P.G. and McDermott, J.J. (2004b). Assessing the patterns of health-seeking behaviour and awareness among sleeping-sickness patients in eastern Uganda. *Annals of Tropical Medicine and Parasitology* **98**, 339–348.

Okia, M., Mbulamberi, D.B. and de Muynck, A. (1994). Risk factors assessment for *T.b. rhodesiense* sleeping sickness acquisition in S.E. Uganda: a case control study. *Annales de la Société Belge de Médecine Tropicale* **74**, 105–112.

Okoth, J.O. (1991). Description of a mono-screen trap for *Glossina fuscipes fuscipes* Newstead in Uganda. *Annals of Tropical Medicine and Parasitology* **85**, 309–315.

Okoth, J.O. and Kapaata, R. (1988). The hosts of *Glossina fuscipes fuscipes*. *Annals of Tropical Medicine and Parasitology* **82**, 517–518.

Okoth, J.O., Kirumira, E.K. and Kapaata, R. (1991). A new approach to community participation in tsetse control in the Busoga sleeping sickness focus, Uganda. A preliminary report. *Annals of Tropical Medicine and Parasitology* **85**, 315–322.

Olaho-Mukani, W., Nyang'ao, J.M.N., Ngaira, J.M., Omuse, J.K., Mbwabi, D., Tengekyon, K.M., Njenga, J.N. and Igweh, A.C. (1994). Immunoassay of circulating trypanosomal antigens in sleeping sickness patients undergoing treatment. *Journal of Immunoassay* **15**, 69–77.

Ollivier, G. and Legros, D. (2001). Trypanosomiase humaine africaine: historique de la thérapeutique et de ses échecs. *Tropical Medicine and International Health* **6**, 855–863.

Onyango, R.J., van Hoeve, K. and de Raadt, P. (1966). The epidemiology of *Trypanosoma rhodesiense* sleeping sickness in Alego location, central Nyanza, Kenya. I. Evidence that cattle may act as reservoir hosts of trypanosomes infective to man. *Transactions of the Royal Society of Tropical Medicine and Hygiene* **60**, 175–182.

Papadopoulos, M.C., Abel, P.M., Agranoff, D., Stich, A., Tarelli, E., Bell, B.A., Planche, T., Loosemore, A., Saadoun, S., Wilkins, P. and Krishna, S. (2004). A novel and accurate diagnostic test for human African trypanosomiasis. *Lancet* **363**, 1358–1363.

Paquet, C., Castilla, J., Mbulamberi, D., Beaulieu, M.F., Etchegorry, M.G. and Moren, A. (1995). La trypanosomiase à *Trypanosoma brucei gambiense* dans le foyer du Nord-Ouest de l'Ouganda. Bilan de 5 années de lutte (1987–1991). *Bulletin de la Société de Pathologie Exotique* **88**, 38–41.

Pécoul, B. (2004). New drugs for neglected diseases: from pipeline to patients. *Public Library of Science Medicine* **1**, 19–22.

Pépin, J., Khonde, N., Maiso, F., Doua, F., Jaffar, S., Ngampo, S., Mpia, B., Mbulamberi, D. and Kuzoe, F. (2000). Short-course eflornithine in Gambian trypanosomiasis: a multicentre randomized controlled trial. *Bulletin of the World Health Organization* **78**, 1284–1295.

Pépin, J. and Méda, H.A. (2001). The epidemiology and control of human African trypanosomiasis. *Advances in Parasitology* **49**, 71–132.

Pépin, J. and Milord, F. (1994). The treatment of human African trypanosomiasis. *Advances in Parasitology* **33**, 1–47.

Pépin, J., Milord, F., Khonde, A., Niyonsenga, T., Loko, L. and Mpia, B. (1994). Gambiense trypanosomiasis: frequency of, and risk factors for, failure of melarsoprol therapy. *Transactions of the Royal Society of Tropical Medicine and Hygiene* **88**, 447–452.

Pépin, J., Milord, F., Khonde, A.N., Niyonsenga, T., Loko, L., Mpia, B. and De Wals, P. (1995). Risk factors for encephalopathy and mortality during melarsoprol treatment of *Trypanosoma brucei gambiense* sleeping sickness. *Transactions of the Royal Society of Tropical Medicine and Hygiene* **89**, 92–97.

Perez-Martin, O., Lastre-Gonzalez, M., Urban, M. and Shwalbach, J. (1991). Resistencia *in vivo* de estirpes de *Trypanosoma rhodesiense*, Mozambique, 1985. *Revista Cubana de Medicina Tropical* **43**, 189–193.

Phiri, I.K., Ngowi, H., Afonso, S., Matenga, E., Boa, M., Mukaratirwa, S., Githigia, S., Saimo, M., Sikasunge, C. and Maingi, N. (2003). The emergence of *Taenia solium* cysticercosis in Eastern and Southern Africa as a serious agricultural problem and public health risk. *Acta Tropica* **87**, 13–23.

Potts, W.H. and Jackson, C.H.N. (1952). The Shinyanga game destruction experiment. *Bulletin of Entomological Research* **43**, 365–374.

Radwanska, M., Claes, F., Magez, S., Magnus, E., Perez-Morga, D., Pays, E. and Büscher, P. (2002a). Novel primer sequences for polymerase chain reaction-based detection of *Trypanosoma brucei gambiense*. *American Journal of Tropical Medicine and Hygiene* **67**, 289–295.

Radwanska, M., Magez, S., Perry-O'Keefe, H., Stender, H., Coull, J., Sternberg, J.M., Büscher, P. and Hyldig-Nielsen, J.J. (2002b). Direct detection and identification of African trypanosomes by fluorescence *in situ* hybridization with peptide nucleic acid probes. *Journal of Clinical Microbiology* **40**, 4295–4297.

Reichard, R. (1999). Case studies of emergency management of screwworm. *Revue Scientifique et Technique de l'Office International des Epizooties* **18**, 145–163.

Reid, S.E., Reid, C.A. and Vermund, S.H. (2004). Antiretroviral therapy in sub-Saharan Africa: adherence lessons from tuberculosis and leprosy. *International Journal of STD & AIDS* **15**, 713–716.

Rickman, L.R., Ernest, A., Kanyangala, S. and Kunda, E. (1991). Human serum sensitivities of *Trypanozoon* isolates from naturally infected hosts in the Luangwa Valley, Zambia. *East African Medical Journal* **68**, 880–892.

Rickman, L.R. and Robson, J. (1970a). The blood incubation infectivity test: a simple test which may serve to distinguish *Trypanosoma brucei* from *T. rhodesiense*. *Bulletin of the World Health Organization* **42**, 650–651.

Rickman, L.R. and Robson, J. (1970b). The testing of proven *Trypanosoma brucei* and *T. rhodesiense* strains by the blood incubation infectivity test. *Bulletin of the World Health Organization* **42**, 911–916.

Robays, J., Bilengue, M.M., Van der Stuyft, P. and Boelaert, M. (2004). The effectiveness of active population screening and treatment for sleeping sickness control in the Democratic Republic of Congo. *Tropical Medicine and International Health* **9**, 542–550.

Robson, J., Rickman, L.R., Allsopp, R. and Scott, D. (1972). The composition of the *Trypanosoma brucei* subgroup in nonhuman reservoirs in the Lambwe Valley, Kenya, with particular reference to the distribution of *T. rhodesiense*. *Bulletin of the World Health Organization* **46**, 765–770.

Rocha, G., Martins, A., Gama, G., Brandao, F. and Atouguia, J. (2004). Possible cases of sexual and congenital transmission of sleeping sickness. *Lancet* **363**, 247.

Rodriques Coura, J. and de Castro, S.L. (2002). A critical review on Chagas disease chemotherapy. *Memórias do Instituto Oswaldo Cruz* **97**, 3–24.

Rogers, D. and Boreham, P.F. (1973). Sleeping sickness survey in the Serengeti area (Tanzania) 1971. II. The vector role of *Glossina swynnertoni* Austen. *Acta Tropica* **30**, 24–35.

Rogers, D.J. (1988). A general model for the African trypanosomiases. *Parasitology* **97**, 193–212.

Rogers, D.J., Hendrickx, G. and Slingenbergh, J.H. (1994). Tsetse flies and their control. *Revue Scientifique et Technique de l'Office International des Epizooties* **13**, 1075–1124.

Rogers, D.J. and Randolph, S.E. (2002). A response to the aim of eradicating tsetse from Africa. *Trends in Parasitology* **18**, 534–536.

Rogers, D.J. and Robinson, T.P. (2004). Tsetse distribution. In: *The Trypanosomiases* (I. Maudlin, P.H. Holmes and M.A. Miles, eds), pp. 139–179. Wallingford: CABI.

Rowland, M., Durrani, N., Kenward, M., Mohammed, N., Urahman, H. and Hewitt, S. (2001). Control of malaria in Pakistan by applying deltamethrin insecticide to cattle: a community-randomised trial. *Lancet* **357**, 1837–1841.

Sachs, R., Schaller, G.B. and Baker, J.R. (1967). Isolation of trypanosomes of the *T. brucei* group from lion. *Acta Tropica* **24**, 109–112.

Sane, B., Laveissiere, C. and Meda, H.A. (2000). Diversité du régime alimentaire de *Glossina palpalis palpalis* en zone forestière de Côte d'Ivoire: relation avec la prévalence de la trypanosomiase humaine africaine. *Tropical Medicine and International Health* **5**, 73–78.

Schares, G. and Mehlitz, D. (1996). Sleeping sickness in Zaire: a nested polymerase chain reaction improves the identification of *Trypanosoma* (*Trypanozoon*) *brucei gambiense* by specific kinetoplast DNA probes. *Tropical Medicine and International Health* **1**, 59–70.

Schmid, C., Nkunku, S., Merolle, A., Vounatsou, P. and Burri, C. (2004). Efficacy of 10-day melarsoprol schedule 2 years after treatment for late-stage gambiense sleeping sickness. *Lancet* **364**, 789–790.

Schonefeld, A., Rottcher, D. and Moloo, S.K. (1987). The sensitivity to trypanocidal drugs of *Trypanosoma vivax* isolated in Kenya and Somalia. *Tropical Medicine and Parasitology* **38**, 177–180.

Shaw, A.P.M. (2004). Economics of African trypanosomiasis. In: *The Trypanosomiases* (I. Maudlin, P.H. Holmes and M.A. Miles, eds), pp. 369–402. Wallingford: CABI.

Simarro, P.P., Franco, J.R. and Asumu, P.N. (2001). Le foyer de trypanosomiase humaine Africaine de Luba en Guinée Equatoriale: a-t-il été éradique? *Médecine Tropicale* **61**, 441–444.

Simarro, P.P., Ruiz, J.A., Franco, J.R. and Josenando, T. (1999). Attitude towards CATT-positive individuals without parasitological confirmation in the African Trypanosomiasis (*T.b. gambiense*) focus of Quicama (Angola). *Tropical Medicine and International Health* **4**, 858–861.

Sinha, A., Grace, C., Alston, W.K., Westenfeld, F. and Maguire, J.H. (1999). African trypanosomiasis in two travelers from the United States. *Clinical Infectious Diseases* **29**, 840–844.

Sloof, P., Bos, J.L., Konings, A., Menke, H.H., Borst, P., Gutteridge, W.E. and Leon, W. (1983). Characterization of satellite DNA in *Trypanosoma brucei* and *Trypanosoma cruzi*. *Journal of Molecular Biology* **167**, 1–21.

Smith, R., Woodward, D., Acharya, A., Beaglehole, R. and Drager, N. (2004). Communicable disease control: a 'Global Public Good' perspective. *Health Policy and Planning* **19**, 271–278.

Snow, W.F., Declercq, J. and van Nieuwenhove, S. (1991). Watering sites in *Glossina fuscipes* habitat as the major foci for the transmission of Gambiense sleeping sickness in an endemic area of southern Sudan. *Annales de la Société Belge de Médecine Tropicale* **71**, 27–38.

Spath, J. (2000). Feeding patterns of three sympatric tsetse species (*Glossina* spp.) (Diptera : Glossinidae) in the preforest zone of Côte d'Ivoire. *Acta Tropica* **75**, 109–118.

Stanghellini, A. and Josenando, T. (2001). The situation of sleeping sickness in Angola: a calamity. *Tropical Medicine and International Health* **6**, 330–334.

Stephen, L.E. (1970). Clinical manifestations of the trypanosomiases in livestock and other domestic animals. In: *The African Trypanosomiases* (H.W. Mulligan, W.H. Potts and W.E. Kershaw, eds), pp. 774–794. London: George Allen and Unwin.

Stephen, L.E. (1986). *Trypanosomiasis: a Veterinary Perspective.* Oxford: Pergamon Press.

Stephens, J.W.W. and Fantham, H.B. (1910). On the peculiar morphology of a trypanosome from a case of sleeping sickness and the possibility of its being a new species (*T. rhodesiense*). *Annals of Tropical Medicine and Parasitology* **4**, 343–350.

Steverding, D. and Troscianko, T. (2004). On the role of blue shadows in the visual behaviour of tsetse flies. *Proceedings of the Royal Society of London Series B—Biological Sciences* **271**, S16–S17.

Stich, A., Abel, P.M. and Krishna, S. (2002). Human African trypanosomiasis. *British Medical Journal* **325**, 202–206.

Swynnerton, C.F.M. (1925). An experiment in the control of tsetse flies at Shinyanga, Tanganyika Territory. *Bulletin of Entomological Research* **15**, 313–363.

Taelman, H., Schechter, P.J., Marcelis, L., Sonnet, J., Kazyumba, G., Dasnoy, J., Haegele, K.D., Sjoerdsma, A. and Wéry, M. (1987). Difluoromethylornithine, an effective new treatment of Gambian trypanosomiasis. Results in five patients. *American Journal of Medicine* **82**, 607–614.

Taylor, K. and Authié, M.-L. (2004). Pathogenisis of animal trypanosomiasis. In: *The Trypanosomiases* (I. Maudlin, P.H. Holmes and M.A. Miles, eds), pp. 331–353. Wallingford: CABI.

Thi, C.D.D., Aerts, D., Steinert, M. and Pays, E. (1991). High homology between variant surface glycoprotein gene-expression sites of *Trypanosoma brucei* and *Trypanosoma gambiense*. *Molecular and Biochemical Parasitology* **48**, 199–210.

Traub, N., Hira, P.R., Chintu, C. and Mhango, C. (1978). Congenital trypanosomiasis: report of a case due to *Trypanosoma brucei rhodesiense*. *East African Medical Journal* **55**, 477.

Triolo, N., Trova, P., Fusco, C. and Le Bras, J. (1985). Bilan de 17 années d'étude de la trypanosomiase humaine africaine à *T. gambiense* chez les enfants de 0 a 6 ans. A propos de 227 cas. *Médecine Tropicale* **45**, 251–257.

Truc, P., Jamonneau, V., Cuny, G. and Frézil, J.L. (1999). Use of polymerase chain reaction in human African trypanosomiasis stage determination and follow-up. *Bulletin of the World Health Organization* **77**, 745–748.

Truc, P., Lejon, V., Magnus, E., Jamonneau, V., Nangouma, A., Verloo, D., Penchenier, L. and Büscher, P. (2002). Evaluation of the micro-CATT,

CATT/*Trypanosoma brucei gambiense*, and LATEX/*T.b.gambiense* methods for serodiagnosis and surveillance of human African trypanosomiasis in West and Central Africa. *Bulletin of the World Health Organization* **80**, 882–886.

Vale, G.A. (1982). The trap-orientated behaviour of tsetse flies (Glossinidae) and other Diptera. *Bulletin of Entomological Research* **72**, 71–93.

Vale, G.A., Lovemore, D.F., Flint, S. and Cockbill, G.F. (1988). Odor-baited targets to control tsetse flies, *Glossina* spp. (Diptera, Glossinidae), in Zimbabwe. *Bulletin of Entomological Research* **78**, 31–49.

Vale, G.A., Mutika, G. and Lovemore, D.F. (1999). Insecticide-treated cattle for controlling tsetse flies (Diptera: Glossinidae): some questions answered, many posed. *Bulletin of Entomological Research* **89**, 569–578.

Van Hoof, L., Lewillon, R., Henrard, C., Péel, E. and Rodjestvensky, B. (1946). A field experiment on the prophylactic value of pentamidine in sleeping sickness. *Transactions of the Royal Society of Tropical Medicine and Hygiene* **39**, 327–329.

Van Nieuwenhove, S. (1999). Present strategies in the treatment of human African trypanosomiasis. In: *Progress in Human African Trypanosomiasis, Sleeping Sickness* (M. Dumas, B. Bouteille and A. Buguet, eds), pp. 235–280. Paris: Springer.

Van Nieuwenhove, S. (2000). Gambiense sleeping sickness: re-emerging and soon untreatable? *Bulletin of the World Health Organization* **78**, 1283.

Vickerman, K. (1985). Developmental cycles and biology of pathogenic trypanosomes. *British Medical Bulletin* **41**, 105–114.

Vreysen, M.J.B., Saleh, K.M., Ali, M.Y., Abdulla, A.M., Zhu, Z.R., Juma, K.G., Dyck, V.A., Msangi, A.R., Mkonyi, P.A. and Feldmann, H.U. (2000). *Glossina austeni* (Diptera : Glossinidae) eradicated on the Island of Unguja, Zanzibar, using the sterile insect technique. *Journal of Economic Entomology* **93**, 123–135.

Wacher, T.J., Milligan, P.M., Rawlings, P. and Snow, W.F. (1994). *Spatial Factors in the Assessment of Trypanosomiasis Challenge*. Paper presented at the Symposium on Modelling Vector-borne and other Parasitic Diseases: Proceedings of a Workshop Organized by ILRAD in Collaboration with FAO, Nairobi, Kenya.

Waiswa, C., Olaho-Mukani, W. and Katunguka-Rwakishaya, E. (2003). Domestic animals as reservoirs for sleeping sickness in three endemic foci in south-eastern Uganda. *Annals of Tropical Medicine and Parasitology* **97**, 149–155.

Welburn, S.C., Maudlin, I. and Ellis, D.S. (1989). Rate of trypanosome killing by lectins in midguts of different species and strains of *Glossina*. *Medical and Veterinary Entomology* **3**, 77–82.

Welburn, S.C. and Maudlin, I. (1999). Tsetse–trypanosome interactions: rites of passage. *Parasitology Today* **15**, 399–403.

Welburn, S.C., Fèvre, E.M., Coleman, P.G., Odiit, M. and Maudlin, I. (2001a). Sleeping sickness: a tale of two diseases. *Trends in Parasitology* **17**, 19–24.

Welburn, S.C., Picozzi, K., Fèvre, E.M., Coleman, P.G., Odiit, M., Carrington, M. and Maudlin, I. (2001b). Identification of human-infective trypanosomes in animal reservoir of sleeping sickness in Uganda by means of serum-resistance-associated (*SRA*) gene. *Lancet* **358**, 2017–2019.

Welburn, S.C., Fèvre, E.M., Coleman, P.G. and Maudlin, I. (2004). Epidemiology of human African trypanosomiasis. In: *The Trypanosomiases* (I. Maudlin, P.H. Holmes and M.A. Miles, eds), pp. 219–232. Wallingford: CABI.

Wellde, B.T., Reardon, M.J., Chumo, D.A., Kovatch, R.M., Waema, D., Wykoff, D.E., Mwangi, J., Boyce, W.L. and Williams, J.S. (1989a). Cerebral trypanosomiasis in naturally infected cattle in the Lambwe Valley, South-Nyanza, Kenya. *Annals of Tropical Medicine and Parasitology* **83**, 151–160.

Wellde, B.T., Reardon, M.J., Kovatch, R.M., Chumo, D.A., Williams, J.S., Boyce, W.L., Hockmeyer, W.T. and Wykoff, D.E. (1989b). Experimental infection of cattle with *Trypanosoma brucei rhodesiense*. *Annals of Tropical Medicine and Parasitology* **83**, 133–150.

White, N.J. and Olliaro, P.L. (1996). Strategies for the prevention of antimalarial drug resistance: rationale for combination chemotherapy for malaria. *Parasitology Today* **12**, 399–401.

White, S.C. (1996). Depoliticising development: the uses and abuses of participation. *Development in Practice* **6**, 6–15.

Wickware, P. (2002). Resurrecting the resurrection drug. *Nature Medicine* **8**, 908–909.

Wilde, J.K.H. and French, M.H. (1945). An experimental study of *Trypanosoma rhodesiense* infection in zebu cattle. *Journal of Comparative Pathology* **55**, 206–228.

Woo, P.T.K. (1970). The haematocrit centrifuge technique for the diagnosis of African trypanosomiasis. *Acta Tropica* **27**, 384–386.

Woolhouse, M.E.J., Taylor, L.H. and Haydon, D.T. (2001). Population biology of multihost pathogens. *Science* **292**, 1109–1112.

World Health Organization (1995). *WHO Model Prescribing Information: Drugs Used in Parasitic Diseases*, 2nd edn. Geneva: WHO.

World Health Organization (1998). *Control and Surveillance of African Trypanosomiasis*. WHO Technical Report Series 881. Geneva: WHO.

World Health Organization (2003). *Report of the Scientific Working Group Meeting on African Trypanosomiasis (Sleeping Sickness)*. TDR/SWG/01 Geneva: WHO/TDR.

Wurapa, F.K., Bulsara, M.K., Chen, M.G. and Wyatt, G.B. (1984). The public health importance of African trypanosomiasis in north east Zambia. *Tropical and Geographical Medicine* **36**, 329–333.

Zumla, A. (2002). Drugs for neglected diseases. *Lancet Infectious Diseases* **2**, 393.

Chemotherapy in the Treatment and Control of Leishmaniasis

Jorge Alvar[1], Simon Croft[2] and Piero Olliaro[3]

[1]*Department for Control of Neglected Tropical Diseases, World Health Organization, 20 Avenue Appia CH-1211 Geneva 27, Switzerland*
[2]*Drugs for Neglected Diseases Initiative (DNDi), 1 Place St. Gervais, CH-1201 Geneva, Switzerland*
[3]*UNICEF/UNDP/WB/WHO Special Programme for Research & Training in Tropical Diseases (TDR), World Health Organization, 20 Avenue Appia CH-1211 Geneva 27, Switzerland*

ADVANCES IN PARASITOLOGY VOL 61
ISSN: 0065-308X
DOI: 10.1016/S0065-308X(05)61006-8

ABSTRACT

Drugs remain the most important tool for the treatment and control of both visceral and cutaneous leishmaniasis. Although there have been several advances in the past decade, with the introduction of new therapies by liposomal amphotericin, oral miltefosine and paromomycin (PM), these are not ideal drugs, and improved shorter duration, less toxic and cheaper therapies are required. Treatments for complex forms of leishmaniasis and HIV co-infections are inadequate. In addition, full deployment of drugs in treatment and control requires defined strategies, which can also prevent or delay the development of drug resistance.

1. INTRODUCTION

The recommended drugs for the treatment of both visceral leishmaniasis (VL) and cutaneous leishmaniasis (CL), the pentavalent antimonials, were first introduced 60 years ago. During the 1950s, pentamidine was added to the list of treatments, followed by amphotericin B (ampB) in the 1960s (Croft and Yardley, 2002). Over the past two decades alternative drugs or new formulations of other standard drugs have become available and registered for use in some countries and a limited number remain in clinical trial. The advances in chemotherapy have been significant and the concept of choice for treatment in VL is now real. However, this is not to state that the drugs available are ideal; the aim remains to identify cheap and safe drugs or formulations that can be used in the treatment and disease control. It is unlikely that one single drug or drug formulation will be effective against all forms of leishmaniasis since (a) the visceral and cutaneous sites of infection impose varying pharmacokinetic requirements on the drugs to be used and (b) there is an intrinsic variation in the drug sensitivity of the 17 *Leishmania* species known to infect humans. In addition, depending on the *Leishmania* species involved, a complicated form of leishmaniasis may develop that merits a specific treatment (Figure 1, which is Plate 6.1 in separate colour plate section). In addition, there are other new problems to be surmounted by novel treatments, namely: (i) the need for drugs for treatment of VL in Bihar State, India, where there is acquired resistance to the pentavalent antimonials (Sundar, 2001), and (ii) the need for treatments for VL and CL in immunosuppressed patients, in particular due to HIV co-infection, where there is exacerbation of disease or emergence from latent infection due to the depleted immune response. In this latter case standard chemotherapy is frequently unsuccessful (Dereure *et al.*, 2003; Pagliano *et al.*, 2003; Mira *et al.*, 2004).

2. THE CURRENT EPIDEMIOLOGIC SITUATION AND REQUIREMENTS FOR NEW CONTROL STRATEGIES

2.1. Epidemiology

Leishmaniasis is one of the most neglected tropical diseases, with a major burden among the poorest segments of impoverished populations in Asia, Africa, South America and, in less degree, Europe (Yamey and Torreele, 2002). Leishmaniasis is in fact a complex of visceral and cutaneous diseases (Figure 1), caused by protozoa of the genus *Leishmania* that live and multiply in macrophages of certain mammals. The mammalian reservoir can act as carriers of the parasite without necessarily having the disease. The parasite is transmitted to humans through the bite of female haematophagous sandflies (*Phlebotomus* and *Lutzomyia*), which have previously fed on an infected reservoir. The zoonotic cycle includes the infected reservoir–sandfly–susceptible human whereas the anthroponotic one involves the infected human–sandfly–susceptible human; this consideration is crucial in the control programmes.

The severity of the two basic forms of disease, CL and VL, depends on the infecting *Leishmania* species and on the host immune response that develops; the outcome is, in most cases, species-dependent (Figure 2). Around 15 species cause the cutaneous form, which normally heals spontaneously leaving scars. However, if caused by *Leishmania tropica*, it may evolve into recidivans cutaneous leishmaniasis (RCL), which is difficult to treat and leaves extensive scars. In Latin America, CL may develop into one of two possible forms, depending on the

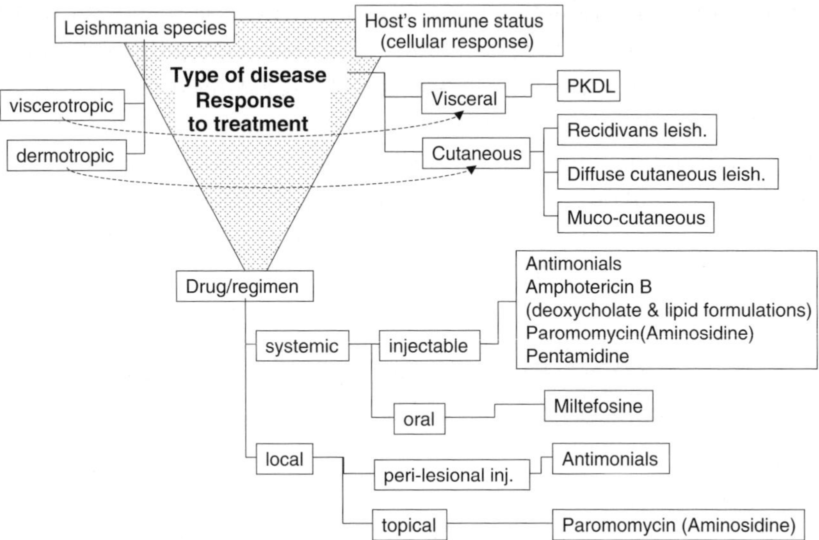

Figure 2 Interaction between *Leishmania* species, host and treatment. Clinical manifestation and response to treatment in leishmaniasis result from a complex interplay between parasite species, host response and treatment. Visceral disease requires systemic treatment and may result in PKDL. Cutaneous forms are treated either systemically or locally. They may evolve towards recidivans, diffuse or mucosal complications.

species, namely: (1) diffuse CL (DCL, if *Leishmania guyanensis* or *Leishmania amazonensis* are involved), which occurs in patients whose immune system is weak, and who thus fail to heal spontaneously and relapse after treatment, with disastrous consequences for the patient; or (2) mucocutaneous leishmaniasis (MCL, known as "espundia" in South America), characterized by the destruction of the mucosa and cartilage of the mouth and pharynx followed by the facial tissue (several species are able to cause MCL, the most important being *Leishmania braziliensis*). VL, or "kala-azar", is caused by two species, *Leishmania donovani* and *Leishmania infantum* (this latter also known as *Leishmania chagasi* in South America); VL is the most severe form and is fatal in almost all cases if left untreated. It may cause epidemic outbreaks with a high mortality rate. A varying proportion of visceral cases due to *L. donovani* may evolve into a cutaneous form known as post-kala-azar dermal leishmaniasis (PKDL), requiring lengthy and costly treatment (Herwaldt, 1999).

From an epidemiological point of view, leishmaniasis is divided into two categories depending on the life cycle: anthoponotic leishmaniasis where infected humans act as the reservoir, being fed upon by the sandfly that will eventually infect another susceptible person, and zoonotic leishmaniasis where the reservoir is a non-human mammal. Although the majority of leishmaniasis is zoonotic, anthroponotic leishmaniasis has the largest impact—namely in *L. donovani* VL and *L. tropica* CL, including PKDL and recidivans cases, respectively. This is a critical factor in epidemiology in relation to the control. For anthroponoses this is focused on early diagnosis, treatment and interruption/reduction of the accessibility of sandflies to the infected human that are the reservoirs by using mechanical barriers (normally, insecticide-impregnated bed nets). In contrast, the control of zoonotic leishmaniasis is focused on the animal reservoir by reducing the reservoir capacity through a number of approaches (sacrifice, treatment, vaccination, etc.), or the contacts with the vector (insecticide spraying, bed nets, repellents, etc.). Moreover, drug resistance is much more important in anthroponotic disease, taking into account that the multiplication of this parasite is mostly clonal, meaning that resistance is inherited in parasites transmitted directly between humans, whereas in zoonoses drug-resistant parasites can be diluted in the mammalian reservoir hosts where there is no selection pressure.

The leishmaniases are prevalent in 88 countries, affecting an estimated 12–14 million people with roughly 1.5–2 million new cases per year, 400 000–500 000 of which are visceral (90% of them in Bangladesh, Brazil, India, Nepal and Sudan) and 1 000 000 to 1 500 000 cutaneous (90% of them in Afghanistan, Algeria, Brazil, Iran, Peru, Saudi Arabia and Sudan) (Desjeux, 1996; Murray and Lopez, 1996). However, there are no accurate studies on the disease mainly because the transmission is in remote and poor areas with difficult health access, in patches and many cases are mild or asymptomatic. All this leads to the use of extrapolated figures derived from estimations. MCL is almost specific to Central and South America (essentially Bolivia, Brazil and Peru) but also can be found in Ethiopia. Many more subjects are asymptomatically infected among the 350 million people living at risk in endemic areas (le Fichoux *et al.*, 1999; Gama *et al.*, 2004). According to official figures, global mortality from VL is estimated at 59 000 (35 000 men and 24 000 women) (Desjeux, 2004). It is globally accepted that these figures are an underestimation since the reporting of the disease is compulsory in only one-third of the endemic countries. In addition, it is often not diagnosed or misdiagnosed where there is no proper access to diagnostic or treatment. The case fatality rate despite the treatment (normally around 5%) can be three times higher in women than in men in some areas due to cultural reasons and access to drugs (Ahluwalia *et al.*, 2004). The disease burden is calculated at 2 357 000 disability-adjusted life years (DALYs: 946 000 in men and 1 410 000 in women), a significant ranking among communicable diseases and the third one among parasitic diseases, after malaria and lymphatic filariasis (Desjeux, 2004).

In immunocompetent patients, VL is considered principally as a childhood disease in historical foci (Aggarwal and Wali, 1991; Evans *et al.*, 1992), more specifically in the Mediterranean countries where the average patient is 3 years old (Kafetzis, 2003). However, in the case of *Leishmania* and HIV co-infection, the age average is 31–50 years, coinciding with the principal group at risk in Southern Europe, the intravenous drug users (IVDUs) (Alvar *et al.*, 1997; Desjeux and Alvar, 2003).

In areas where leishmaniasis is spreading, it affects all ages—the major factors being environmental, social and individual, such as displacement of non-immune people to endemic areas, new irrigation infrastructures for agriculture, disruption of social and health facilities in suburbs of cities where new settlers overcrowd, the trend from rural to urban transmission, malnutrition weakening of the immune system and, lastly, the overlapping of VL and AIDS (Ashford, 2000; Desjeux, 2001).

Effective treatment remains the most important challenge in leishmaniasis: (i) there are few drugs available and are expensive and toxic; (ii) the patients live in remote rural areas and have limited access to treatment centres; (iii) there are frequent drug shortages making the price even higher on the black market; and the treatments are of long duration interrupting the income of the families, etc. As a result, the patients often fail to complete a whole course of treatment (if started) creating a situation where drug resistance can develop. Information on the social cost of leishmaniasis is scarce; in Bangladesh a family with a case of kala-azar is three times more likely to have sold the cow or the rice field, leading into a vicious circle of disease–poverty–malnutrition–disease (Sharma *et al.*, in press; Ahluwalia *et al.*, 2004).

2.2. HIV–*Leishmania* co-infection

In the past two decades more than 2000 HIV–*Leishmania* co-infection cases have been reported from southern Europe (Desjeux and Alvar, 2003). This co-infection is more than the mere spatial coincidence of two pathogens. Both share the same host cell, facilitate their own multiplication and replication of the parasite and virus, respectively, and both provoke the impairment of the T-cell response. The clinical and epidemiological features are noteworthy. A total of 34 of the 88 countries in which the disease is endemic have reported cases of co-infection. Before the introduction of high activity antiretroviral therapy (HAART) for all AIDS patients in European countries in 1997, two-thirds of all the cases of VL were associated with HIV infection. Up to 1.5–9% of AIDS patients suffered a bout of leishmaniasis, either as a new infection or as reactivation of a latent infection (Alvar *et al.*, 1997; Cruz *et al.*, in press). Being infected with HIV/AIDS increases (by 100–2320 fold) the risk of developing leishmaniasis (López-Vélez *et al.*, 1998). In Spain, 60–85% of the co-infected cases were IVDUs (male/female ratio = 8:2), the most important risk group of acquiring HIV, while in East Africa and southern Asia co-infection affects seasonal workers, displaced people, sex workers and truckers. Co-infection increases the mortality rate up to 20–25% during treatment, and most of the patients die within 1–2 years after several relapses. Life expectancy is two-thirds lower than it is for AIDS patients who do not have leishmaniasis.

In Humera (Tigray region, Ethiopia), an endemic area of leishmaniasis bordering Eritrea and Sudan with both soldiers and migrant workers, HIV prevalence is high leading to the highest prevalence of co-infection known (up to 25% of all kala-azar cases). The risk factor has been identified as due to seasonal workers sleeping under the *Acacia* and *Balanites* trees where the sandflies rest, exposing themselves to the bites (Lyons *et al.*, 2003; Elnaiem *et al.*, 1999). In similar areas of Sudan this percentage is 5–9.4% depending on the areas (El-Safi *et al.*, in preparation). In Addis Ababa (Ethiopia), 35% of all the cases of leishmaniasis are found in HIV-infected patients (Berhe *et al.*, 1999). In Africa mass migration and wars are considered to be factors responsible for spreading co-infection (Guiguemde *et al.*, 2003). Less documented information from the subcontinent of India suggests that the problem is increasing, and is aggravated by the resistance to pentavalent antimonials (Sundar, 2001; Sinha *et al.*, 2003). In South America most of the cases are reported from Brazil due to the increase in the incidence of AIDS up to 12.3 every 100 000 inhabitants in 2001 and the urbanization of leishmaniasis transmission (Sampaio *et al.*, 2002; Rabello *et al.*, 2003). The real impact of the problem is probably underestimated on the global scale due to deficiencies in the surveillance systems.

In general, HAART has sharply reduced the prevalence of co-infection and the patients have a better rate of survival than those who do not receive it (Pintado *et al.*, 2001; de la Rosa *et al.*, 2002). These medicines greatly benefit patients in developed countries since the mean coverage is 15% (8% for African countries) (UNAIDS, 2005). Two situations, prime attack and relapses, are under consideration. By increasing the CD4+ count thanks to HAART there is a greater chance to control the initial *Leishmania* infection (López-Vélez, 2003). In contrast, the patient not receiving HAART has a greater chance of developing a bout of leishmaniasis with later clinical and parasitological relapses (Pintado and López-Vélez, 2001; Pintado *et al.*, 2001). The response seems to be inversely related to the viral load before treatment (Berhe *et al.*, 1999). However, if the patient has already had a prime attack of leishmaniasis, HAART seems to be insufficient to prevent relapses, although these can be delayed. In 38–70% of the co-infected patients, it will relapse within 24 months after the anti-*Leishmania* treatment independent of the CD4+ increase and even with undetectable viral load (López-Vélez, 2003; Mira *et al.*, 2004).

2.3. Canine Leishmaniasis

Among the zoonotic leishmaniases, the only case in which the reservoir is treated is canine leishmaniasis since the dog plays an important role in the family, society and even in economic terms, being a major target for the veterinary companies. The dog is the reservoir but also a victim of leishmaniasis and the impact cannot be ignored. Infected dogs are treated with the same drug armamentarium which is used for human leishmaniasis, although the method of administration and posology differ. The drugs of first choice are the pentavalent antimonials in combination with either allopurinol, or, as a second choice, ampB (Alvar *et al.*, 2004). Although initially a good response is seen, even with loss of infectivity to the sandflies, in most of the dogs it relapses, and they become infective to the sandfly again and, normally, are re-treated with the same or an alternative drug (Alvar *et al.*, 1994). The response and infectivity have been proven to be dependent on the CD4+ count restored after chemotherapy (Moreno *et al.*, 1999). As infected dogs are treated with the same drugs as humans, their misuse could eventually lead to resistance with implications in human leishmaniasis.

2.4. Control Components: Epidemiological Information, Diagnosis, Treatment and Prevention

Improved control reduces both mortality (in the case of VL) and morbidity (in the case of both the VL and CL). It also reduces the role of humans as a reservoir in anthroponotic cycles (*L. tropica* and *L. donovani*) and makes it possible to avert progression to complicated clinical presentations (DCL, RCL, MCL and PKDL). The combination of active case detection and treatment is the key to control. Nevertheless, there are huge obstacles even to something that is apparently so simple. During their initial phases, leishmaniases (visceral and cutaneous) respond better to treatment, but patients are unaware of the initial symptoms or health systems are poorly staffed, lack equipment or do not exist in remote rural areas, where contact with sandflies is most common.

Prevalence and incidence data on the real impact of leishmaniasis are unreliable because no prospective and broad study has ever been carried out; figures have always been extrapolated from the fragmentary data that exist (Ashford *et al.*, 1992). This makes it virtually impossible to set up a control programme with objectively determined aims and time frames. It is possible to make only an approximate estimate of prevalence and incidence and there are no objective data because: (i) transmission of the disease occurs in remote rural areas in many cases not homogeneously distributed but in patches; (ii) many cases are not diagnosed because they do not receive medical care and have no access to diagnosis or to medication; and (iii) because leishmaniasis notification is compulsory in only 33 of the 88 countries in which it is endemic (Desjeux, 2004). Classifying leishmaniasis as a notifiable disease would imply greater commitment to the control effort on the part of health authorities. Currently, the figures used by countries are mere approximations, and this is shown by the difference between the results of active and passive case detection (Copeland *et al.*, 1990). Lastly, there are far more asymptomatic and mild than clinically declared cases.

Currently, there is no well-defined scheme for cost-effective control (Boelaert *et al.*, 1999). There is a clear need to strengthen active case detection, of both cutaneous and VL cases, and to strengthen diagnosis at peripheral health centres where patients are usually treated on the basis of presumptive diagnosis. So far, definitive diagnosis has relied on visual identification of the parasite under the microscope. The fact is that in most district hospitals there are no resources to collect and interpret bone marrow aspirates or even to perform skin tests, and hence the need for rapid and easy-to-interpret techniques. At present, three diagnostic methods are available that are sensitive and specific to VL, and that are being compared in field conditions in Africa and Asia (dipstick k39, US\$1.5; DAT freeze-dried antigen, US\$2.5; and a latex agglutination test to detect the antigen in urine, US\$1.5); they are more affordable than the conventional serological tests (El Safi and Evans, 1989; Badaro *et al.*, 1996; Boelaert *et al.*, 1999; Attar *et al.*, 2001).

VL is normally treated with injectable drugs requiring hospitalization, or with an oral medicament (miltefosine), that can be administered in outstations and is only currently registered in few countries. The essential problem is access to treatment, since the cost of hospitalization for several weeks has to be added to the cost of the drug, bed availability, loss of working days, etc. (Boelaert *et al.*, 1999; Murray, 2004). VL patients need to be hospitalized to monitor cardiac and renal functions during treatment. The injectable drugs are toxic and merit a clinical and laboratory examination if possible, including the nutritional status, weight, spleen size, temperature, haemoglobin and leucocytes, platelets and prothrombin time, hepatic enzymes, creatinine, electrocardiogram, serum albumin and other serum proteins. The patients are considered to be cured if 6 months after chemotherapy there is no fever and the splenomegaly has disappeared. Malnutrition is associated with the exacerbation of kala-azar, and, conversely, the infection has a deep effect on the nutritional status of the patient (Harrison *et al.*, 1986).

The first-line drugs are pentavalent antimonials that have to be administered intramuscularly or intravenously for 4 weeks (Table 1); they are cardiotoxic and expensive (Table 2) for developing countries (for example, sodium stibogluconate (SSG) US$180–200). A generic SSG is now available at a cost of US$30. Poor use and compliance with the latter have resulted in the emergence of resistance in 40–65% of patients in some areas of Bihar, India, spreading now to adjacent districts in Nepal. An alternative drug is ampB deoxycholate (US$60), which is highly nephrotoxic if administered without supervision, and hence it is necessary that the patients are hospitalized for the 4 weeks during treatment. Liposomal ampB is unaffordable (US$450 preferential price for NGOs in East Africa, to US$2080 or more per course elsewhere) in developing countries although there are almost no side effects. Miltefosine, the only drug administered orally for 28 days (Table 1), is licensed in India, Germany and Colombia at present (US$167 in India, US$270 in Colombia); the possibility of a teratogenic effect has not been excluded (Table 2) and it should be considered for use in combination to avert the emergence of resistance (Sundar and Murray, 2005).

CL caused by species that do not tend to evolve into complicated disease forms (i.e. *Leishmania major*, *Leishmania peruviana* and *Leishmania mexicana*) can be treated intralesionally with antimonials (intermittent injections until healing) if (i) they are not open ulcers, (ii) if they are not multiple lesions, (iii) if there is no proximity to a lymphatic duct and (iv) if they are not in areas difficult to heal (joints). As a general rule, the crust should be kept to avoid secondary infections, and antiseptics applied only if the ulcer is infected. Under other circumstances, all lesions should be treated systemically with

Table 1 Current drugs used in the treatment of leishmaniasis

Drug	Doses in adults and children	First line drug	Second line drug
Visceral leishmaniasis (*L. donovani* and *L. infantum*)			
SSG (Pentostam[®]; generic SSG, Albert David, Kolkata)	20 mg Sb^V/kg/d IM, 4 weeks	East Africa, South Asia (excluding Bihar State, India)	
Meglumine antimoniate (Glucantime[®])[a]		Mediterranean countries, Central and South America	
Amphotericin B-liposomal (AmBisome[®])	2 mg/kg/d IV, e.o.d. × 5 doses over 10 days	Mediterranean countries	India, Kenya
Amphotericin B-deoxycholate (Fungizone[®])	2 mg/kg/d IV, 4 weeks or 1 mg/kg/d IV e.o.d. × 15 doses over 4 weeks	India	Rescue treatment elsewhere
Pentamidine (Pentacarinat[®])	4 mg/kg/d IM, 15–20 doses every other day		Rescue treatment
Paramomycin	15 mg/kg/d 21 days	Phase IV, India	
Miltefosine (Impavido[®])	100 mg/d for >25 kg or 50 mg/kg if <25 kg p.o. × 28 days	Potential tool in elimination program in India, Bangladesh and Nepal (see text)	
Cutaneous leishmaniasis (except *L. braziliensis* and *L. guyanensis*)			
Local			
SSG (Pentostam[®])[b]	Local therapy in single lesion: injection of 1–5 ml in the basis and margins of the lesion, daily or every other day until healing the lesion	East Africa, South Asia (excluding India)	
Meglumine antimoniate (Glucantime[®])[a]		Mediterranean countries, Central and South America	
Thermotherapy	Local therapy in single lesion: 1 treatment of ≥ consecutive application at 50°C for 30 s.	Afghanistan	
Paramomycin topical formulations	Application up to 28 days	Iran, Israel	

Drug	Dose		
Parenteral			
SSG (Pentostam®)[b]	20 mg Sb^V/kg/d IM, 21 days	East Africa, South Asia (excluding India)	
Meglumine antimoniate (Glucantime®)[a]		Mediterranean countries, Central and South America	
Oral			
Miltefosine (Impavido®)	150 mg/kg/d × 28 days		Colombia (only *L. panamensis*)
Cutaneous leishmaniasis by *L. braziliensis* and *L. guyanensis*			
Meglumine antimoniate (Glucantime®)[a]	20 mg Sb^V/kg/d IM, 21 days	Central and South America	
Mucocutaneous leishmaniasis			
Meglumine antimoniate (Glucantime®)[a]	20 mg Sb^V/kg/d IM, 4 weeks	Central and South America	
Amphotericin B-liposomal (AmBisome®)	3 mg/kg/d IV, days 0, 1, 2, 3, 4 and 10		Central and South America
Amphotericin B-deoxycholate (Fungizone®)	0.5–1 g/kg/d IV, 4 weeks	Central and South America	
Pentamidine (Pentacarinat®)	4 mg/kg/d IM, 15–20 doses every other day	MCL by *L. guyanensis* (South America) and by *L. aethiopica* (Ethiopia)	
Miltefosine (Impavido®)	2–2.5 mg/kg/d total dose		Bolivia
Diffuse cutaneous leishmaniasis			
Meglumine antimoniate (Glucantime®)[a]	20 mg Sb^V/kg/d IM from 2 to several months, until recovery	DCL caused by *L. amazonensis* (South America)	
Pentamidine (Pentacarinat®)	4 mg/kg/d IM, every other day, not less than 4 months	DCL caused by *L. aethiopica* (Ethiopia)	DCL caused by *L. amazonensis* (South America)
Miltefosine (Impavido®)	2–2.5 mg/kg/d total dose		Venezuela
Recidivans cutaeous leishmaniasis			
SSG (Pentostam®)[b]	20 mg Sb^V/kg/d IM, 4–8 weeks		
Post-kala-azar dermal leishmaniasis			

Table 1 (*Continued*)

Drug	Doses in adults and children	First line drug	Second line drug
SSG (Pentostam[®])[b] for PKDL with conjunctiva involvement or severe PKDL	20 mg Sb^V/kg/d IM, 4–8 weeks or until recovery	East Africa, Bangladesh, Nepal	
Amphotericin B-deoxicholate (Fungizone[®])	0.5–1 g/kg/d IV, 3 weeks, 10 days off, 3 weeks, 10 days off, 3 weeks	India	
Pentamidine (Pentacarinat[®])	4 mg/kg/d IM, every other day, 4–8 weeks		India

[a] 1 ml of Glucantime contains 85 mg of antimony (Sb^V). The normal dose for an adult is 10 mm^3 (2 vials) per day.
[b] 1 ml of Pentostam contains 100 mg of antimony (Sb^V). Maximum dose: 800 mg/d.

Table 2 Summary characteristics of regimens considered

Drug	Status	Average cure rate %	Toxicity	Main issues
Antimony	First-line treatment worldwide except Bihar (India) due to resistance	50% Bihar	GI; cutaneous (rash); myalgia, arthralgia; renal; cardiac. Dose-related. Drug quality-related?	Resistance in India
SSG		90% Elsewhere		Variable quality of generics
Meglumine antimoniate				
Amphotericin B deoxycholate (Fungizone®)	Variably used; replaces antimony as first-line in Bihar	>95%	Infusion-related (fever, chills, bone pain, rarely cardiac arrest) Delayed (hypokalaemia, renal functions)	Toxicity
Liposomal amphoB AmBisome®	Widely registered, minimal use due to cost	>95% (India, Africa)	Rare and minor (fever, rigor, backache)	Cost (even with MSF-negotiated price US$ 0.4/ampoule)
AmphoB lipid complex (ABLC)	Little data	ca. 90% (India) 90	Like AmBisome but more frequent	Cost, availability
Pentamidine	Little use		Diabetes Rare in VL: shock, myocarditis, death	Not a valid option today: availability, toxicity, declining efficacy in India
Paromomycin	PhIII regulatory studies completed in India, underway in Africa	>90%	Generally safe in VL; ototoxicity	Will be cheap (10$)

Table 2 (*continued*)

Drug	Status	Average cure rate %	Toxicity	Main issues
		>90%		Data limited to India, some use also in Sudan
Miltefosine	Registered in India, Colombia, Germany; regularoty filing in Nepal, Bangladesh	*c.* 95% (India)	GI (vomiting, diarrhoea, elevated liver enzymes); rash, nephrotoxicity;	Teratogenic (may not be used in women of childbearing age without contraception including treatment plus 2 months)
Sitamaquine	PhII underway	<90%	Dose-limiting renal toxicity, metheglobinemia	Slow development
				Unclear dosage

the same drugs and schedules as VL, or even more if they are caused by *Leishmania braziliensis*.

An assessment of cost and cost-effectiveness of interventions, recently carried out in India, compared the cost of the drug, of hospitalization and evolution after treatment (cure, relapse, treatment failure and interruption). The results showed that the final cost of successful treatment varied considerably from US$175 using miltefosine, US$467 using ampB, to US$1613 using liposomal ampB. Assuming that there are 100 000 new cases each year in Bihar State, India, and that these need treatment using miltefosine as first line drug or ampB as second line drug, the cost of treating all the patients would amount to around US$11 million.

Active case detection has proved cheaper than passive detection. Each case detected actively costs US$25 as opposed to US$145 for passive case detection, and comparison of the cost of preventing death results in US$131 for active case detection and US$200 for passive case detection. In other words, passive case detection implies the unforeseen death of some patients, and hence a greater disease burden. With regard to case management of VL, the most cost-effective combination for early case detection is systematic serological screening in endemic areas using one of the recommended techniques, leaving parasitological diagnosis for cases in which serological diagnosis is doubtful. Following an epidemic of VL in Africa, it was possible to carry out a comparative retrospective study of data for "excess mortality", the cost of the control measures and the results obtained. In cost-effectiveness terms the cost of each DALY saved amounted to US$18.40, making treatment a measure of "high return on investment" (Boelaert *et al.*, 1999; Griekspoor *et al.*, 1999). This should be noted in case of future epidemics.

Vector control using indoor spraying of insecticides is always determined by the endo/exophilic and endo/exophagous behaviour of the species of sandfly present in each area. Irrespective of the case, for logistic and cost reasons, periodic spraying of walls is difficult to sustain over time. However, combined campaigns targeting *Anopheles* mosquitoes and sandflies are more cost-effective. A suitable alternative is the use of bed nets impregnated with long-lasting insecticide at an estimated cost of US$5 per unit; on average, the nets last for 5 years.

3. CURRENT DRUGS USED FOR THE TREATMENT OF LEISHMANIASIS

For the first time there are options for the treatment of leishmaniasis, including one oral drug. The chemical structures of the main drugs are given in Figure 3. Standard regimens for the different forms of disease are shown in Table 1. Although this is progress, it must still be seen within the context of the limitations of these drugs, namely, long courses, parenteral administration (except miltefosine), toxicity, variable efficacies and/or high cost and limitations in deployment. The following section briefly reviews the drugs currently in use or in development.

3.1. Treatments for VL

The summary characteristics of current and future options for the treatment of VL are given in Table 2.

3.1.1. Pentavalent Antimonials

The pentavalent antimonials (meglumine antimoniate and SSG) were first introduced for the treatment of leishmaniasis in 1940s and remain effective treatments for most forms of this disease. However, the requirement of up to 28 days of parenteral administration, increasing concern about toxicity, the variable efficacy against VL and CL, and the emergence of significant resistance in the major VL focus (India and Nepal) are all factors limiting the drugs' usefulness. There are two major issues relating to treatment and control with antimonials:

- Confirmation of the efficacy, consistent formulation and side effects of low-cost generic drugs
- Elucidation of the mechanism of drug resistance, understanding the cause of resistance, markers for resistance and restriction of spread of resistance

With respect to the first point, the studies with generic SSG in India and East Africa (Ritmeijer *et al.*, 2001), manufactured by Albert David

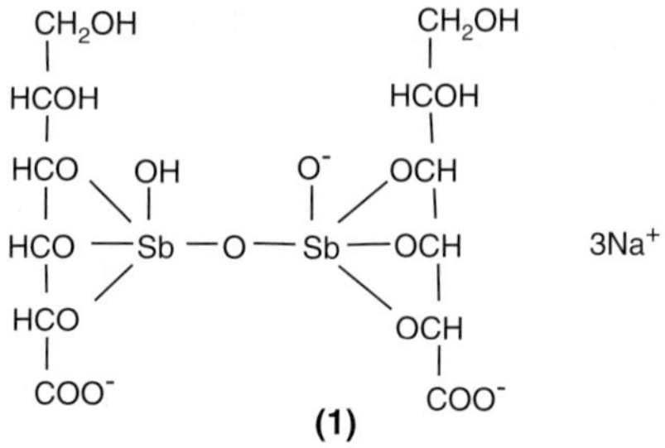

(1)

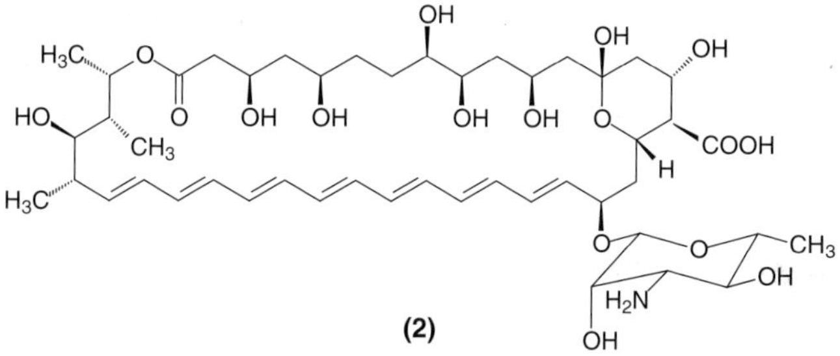

(2)

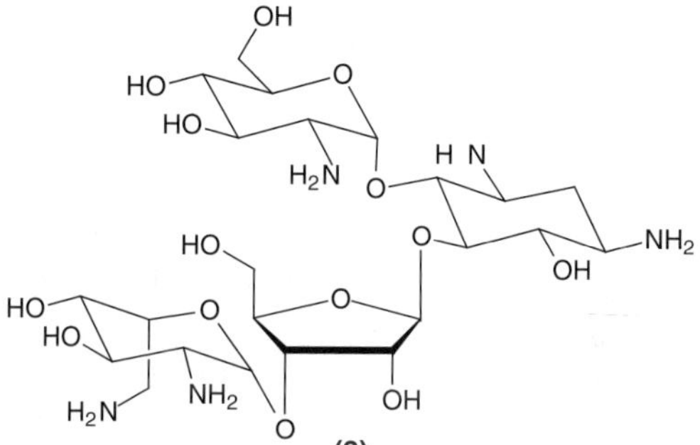

(3)

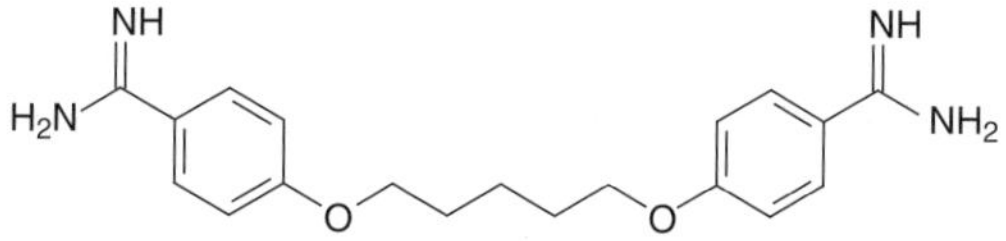

(4)

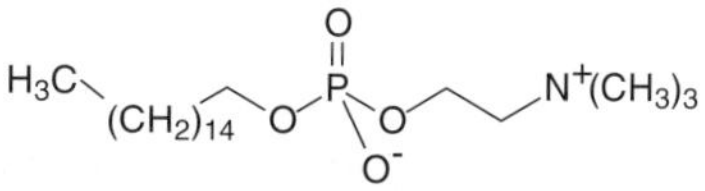

(5)

Figure 3 Structures of drugs used in the treatment of leishmaniasis: (1) SSG (Pentostam), (2) ampB, (3) PM, (4) pentamidine and (5) miltefosine.

(Kolkata, India) and marketed at 1/14th cost of formulations from GSK (Pentostam^{TM}), has offered major advantage to health systems and NGOs involved in treating patients. While these studies have also helped to allay some concerns about the consistency and associated toxicities of some generic products, there is no guarantee that all products have been consistently good all the time. It is difficult to establish with certainty whether substandard products may have had a role in the generation of resistance in India, but there is some evidence that it has added to toxicity (Sundar *et al.*, 1998; Rijal *et al.*, 2003).

Regarding the second point, studies over the past two decades have demonstrated an ever decreasing response rate of VL cases to antimonial treatment in Bihar, India (Figure 4). The erosion of response to SSG has been documented in this major focus by some 13 studies conducted during 1980–2004, enrolling over 1500 patients (Olliaro *et al.*, 2005). In two major studies conducted in the late 1990s (Sundar *et al.*, 2004; Thakur *et al.*, 2004) over 60% VL cases fail to respond to 20 mg/kg/d of SSG over 28 days at 6-month follow-up (Sundar, 2001).

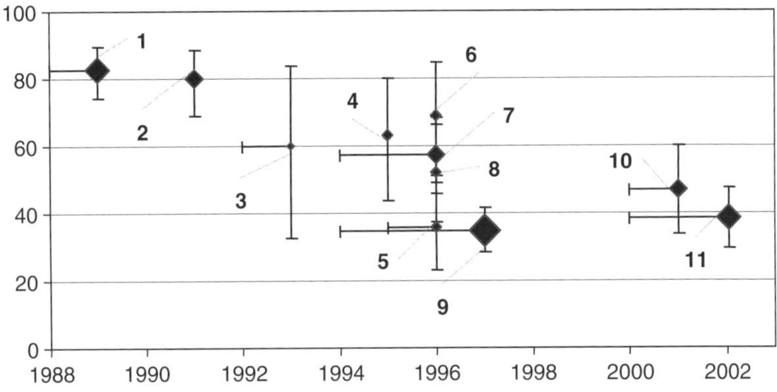

Figure 4 Efficacy (%) at 6-month follow-up of treatment with antimony at 20 mg/kg/d for 4 weeks in Bihar, India, during 1988–2002. Mean efficacy with 95%CI (bar on the *Y* axis); the bar on the *X* axis is duration of study; marker size is proportional to study size. 1: Thakur *et al.* (1993a), 2: Thakur *et al.* (1993b), 3: Sundar *et al.* (1995), 4: Jha *et al.* (1998), 5: Sundar *et al.* (1997), 6: Thakur *et al.* (2000a), 7: Thakur *et al.* (1998), 8: Thakur *et al.* (2000b), 9: Sundar *et al.* (2000), 10: Thakur and Narayan (2004), 11: Thakur *et al.* (2004).

The focus of resistance is geographically restricted to districts of Bihar north of the Ganges up to Nepal, yet affecting 50% of the total burden of kala-azar (Figure 5). An *in vitro* survey of parasite sensitivities across Bihar showed varying levels of resistance, although sampling varied greatly in the different districts (Figure 3) (Thakur *et al.*, 2004).

The failure of response appears to be due to acquired resistance, i.e. selection of resistant mutants. In one study, *L. donovani* isolates were taken from patients who responded to antimonial treatment and those who were non-responders in Bihar, India (Lira *et al.*, 1999). The sensitivity of clinical isolates to SSG was tested in an *in vitro* amastigote–macrophage model, where isolates from responder patients were three-fold more sensitive (ED_{50} values around 2.5 µg Sb/ml) than isolates from non-responder patients (ED_{50} values around 7.5 µg Sb/ml). There was no difference in the sensitivity of isolates when the promastigote assay was used (Lira *et al.*, 1999; Dube *et al.*, 2005). The significant difference in amastigote sensitivity and the correlation is consistent with the concept of acquired resistance. However, the

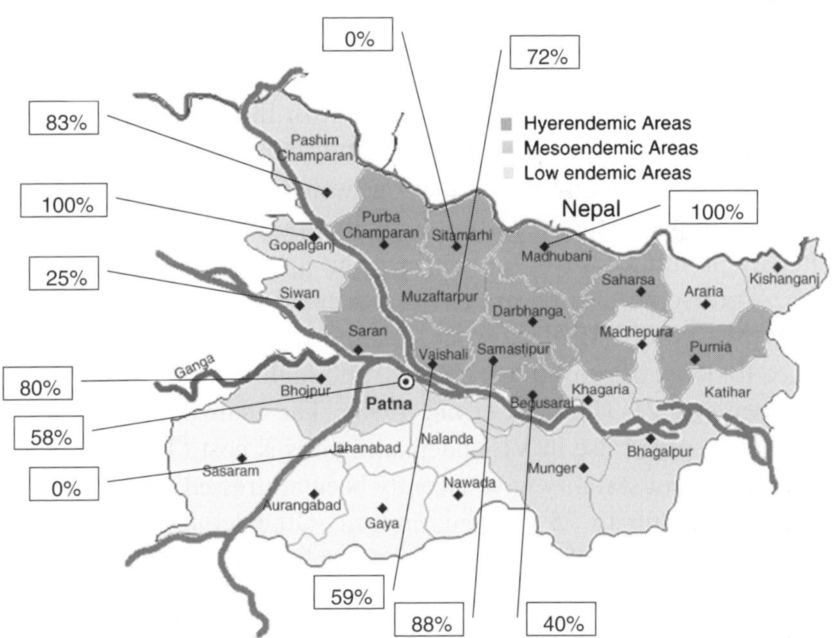

Figure 5 Distribution of resistance of visceral leishmaniasis to antimony in Bihar and Nepal. From Thakur *et al.* (2004).

sample size was small (15 non-responders, 9 responders), and a three-fold difference in sensitivity can be seen between experiments in this model (Croft and Brun, 2003). In addition, it is known that there are strains in circulation that show intrinsic lack of sensitivity to pent-avalent antimonials in *in vitro* assays. Other reports on VL isolates from Sudan also showed that there was an apparent association be-tween clinical response to Pentostam and sensitivity in the amasti-gote–macrophage model (but not in promastigotes) in an area where there was only a 5% failure to respond to antimonials (Ibrahim *et al.*, 1994; Abdo *et al.*, 2003). Sundar (2001) has suggested that inadequate treatment due to use of unqualified practitioners, failure to follow WHO guidelines, or use of poor quality drug, are the reasons for the increasing levels of drug failure.

3.1.2. Amphotericin B

Amphotericin B deoxycholate (Fungizone®) has been a second-line treatment for VL for over two decades. With the profound failure in pentavalent antimonial therapy in Bihar State, it has assumed front line status. Originally developed as a systemic anti-fungal, ampB is a highly active antileishmanial agent, but with the major drawback of being acutely toxic and requiring careful and slow intravenous ad-ministration. Lipid ampB formulations were initially developed in the 1980s to improve the toxic profile of this polyene antibiotic and to alter its pharmacokinetic properties. The liposomal ampB formula-tion, AmBisome®, is an approved treatment of VL in Europe and USA (Meyerhoff, 1999), and has all the requisite properties of re-duced toxicity, improved half-life $t_{1/2}$, and high level of efficacy in the treatment of VL (Berman *et al.*, 1998). The main limitation to its more widespread use in VL-endemic regions is cost (Table 1). Some concerns about stability have recently been addressed and stability at temperatures up to 25°C is guaranteed. Other commercial ampB–lipid formulations, the ampB–lipid complex (Abelcet®), an ampB colloidal dispersion (Amphocil™) and a multilamellar liposomal formulation, have also been used in the treatment of VL, although less extensively than AmBisome®, and with less efficacy and higher toxicity (Bodhe *et al.*, 1999; Sundar *et al.*, 2004).

Perhaps the most important recent observation for the treatment of VL is that a single dose of AmBisome can produce a 90% cure rate (Sundar, 2001), an important finding for future development of co-administrations. The development of alternative nanoparticle/lipid formulations or chemical derivatives has been limited to experimental models (Petit *et al.*, 1999; Zvulunov *et al.*, 2003). Of these the use of "heated" ampB deoxycholate, with the formation of superaggregates with reduction in toxicity and without loss of efficacy, is an option for further investigation as a cheaper alternative to the lipid formulations (Kwong *et al.*, 2001; Fukui *et al.*, 2003).

In conclusion, ampB is highly potent, and if better (safer and more convenient) alternatives were available at low cost it would make an ideal treatment alone or in combination.

3.1.3. Miltefosine

Miltefosine (hexadecylphosphocholine), originally developed as an anticancer drug, is the first effective oral treatment for VL and the most recent antileishmanial drug to enter the market. The antileishmanial activity of miltefosine was initially discovered in the mid-1980s, following which efficacy was demonstrated in a number of experimental models *in vitro* and *in vivo* (Croft *et al.*, 1987, 1996; Kuhlencord *et al.*, 1992). Clinical trials in the mid-to-late 1990s, part of a co-development partnership between Asta Medica (now Zentaris) and WHO/TDR, showed oral activity in VL patients including those who were not responsive to antimonial treatment. After a Phase III trial, in which 282 out of 299 (94%) VL patients were cured with an oral dose of 2.5 mg/kg of miltefosine daily for 28 days (Sundar *et al.*, 2002), miltefosine was registered in India in March 2002 for oral treatment of VL. A Phase IV study has been completed and analysis should be available in 2006.

The potential of oral miltefosine in the treatment of VL/HIV-co-infected patients has also been investigated. In a compassionate use programme an initial response was achieved in 25 out of 39 (64%) patients, including 16 patients (43%) with initial parasitological cure. Median duration of treatment was 1 month but considerably longer in some cases (Sindermann *et al.*, 2004).

The major limitation on the use of miltefosine is teratogenicity; this means that women of child-bearing age must be ensured contraception for the period of treatment and, due to the long half-life ($t_{1/2} = 120\,h$), an additional 2 months. The long half-life and uncontrolled availability of this drug has also raised concerns about the emergence of resistance (Bryceson, 2001; Sundar and Murray, 2005). Laboratory studies on *L. donovani* promastigote cultures showed that miltefosine-resistant clones could be readily selected (Seifert *et al.*, 2003) and that the resistance is related to two point mutations on an aminophospholipid translocase (Pérez-Victoria *et al.*, 2003). Thus, oral bioavailability has in practice both advantages and disadvantages. It increases the treatment base in the population and hence potential coverage of otherwise untreated cases (due to inconvenience, bed capacity, etc.) yet reducing costs to and burden on the health sector. However, the current uncontrolled release of the drug at a high price through the private sector by untrained sellers creates misuse and exposes to the risk of toxicity (inadvertent exposure during pregnancy) and resistance (subcurative doses). Miltefosine has great potential if properly used (e.g. subsidized and via DOT-type systems, see Section 4) (Sundar and Murray, 2005).

3.1.4. Paromomycin

The antileishmanial activity of PM, an aminoglycoside antibiotic, was identified in the 1960s but it has taken several decades for this known anti-microbial agent to move through clinical trials for both VL and CL to become a useful treatment. Although a parenteral formulation of PM, a drug with poor oral bioavailability, had been in use for anti-bacterial infections for decades worldwide, the full potential for treatment of VL has been painfully slow. Several Phase II trials in India in the 1990s showed promising results, with >90% of patients cured of VL following treatment with 16–20 mg/kg daily for 20 days alone (Jha *et al.*, 1998; Thakur *et al.*, 2000b) or 12–20 mg/kg/d combined with antimony (Thakur *et al.*, 2000b).

A prospective, randomized, comparative, open-label trial of the safety and efficacy of PM (aminosidine) plus SSG versus SSG alone for the treatment of VL has been made. A Phase III multi-centre, randomized, controlled, comparative trial to provide data on efficacy and safety of PM for VL has been completed in India (Jha *et al.*, 2005a) with an aim for registration in India in 2006 (www.iowh.com). Phase IV trials are already planned. Clinical trials with PM for VL are currently ongoing in East Africa through DNDi and partner institutes (www.dndi.org). PM is off-patent and has received Orphan Drug status by the US FDA and the EU EMEA. It is expected to be very cheap. The possibility of resistance must also be considered. PM-resistant *L. donovani* promastigotes were generated experimentally (Maarouf *et al.*, 1998) and with PM moving towards clinical use, more studies on mechanism of action and resistance are needed. Although there are concerns about monotherapy and the development of resistance, the necessity for parenteral administration by trained medical staff probably makes this less of a concern than for miltefosine.

3.1.5. Other Treatments for VL

Another candidate for oral treatment is the 8-aminoquinoline discovered by the Walter Reed Army Institute of Research (WRAIR, USA) and under development with GSK, UK. Progress has been very slow. Phase II studies were conducted in Kenya, Brazil and India. In Kenya, 4 out of 8 patients were cured with 1 mg/kg/d for 28 d; treatment was well tolerated expect minor GI events and methaemoglobinaemia (Sherwood *et al.*, 1994). In a dose-escalating trial in Brazil, results were inconclusive for efficacy in the dose range 1–3.25 mg/kg/d for 28 d, but previously unreported nephrotoxicity occurred from 2.3 mg/kg/d (Dietze *et al.*, 2001). More recently reported trials in Bihar and Kenya showed that there was a dose effect in terms of both efficacy and toxicity between 1.5 and 2.5 mg/kg/d for 28 days. Treatment was 100% effective at 2 mg/kg/d and safe up to a dose of 1.75 mg/kg/d for 28 days except methaemoglobinaemia. Nephrotoxicity occurred from 2 mg/kg/d (Jha *et al.*, 2005b; Wasunna *et al.*, 2005).

3.2. Treatments for CL

Although a variety of drugs have been used in the treatment of CL, many (Table 1) have proved to give equivocal results or proved active against some forms of CL and not others. There is a current re-interest in cryo- and heat therapies to treat this disease. However, it is unlikely that these alternative therapies will play a major role in the treatment and control. Drugs in current use and on trial are described below.

3.2.1. Pentavalent Antimonials

The variation in clinical response to the standard pentavalent antimonials, SSG (Pentostam) and meglumine antimoniate (Glucantime) has been a persistent problem in the treatment of leishmaniasis over the past 50 years. The absence of controlled clinical trials that actually confirm the efficacy of these drugs has been compounded by problems associated with species variation in drug sensitivity. The potential advantage of intralesional injection over parenteral administration has been the subject of investigation in clinical practice over the past two decades. Intrinsic variation in the sensitivity of *Leishmania* species to pentavalent antimonials has been shown *in vitro* using the amastigote–macrophage model, where *L. donovani* and *L. brasiliensis* were >five-fold more sensitive than *L. major*, *L. tropica* and *L. mexicana* (Allen and Neal, 1989; Neal *et al.*, 1995). In other studies by Berman *et al.* (1982), using a different amastigote–macrophage model, and Grogl *et al.* (1992), using promastigote cultures, a wide variation in the sensitivity of clinical isolates from CL cases was demonstrated, which was suggested to be correlated to subcurative treatment. In one of the few controlled clinical trials that compared the cure rate of antimonials in CL caused by different species, Pentostam produced a significantly higher cure rate for *L. braziliensis* lesions than for *L. mexicana* lesions (Navin *et al.*, 1992).

3.2.2. Amphotericin B

AmpB deoxycholate is also a second-line drug for CL, and especially for mucocutaneous disease unresponsive to other drugs. Novel ampB formulations have been used successfully to treat CL, for example in immunocompromised patients (Amato *et al.*, 2004) and paediatric CL (Zvulunov *et al.*, 2003). However as CL is usually a self-limiting syndrome, parental administration, cost and toxicity have limited the evaluation of ampB as a wider treatment for CL.

3.2.3. Miltefosine

Miltefosine was first shown to be active against CL in a Phase II trial in Colombia. A more recent study against CL was carried out in Colombia and Guatemala with oral miltefosine at 2.5 mg/kg/d for 28 days (Soto *et al.*, 2004). In Colombia, a region where *Leishmania panamensis* is common, the cure rates for miltefosine were 91% (40 of 44 patients), whereas in Guatemala (regions where *L. braziliensis* and *L. mexicana* are common) cure rates achieved were only 53% (20 of 38 patients) and were lower than the historic antimony cure rates of >90%. This pattern of variable response could be related to species sensitivity, which has been shown in laboratory studies (Escobar *et al.*, 2001; Yardley *et al.*, 2005).

3.2.4. Paromomycin

PM in topical formulations has been shown to be a suitable treatment of CL. The work of El-On and colleagues in the early 1980s (El-On *et al.*, 1984) showed that a topical formulation containing 15% PM and 12% methyl benzethonium chloride (a skin-penetrating agent) was effective against experimental CL. In subsequent clinical trials 77% patients were cured after 20 days treatment compared with 27% cured in the placebo group (El-On *et al.*, 1992). This formulation is available through TEVA (Israel) but has not been widely used because of cost and irritancy. Other topical formulations with a lower skin irritancy have also been on clinical trial, including one containing 15% PM with 10% urea. A recent trial in an endemic *L. major* area of Iran showed no improved cure rate for PM with this formulation: rather, accelerated cure was demonstrated (Iraji and Sadeghinia, 2005). This formulation is available through Razak Labs (Tehran). A third PM topical formulation containing 15% PM with 0.5% gentamicin in a 10% surfactant vehicle (WR279,396) is also in development. The formulation cured 64% of CL patients after 20 days treatment in Colombia (Soto *et al.*, 2002) and 92% more recently in trials in Tunisia (Ben Salah *et al.*, 2005a).

3.2.5. Other Treatments for CL

Imiquimod (Aldara, 3 M Pharmaceuticals) is an immunomodulatory imidazoquinoline derivative that is used for the topical treatment of genital warts caused by the human papillomavirus. Imiquimod stimulates a local immune response at the site of application, induces the production of cytokines and nitric oxide in macrophages and has been shown to have an effect in experimental infections of CL (Buates and Matlashewski, 1999). In conjunction with standard antimonial chemotherapy it has been used to successfully treat patients with cutaneous lesions, which did not respond to antimonial therapy alone (Arevalo *et al.*, 2001). Other studies on Old World CL failed to show that imiquimod was effective as a topical agent alone (Seeberger*et al.*, 2003) and further clinical studies on combinations are required.

3.3. Treatment of Complicated Forms

3.3.1. Leishmania– HIV Co-infections and Secondary Prophylaxis

From a clinical point of view, *Leishmania*–HIV co-infection is similar to conventional VL, with four peculiarities: (a) DCL is often seen, with or without granulomas, but skin biopsy shows frequent amastigotes with a negative skin test; (b) unusual organs can be affected, such as lungs, larynx, intestine, etc., the reason why the clinical signs can be unspecific or even unnoticed; (c) in the great majority, patients relapse despite correct treatment; and (d) more than 40% of the co-infected patients do not exhibit anti-*Leishmania* antibodies despite parasites being present in bone marrow and spleen.

In *Leishmania*–HIV co-infected patients, antimonials and ampB are the drugs of choice, using the same schedules and doses as in immunocompetent patients, although there are few clinical trials supporting recommendations. In an open, randomized and multi-centred study comparing meglumine antimoniate versus ampB deoxycholate with overdose of serum saline, no differences were found among both drugs. Within 6 months after chemotherapy (Laguna *et al.*, 1999) 17% relapsed in the antimonial branch and 24% in the ampB group, and within 12 months 73 and 61%, respectively. The survival rate was 52 weeks for the patients enrolled in the antimonial arm and 44 in the ampB group. The first cohort had higher cardiotoxicity and chemical pancreatitis, the second one exhibited nephrotoxicity and a trend to develop anaemia. Similar results were obtained in a second open, randomized and multicentre clinical trial comparing lipid complex ampB (ABCL) given at dose of 3 mg/kg/d during 5 or 10 days, with meglumine antimoniate; the cure rate was 35% (Laguna *et al.*, 2003). The high rate of side effects is avoided if liposomal ampB is used for 21 days (Davidson *et al.*, 1994) although a shorter duration treatment has the same efficacy (4 mg/kg/d given 5 consecutive days plus days 10, 17, 24, 31 and 28) (Russo *et al.*, 1996); however relapses are not prevented in either case.

Secondary prophylaxis is recommended in co-infected patients for life to avoid relapses, although for others it can be discontinued when the CD4+ count is restored thanks to highly active antiretroviral therapy (HAART) (Soriano *et al.*, 2000; Berenguer *et al.*, 2000). Pentamidine every three or 4 weeks was initially used to prevent relapses and additional infections by *Pneumocystis carinii* (*P. jirovecii*), despite the risk of creating an insulin-dependent diabetes. Monthly meglumine antimoniate or liposomal ampB given every 2 or 4 weeks are very commonly used and lead to a lower proportion of relapses (Ribera *et al.*, 1996; Pintado and López-Vélez, 2001). The only open, randomized, comparative study of secondary prophylaxis, compared lipidic complex ampB (3 mg/kg every 21 days) with a co-infected group of patients not getting secondary prophylaxis, showed a relapse rate of 50 and 78%, respectively after 1-year follow-up (López-Vélez *et al.*, 2004).

In general, HAART has sharply reduced the prevalence of co-infection and the patients have a better survival rate than those that do not receive it (Pintado *et al.*, 2001; de la Rosa *et al.*, 2002). Two situations are under consideration: prime attack and relapses. By increasing the CD4+ count, thanks to HAART, there is a greater chance to control the initial *Leishmania* infection (López-Vélez *et al.*, 2003). In contrast, patients not receiving HAART have a greater chance of developing a bout of leishmaniasis with later clinical and parasitological relapses (Pintado and López-Vélez, 2001; Pintado *et al.*, 2001). The response seems to be inversely related to the viral load before treatment (Berhe *et al.*, 1999). However, if the patient has already had a prime attack of leishmaniasis, HAART seems not to be so efficient in the prevention of relapses, although these can be delayed. 38–70% of the co-infected patients will relapse within 24 months after the anti-*Leishmania* treatment independently of the CD4+ increase and even with undetectable viral load (López-Vélez, 2003; Mira *et al.*, 2004).

In brief, the use of antiretrovirals has modified the outcome of co-infection as (i) the incidence has dropped sharply since they were introduced and given freely in Europe in 1997, (ii) the prime attack by leishmaniasis appears only when there is a clear failure of the antiretroviral therapy, and (iii) relapses can appear despite the increase of CD4+ and non-detectable viral load, meaning that the success in virus control does not necessarily avoids relapses. Unfortunately, antiretrovirals do not greatly benefits patients in developing countries since the mean coverage is 15% (8% for African countries) (UNAIDS, 2005).

3.3.2. Recidivans Cutaneous Leishmaniasis

RCL due to *L. tropica* needs antimonial treatment for long periods and relapses are common leading to the use of combined treatments (Momeni and Aminjavaheri, 1995) or surgical interventions; thermotherapy is effective only in primary lesions of reduced size (Reithinger *et al.*, 2005).

3.3.3. Diffuse Cutaneous Leishmaniasis

DCL due to *L. amazonensis* can be treated with antimonials associated with isoniazid and rifampicin due to the synergistic effect, or immunotherapy combining killed *Leishmania* promastigotes and BCG (Convit *et al.*, 1989). CL due to *Leishmania aethiopica* normally does not respond to meglumine antimoniate but to SSG (3–4 mg/kg once a week). Without this healing is not ensured and relapses can be seen months later. It has been suggested to combine sodium stiblogluconate with PM (Teklemariam *et al.*, 1994).

3.3.4. Mucocutaneous Leishmaniasis

MCL is normally treated with meglumine antimoniate (20 mg/kg/d for 28 days); non-healing lesions are susceptible, and have to be treated for 2 months instead or, eventually, with ampB. Immunotherapy is a promising method to treat MCL although more experience is needed (Convit *et al.*, 2003).

3.3.5. PKDL

This syndrome, characterized as skin lesions, nodules or papules, frequently on the face, has been well characterized in India and Sudan. PKDL often appears in patients 2–7 years after apparently successful antimonial treatment of VL. Treatment of PKDL has long been a problem, and formal recommendations for this treatment, based upon studies in India and Sudan, have been using SSG (20 mg/kg for at least 120 days) (Thakur and Kumar, 1990; Zijlstra and El-Hassan, 2001). A reconsideration of the recommended treatment is required due to antimonial resistance in India, making ampB the preferred drug (Thakur *et al.*, 1997). AmBisome, very effective in treatment of VL, has also proved to be an effective treatment for PKDL at 2.5 mg/kg for 20 days (Musa *et al.*, 2005), with the same caveat of high cost restricting its use.

3.3.6. Pregnancy

Although very little information regarding treatment of VL in pregnancy is available, there is no discussion that the threat of a fatal outcome of leishmaniasis for the mother, the foetus and the newborn is much higher than the risk of drug side effects (Pagliano *et al.*, 2005). If untreated, abortion, small-for-date and congenital leishmaniasis have been often described. Antimonials are considered less safe because of embryotoxicity in experimental models (Paumgartten and Chahoud, 2001), and the fact that in one Sudanese case Pentostam did not avoid kala-azar in the newborn with a fatal outcome (Eltoum *et al.*, 1992). Amphotericin deoxycholate has been used successfully in six pregnant women; however, the renal toxicity risk cannot be ruled out, although it can be circumvented using liposomal ampB. In fact, it has been fully effective in seven women suffering VL during pregnancy (Pagliano *et al.*, 2005).

4. CONTROL OF LEISHMANIASIS—NEEDS

4.1. Visceral Leishmaniasis

While more treatment options are and will be available, there remain several operational issues to tackle for successful control of VL:

- Coverage remains the greatest challenge. For instance, only around 15 000 cases are treated at health facilities in Bihar per annum out of an estimated 100 000 cases or more every year. Cost and access to proper medical care are limiting factors.
- The majority of treatments are parenteral. Where hospital facilities exist, treatment may be given by injection (venous drip or i.m.), but bed occupancy remains a limiting factor and hospitalization costs add to the overall treatment costs. In other cases, i.m. treatment can be provided on outpatient basis at a lower cost.
- Even with an oral medication, optimal prescriber and patient adherence must be guarded. Misuse will lead to untoward toxicity and parasite resistance. Conditions for directly observing treatment have to be set in place.

4.2. Cutaneous Leishmaniasis

Current treatment and control of CL are inadequate. There are two areas where changes in approach are required to provide significant improvements: in the methodology for determining the efficacy of known and novel drugs, and improvement in simplified treatment regimes and formulations to treat simple CL.

The problems associated with measurement of rate of cure following treatment, in a self-curing disease, with high variation of self-cure rate and drug response, have made CL a difficult disease for which to measure drug efficacy. Ideally, a clinical trial should include:

- randomized double-blind controlled treatment regime,
- species identification,
- measurement of cure in relation to clinical signs (lesion measurement) as well as parasitological load (by PCR) and

- an integrated model of analysis to measure rates of regression in lesion size in treated versus placebo groups.

Recent trials have started to address these problems (Iraji and Sadeghinia, 2005; Ben Salah *et al.*, 2005b).

Secondly, there is a need for rational pharmaceutical design of formulations optimal for CL (Garnier and Croft, 2002). Topical formulations offer significant advantages over systemic therapy, such as ease of administration, lower adverse effects and cost effectiveness. As a local treatment, it is an attractive approach for simple forms of CL without the risk of developing complications that require systemic therapy.

However, further studies are required to investigate the topical potential for a number of candidate antileishmanial drugs. Many antileishmanial drugs have undesirable physicochemical properties for transdermal delivery and so novel strategies are required to enhance absorption. Total flux depends on drug physicochemical properties, combined with vehicle influence on altering penetration profiles. Future topical development must employ rational drug design to take into account physicochemical properties of drugs, their effect on percutaneous absorption and their retention or drug release at the sites of infection in the dermis. Therapeutic efficacy depends on both adequate permeation and pharmacological potency.

4.3. Test of Cure

For both VL and CL, monitoring of the efficacy of treatments is limited by diagnosis through out-of-date difficult and invasive techniques—spleen or bone marrow puncture for VL and lesion biopsy for CL. The development of non-invasive serological diagnostic methods with high sensitivity and specificity, for example DAT, K39 and Katex (urine dipstick), is a major advance in control of leishmaniasis (Guerin *et al.*, 2002). In the context of monitoring the drug response in patients, antigen detection methods must be developed. The antigen-detecting Katex (Sarkari *et al.*, 2002; Boelaert *et al.*, 2004) is an example of this approach. However, other antigen methods are in development and research in this area needs to be encouraged.

4.4. A Policy for Drug Resistance

There is no current policy at a national or international level to prevent the emergence of resistance to antileishmanial drugs (Bryceson, 2001). The seriousness of the threat is not the same in anthroponotic and zoonotic foci of leishmaniasis. In zoonotic diseases, most CL and also VL caused by *L. infantum* (or *L. chagasi*), the parasite is primarily an infection of a feral or domestic mammalian host and only occasionally humans. In zoonotic foci, the time that a parasite population is exposed to the drug, when resistant forms can be selected, is insignificant unless the mammalian host is also treated. This is also true for those leishmaniases where most infections cause asymptomatic infections that do not receive treatment. In relation to zoonotic leishmaniasis the most important consideration is where control methods for canine leishmaniasis are implemented using the same drugs used in the treatment of human disease. It has been shown that treatment of the domestic canine host with pentavalent antimonials can lead to changes in sensitivity of parasites as determined in isolates taken before and after treatment (Gramiccia *et al.*, 1992; Gradoni *et al.*, 2003). Presently, it is only possible to speculate upon the implications of these observations that any drug used in dogs might select for resistant parasites. The spread of resistant parasites has to be related to a number of parameters that are currently unknown. For example, little is known about the effects of drug resistance on the fitness and virulence of *Leishmania* parasites, including ability to transform, establish an infection in the vector or outgrow a nonresistant wild type and R_0 of *Leishmania*. Unlike anti-bacterial drug resistance, no mathematical model has been developed to model the spatio-temporal spread of drug-resistant *Leishmania* parasites. Such a model would both help in our understanding, as has been shown for antibiotic resistance (McCormick *et al.*, 2003), and provide a tool for evaluating control strategies to contain or prevent the development of drug resistance.

Current knowledge of the epidemiology and transmission of leishmaniasis would suggest that the spread of acquired drug resistance need not be considered as a factor in CL, except in anthroponotic foci of *L. tropica*. However, an additional factor that requires consideration is the potential transmission of *L. infantum* by needle (Alvar *et al.*, 1997). Apart from the acquired resistance in these foci, it is clear that even among populations of zoonotic *Leishmania* there are parasites that are highly insensitive to antimonials (Grogl *et al.*, 1992), and these parasites may have a common "resistance" phenotype that can be transmitted from host to host.

Acquired resistance is a major concern in anthroponotic disease foci, for example *L. donovani* in Bihar State, India (Sundar, 2001), and in the Sudan where, with respect to pentavalent antimonials, the evidence for increasing number of treatment failures has been well documented (see above). Considering the two elements of drug resistance, "intrinsic variation in sensitivity" and "acquired drug resistance" separately, there are several different strategies that can be employed.

For zoonotic disease, improved field methods for species identification are essential. This is of greatest clinical significance in Central and South America, where the distribution of *L. mexicana*, *L. amazonensis*, *L. panamensis*, *L. braziliensis* and other members of these complexes overlap. However, the molecular tools, for example PCR, that have been developed have to be implemented on a wider scale.

For anthroponotic disease a number of measures can be introduced, as shown in other infectious diseases, for the control of drug resistance. These measures would include monitoring/surveillance of clinical isolates, improved methods to observe patient adherence to treatment regimes, use of drug combinations and legal restrictions on drug accessibility, for example through the private sector. For implementation of any policy, improved diagnostic methods and a wider range of drugs are also of importance.

As a first step in developing a strategy, a policy and structure are needed to monitor drug resistance through either (i) phenotypic sensitivity of parasite isolates, or (ii) molecular changes that indicate alterations in either the drug target or mechanisms that alter the intra-parasite level of active drug. There are problems with both approaches. First, after isolation from the patient, drug sensitivity of clinical isolates must be tested as soon as possible using carefully defined protocols. Although promastigote assays are the simplest, this assay is not predictive and should be avoided (Croft and Brun, 2003).

The amastigote–macrophage assay is currently the only model able to correlate clinical response to the sensitivity of the isolate, as demonstrated with respect to pentavalent antimonials (Ibrahim *et al.*, 1994; Lira *et al.*, 1999; Dube *et al.*, 2005). Axenic amastigotes are sensitive but adaptation of isolates is both a selective and long process for this type of assay (Ephros *et al.*, 1997; Sereno and Lemesre, 1997). Secondly, the development of molecular probes or PCR-based diagnostics to monitor the development and spread of drug resistance is severely limited by a lack of knowledge of the molecular and biochemical mechanisms of action and resistance of antileishmanial drugs. So far molecular techniques have been successfully used to identify resistance loci to antifolates, pentamidine, miltefosine and sterol biosynthesis inhibitors in some *Leishmania* (Cotrim *et al.*, 1999; Coelho *et al.*, 2003; Pérez-Victoria *et al.*, 2003). But these laboratory studies are a long way from application in the field.

The introduction of oral drugs for leishmaniasis offers advantages of improved compliance, self-administration and reduced costs. In the Phase IV trial of miltefosine a 7-day supply was issued to patients who had to return to the clinic each week for 4 weeks for examination and re-supply. For drugs like miltefosine, which have a long half-life and a propensity for selection of resistant forms, the monitoring of daily dosing and the completion of a course of treatment is essential. The directly observed treatment strategy (DOTS) for TB chemotherapy has been successfully introduced in India by the Revised National TB Control Programme (RNTCP) in 1997 (see WHO Report, 2003, Global Tuberculosis Control—www.who.int/gtb/publications/globerep/index.html). The potential for use of a parallel system in the deployment of antileishmanials like miltefosine, and hopefully other drugs in the future, needs to be considered urgently (Sundar and Murray, 2005).

In addition to having strategies for monitoring and surveillance, there is a need to prevent the problem, for example through use of drug combinations. Combinations have proved to be an essential feature in antimicrobial chemotherapy through design or use to (i) increase activity through use of compounds with synergistic or additive activity, (ii) prevent the emergence of drug resistance, (iii) lower required doses, reducing chances of toxic side effects and cost or (iv) increase the spectrum of activity, for example antileishmanial and anti-inflammatory or immunodulator in CL. Previous studies on drug combinations for VL, for example, allopurinol plus SSG (Chunge *et al.*, 1985) and PM plus SSG (Neal *et al.*, 1985, 1995; Chunge *et al.*, 1990; Thakur *et al.*, 2000) have aimed at improving efficacy. The use of combinations to combat resistance has been well rehearsed in antimalarials; for example, with resistance due to point mutations it has been estimated that symptomatic individuals harbour up to about 10^{12} parasites. If a target enzyme has a mutation rate of 10^{-7}, the chance of developing resistance to a single agent is high, but the likelihood of resistance to two compounds with different targets is very low (White and Pongtavornpinyo, 2002). Studies to fully explore and provide a rational basis for drug combinations are rare for leishmaniasis (Seifert and Croft, 2006). Bryceson (2001) argued the case for examining combinations of strong antileishmanials with "weak" drugs (e.g. azoles). This is an approach also used in malaria treatment, for example the inclusion of clindamycin or azithromycin in drug combinations. In the context of leishmaniasis, considering the properties of established therapies, the use of both simultaneous and sequential combination therapies needs to be investigated. Ultimately, improved combinations will come with an improved armoury of drugs that have different targets and have no cross-resistance. In this respect, the omens are not good (Croft and Coombs, 2003). Apart from PM, which is in the last stages of development, the only other drug on the horizon for leishmaniasis is sitamaquine.

4.5. Elimination Programme

A major event in 2005 has been the decision of three countries in the Indian subcontinent (Bangladesh, India and Nepal) to sign an agreement towards elimination of VL as a public health problem. Indeed the political backing will ignite the effort to reduce the disease burden. This will be a gigantic endeavour. For it to succeed, the campaign must reach out to the large number of patients who are currently without treatment, but the tools available are few (Guerin *et al.*, 2002). Current tools for early diagnosis are limited. Options for large-scale treatment are restricted to miltefosine and soon PM, and both have limitations (see respective sections), which will be amplified by mass use. With time, parasites in Bihar have become increasingly tolerant and resistant to antimony deployed as single agent (Olliaro *et al.*, 2005); new drugs must be protected through combinations, but these are yet to be tested. In summary, research has not produced the tools for control to operate efficiently. We must step up coordinated efforts for development and applied research in support of control programmes (Figure 6, which is Plate 6.6 in the separate colour plate section).

5. CONCLUSIONS

The current analysis of drugs in the treatment and control of leishmaniasis show that despite several improvements in therapeutic options in India, on the whole the situation is unsatisfactory. Adjuncts to improved therapies must include better markers of cure, deployment and monitoring strategies. In summary:

- Drugs remain the major method for treatment and control of leishmaniasis.
- Despite the much heralded arrival of new drugs, e.g. miltefosine and PM, long courses, parenteral administration and various toxicities, show that we still have some way to go in terms of having "ideal" drugs.
- HIV co-infections are increasing on a worldwide basis, but we have no treatment and no specific initiatives to find new therapies.
- Resistance to current drugs is increasing, especially in India, and concerns were expressed elsewhere, but we have no policy. This is also relevant in the treatment of canine leishmaniasis with the same drugs than human leishmaniasis.
- Cost of drugs in treatment and control is now being analysed and implications for the rural poor need to be confirmed. It is unlikely that most patients with VL will ever be able to afford the drugs required. An initiative is needed to extend the support for purchase of these essential drugs, similar to that for malaria, TB, HIV and other diseases.

There are options to improve drug treatment of patients with VL and CL. There are ways in which these treatments could be incorporated into national policies. There are organisations that could support the purchase of these tools for treatment and control. The next 3 years will see if there is the will to implement the possible.

DISCLAIMER

The opinions expressed by the authors in this article do not necessarily reflect the opinions of the institution to which the authors are affiliated. The use of trade names is for identification only and does not constitute endorsement by the authors or their institutions. The authors declare no conflicting interests.

ACKNOWLEDGEMENT

We thank Elodie Namer for assisting with preparation of the manuscript.

REFERENCES

Abdo, M.G., Elamin, W.M., Khalil, E.A. and Mukhtar, M.M. (2003). Antimony-resistant *Leishmania donovani* in eastern Sudan: incidence and in vitro correlation. *East Mediterranean Health Journal* **9**, 837–843.

Aggarwal, P. and Wali, J.P. (1991). Profile of kala-azar in north India. *Asia Pacific Journal of Public Health* **5**, 90–93.

Ahluwalia, I.B., Bern, C., Wagatsuma, Y., Costa, C., Chowdhury, R., Ali, M., Amann, J., Haque, R., Breiman, R. and Maguire, J.H. (2004). Visceral leishmaniasis: consequences to women in a Bangladeshi community. *Journal of Women's Health (Larchmt)* **13**, 360–364.

Allen, S. and Neal, R.A. (1989). The *in vitro* susceptibility of macrophages infected with amastigotes of *Leishmania* spp. to pentavalent antimonial drugs and other compounds with special relevance to cutaneous isolates. In: *Leishmaniasis* (D.T. Hart, ed.). New York: Plenum Press.

Alvar, J., Canavate, C., Gutierrez-Solar, B., Jimenez, M., Laguna, F., López-Vélez, R., Molina, R. and Moreno, J. (1997). *Leishmania* and human immunodeficiency virus coinfection: the first 10 years. *Clinical Microbiology Reviews* **10**, 298–319.

Alvar, J., Canavate, C., Molina, R., Moreno, J. and Nieto, J. (2004). Canine leishmaniasis. *Advances in Parasitology* **57**, 1–88.

Alvar, J., Molina, R., San Andres, M., Tesouro, M., Nieto, J., Vitutia, M., Gonzalez, F., San Andres, M.D., Boggio, J., Rodriguez, F., Saïnz, A. and Escacena, C. (1994). Canine leishmaniasis: clinical, parasitological and entomological follow-up after chemotherapy. *Annals of Tropical Medicine and Parasitology* **88**, 371–378.

Amato, V.S., Rabello, A., Rotondo-Silva, A., Kono, A., Maldonado, T.P., Alves, I.C., Floeter-Winter, L.M., Neto, V.A. and Shikanai-Yasuda, M.A. (2004). Successful treatment of cutaneous leishmaniasis with lipid formulations of amphotericin B in two immunocompromised patients. *Acta Tropica* **92**, 127–132.

Arevalo, I., Ward, B., Miller, R., Meng, T.C., Najar, E., Alvarez, E., Matlashewski, G. and Llanos-Cuentas, A. (2001). Successful treatment of drug-resistant cutaneous leishmaniasis in humans by use of imiquimod, an immunomodulator. *Clinical Infectious Disease* **33**, 1847–1851.

Ashford, R.W. (2000). The leishmaniases as emerging and reemerging zoonoses. *International Journal for Parasitology* **30**, 1269–1281.

Ashford, R.W., Desjeux, P. and de Raadt, P. (1992). Estimation of population at risk of infection and number of cases of leishmaniasis. *Parasitology Today* **8**, 104–105.

Attar, Z.J., Chance, M.L., El-Safi, S., Carney, J., Azazy, A., El-Hadi, M., Dourado, C. and Hommel, M. (2001). Latex agglutination test for the detection of urinary antigens in visceral leishmaniasis. *Acta Tropica* **78**, 11–16.

Badaro, R., Benson, D., Eulalio, M.C., Freire, M., Cunha, S., Netto, E.M., Pedral-Sampaio, D., Madureira, C., Burns, J.M., Houghton, R.L., David, J.R. and Reed, S.G. (1996). rK39: a cloned antigen of *Leishmania chagasi* that predicts active visceral leishmaniasis. *Journal of Infectious Disease* **173**, 758–761.

Ben Salah, A., Buffet, P.A., Louzir, H., Morizot, G., Zaâtour, A., Ben Alaya, N., Bel Hajhmida, N., Elahmadi, S., Chlif, S., Lehnert, E., Doughty, S., Dellagi, K., and Grögl, M. (2005a). WR279396 an efficient non toxic topical treatment of old world cutaneous leishmaniasis. *Abstract Book, Third World Congress on Leishmaniosis*, 10–15 April, Sicily, Italy.

Ben Salah, A., Ben Alaya, N., Mokni, M., Morizot, G., Lehnert, E., doughty, S., Grögl, M., and Buffet, P.A. (2005b). Determining treatment efficacy in cutaneous leishmaniasis: an optimized clinical score based on both ulceration and induration outcomes. *Abstract Book, Third World Congress on Leishmaniasis*, 10–15 April, Sicily.

Berenguer, J., Cosin, J., Miralles, P., López, J.C. and Padilla, B. (2000). Discontinuation of secondary anti-leishmania prophylaxis in HIV-infected patients who have responded to highly active antiretroviral therapy. *AIDS* **14**, 2946–2948.

Berhe, N., Wolday, D., Hailu, A., Abraham, Y., Ali, A., Gebre-Michael, T., Desjeux, P., Sonnerborg, A., Akuffo, H. and Britton, S. (1999). HIV viral load and response to antileishmanial chemotherapy in co-infected patients. *AIDS* **13**, 1921–1925.

Berman, J.D., Badaro, R., Thakur, C.P., Wasunna, K.M., Behbehani, K., Davidson, R., Kuzoe, F., Pang, L., Weerasuriya, K. and Bryceson, A.D. (1998). Efficacy and safety of liposomal amphotericin B (AmBisome) for visceral leishmaniasis in endemic developing countries. *Bulletin of the World Health Organization* **76**, 25–32.

Berman, J.D., Chulay, J.D., Hendricks, L.D. and Oster, C.N. (1982). Susceptibility of clinically sensitive and resistant *Leishmania* to pentavalent antimony in vitro. *American Journal of Tropical Medicine and Hygiene* **31**, 459–465.

Bodhe, P.V., Kotwani, R.N., Kirodian, B.G., Pathare, A.V., Pandey, A.K., Thakur, C.P. and Kshirsagar, N.A. (1999). Dose-ranging studies on liposomal amphotericin B (L-AMP-LRC-1) in the treatment of visceral leishmaniasis. *Transactions of the Royal Society of Tropical Medicine and Hygiene* **93**, 314–318.

Boelaert, M., Lynen, L., Desjeux, P. and Van der Stuyft, P. (1999). Cost-effectiveness of competing diagnostic-therapeutic strategies for visceral leishmaniasis. *Bulletin of the World Health Organization* **77**, 667–674.

Boelaert, M., Rijal, S., Regmi, S., Singh, R., Karki, B., Jacquet, D., Chappuis, F., Campino, L., Desjeux, P., Le Ray, D., Koirala, S. and Van der Stuyft, P. (2004). A comparative study of the effectiveness of diagnostic tests for visceral leishmaniasis. *American Journal of Tropical Medicine and Hygiene* **70**, 72–77.

Bryceson, A. (2001). A policy for leishmaniasis with respect to the prevention and control of drug resistance. *Tropical Medicine & International Health* **6**, 928–934.

Buates, S. and Matlashewski, G. (1999). Treatment of experimental leishmaniasis with the immunomodulators imiquimod and S-28463: efficacy and mode of action. *Journal of Infectious Disease* **179**, 1485–1494.

Chunge, C.N., Gachihi, G., Muigai, R., Wasunna, K., Rashid, J.R., Chulay, J.D., Anabwani, G., Oster, C.N. and Bryceson, A.D. (1985). Visceral leishmaniasis unresponsive to antimonial drugs. III. Successful treatment using a combination of sodium stibogluconate plus allopurinol. *Transactions of the Royal Society of Tropical Medicine and Hygiene* **79**, 715–718.

Chunge, C.N., Owate, J., Pamba, H.O. and Donno, L. (1990). Treatment of visceral leishmaniasis in Kenya by aminosidine alone or combined with sodium stibogluconate. *Transactions of the Royal Society of Tropical Medicine and Hygiene* **84**, 221–225.

Coelho, A.C., Beverley, S.M. and Cotrim, P.C. (2003). Functional genetic identification of PRP1, an ABC transporter superfamily member conferring pentamidine resistance in *Leishmania major*. *Molecular and Biochemical Parasitology* **130**, 83–90.

Convit, J., Castellanos, P.L., Ulrich, M., Castes, M., Rondon, A., Pinardi, M.E., Rodriquez, N., Bloom, B.R., Formica, S., Valecillos, L., et al. (1989). Immunotherapy of localized, intermediate, and diffuse forms of American cutaneous leishmaniasis. *Journal of Infectious Disease* **160**, 104–115.

Convit, J., Ulrich, M., Zerpa, O., Borges, R., Aranzazu, N., Valera, M., Villarroel, H., Zapata, Z. and Tomedes, I. (2003). Immunotherapy of American cutaneous leishmaniasis in Venezuela during the period 1990–99. *Transactions of the Royal Society of Tropical Medicine and Hygiene* **97**, 469–472.

Copeland, H.W., Arana, B.A. and Navin, T.R. (1990). Comparison of active and passive case detection of cutaneous leishmaniasis in Guatemala. *American Journal of Tropical Medicine and Hygiene* **43**, 257–259.

Cotrim, P.C., Garrity, L.K. and Beverley, S.M. (1999). Isolation of genes mediating resistance to inhibitors of nucleoside and ergosterol metabolism in *Leishmania* by overexpression/selection. *Journal of Biological Chemistry* **274**, 37723–37730.

Croft, S.L., and Brun, R. (2003). *In vitro* and *in vivo* models for the identification and evaluation of drugs active against *Trypanosoma* and *Leishmania*. In: *Drugs Against Parasitic Diseases: R&D Methodologies and Issues* (A.H. Fairlamb, R. Ridley, and H. Vial, eds), UNDP/World Bank/ WHO Special Program for Research and Training in Tropical Diseases (TDR, Geneva), pp. 165–173.

Croft, S.L. and Coombs, G.H. (2003). Leishmaniasis—current chemotherapy and recent advances in the search for novel drugs. *Trends in Parasitology* **19**, 502–508.

Croft, S.L., Neal, R.A., Pendergast, W. and Chan, J.H. (1987). The activity of alkyl phosphorylcholines and related derivatives against *Leishmania donovani*. *Biochemical Pharmacology* **36**, 2633–2636.

Croft, S.L., Snowdon, D. and Yardley, V. (1996). The activities of four anticancer alkyllysophospholipids against *Leishmania donovani, Trypanosoma cruzi* and *Trypanosoma brucei*. *Journal of Antimicrobial Chemotherapy* **38**, 1041–1047.

Croft, S.L. and Yardley, V. (2002). Chemotherapy of leishmaniasis. *Current Pharmaceutical Design* **8**, 319–342.

Cruz, I., Moreno, J., Cañavate, C., Desjeux, P. and Alvar, J. (in press). *Leishmania*/HIV co-infections in the second decade. *Indian Journal of Medical Research*.

Davidson, R.N., Di Martino, L., Gradoni, L., Giacchino, R., Russo, R., Gaeta, G.B., Pempinello, R., Scott, S., Raimondi, F., Cascio, A., Prestileo, T., Caldeira, L., Wilkinson, R.J. and Bryceson, A.D.M. (1994). Liposomal amphotericin B (AmBisome) in Mediterranean visceral leishmaniasis: a multi-centre trial. *Quarterly Journal of Medicine* **87**, 75–81.

de la Rosa, R., Pineda, J.A., Delgado, J., Macias, J., Morillas, F., Mira, J.A., Sánchez-Quijano, A., Leal, M. and Lissen, E. (2002). Incidence of and risk factors for symptomatic visceral leishmaniasis among human immunodeficiency virus type 1-infected patients from Spain in the era of highly active antiretroviral therapy. *Journal of Clinical Microbiology* **40**, 762–767.

Dereure, J., Duong Thanh, H., Lavabre-Bertrand, T., Cartron, G., Bastides, F., Richard-Lenoble, D. and Dedet, J.P. (2003). Visceral leishmaniasis. Persistence of parasites in lymph nodes after clinical cure. *Journal of Infection* **47**, 77–81.

Desjeux, P. (1996). Leishmaniasis. Public health aspects and control. *Clinics in Dermatology* **14**, 417–423.

Desjeux, P. (2001). The increase in risk factors for leishmaniasis worldwide. *Transactions of the Royal Society of Tropical Medicine and Hygiene* **95**, 239–243.

Desjeux, P. (2004). Leishmaniasis: current situation and new perspectives. *Comparative Immunology Microbiology and Infectious Diseases* **27**, 305–318.

Desjeux, P. and Alvar, J. (2003). *Leishmania*/HIV co-infections: epidemiology in Europe. *Annals of Tropical Medicine and Parasitology* **97** (supplement 1), 3–15.

Dietze, R., Carvalho, S.F., Valli, L.C., Berman, J., Brewer, T., Milhous, W., Sánchez, J., Schuster, B. and Grogl, M. (2001). Phase 2 trial of WR6026, an orally administered 8-aminoquinoline, in the treatment of visceral leishmaniasis caused by *Leishmania chagasi*. *American Journal of Tropical Medicine and Hygiene* **65**, 685–689.

Dube, A., Singh, N., Sundar, S. and Singh, N. (2005). Refractoriness to the treatment of sodium stibogluconate in Indian kala-azar field isolates persist in *in vitro* and *in vivo* experimental models. *Parasitology Research* **96**, 216–223.

Elnaiem, D.A., Hassan, H.K. and Ward, R.D. (1999). Associations of *Phlebotomus orientalis* and other sandflies with vegetation types in the eastern Sudan focus of kala-azar. *Medical and Veterinary Entomology* **13**, 198–203.

El-On, J., Jacobs, G.P., Witztum, E. and Greenblatt, C.L. (1984). Development of topical treatment for cutaneous leishmaniasis caused by *Leishmania major* in experimental animals. *Antimicrobial Agents and Chemotherapy* **26**, 745–751.

El-On, J., Halevy, S., Grunwald, M.H. and Weinrauch, L. (1992). Topical treatment of Old World cutaneous leishmaniasis caused by *Leishmania major*: a double-blind control study. *Journal of the American Academy of Dermatology* **27**, 227–231.

El-Safi, S.H. and Evans, D.A. (1989). A comparison of the direct agglutination test and enzyme-linked immunosorbent assay in the serodiagnosis of leishmaniasis in the Sudan. *Transactions of the Royal Society of Tropical Medicine and Hygiene* **83**, 334–337.

Eltoum, I.A., Zijlstra, E.E., Ali, M.S., Ghalib, H.W., Satti, M.M., Eltoum, B. and el-Hassan, A.M. (1992). Congenital kala-azar and leishmaniasis in the placenta. *American Journal of Tropical Medicine and Hygiene* **46**, 57–62.

Ephros, M., Waldman, E. and Zilberstein, D. (1997). Pentostam induces resistance to antimony and the preservative chlorocresol in *Leishmania donovani* promastigotes and axenically grown amastigotes. *Antimicrobial Agents and Chemotherapy* **41**, 1064–1068.

Escobar, P., Yardley, V. and Croft, S.L. (2001). Activities of hexadecylphosphocholine (miltefosine), AmBisome, and sodium stibogluconate (Pentostam) against *Leishmania donovani* in immunodeficient SCID mice. *Antimicrobial Agents and Chemotherapy* **45**, 1872–1875.

Evans, T.G., Teixeira, M.J., McAuliffe, I.T., Vasconcelos, I., Vasconcelos, A.W., Sousa Ade, A., Lima, J.W. and Pearson, R.D. (1992). Epidemiology of visceral leishmaniasis in northeast Brazil. *Journal of Infectious Disease* **166**, 1124–1132.

Fukui, H., Koike, T., Nakagawa, T., Saheki, A., Sonoke, S., Tomii, Y. and Seki, J. (2003). Comparison of LNS-AmB, a novel low-dose formulation of amphotericin B with lipid nano-sphere (LNS), with commercial lipid-based formulations. *International Journal of Pharmaceutics* **267**, 101–112.

Gama, M.E., Costa, J.M., Gomes, C.M. and Corbett, C.E. (2004). Subclinical form of the American visceral leishmaniasis. *Memórias do Instituto Oswaldo Cruz* **99**, 889–893.

Garnier, T. and Croft, S.L. (2002). Topical treatment for cutaneous leishmaniasis. *Current Opinion in Investigative Drugs* **3**, 538–544.

Gradoni, L., Gramiccia, M. and Scalone, A. (2003). Visceral leishmaniasis treatment, Italy. *Emerging Infectious Disease* **9**, 1617–1620.

Gramiccia, M., Gradoni, L. and Orsini, S. (1992). Decreased sensitivity to meglumine antimoniate (Glucantime) of *Leishmania infantum* isolated from dogs after several courses of drug treatment. *Annals of Tropical Medicine and Parasitology* **86**, 613–620.

Griekspoor, A., Sondorp, E. and Vos, T. (1999). Cost-effectiveness analysis of humanitarian relief interventions: visceral leishmaniasis treatment in the Sudan. *Health Policy and Planning* **14**, 70–76.

Grogl, M., Thomason, T.N. and Franke, E.D. (1992). Drug resistance in leishmaniasis: its implication in systemic chemotherapy of cutaneous and mucocutaneous disease. *American Journal of Tropical Medicine and Hygiene* **47**, 117–126.

Guerin, P.J., Olliaro, P., Sundar, S., Boelaert, M., Croft, S.L., Desjeux, P., Wasunna, M.K. and Bryceson, A.D. (2002). Visceral leishmaniasis: current status of control, diagnosis, and treatment, and a proposed research and development agenda. *Lancet Infectious Disease* **2**, 494–501.

Guiguemde, R.T., Sawadogo, O.S., Bories, C., Traore, K.L., Nezien, D., Nikiema, L., Pratlong, F., Marty, P., Houin, R. and Deniau, M. (2003). *Leishmania major* and HIV co-infection in Burkina Faso.

Transactions of the Royal Society of Tropical Medicine and Hygiene **97**, 168–169.

Harrison, L.H., Naidu, T.G., Drew, J.S., de Alencar, J.E. and Pearson, R.D. (1986). Reciprocal relationships between undernutrition and the parasitic disease visceral leishmaniasis. *Review of Infectious Disease* **8**, 447–453.

Herwaldt, B.L. (1999). Leishmaniasis. *Lancet* **354**, 1191–1199.

Ibrahim, M.E., Hag-Ali, M., el-Hassan, A.M., Theander, T.G. and Kharazmi, A. (1994). *Leishmania* resistant to sodium stibogluconate: drug-associated macrophage-dependent killing. *Parasitology Research* **80**, 569–574.

Iraji, F. and Sadeghinia, A. (2005). Efficacy of paromomycin ointment in the treatment of cutaneous leishmaniasis: results of a double-blind, randomized trial in Isfahan, Iran. *Annals of Tropical Medicine and Parasitology* **99**, 3–9.

Jha, T.K., Olliaro, P., Thakur, C.P., Kanyok, T.P., Singhania, B.L., Singh, I.J., Singh, N.K., Akhoury, S. and Jha, S. (1998). Randomised controlled trial of aminosidine (paromomycin) v. sodium stibogluconate for treating visceral leishmaniasis in North Bihar, India. *British Medical Journal* **316**, 1200–1205.

Jha, T.K., Sundar, S., Bhattacharya, S.K., Sinha, P.K., and Thakur, C.P. (2005a). Paromomycin as a new cure for visceral leishmaniasis: preliminary results of a Phase III randomized controlled trial of efficacy and safety. *Abstract Book, Third World Congress on Leishmaniasis*, 10–15 April 2005, Sicily, Italy.

Jha, T.K., Sundar, S., Thakur, C.P., Sabin, A.J., Horton, J. and Felton, J.M. (2005b). A phase II dose-ranging study of sitamaquine for the treatment of visceral leishmaniasis in India. *American Journal of Tropical Medicine and Hygiene* **73**, 1005–1111.

Kafetzis, D.A. (2003). An overview of paediatric leishmaniasis. *Journal of Postgraduate Medicine* **49**, 31–38.

Kuhlencord, A., Maniera, T., Eibl, H. and Unger, C. (1992). Hexadecylphosphocholine: oral treatment of visceral leishmaniasis in mice. *Antimicrobial Agents and Chemotherapy* **36**, 1630–1634.

Kwong, E.H., Ramaswamy, M., Bauer, E.A., Hartsel, S.C. and Wasan, K.M. (2001). Heat treatment of amphotericin B modifies its serum pharmacokinetics, tissue distribution, and renal toxicity following administration of a single intravenous dose to rabbits. *Antimicrobial Agents and Chemotherapy* **45**, 2060–2063.

Laguna, F., López-Vélez, R., Pulido, F., Salas, A., Torre-Cisneros, J., Torres, E., Medrano, F.J., Sanz, J., Pico, G., Gómez-Rodrigo, J., Pasquau, J. and Alvar, J. (1999). Treatment of visceral leishmaniasis in HIV-infected patients: a randomized trial comparing meglumine antimoniate with amphotericin B. *AIDS* **13**, 1063–1069.

Laguna, F., Videla, S., Jiménez-Mejias, M.E., Sirera, G., Torre-Cisneros, J., Ribera, E., Prados, D., Clotet, B., Sust, M., López-Vélez, R. and Alvar, J.

(2003). Amphotericin B lipid complex versus meglumine antimoniate in the treatment of visceral leishmaniasis in patients infected with HIV: a randomized pilot study. *Journal of Antimicrobial Chemotherapy* **52**, 464–468.

le Fichoux, Y., Quaranta, J.F., Aufeuvre, J.P., Lelievre, A., Marty, P., Suffia, I., Rousseau, D. and Kubar, J. (1999). Occurrence of *Leishmania infantum* parasitemia in asymptomatic blood donors living in an area of endemicity in southern France. *Journal of Clinical Microbiology* **37**, 1953–1957.

Lira, R., Sundar, S., Makharia, A., Kenney, R., Gam, A., Saraiva, E. and Sacks, D. (1999). Evidence that the high incidence of treatment failures in Indian kala-azar is due to the emergence of antimony-resistant strains of *Leishmania donovani*. *Journal of Infectious Disease* **180**, 564–567.

López-Vélez, R. (2003). The impact of highly active antiretroviral therapy (HAART) on visceral leishmaniasis in Spanish patients who are co-infected with HIV. *Annals of Tropical Medicine and Parasitology* **97** (supplement 1), 143–147.

López-Vélez, R., Perez-Molina, J.A., Guerrero, A., Baquero, F., Villa-rrubia, J., Escribano, L., Bellas, C., Pérez-Corral, F. and Alvar, J. (1998). Clinicoepidemiologic characteristics, prognostic factors, and survival analysis of patients coinfected with human immunodeficiency virus and *Leishmania* in an area of Madrid, Spain. *American Journal of Tropical Medicine and Hygiene* **58**, 436–443.

López-Vélez, R., Videla, S., Márquez, M., Boix, V., Jiménez-Mejias, M.E., Gorgolas, M., Arribas, J.R., Salas, A., Laguna, F., Sust, M., Cãnavate, C. and Alvar, J. (2004). Amphotericin B lipid complex versus no treatment in the secondary prophylaxis of visceral leishmaniasis in HIV-infected patients. *Journal of Antimicrobial Chemotherapy* **53**, 540–543.

Lyons, S., Veeken, H. and Long, J. (2003). Visceral leishmaniasis and HIV in Tigray, Ethiopia. *Tropical Medicine & International Health* **8**, 733–739.

Maarouf, M., Adeline, M.T., Solignac, M., Vautrin, D. and Robert-Gero, M. (1998). Development and characterization of paromomycin-resistant *Leishmania donovani* promastigotes. *Parasite* **5**, 167–173.

McCormick, A.W., Whitney, C.G., Farley, M.M., Lynfield, R., Harrison, L.H., Bennett, N.M., Schaffner, W., Reingold, A., Hadler, J., Cieslak, P., Samore, M.H. and Lipsitch, M. (2003). Geographic diversity and temporal trends of antimicrobial resistance in *Streptococcus pneumoniae* in the United States. *Nature Medicine* **9**, 424–430.

Meyerhoff, A. (1999). U.S. Food and Drug Administration approval of AmBisome (liposomal amphotericin B) for treatment of visceral leishmaniasis. *Clinical Infectious Disease* **28**, 42–48 (discussion 49–51).

Mira, J.A., Corzo, J.E., Rivero, A., Macias, J., de Leon, F.L., Torre-Cisneros, J., Gomez-Mateos, J., Jurado, R. and Pineda, J.A. (2004). Frequency of visceral leishmaniasis relapses in human immunodeficiency virus-infected patients receiving highly active antiretroviral therapy. *American Journal of Tropical Medicine and Hygiene* **70**, 298–301.

Momeni, A.Z. and Aminjavaheri, M. (1995). Treatment of recurrent cutaneous leishmaniasis. *International Journal of Dermatology* **34**, 129–133.

Moreno, J., Nieto, J., Chamizo, C., Gonzalez, F., Blanco, F., Barker, D.C. and Alvar, J. (1999). The immune response and PBMC subsets in canine visceral leishmaniasis before, and after, chemotherapy. *Veterinary Immunology and Immunopathology* **71**, 181–195.

Murray, H.W. (2004). Treatment of visceral leishmaniasis in 2004. *American Journal of Tropical Medicine and Hygiene* **71**, 787–794.

Murray, C.J.L. and Lopez, A. (1996). *Global Health Statistics: A Compendium of Incidence, Prevalence and Mortality Estimates for over 200 Conditions*. Boston, MA: Harvard School of Public Health on behalf of World Health Organization and World Bank (Global Burden of Disease and Injury Series).

Musa, A.M., Khalil, E.A., Mahgoub, F.A., Hamad, S., Elkadaru, A.M. and el-Hassan, A.M. (2005). Efficacy of liposomal amphotericin B (AmBisome) in the treatment of persistent post-kala-azar dermal leishmaniasis (PKDL). *Annals of Tropical Medicine and Parasitology* **99**, 563–569.

Navin, T.R., Arana, B.A., Arana, F.E., Berman, J.D. and Chajon, J.F. (1992). Placebo-controlled clinical trial of sodium stibogluconate (Pentostam) versus ketoconazole for treating cutaneous leishmaniasis in Guatemala. *Journal of Infectious Disease* **165**, 528–534.

Neal, R.A., Allen, S., McCoy, N., Olliaro, P. and Croft, S.L. (1995). The sensitivity of *Leishmania* species to aminosidine. *Journal of Antimicrobial Chemotherapy* **35**, 577–584.

Neal, R.A., Croft, S.L. and Nelson, D.J. (1985). Anti-leishmanial effect of allopurinol ribonucleoside and the related compounds, allopurinol, thiopurinol, thiopurinol ribonucleoside, and of formycin B, sinefungin and the lepidine WR6026. *Transactions of the Royal Society of Tropical Medicine and Hygiene* **79**, 122–128.

Olliaro, P.L., Guerin, P.J., Gerstl, S., Haaskjold, A.A., Rottingen, J.A. and Sundar, S. (2005). Treatment options for visceral leishmaniasis: a systematic review of clinical studies done in India, 1980–2004. *Lancet Infectious Disease* **5**, 763–774.

Pagliano, P., Carannante, N., Rossi, M., Gramiccia, M., Gradoni, L., Faella, F.S. and Gaeta, G.B. (2005). Visceral leishmaniasis in pregnancy: a case series and a systematic review of the literature. *Journal of Antimicrobial Chemotherapy* **55**, 229–233.

Pagliano, P., Rossi, M., Rescigno, C., Altieri, S., Coppola, M.G., Gramiccia, M., Scalone, A., Gradoni, L. and Faella, F. (2003). Mediterranean visceral leishmaniasis in HIV-negative adults: a retrospective analysis of 64 consecutive cases (1995–2001). *Journal of Antimicrobial Chemotherapy* **52**, 264–268.

Paumgartten, F.J. and Chahoud, I. (2001). Embryotoxicity of meglumine antimoniate in the rat. *Reproductive Toxicology* **15**, 327–331.

Pérez-Victoria, F.J., Gamarro, F., Ouellette, M. and Castanys, S. (2003). Functional cloning of the miltefosine transporter. A novel P-type phospholipid translocase from *Leishmania* involved in drug resistance. *Journal of Biological Chemistry* **278**, 49965–49971.

Petit, C., Yardley, V., Gaboriau, F., Bolard, J. and Croft, S.L. (1999). Activity of a heat-induced reformulation of amphotericin B deoxycholate (fungizone) against *Leishmania donovani*. *Antimicrobial Agents and Chemotherapy* **43**, 390–392.

Pintado, V. and López-Vélez, R. (2001). Visceral leishmaniasis associated with human immunodeficiency virus infection. *Enfermedades Infecciosas y Microbiologia Clinica* **19**, 353–357.

Pintado, V., Martín-Rabadán, P., Rivera, M.L., Moreno, S. and Bouza, E. (2001). Visceral leishmaniasis in human immunodeficiency virus (HIV)-infected and non-HIV-infected patients. A comparative study. *Medicine (Baltimore)* **80**, 54–73.

Rabello, A., Orsini, M. and Disch, J. (2003). *Leishmania*/HIV co-infection in Brazil: an appraisal. *Annals of Tropical Medicine and Parasitology* **97** (supplement 1), 17–28.

Reithinger, R., Mohsen, M., Wahid, M., Bismullah, M., Quinnell, R.J., Davies, C.R., Kolaczinski, J. and David, J.R. (2005). Efficacy of thermotherapy to treat cutaneous leishmaniasis caused by *Leishmania tropica* in Kabul, Afghanistan: a randomized, controlled trial. *Clinical Infectious Disease* **40**, 1148–1155.

Ribera, E., Ocaña, I., de Otero, J., Cortés, E., Gasser, I. and Pahissa, A. (1996). Prophylaxis of visceral leishmaniasis in human immunodeficiency virus-infected patients. *American Journal of Medicine* **100**, 496–501.

Rijal, S., Chappuis, F., Singh, R., Boelaert, M., Loutan, L. and Koirala, S. (2003). Sodium stibogluconate cardiotoxicity and safety of generics. *Transactions of the Royal Society of Tropical Medicine and Hygiene* **97**, 597–598.

Ritmeijer, K., Veeken, H., Melaku, Y., Leal, G., Amsalu, R., Seaman, J. and Davidson, R.N. (2001). Ethiopian visceral leishmaniasis: generic and proprietary sodium stibogluconate are equivalent; HIV co-infected patients have a poor outcome. *Transactions of the Royal Society of Tropical Medicine and Hygiene* **95**, 668–672.

Russo, R., Nigro, L.C., Minniti, S., Montineri, A., Gradoni, L., Caldeira, L. and Davidson, R.N. (1996). Visceral leishmaniasis in HIV infected patients: treatment with high dose liposomal amphotericin B (AmBisome). *Journal of Infection* **32**, 133–137.

Sampaio, R.N., Salaro, C.P., Resende, P. and de Paula, C.D. (2002). American cutaneous leishmaniasis associated with HIV/AIDS: report of four clinical cases. *Revista da Sociedade Brasileira de Medicina Tropical* **35**, 651–654.

Sarkari, B., Chance, M. and Hommel, M. (2002). Antigenuria in visceral leishmaniasis: detection and partial characterisation of a carbohydrate antigen. *Acta Tropica* **82**, 339–348.

Seeberger, J., Daoud, S. and Pammer, J. (2003). Transient effect of topical treatment of cutaneous leishmaniasis with imiquimod. *International Journal of Dermatology* **42**, 576–579.

Seifert, K. and Croft, S.L. (2006). In vitro and in vivo interactions between miltefosine and anti-leishmanial drugs. *Antimicrobial Agents and Chemotherapy* **50**, 73–79.

Seifert, K., Matu, S., Pérez-Victoria, F.J., Castanys, S., Gamarro, F. and Croft, S.L. (2003). Characterisation of *Leishmania donovani* promastigotes resistant to hexadecylphosphocholine (miltefosine). *International Journal of Antimicrobial Agents* **22**, 380–387.

Sereno, D. and Lemesre, J.L. (1997). Axenically cultured amastigote forms as an *in vitro* model for investigation of antileishmanial agents. *Antimicrobial Agents and Chemotherapy* **41**, 972–976.

Sharma, D., Bern, C., Varghese, B., Chowdhury, R., Haque, R., Ali, M., Amann, J., Ahluwalia, I.B., Wagatsuma, Y., Breiman, R., Maguire, J.H., and McFarland, D.A. (in press). The economic impact of visceral leishmaniasis on households in Bangladesh. *Tropical Medicine & International Health*.

Sherwood, J.A., Gachihi, G.S., Muigai, R.K., Skillman, D.R., Mugo, M., Rashid, J.R., Wasunna, K.M., Were, J.B., Kasili, S.K. and Mbugua, J.M. (1994). Phase 2 efficacy trial of an oral 8-aminoquinoline (WR6026) for treatment of visceral leishmaniasis. *Clinical Infectious Disease* **19**, 1034–1039.

Sindermann, H., Engel, K.R., Fischer, C. and Bommer, W. (2004). Oral miltefosine for leishmaniasis in immunocompromised patients: compassionate use in 39 patients with HIV infection. *Clinical Infectious Disease* **39**, 1520–1523.

Sinha, P.K., Rabidas, V.N., Pandey, K., Verma, N., Gupta, A.K., Ranjan, A., Das, P. and Bhattacharya, S.K. (2003). Visceral leishmaniasis and HIV coinfection in Bihar, India. *Journal of Acquired Immune Deficiency Syndromes* **32**, 115–116.

Soriano, V., Dona, C., Rodríguez-Rosado, R., Barreiro, P. and Gonzalez-Lahoz, J. (2000). Discontinuation of secondary prophylaxis for opportunistic infections in HIV-infected patients receiving highly active antiretroviral therapy. *AIDS* **14**, 383–386.

Soto, J., Arana, B.A., Toledo, J., Rizzo, N., Vega, J.C., Díaz, A., Luz, M., Gutiérrez, P., Arboleda, M., Berman, J.D., Junge, K., Engel, J. and Sindermann, H. (2004). Miltefosine for new world cutaneous leishmaniasis. *Clinical Infectious Disease* **38**, 1266–1272.

Soto, J.M., Toledo, J.T., Gutíerrez, P., Arboleda, M., Nicholls, R.S., Padilla, J.R., Berman, J.D., English, C.K. and Grogl, M. (2002).

Treatment of cutaneous leishmaniasis with a topical antileishmanial drug (WR279396): phase 2 pilot study. *American Journal of Tropical Medicine and Hygiene* **66**, 147–151.

Sundar, S. (2001). Drug resistance in Indian visceral leishmaniasis. *Tropical Medicine & International Health* **6**, 849–854.

Sundar, S., Jha, T.K., Thakur, C.P., Engel, J., Sindermann, H., Fischer, C., Junge, K., Bryceson, A. and Berman, J. (2002). Oral miltefosine for Indian visceral leishmaniasis. *New England Journal of Medicine* **347**, 1739–1746.

Sundar, S., Mehta, H., Suresh, A.V., Singh, S.P., Rai, M. and Murray, H.W. (2004). Amphotericin B treatment for Indian visceral leishmaniasis: conventional versus lipid formulations. *Clinical Infectious Disease* **38**, 377–383.

Sundar, S., More, D.K., Singh, M.K., Singh, V.P., Sharma, S., Makharia, A., Kumar, P.C. and Murray, H.W. (2000). Failure of pentavalent antimony in visceral leishmaniasis in India: report from the center of the Indian epidemic. *Clinical Infectious Disease* **31**, 1104–1107.

Sundar, S. and Murray, H.W. (2005). Availability of miltefosine for the treatment of kala-azar in India. *Bulletin of the World Health Organization* **83**, 394–395.

Sundar, S., Rosenkaimer, F., Lesser, M.L. and Murray, H.W. (1995). Immunochemotherapy for a systemic intracellular infection: accelerated response using interferon-gamma in visceral leishmaniasis. *Journal of Infectious Diseases* **171**, 992–996.

Sundar, S., Singh, V.P., Sharma, S., Makharia, M.K. and Murray, H.W. (1997). Response to interferon-gamma plus pentavalent antimony in Indian visceral leishmaniasis. *Journal of Infectious Disease* **176**, 1117–1119.

Sundar, S., Sinha, P.R., Agrawal, N.K., Srivastava, R., Rainey, P.M., Berman, J.D., Murray, H.W. and Singh, V.P. (1998). A cluster of cases of severe cardiotoxicity among kala-azar patients treated with a high-osmolarity lot of sodium antimony gluconate. *American Journal of Tropical Medicine and Hygiene* **59**, 139–143.

Teklemariam, S., Hiwot, A.G., Frommel, D., Miko, T.L., Ganlov, G. and Bryceson, A. (1994). Aminosidine and its combination with sodium stibogluconate in the treatment of diffuse cutaneous leishmaniasis caused by *Leishmania aethiopica*. *Transactions of the Royal Society of Tropical Medicine and Hygiene* **88**, 334–339.

Thakur, C.P., Kanyok, T.P., Pandey, A.K., Sinha, G.P., Messick, C. and Olliaro, P. (2000a). Treatment of visceral leishmaniasis with injectable paromomycin (aminosidine). An open-label randomized phase-II clinical study. *Transactions of the Royal Society of Tropical Medicine and Hygiene* **94**, 432–433.

Thakur, C.P., Kanyok, T.P., Pandey, A.K., Sinha, G.P., Zaniewski, A.E., Houlihan, H.H. and Olliaro, P. (2000b). A prospective randomized, comparative, open-label trial of the safety and efficacy of paromomycin (aminosidine) plus sodium stibogluconate versus sodium stibogluconate alone for the treatment of visceral leishmaniasis. *Transactions of the Royal Society of Tropical Medicine and Hygiene* **94**, 429–431.

Thakur, C.P. and Kumar, K. (1990). Efficacy of prolonged therapy with stibogluconate in post kala-azar dermal leishmaniasis. *Indian Journal of Medical Research* **91**, 144–148.

Thakur, C.P., Narain, S., Kumar, N., Hassan, S.M., Jha, D.K. and Kumar, A. (1997). Amphotericin B is superior to sodium antimony gluconate in the treatment of Indian post-kala-azar dermal leishmaniasis. *Annals of Tropical Medicine and Parasitology* **91**, 611–616.

Thakur, C.P. and Narayan, S. (2004). A comparative evaluation of amphotericin B and sodium antimony gluconate, as first-line drugs in the treatment of Indian visceral leishmaniasis. *Annals of Tropical Medicine and Parasitology* **98**, 129–138.

Thakur, C.P., Narayan, S. and Ranjan, A. (2004). Epidemiological, clinical & pharmacological study of antimony-resistant visceral leishmaniasis in Bihar, India. *Indian Journal of Medical Research* **120**, 166–172.

Thakur, C.P., Sinha, G.P., Pandey, A.K., Barat, D. and Sinha, P.K. (1993a). Amphotericin B in resistant kala-azar in Bihar. *National Medical Journal of India* **6**, 57–60.

Thakur, C.P., Sinha, G.P., Pandey, A.K., Kumar, N., Kumar, P., Hassan, S.M., Narain, S. and Roy, R.K. (1998). Do the diminishing efficacy and increasing toxicity of sodium stibogluconate in the treatment of visceral leishmaniasis in Bihar, India, justify its continued use as a first-line drug? An observational study of 80 cases. *Annals of Tropical Medicine and Parasitology* **92**, 561–569.

Thakur, C.P., Sinha, G.P., Sharma, V., Pandey, A.K., Kumar, M. and Verma, B.B. (1993b). Evaluation of amphotericin B as a first line drug in comparison to sodium stibogluconate in the treatment of fresh cases of kala-azar. *Indian Journal Medical Research* **97**, 170–175.

UNAIDS (2005). *AIDS Epidemic Update 2005* (www.unaids.org).

Wasunna, M.K., Rashid, J.R., Mbui, J., Kirigi, G., Kinoti, D., Lodenyo, H., Felton, J.M., Sabin, A.J. and Horton, J. (2005). A phase II dose-rising study of sitamaquine for the treatment of visceral leishmaniasis in Kenya. *American Journal of Tropical Medicine and Hygiene* **73**, 871–876.

White, N.J. and Pongtavornpinyo, W. (2002). The *de novo* selection of drug-resistant malaria parasites. *Proceedings of the Royal Society of London Series B* **270**, 545–554.

Yamey, G. and Torreele, E. (2002). The world's most neglected diseases. *British Medical Journal* **325**, 176–177.

Yardley, V., Croft, S.L., De Doncker, S., Dujardin, J.C., Koirala, S., Rijal, S., Miranda, C., Llanos-Cuentas, A. and Chappuis, F. (2005). The sensitivity of clinical isolates of *Leishmania* from Peru and Nepal to miltefosine. *American Journal of Tropical Medicine and Hygiene* **73**, 272–275.

Zijlstra, E.E. and el-Hassan, A.M. (2001). Leishmaniasis in Sudan. Post kala-azar dermal leishmaniasis. *Transactions of the Royal Society of Tropical Medicine and Hygiene*, **95** (supplement 1), S59–S76.

Zvulunov, A., Cagnano, E., Frankenburg, S., Barenholz, Y. and Vardy, D. (2003). Topical treatment of persistent cutaneous leishmaniasis with ethanolic lipid amphotericin B. *Pediatric Infectious Disease Journal* **22**, 567–569.

Dracunculiasis (Guinea Worm Disease) Eradication

Ernesto Ruiz-Tiben[1] and Donald R. Hopkins[2]

[1]*Dracunculiasis Eradication, The Carter Center, 453 Freedom Parkway, Atlanta, GA 30307, USA*
[2]*The Carter Center, 453 Freedom Parkway, Atlanta, GA 30307, USA*

ADVANCES IN PARASITOLOGY VOL 61
ISSN: 0065-308X
DOI: 10.1016/S0065-308X(05)61007-X

ABSTRACT

Since the seminal review by Ralph Muller about *Dracunculus* and dracunculiasis in this serial publication in 1971, the Centers for Disease Control and Prevention and The Carter Center forged, during the 1980s, a coalition of organizations to support a campaign to eradicate dracunculiasis. Eighteen of 20 countries were known in 1986 to have endemic dracunculiasis, i.e., Benin, Burkina Faso, Cameroon, Chad, Côte d'Ivoire, Ethiopia, Ghana, India, Kenya, Mali, Mauritania, Niger, Nigeria, Pakistan, Senegal, Sudan, Togo, and Uganda. Transmission of the disease in Yemen was documented in 1995, and the World Health Organization (WHO) declared Central African Republic endemic in 1995. As of the end of 2004, a total of 16 026 cases of dracunculiasis were reported from 12 endemic countries (91% of these cases were reported from Ghana and Sudan, combined), a reduction greater than 99% from the 3.5 million cases of dracunculiasis estimated in 1986 to occur annually; the number of endemic villages has been reduced by >91%, from the 23 475 endemic villages in 1991; disease transmission has been interrupted in 9 of the 20 endemic countries; and WHO has certified 168 countries free of dracunculiasis, including Pakistan (1996), India (2000), Senegal and Yemen (2004). Asia is now free of dracunculiasis.

"The public interest requires doing today those things that men of intelligence and good will would wish, five or ten years hence, had been done"

Edmund Burke

1. INTRODUCTION

A seminal review by Ralph Muller about *Dracunculus* and dracunculiasis appeared in *Advances in Parasitology* in 1971 and since then comprehensive reviews about the Dracunculiasis Eradication Program (DEP) have been published (Hopkins *et al.*, 2002; Cairncross *et al.*, 2002; Greenaway, 2004; CDC/MMWR, 2004; WHO/WER, 2004). Our intent here, besides describing the life cycle of the parasite, the disease, and its epidemiology, is to provide a chronology of the events that created momentum for the campaign to eradicate dracunculiasis, discuss the strategy for eradication, and the progress so far, including the final stage of the campaign to eradicate this ancient scourge of mankind.

2. LIFE CYCLE

Dracunculiasis (Guinea worm disease) is caused by the nematode parasite *Dracunculus medinensis* (Linnaeus, 1758) (Figure 1). Persons become infected by drinking water from stagnant ponds, pools, cisterns, or open wells containing fresh water copepods ("Cyclops" or "water fleas") harbouring infective larvae of the parasite (Figure 2).

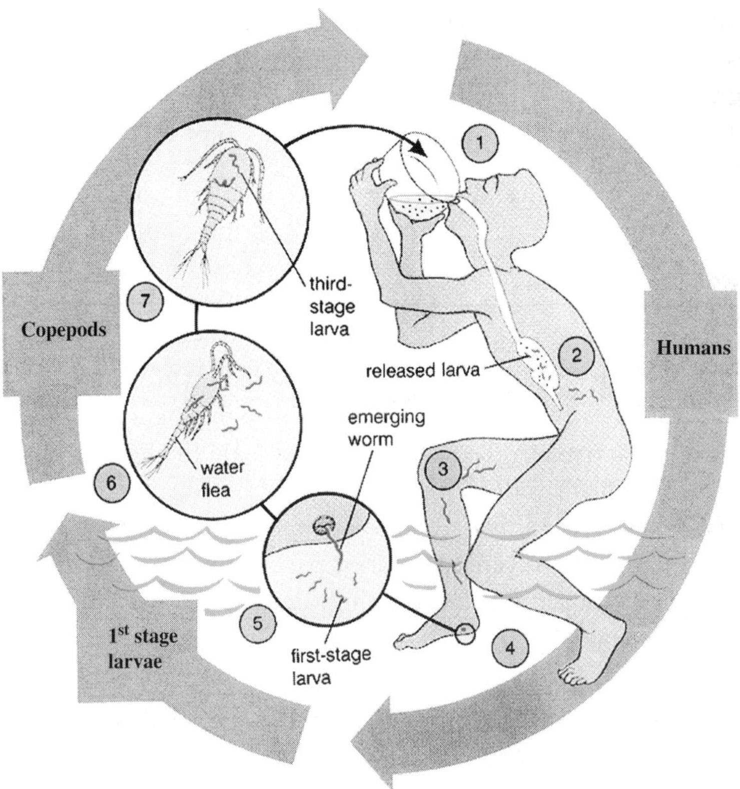

Figure 1 Life Cycle of *D. medinensis.* By courtesy of Encyclopedia Britannica, Inc., © 1996.

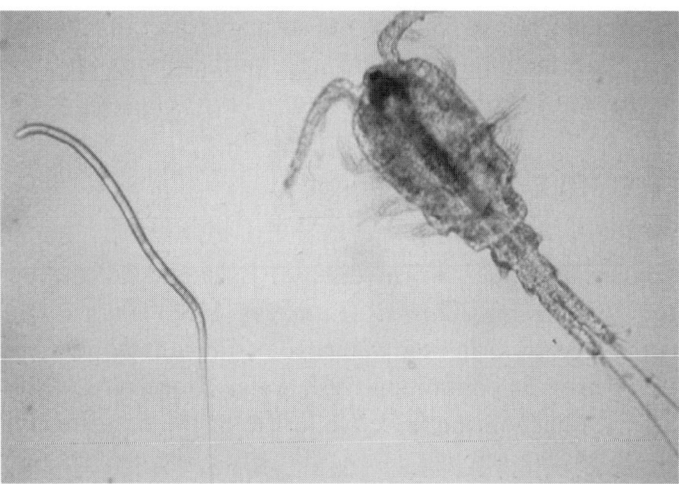

Figure 2 Fresh water copepod and first-stage larvae of *D. medinensis.* WHO CCRTED archives.

The digestive juices in the stomach kill the copepods, allowing the larvae to be released and to move to the small intestine, where they penetrate the intestinal wall and migrate to the connective tissues of the thorax (Muller, 1971). Male and female larvae mature and mate 60–90 days after infection (Muller, 1971). Infected people do not experience symptoms until 10–14 months later when the gravid adult female worm(s), measuring up to 70–100 centimetres long, causes a painful lesion to form on the skin and through which it may extrude to become exposed to the environment outside the human body. On contact with fresh water, powerful contractions cause a loop of the worm's uterus, containing a million or more larvae (Muller, 1971) to prolapse through a ruptured anterior part of the body or through the mouth, and discharge a swarm (hundreds of thousands) of motile larvae. Contraction of the worm and discharge of larvae may be repeated if the lesion is again submerged in water, until the entire brood of larvae is discharged. These larvae (first-stage) must then be ingested whole by certain species of water copepods, invade the copepod body cavity (Figure 3) and become infective (third-stage) after 14 days of development. People drinking water from such sources ingest the infected copepods, thus repeating the life cycle.

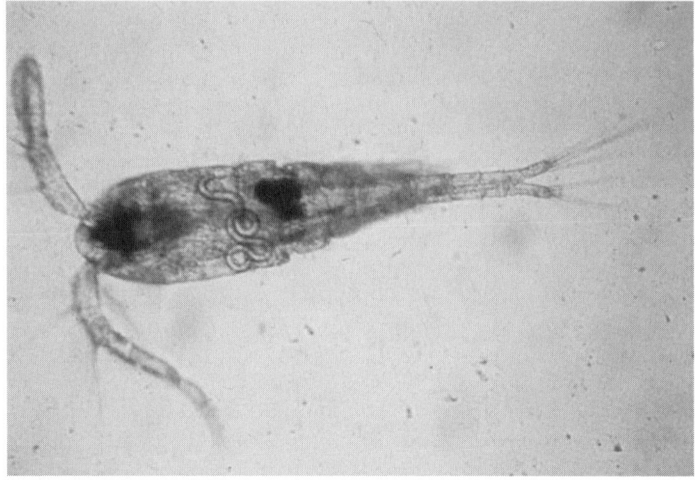

Figure 3 Larva of *D. medinensis* ingested by a fresh water copepod. WHO CCRTED archives.

Stagnant sources of drinking water such as ponds, cisterns, pools in dried-up riverbeds, and shallow unprotected hand-dug wells commonly harbour populations of copepods, and are the usual sites where infection is transmitted. The life cycle of the parasite was first fully described 135 years ago (Fedchenko, 1870).

3. DRACUNCULIASIS

3.1. Clinical Impact

Dracunculiasis has been known as a human parasitic disease since at least ancient Egypt (Muller, 1971; Hopkins and Hopkins, 1992). Acute systemic symptoms begin 10–14 months after infection and are related to the formation of a blister (Figure 4) and the subsequent skin lesion that allows the Guinea worm to become exposed to the environment outside of the human body. The blister is accompanied by redness and induration and is preceded by fever and allergic symptoms. These are local erythema and an urticarial rash with intense itching, nausea, vomiting, diarrhoea, and dizziness. Guinea worms emerge from the lower extremities in about 80–90% of cases,

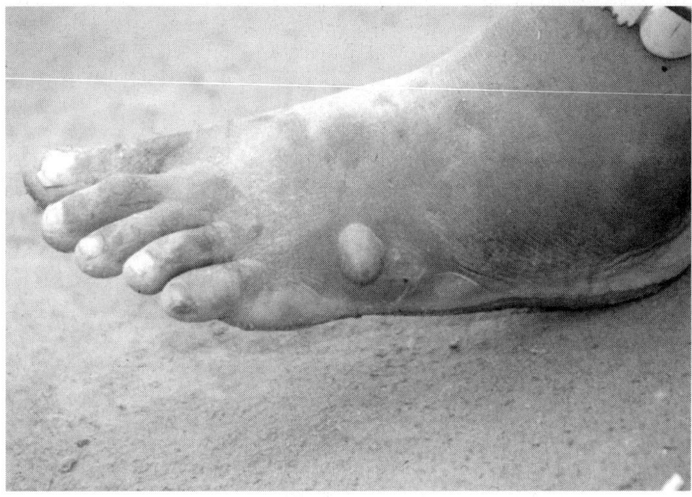

Figure 4   Blister caused by *D. medinensis*. WHO CCRTED archives.

but they can also emerge from other parts of the body, including the head, torso, upper extremities, buttocks, and genitalia. The formation of the blister induces irritation and a burning sensation, causing the patient to seek relief by immersing the affected limb or by pouring water over the lesion, which expedites the sloughing-off of the skin over the blister, allowing exposure of the anterior end of the Guinea worm to the environment outside its human host, and the discharge of larvae into water. As the Guinea worm extrudes through the skin, experienced patients invariably seek to pull it out, usually by winding a few centimetres of the worm each day on a small stick (Figure 5). This painful process is exacerbated by the secondary bacterial infections that usually ensue (Figure 6). If untreated, these lesions cause severe local inflammation and pain, and may lead to abscesses, septic arthritis, ankylosis of the joint, or even tetanus. If the Guinea worm breaks during manual extraction, an intense inflammatory reaction ensues, with more pain, swelling, and cellulitis along the worm tract. Based on several studies, the reported period of incapacitation averages about 8.5 weeks (Belcher *et al.*, 1975; Kale, 1977; Nwosu *et al.*, 1982; Edungbola, 1983; Adeyeba, 1985; Khan *et al.*, 1986; Smith *et al.*, 1989; Watts *et al.*, 1989; Suleiman and Abdullahi, 1990; Adeyeba and Kale, 1991; Ilegbodu *et al.*, 1991; Chippaux *et al.*, 1992;

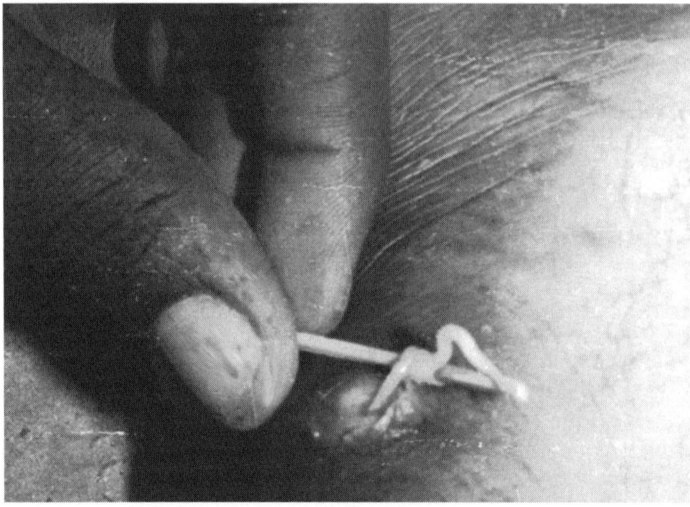

Figure 5 Skin lesions with *D. medinensis* emerged and being manually extracted by rolling it on a stick. TCC archives/E. Staub.

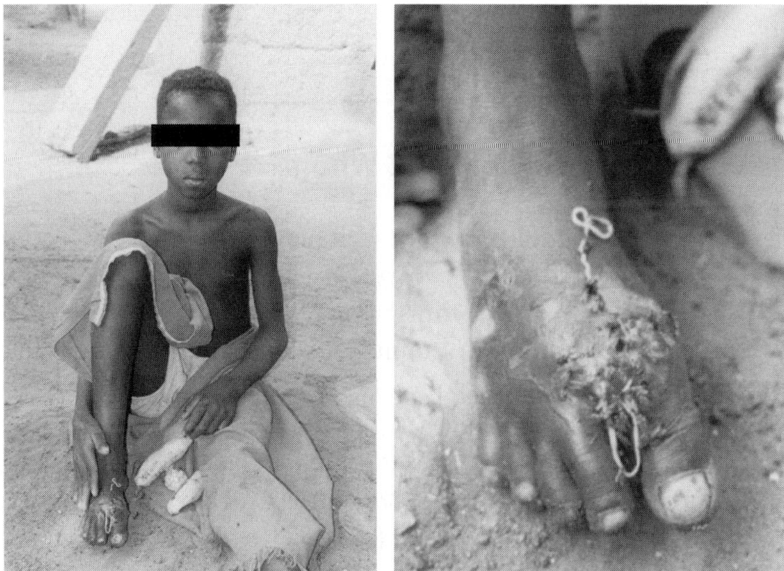

Figure 6 Young boy from Benin with dracunculiasis complicated by a severe secondary bacterial infection. WHO CCRTED archives.

Rhode *et al.*, 1993), with a range from 2 to 16 weeks, depending on the number of Guinea worms that emerge, their location, the complications that ensue, and the degree of medical care that may be available to the patient.

3.2. Treatment

There is no curative drug or vaccine against dracunculiasis. Infected persons do not develop immunity. Applying wet compresses to the lesion may relieve pain during the worm's emergence. Placing an occlusive bandage on the wound keeps it clean and counselling at this stage may help prevent the patient from contaminating sources of drinking water. Oral medications to alleviate the associated pain, and topical antiseptics or antibiotic ointment to minimize the risk of secondary bacterial infections also help reduce inflammation, and may permit removal of the worm by gentle traction over several days, instead of weeks (Figure 7).

4. EPIDEMIOLOGY

4.1. Where, Why, When, and Whom

During the 19th and 20th centuries, dracunculiasis was common in much of southern Asia, and in North, West, and East Africa. During the 1980s and 1990s endemic transmission of the disease was confined to 17 African and 3 Asian countries, i.e., Benin, Burkina Faso, Cameroon, Chad, Côte d'Ivoire, Ethiopia, Ghana, India, Kenya, Mali, Mauritania, Niger, Nigeria, Pakistan, Senegal, Sudan, Togo, and Uganda. Transmission of the disease in Yemen was documented in 1995, and the World Health Organization (WHO) declared Central African Republic endemic in 1995 (Figure 8).

Dracunculiasis is a disabling disease of poor people in remote rural areas who do not have access to safe drinking water and instead use stagnant sources of drinking water such as ponds, cisterns, pools in dried-up riverbeds, and shallow unprotected wells, which commonly

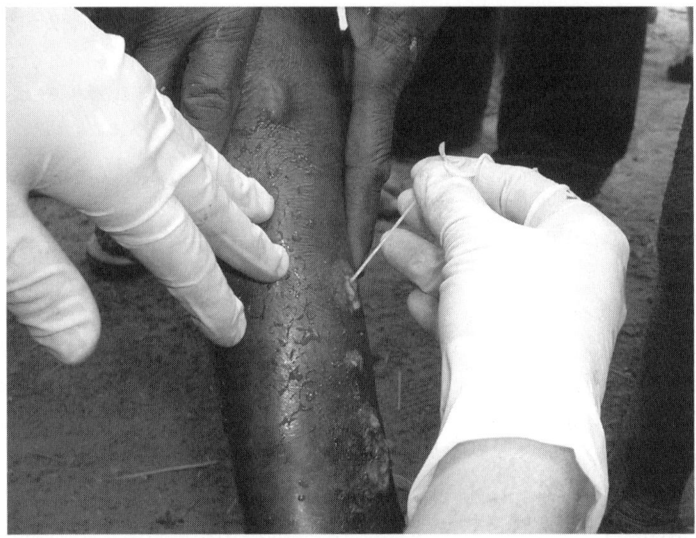

Figure 7   Traction being applied to a Guinea worm, after application of wet compresses. TCC archives/E. Staub.

harbour populations of copepods and are the usual sites from which infection is acquired. Local beliefs and ignorance about the origin and cause of dracunculiasis are important determinants of disease transmission and part of the insidious cycle of poor education associated with extreme poverty in the remote rural areas where the disease is common. Seasonality of disease occurrence varies according to location (Figure 9). In endemic areas on the southern fringes of the Sahara Desert (e.g., Mauritania, Mali, Niger, Burkina Faso, southern Sudan, and Ethiopia) transmission usually peaks during the rainy season at mid-year (May–October). This is because stagnant surface sources of water are only present during the relatively brief rainy season in such areas. In areas near the Gulf of Guinea (e.g., Côte d'Ivoire, Ghana, Togo, and Benin), the disease peaks during the dry season, from October to March, when surface sources of drinking water are scarcest and most concentrated, in contrast to abundant and often flowing surface water sources during the rest of the year. Nigeria has two peak transmission seasons, one in the southern half of the country during November–February and another in the more arid northern half during May–August.

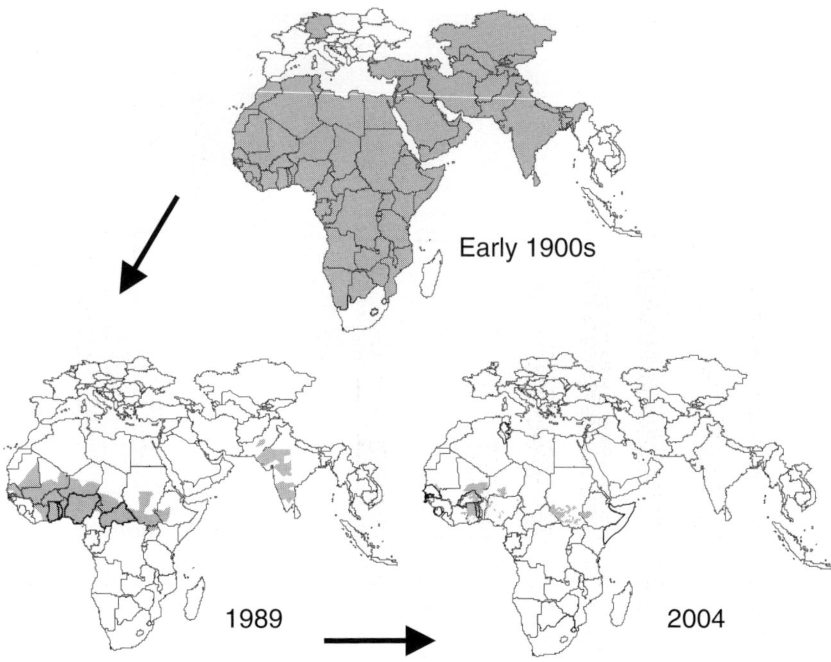

Figure 8   Historical distribution of reported cases of dracunculiasis in the early 1900s, known distribution in 1989, and in 2004. WHO CCRTED archives.

Cases of dracunculiasis occur in all age groups, but in general, it is most common among young adults (ages 15–45), and is distributed roughly equally among males and females. However, significant exceptions to the rule have been documented during the eradication campaign, e.g., the ratio of female to males with dracunculiasis in northeastern Uganda was 3:1 (J. B. Rwakimari, personal communication). Occupation is an important determinant of infection. Farmers and those who fetch drinking water are those most frequently infected. In certain endemic areas the preponderance of disease is often a burden of a particular ethnic group, e.g., the Bella people or "Black Tuaregs" in areas of Mali, Niger, and Burkina Faso, the Konkomba people in the northern parts of Ghana dond Togo, and the Karamajong people in northeastern Uganda. The frequent movement of people for social events such as funerals, the seasonal search for water and pasture for cattle, and itinerant farmers and traders often

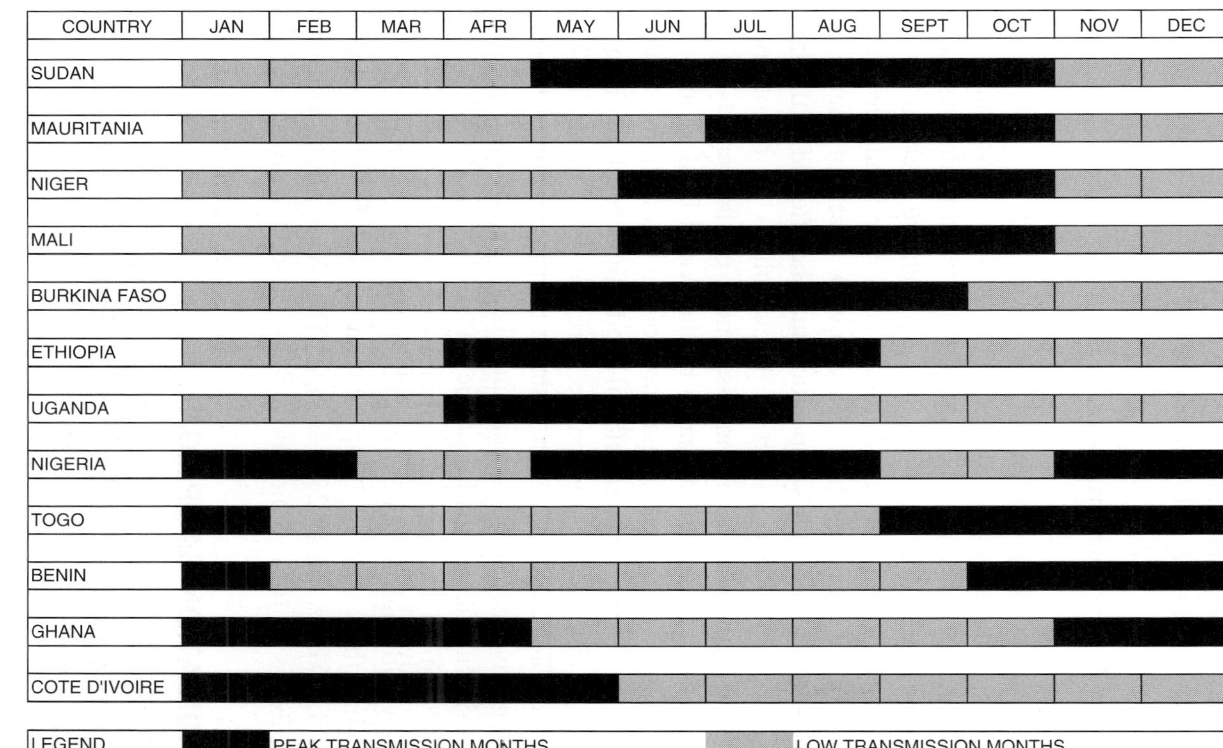

Figure 9 Country and months of peak and low transmission months for dracunculiasis. Based on historical data 1988–2000. Number of reported cases of dracunculiasis by country and year: 1983–2004. WHO CCRTED archives.

disseminate the infection over long distances. Persons in northern Ghana suffering dracunculiasis during a given year were found to be five times more likely than those not affected by the disease, to suffer dracunculiasis again the following year (Tayeh *et al.*, 1993).

4.2. Socio-Economic Impact

The seasonal occurrence of cases of the disease often coincides with harvest or planting seasons and significantly affects agricultural productivity, school attendance, and maternal and child health. As adults are incapacitated by dracunculiasis their children are likely to have to take over farming and household duties; and when incidence is high among children it precludes their ability to walk to school (Figure 10). More than 50% of a village's population may be affected at the same time. The socio-economic impact of dracunculiasis on remote rural villages have been qualified in an assessment of the benefits of the Dracunculiasis Eradication Campaign by the World Bank (Kim *et al.*, 1997). This study compared expenditures of the eradication campaign with estimates of increased agricultural productivity resulting from the prevention of disease transmission, i.e., prevention of morbidity as a result of the eradication campaign. Using a project horizon of 10 years and conservative assumptions regarding the degree of incapacitation caused by dracunculiasis, the Economic Rate of Return (ERR) is 11%, 29% or 44%, if the average period of incapacitation is 4, 5, or 6 weeks, respectively (although estimates from 12 published studies (cited above) indicate that the extent of incapacitation caused by dracunculiasis averages 8.5 weeks, range 2–16 weeks). The World Bank considers ERRs in excess of 10% to indicate a sound economic investment.

5. ERADICATION CAMPAIGN

5.1. Genesis and Initial Efforts to Gain Traction on Eradicating the Disease

In 1980, shortly after WHO declared the world free of smallpox, the idea of eradicating dracunculiasis globally was kindled when Drs

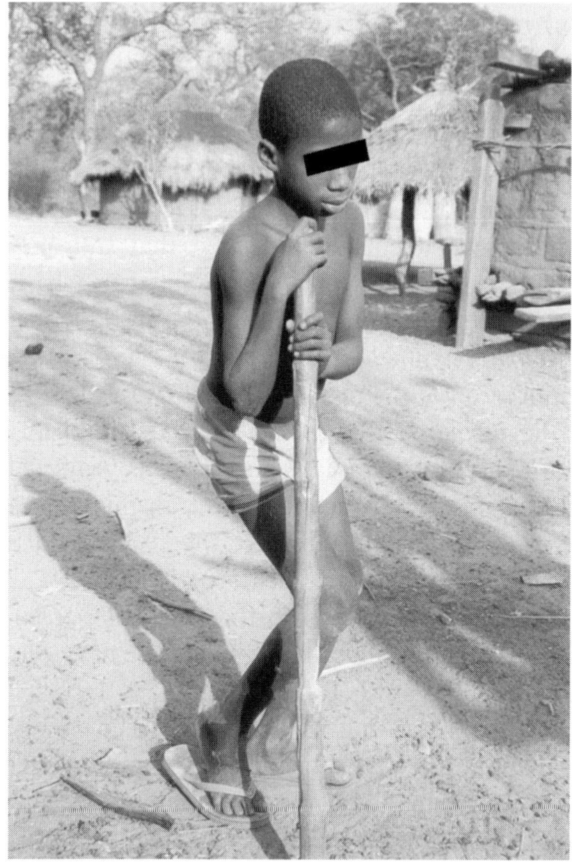

Figure 10 School-age young boy incapacitated by dracunculiasis. WHO CCRTED archives.

Donald Hopkins and William Foege of the Centers for Disease Control and Prevention (CDC) wrote a letter to the editor of the journal *Science* (Hopkins and Foege, 1981), suggesting that the eradication of dracunculiasis, a disease transmitted only via drinking water, would be an ideal indicator of the success of the International Drinking Water Supply and Sanitation Decade (IDWSSD) 1981–1990 (which the UN was about to launch). In 1981 the steering committee of the IDWSSD adopted dracunculiasis eradication as a sub-goal of their efforts (Hopkins, 1990).

5.2. Workshop on Opportunities to Control Dracunculiasis: 1982

Leading authorities from around the world met in June 1982 for the first international meeting devoted to dracunculiasis, entitled Workshop on Opportunities for Control of Dracunculiasis. A review of knowledge about dracunculiasis indicated that transmission of the disease was confined to only parts of sub-Saharan Africa, and India and Pakistan (in 1994 endemic transmission was documented to occur in Yemen). This seminal meeting provided information about the deliberate elimination of the disease from parts of the southern tier of republics in the former USSR during the 1920s and absence of the transmission of disease in humans for over 50 years (Litvinov and Lysenko, 1982). Moreover, dracunculiasis transmission had also been stopped in endemic areas of Iran since the 1970s, as a result of extensive use of dichloro-diphenyl-trichloroethane (DDT) for malaria control and chlorination of water in the "birkehs" or large, covered concrete cisterns storing rainwater, where malaria mosquitoes bred and where dracunculiasis was transmitted.

A review of the disease and its transmission concluded that there was no known animal reservoir for the disease; no human carrier state beyond the 1-year incubation period; no immunity to the infection; and the disease could not be cured with available anthelminthics. Additionally the occurrence of disease was known to be seasonal and its clinical presentation unique, and wherever dracunculiasis transmission was endemic it had a well-known name in the local language, thus facilitating the identification of localities with endemic transmission, including the ideal timing for prevalence surveys.

Participants concluded that dracunculiasis could be prevented completely by teaching people about the origin of the disease and how to prevent the infection, e.g., by keeping persons with emerging worms from entering sources of drinking water, and by filtering all drinking water through a cloth filter. Other available interventions to prevent transmission included the provision of safe sources of drinking water to affected villages, and treatment of unsafe sources of drinking water with 1 ppm concentration of ABATE® larvicide (temephos). Experts from India indicated they would officially launch their national eradication programme in 1983, after three consecutive annual case searches to ascertain the extent of dracunculiasis.

5.3. The WHO Collaborating Center for Research, Training, and Eradication of Dracunculiasis at the CDC

In 1984, CDC was designated the WHO Collaborating Center for Research, Training, and Eradication of Dracunculiasis (CCRTED), and charged with monitoring the status of efforts of the DEP, as well as providing technical assistance to national eradication programmes. CCRTED continued to publish quarterly issues of the *Guinea Worm Wrap-Up*, which chronicled the initiative, beginning in 1983, established the life cycle of *Dracunculus insignis* in raccoons and ferrets, and evaluated the effectiveness of existing anthelminthics against this parasite. None of the selected off-the-shelf anthelminthics tested had any overt effect on *D. insignis* (Eberhard, 1990). The CCRTED has since provided numerous consultants for national eradication programmes, it continues to monitor the progress of the global campaign, and has worked closely with The Carter Center (TCC) since 1986.

5.4. The First African Regional Conference on Dracunculiasis Eradication and First World Health Assembly Resolution

The first African Regional Conference on Dracunculiasis Eradication was convened in Niamey, Niger on July 1–3, 1986. Reports provided during this meeting revealed that an estimated total of 3.2 million cases occurred annually in Africa and 120 million people were at risk of the infection in the known endemic areas (Watts, 1987). Estimates of the incidence of the disease in Asia (India and Pakistan) brought the estimated global burden of disease to 3.5 million cases annually.

The 39th World Health Assembly (WHA) adopted resolution WHA 39.21 on May 16, 1986 endorsing national efforts to eliminate dracunculiasis country by country, in association with the IDWSSD. However, it was evident by the mid-1980s that the IDWSSD would not be able to muster the funding necessary to meet the enormous challenge of providing safe drinking water and sanitation to all in need of it and to eradicate dracunculiasis in the process.

5.5. The Carter Center

In 1986 former US President Jimmy Carter met with the President and Prime Minister of Pakistan and gained their support for a national eradication programme. A workshop to plan the campaign in Pakistan was held in Atlanta in November 1986 and TCC and CDC immediately began assisting Pakistan to ascertain the extent of the disease and to organize the national programme. With support from TCC and CDC, Pakistan began to implement interventions against the disease in 1988, Ghana and Nigeria in 1989, Uganda in 1991, and Mali and Niger in 1993, respectively. The year of initiation of national eradication efforts country-by-country is shown in Table 1. TCC soon became the lead non-governmental agency advocating for the global campaign to eradicate dracunculiasis, and providing technical and financial assistance to national eradication programmes.

Table 1　National Dracunculiasis Eradication Program start-ups

Year interventions started	Country	Active programs (cumulative)
1983	India	1
1988	Pakistan	2
1989	Nigeria, Ghana	4
1991	Cameroon	5
1992	Togo, Burkina Faso, Senegal, Uganda	9
1993	Benin, Mauritania, Niger, Mali, Côte d'Ivoire	14
1994	Sudan, Kenya, Chad, Ethiopia	18
1995	Yemen, Central African Republic	20

Source: WHO CCRTED archives.

5.6. Other Resolutions

In September 1988 African Ministers of Health passed a resolution calling for the eradication of dracunculiasis from Africa by 1995 (AFR/RC38/R13). However, the WHA passed a second resolution in May 1989 (WHA 42.29) declaring the goal of eliminating dracunculiasis as a public health problem from the world during the 1990s. The WHA adopted a third, and more definitive resolution on May 13, 1991 (WHA 44.5) calling for a global campaign to eradicate the disease by the end of 1995, and urging the Director-General of WHO to immediately initiate country-by-country certification of elimination, so by the end of the 1990s the certification process could be completed.

These resolutions, strong advocacy from TCC, and tangible and credible results from ongoing eradication efforts in Pakistan, India, Ghana, and Nigeria engendered increasing support from bilateral donors, industry, and international organizations that helped the remaining endemic countries to conduct nationwide case searches to assess the extent of the problem, organize national secretariats, and begin implementing of interventions against the disease. By 1992 only 5 of 20 countries had implemented programmes, but the target date for eradication was 1995. Although TCC provided assistance to all endemic countries (except India), it assigned Resident Technical Advisors to Pakistan and the most endemic African countries, i.e., Nigeria, Ghana, Mali, Niger, Uganda, Sudan, and Burkina Faso.

5.7. Strategy for Eradication

The strategy for dracunculiasis eradication includes three phases (Hopkins and Ruiz–Tiben, 1991). During Phase I national programmes conducted nationwide or area-wide case searches to determine the locations of villages with endemic transmission and record the numbers of cases, organized a national secretariat and a programme structure at district and village levels, and developed a national plan of action. In Phase II, programme staff and village-based health workers (village volunteers) were trained to implement interventions against transmission of the disease, conduct active village-based surveillance using case registers, provide health education to mobilize communities to action, provide cloth filters, and educate villagers on their care and proper use. During Phase III, when the incidence of disease had been reduced to far fewer cases per year and halting transmission was imminent, surveillance was intensified to rapidly detect all persons with emerging worms (preferably before or within 24 hours of worm emergence) and to contain transmission from each case by providing care for the wounds, applying occlusive bandages, and counselling the patient not to enter sources of drinking water. In 2001, most national programmes began offering persons with dracunculiasis the option of medical care at "case containment centres". When patients voluntarily attend such case containment centres they are provided a small monetary or in-kind incentive for agreeing to stay at the centre until each Guinea worm is successfully pulled out and are provided medical care, food, sanitation, and shelter. Care of the last cases of dracunculiasis at case containment centres or at established public health clinics permits patients to recover from their incapacity much faster and the programme to contain transmission from each emerging worm much more effectively. All other broad-based interventions continue to be employed until transmission is halted.

5.7.1. Interventions against Disease Transmission

Interventions against the disease include village-based surveillance, maintenance of a village case register and monthly reporting of cases, and community mobilization to educate residents about the origin of the disease and empower them with knowledge to prevent the disease by keeping infected persons from contaminating sources of drinking water, and by using donated cloth and/or pipe filters to make infected drinking water copepod free. ABATE® larvicide is applied monthly in ponds, stagnant pools, and unprotected wells during the transmission season, and listings of known endemic villages are made available to water sector organizations so they can target villages with endemic disease for provision or rehabilitation of sources of drinking water. The strategy of combining early detection of cases and containment of transmission began in 1991 in Pakistan (Kappus *et al.*, 1991), and in the endemic countries in Africa during 1993.

Scaling Up; Using Data; Advocacy by Eminent Persons. Scaling up of the DEP, beyond efforts already underway in Pakistan, Ghana, and Nigeria during the late 1980s, would not have been possible without the US $1.5 million authorized by former Director of UNICEF, Mr James Grant, in 1989 to support national case searches, beginning that year, in the endemic countries in need of determining the extent of dracunculiasis, and the endorsement of the DEP initiative by the World Summit for Children in 1990. The $1.5 million promised by UNICEF was part of nearly $10 million pledged for dracunculiasis eradication at the International Donors Conference that was held in Lagos, Nigeria in July 1989. The 1991 WHA resolution (WHA 44.5) calling for eradication of the disease by 1995 was also a clarion call for galvanizing national and international advocacy and support for the DEP.

Beginning in 1989, the CCRTED in collaboration with TCC and WHO developed, published, and disseminated operational guidelines for the DEP:

* Guidelines on Surveillance of Dracunculiasis (1988)
* Guidelines for Development of National Plans of Action (1989)
* Guidelines for Chemical Control of Copepods (1989)
* Guidelines for Health Education and Social Mobilization (1990)
* Guidelines for Case Containment (1994), in collaboration with UNICEF.

Additionally, in 1990 the CCRTED drafted the first set of Guidelines for Certification of the Eradication of Dracunculiasis. This document was presented to a group of national and international experts at an informal meeting hosted by WHO in 1990, and adopted as amended (WHO/FIL/90.185). The mandate to make this document operational came in May 13, 1991 with the above-mentioned WHA resolution 44.5, which called for a global campaign to eradicate the disease by the end of 1995, and urged the Director-General (of WHO) to immediately initiate country-by-country certification of elimination, so the certification process could be completed by the end of the 1990s. Beginning in 1991, UNICEF and the

CCRTED at CDC and WHO collaborated closely in assisting the endemic countries develop plans of action and budgets for the national case searches and for the initial years of the country-based campaign.

From the very onset of the national eradication efforts, including India's in 1983, the leaders of the DEP gave highest priority to the collection and use of data about the extent and incidence of dracunculiasis in order to plan and take actions against transmission of the disease. Without such a resolve, it would not have been possible to demonstrate quickly the feasibility and effectiveness of interventions against the disease, and the robustness of the strategy for eradication to the national and international public health community, including donor organizations. Keeping everyone who needed to know informed and updated about the DEP was an imperative from the beginning, and sharing the latest data on the campaign through periodic issues of the *Guinea Worm Wrap-Up* was not only critical to gaining supporters for the DEP, but also for providing guidance to national eradication programmes. Updating all who needed to know also engendered healthy competition between national coordinators about their progress of their programmes, often such competition to finish the job at an international level, e.g., the race between India and Pakistan, between Togo and Niger, and between Nigeria and Ghana helped to keep programmes motivated.

One of the outcomes of the Second African Regional Conference on Dracunculiasis Eradication that was held in Accra, Ghana in March 1988, was a call to all countries to begin providing reports on the status of national programmes to WHO and other partner organizations. Monthly reporting of village-based surveillance data did not begin until 1992 when a critical mass of the national eradication programmes had concluded their national case searches, defining the extent of the disease, and implemented village-based surveillance and monthly reporting of cases of dracunculiasis.

During a tour to five French-speaking endemic countries in 1992, President Carter convinced then former Malian head of state General Amadou Toumani Touré, to lead the fight to eradicate dracunculiasis from Mali and to help with national efforts in other francophone countries. With then President Alpha Konare's support, General Touré became President of Mali's National Intersectorial Committee for Dracunculiasis Eradication and a roving ambassador and lead advocate for the DEP in French-speaking Africa, roles he carried out energetically (Figure 11), until he was elected President of the Republic of Mali in 2002. Similarly, in 1998, President Carter asked General Yakubu Gowon, a former head of state in Nigeria, to assist during the final phase of the eradication effort in that country. General Gowon also has been an indefatigable Guinea worm warrior, visiting most of the endemic states and local government areas in Nigeria to advocate for greater involvement of the state and local governments in the eradication effort and particularly with the provision/rehabilitation of sources of safe drinking water (Figure 12).

Since the early years of the DEP, the CCRTED, TCC, WHO, and UNICEF provided technical assistance to the national eradication programmes. However, beginning in 1998 TCC decided as a result of the stagnation of progress in some key endemic countries since 1995, to provide in addition ad hoc technical advisors (TAs) to help the national programmes to improve programme management, monitoring

Figure 11   Malian head of state Amadou Toumani Touré and former US President Jimmy Carter attending the Dracunculiasis Eradication Program Conference in Africa. WHO CCRTED archives.

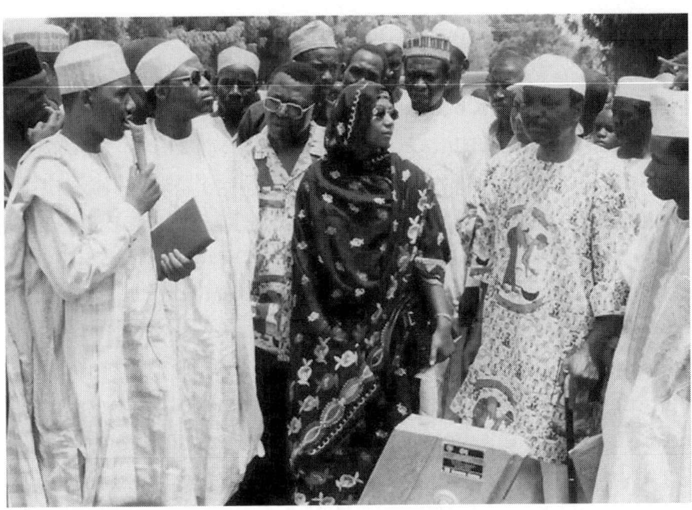

Figure 12 Former Nigerian head of state, General (Dr.) Yakubu Gowon, undertaking advocacy on behalf of the Nigerian DEP while commissioning a bore-hole well in an endemic village in Nigeria. WHO CCRTED archives.

of interventions, including provision and rehabilitation of sources of drinking water, and the quality and frequency of supervision of personnel. Most of these TAs have been former US Peace Corps Volunteers in Africa who had worked with a national eradication programme during their tours of duty with the US Peace Corps. During 1999 a total of 28 person–months of TAs were provided to endemic countries, followed by 88 person–months in 2000, 150 in 2001, 150 in 2002, 139 in 2003, and 127 in 2004. These TAs, placed to work with district level eradication teams, have played a vital role in ensuring that all interventions against dracunculiasis are implemented in the right places at the right times and in the correct way. They actively participate in training, via intense village-based, week-long health education campaigns, i.e., "Guinea Worm Weeks," and in mobilizing communities to take actions to prevent disease transmission in their villages. TAs have also played a key role in intervening during outbreaks of dracunculiasis in unexpected places in many of the endemic countries.

Since 1986, biennial regional conferences have been held (alternating between Francophone and Anglophone endemic countries), and, beginning in 1990, Program Manager meetings in the intervening years. Additionally, annual technical programmes reviews are also held during September–November. Since 1987, an Interagency Coordinating Group for Dracunculiasis Eradication has held quarterly or semi-annual meetings. National DEPs also hold their own annual review meetings, which are often attended by members of the coalition of partner organizations.

Attainment of eradication is not certified until the national programme requests WHO to validate the claim that no cases have occurred during 3 consecutive years since the last indigenous case, and an international certification team confirms that the surveillance system is sensitive and has not detected indigenous cases during the required 3-year period. An International Commission for the Certification of Dracunculiasis Eradication, established by WHO in 1995, reviews the findings of the certification team and recommends to the WHO whether or not to certify the country free of dracunculiasis.

Coalition of Partners. During this campaign TCC has forged a coalition of more than 30 agencies, organizations, governments, bilateral donors, industry, and NGOs that assist national programmes with their eradication efforts (Tables 2 and 3). CDC has played a critical role in helping TCC, WHO, and UNICEF lead this campaign. Advocacy by President Carter at the DuPont Corporation led to donations equivalent to US $17 million during 1990–1998, in nylon cloth for cloth filters from DuPont Corporation and Precision Fabrics Group Inc. Similar efforts resulted in over US $2 million worth in donations of ABATE® larvicide from BASF Corporation (currently the sole producer of ABATE® larvicide obtained from what was American Cyanamid, formerly part of American Home Products). The Bill and Melinda Gates Foundation provided 28.5 million dollars in May 2000 to help accelerate the eradication of dracunculiasis. The grant channelled through The World Bank Trust Fund for Guinea Worm Eradication allocated:

- $15 million to TCC for a 3-year period (2000–2002) to assist the remaining countries (except Mauritania and Uganda for which UNICEF has primary responsibility) to stop transmission.

Table 2 Coalition of organizations, agencies, governments, corporations, and others supporting the DEP

Major partners	Other UN organizations	Ministries of Health	Partners
The Carter Center	Office for the Coordination of Humanitarian Affairs	Benin	Adventist Health International
Centers for Disease Control and Prevention	UNDP	Burkina Faso	Adventist Development and Relief Agency
UNICEF	The World Bank	Cameroon	Aktion Afrike Hilfe
World Health Organization	World Food Programme	Chad	American Refugee Committee
		Cote d'Ivoire Central African Republic	Association of Christian Resource Organizations Serving Sudan
		Ethiopia	CARE International
		Ghana	Catholic Relief Services
		India	Christian Mission Aid
		Kenya	Comitato Collaborazione Medica
		Mali	Coordination Committee for Voluntary Service
		Mauritania	Diocese of Rumbek
		Niger	Diocese of Torit
		Nigeria	Fellowship for African Relief
		Pakistan	Gowon Center
		Senegal	Health & Development International
		Sudan	InterChurch Medical Assistance
		Togo	International Aid Sweden
		Uganda	International Committee of the Red Cross
		Yemen	International Medical Corps
			International Rescue Committee
			Japanese Overseas Cooperation Volunteers
			Map International
			MEDAIR
			Médecins Sans Frontières (Belgium, The Netherlands, Switzerland)

Table 2 (*continued*)

Major partners	Other UN organizations	Ministries of Health	Partners
			Mundri Relief and Development Association
			Norwegian Church Aid
			Nuba Relief, Rehabilitation, and Development Organization
			Okenden International
			Operation Lifeline Sudan/ South
			OXFAM UK
			Ghana Red Cross Society
			Save the Children (UK, Sweden)
			Sudan Medical Care
			Sudan National Water Corporation
			Sudan Production Aid
			Sudan Relief and Rehabilitation Commission
			Tearfund
			U.S. Peace Corps
			Vétérinaires Sans Frontières Belgium
			Voice of America
			World Relief International
			World Vision International
			ZOA Refugee Care

Source: TCC/N. Kruse.

- $8.5 million to the World Bank, TCC, WHO, and UNICEF to provide support for contingencies, and for other expenditures related to the eradication campaign.
- $5 million to the World Health Organization, which has primary responsibility for certification of eradication. For the purposes of this grant WHO assumed primary responsibility for assistance to countries in the pre-certification stage, including still-endemic countries close to interrupting transmission, i.e., reporting fewer than 100 cases of dracunculiasis or less during the calendar year.

Table 3 Coalition of organizations, agencies, governments, corporations, and others supporting the DEP (continuation)

Governments	Foundations	Individuals	Corporations
Canada	A.G. Leventis Foundation	Many individual donors have supported the global campaign to eradicate dracunculiasis.	Ad-Rem Concepts
Denmark	The Hugh J. Andersen Foundation		AGCO Corporation
Finland	Next Generation Fund		American Cyanamid
Japan	Bill & Melinda Gates Foundation		American Home Products
Kuwait Fund for Arab Economic Development	Conrad N. Hilton Foundation		BASF Corporation
Luxembourg	The Diebold Foundation		BellSouth Corporation
The Netherlands	International Humanitarian Foundation		Computer Associates International
Nigeria	The Morningside Foundation		Defined Health
Norway	PPG Industries Foundation		E. A. Juffali & Brothers
OPEC Fund for International Development	United Nations Foundation		E.I. du Pont de Nemours
Qatar	W.B. Haley Foundation		Environmental Systems Research Institute, Inc.
Saudi Arabia			Evergreen International Aviation
Saudi Fund for Development			Georgia-Pacific Corporation
United Arab Emirates			Human Wildlife Productions
United Kingdom			ITOCHU Corporation
United States			Johnson & Johnson
			Nippon Keidanren
			Norsk Hydro
			Perma-Guard, Inc.
			Precision Fabrics Group, Inc.
			Ravenswork
			Society of Plastics Engineers, Inc.
			Tsunami Films
			Vestergaard Frandsen Wyeth

Source: TCC/N. Kruse.

5.8. Progress towards Eradication

5.8.1. Reductions in Cases of Dracunculiasis

During 2004, a total of 16 026 cases of dracunculiasis were reported from the 12 remaining endemic countries cases: 7266 from Sudan, 7275 from Ghana, and 1485 from the other 10 countries reporting cases (Table 4, Figure 13). These 16 026 cases represent a reduction of 99.5% from the estimated 3.5 million cases occurring annually in 1986, or a 98% reduction from the 892 926 cases of dracunculiasis reported by the DEP in 1989, the year when the highest number of cases on record was reported (Table 1). Sudan reported fewer cases of dracunculiasis (7266) than all 11 other countries combined (8760) during 2004, and for the first time since 1996 (Figure 14). The major remaining foci of transmission of dracunculiasis now are in southern Sudan, Ghana, Mali, and Niger (Figure 15, which is Plate 7.15 in the separate colour plate section). The 7257 cases of dracunculiasis reported from Ghana in 2004 represent a 12% reduction in cases from the 8290 cases Ghana reported in 2003, and 83% of all cases reported outside of Sudan in 2004. The overall percent reduction in indigenous cases for all countries combined during 2004, compared with 2003, is 50% (Figure 16). Outside of Sudan the overall percent reduction in 2004 was 60%. These are the largest reductions in cases observed so far between one year and the next during this campaign, and augur well for accelerated progress towards eradication during 2005. Burkina Faso reported only 35 indigenous cases, a reduction of 80% from the 175 indigenous cases it reported in 2003. Nigeria, the most endemic country during this campaign, reported only 495 indigenous cases, a reduction of 99.9% from the 653 492 cases it reported during its first national village-by-village case search in 1988, and a reduction of 66% from the 1459 cases it reported in 2003. Interventions against the disease in Togo and Mali in 2003 were also effective, as demonstrated by the 63% and 57% reductions in cases (from 622 to 230, and from 824 to 349) in 2004, respectively. Forty-six (46) of the 276 cases reported by Togo in 2004 were imported from neighbouring Ghana (Table 5). Niger was able only to reduce its cases from 279 to 233 (16%) between 2003 and 2004. The vast majority of Niger's cases

Table 4 Number of reported cases of dracunculiasis by country and year: 1983–2004

Country	Year and number of cases reported																					
	1983	1984	1985	1986	1987	1988	1989	1990	1991	1992	1993	1994	1995	1996	1997	1998	1999	2000	2001	2002	2003	2004
Sudan				822	399	542	NR	NR	NR	2447	2984	53 271	64 608	118 578	43 596	47 977	66 097	54 890	49 471	41 493	20 299	7266
Nigeria				2821	216 484	653 492	640 008	394 082	281 937	183 169	75 752	39 774	16 374	12 282	12 590	13 420	13 237	7869	5355	3820	1459	495
Ghana			4501	4717	18 398	71 767	179 556	123 793	66 697	33 464	17 918	8432	8894	4877	8921	5473	9027	7402	4739	5611	8290	7275
Togo			1456	1325	NR	178	2749	3042	5118	8179	10 349	5044	2073	1626	1762	2128	1589	828	1354	1502	669	278
Burkina Faso			458	2558	1957	1266	45 004	42 187	NR	11 784	8281	6861	6281	3241	2477	2227	2184	1956	1032	591	203	60
Mali			4072	5640	435	564	1111	884	16 024	NR	12 011	5581	4218	2402	1099	650	410	290	718	861	829	357
Niger			1373	NR	699	NR	288	NR	32 829	500	25 346	18 562	13 821	2956	3030	2700	1920	1166	417	248	293	240
Côte d'ivoire			1889	1177	1272	1370	1555	1360	12 690	NR	8034	5061	3801	2794	1254	1414	476	297	231	198	42	21
Benin					400	33 962	7172	37 414	4006	4315	16 334	4302	2273	1427	855	695	492	186	172	181	30	3
Mauritania			1291		227	608	447	8301	NR	1557	5882	5029	1762	562	388	379	255	136	94	42	13	3
Uganda			4070	NR	NR	1960	1309	4704	NR	126 369	42 852	10 425	4810	1455	1374	1061	321	96	55	24	26	4
Ethiopia				3885	2302	1487	3565	2333	NR	303	1120	1252	514	371	451	366	249	60	29	47	28	17
Central African Republic					1322	NR	871	10	NR	NR	NR	NR	18	9	5	34	26	35	36	NR	0	0
Kenya							5	6	NR	NR	35	53	23	0	6	7	1	4	8	17	12	7
Pakistan					2400	1110	534	160	106	23	2	0	0	0	~	~	~	~	~	~	~	~
India	44 818	40 443	30 950	23 070	17 031	12 023	7881	4798	2185	1081	755	371	60	9	0	0	0	~	~	~	~	~
Cameroon			168	86		752	871	742	393	127	72	30	15	17	19	23	8	5	5	3	0	0
Chad				314	NR	NR	NR	NR	NR	156	1231	640	149	127	25	3	1	3	0	0	0	0
Senegal			62	128	132	138	NR	38	1341	728	815	195	76	19	4	0	0	0	1	0	0	~
Yemen									NR	NR	NR	0	94	82	62	7	0	0	0	0	0	~
Total	44 818	40 443	50 290	46 543	263 458	781 219	892 926	623 854	423 326	374 202	229 773	164 977	129 852	152 814	77 863	78 557	96 293	75 223	63 717	54 638	32 193	16 026

Note: Grey shaded cells indicate cases detected during a national case search. Numbers preceding national case search are from passive surveillance. Numbers after case search are from village-based reporting.
Black cells indicate imported cases only. All other cells include both indigenous and imported cases.
Source: WHO CCRTED.
~ = Country certified free of dracunculiasis by WHO; NR = no report.

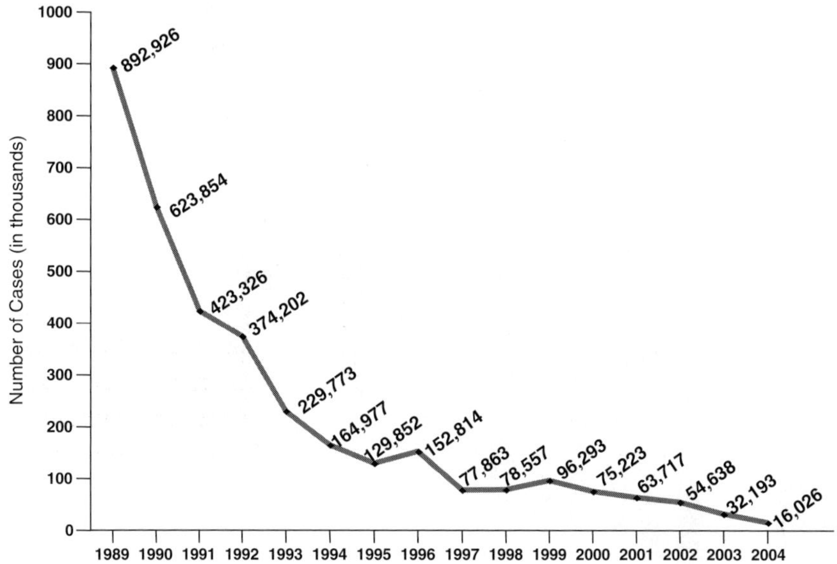

Figure 13 Number of reported cases of dracunculiasis by country during 1989–2004 for Sudan and all other countries. WHO CCRTED archives.

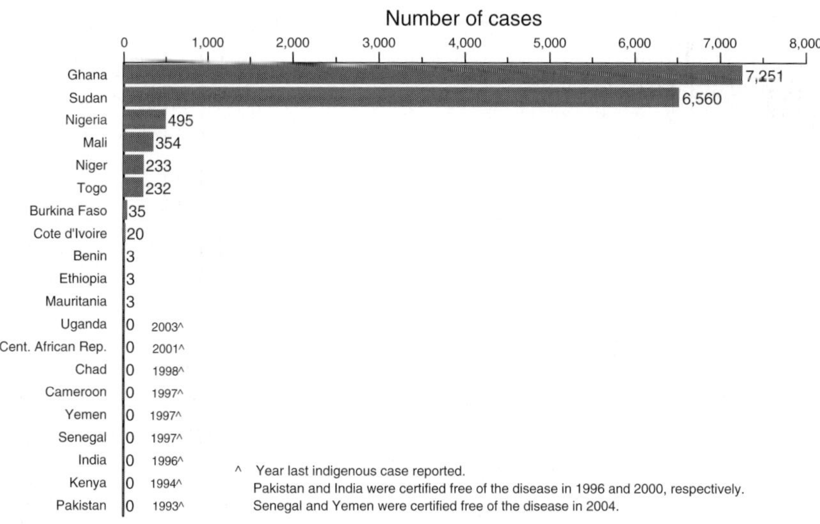

Figure 14 Reported cases of dracunculiasis by country in 2004. WHO CCRTED archives.

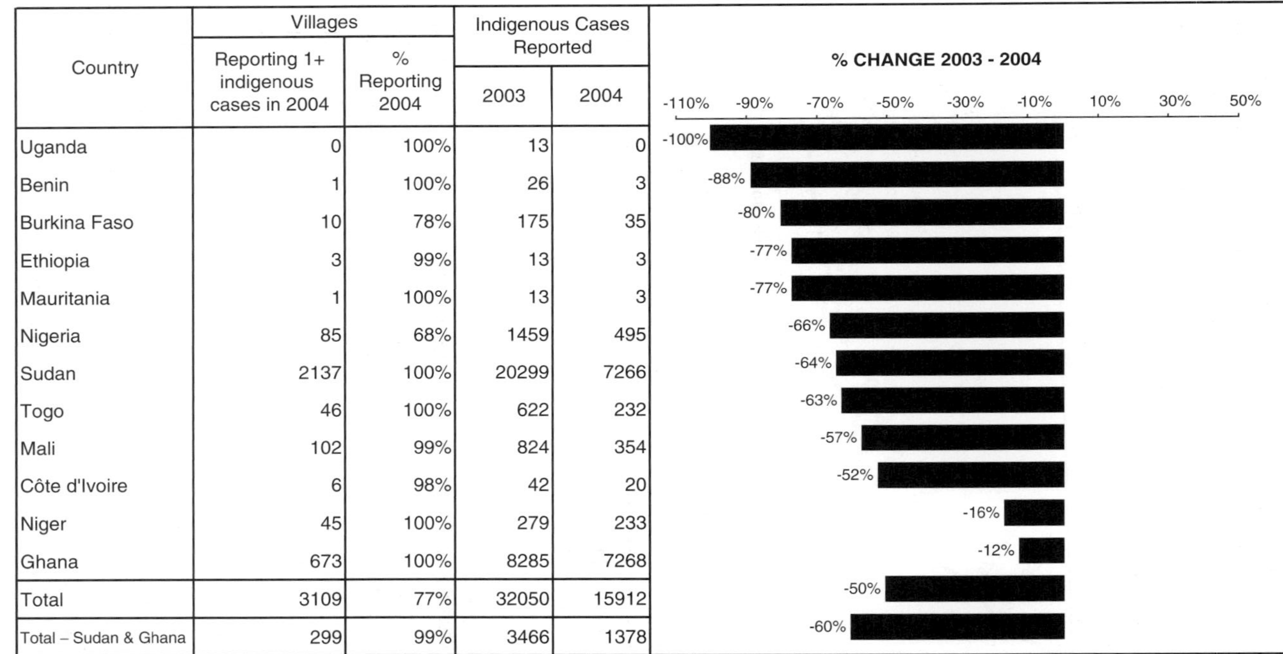

Country	Villages		Indigenous Cases Reported		% CHANGE 2003 - 2004
	Reporting 1+ indigenous cases in 2004	% Reporting 2004	2003	2004	
Uganda	0	100%	13	0	-100%
Benin	1	100%	26	3	-88%
Burkina Faso	10	78%	175	35	-80%
Ethiopia	3	99%	13	3	-77%
Mauritania	1	100%	13	3	-77%
Nigeria	85	68%	1459	495	-66%
Sudan	2137	100%	20299	7266	-64%
Togo	46	100%	622	232	-63%
Mali	102	99%	824	354	-57%
Côte d'Ivoire	6	98%	42	20	-52%
Niger	45	100%	279	233	-16%
Ghana	673	100%	8285	7268	-12%
Total	3109	77%	32050	15912	-50%
Total – Sudan & Ghana	299	99%	3466	1378	-60%

Figure 16 Number of villages/localities reporting cases of dracunculiasis in 2003, percentage of endemic villages reporting in 2004, and number of indigenous cases reported during the specified period in 2003 and 2004, and percent change cases reported. WHO CCRTED archives.

Table 5 Number of reported indigenous and imported cases of dracunculiasis during 2004 by country, and origin of imported cases

Country	Cases of dracunculiasis reported during 2004[a]			Country of origin and number of imported cases
	Indigenous	Imported	Total	
Ghana	7268	7	7275	Togo = 6; Niger = 1
Sudan	7266	0	7266	
Nigeria	495	0	495	
Mali	354	3	357	Burkina Faso = 2; Niger = 1
Nigeria	233	7	240	Nigeria = 3; Mali = 2; Ghana = 1; Togo = 1
Togo	232	46	278	Ghana = 46
Burkina Faso	35	25	60	Mali = 15; Ghana = 8; Benin = 1; Côte d'Ivoire = 1
Côte d'Ivoire	20	1	21	Ghana = 1
Benin	3	0	3	
Ethiopia	3	14	17	Sudan = 14
Mauritania	3	0	3	
Uganda	0	4	4	Sudan = 4
Kenya	0	7	7	Sudan = 7
Total	15912	114	16026	

Source: WHO CCRTED.
[a]Data for 2004 are provisional.

were reported from the districts of Tillaberi and Tera in the western end of the country and adjoining some of the remaining endemic districts in Mali and Burkina Faso. Cases of dracunculiasis in this tri-border area occur among the nomadic Tuaregs, and mostly among the Bella or "Black Tuareg" people. Uganda reported zero indigenous cases during 2004 and has not reported a single indigenous case of dracunculiasis since July 2003. Mauritania and Benin reported only three cases each, and it is possible these two countries may have already stopped transmission during 2004. Ethiopia also reported only three cases, all from Gambella Region. However, Akobo Woreda (district) in Gambella, where endemic transmission of dracunculiasis is likely, continues to be inaccessible to the national eradication programme because of insecurity, and has been so for years. Halting transmission of dracunculiasis in Ethiopia is not likely until its national eradication programme can access Akobo District and implement interventions against the disease there.

5.8.2. Reductions in Endemic Villages

In 2004 there were only 3109 villages in the 12 endemic countries that reported indigenous cases of dracunculiasis. Of these, 2173 (70%) endemic villages were in Sudan and 936 in the other 11 endemic countries, including 673 (22%) in Ghana. These 3109 villages represented a reduction of 87% from the 23 735 endemic villages reporting cases in 1993, when the largest number of endemic villages was recorded.

5.8.3. Reductions in Endemic Countries

As of the end of 2004, 9 of the 20 endemic countries have halted transmission of dracunculiasis (Figure 16), and 4 of those countries (Pakistan in 1996, India in 2000, and Yemen and Senegal in 2004) have been certified free of dracunculiasis by WHO. Uganda stopped transmission of dracunculiasis in 2003 and joined the list of countries now in the pre-certification stage, i.e., Cameroon, Central African Republic, Chad, and Kenya (Figure 17, which is Plate 7.17 in the separate colour plate section). As of March 2004, the International Commission for Certification of Dracunculiasis Eradication had recommended, and WHO had certified, 168 countries as free of dracunculiasis.

5.8.4. Finishing the Job

We estimate the cost of the DEP during 1987–2004 to be circa US $122–125 million, and that an additional US $65 million will be required to finish the job by 2010. Most of these additional funds will be required to stop transmission of dracunculiasis in southern Sudan, a vast country with little infrastructure, including extremely poor transportation and communications, which is just emerging from 21 years of civil war (CDC, 1995; Hopkins and Withers, 2002). The DEP in Sudan, as in other countries, requires implementing a village-based programme in each endemic village, and there may be as many as 5000 villages with endemic transmission of dracunculiasis in southern Sudan. Stopping transmission of dracunculiasis from southern Sudan will be a Herculean task.

In 2004 WHA passed resolution WHA 57.9 urging all remaining endemic countries to stop transmission as soon as possible, and by 2009 in Sudan, which because of the civil conflict that ended on January 9, 2005 will require additional years to halt transmission. The Ministers of Health of endemic countries, or their representatives attending the 2004 WHA, also signed the "Geneva Declaration" in which the ministers pledged to exert their leadership and political will in their countries to accelerate attainment of the goal of eradicating dracunculiasis. With only 16 026 cases of dracunculiasis left in the world as of the end of 2004, high level advocacy with national and international leaders will be vital in order to prevent complacency about the progress made so far. TCC will continue to urge national and international leaders, including President Touré of Mali, and General (Dr) Gowon in Nigeria to do all they can to continue their advocacy until dracunculiasis is eradicated.

Staff of the national DEPs are now very experienced and know well the level of attention to detail and good supervision required to stop transmission of dracunculiasis. Given sufficient resources, and their effective use, and peace in the affected areas, there is no reason why this ancient scourge of mankind cannot be eradicated soon.

REFERENCES

Adeyeba, O.A. (1985). Secondary infections in dracunculiasis: bacteria and morbidity. *International Journal of Zoonoses* **12**, 147.

Adeyeba, O.A. and Kale, O.O. (1991). Epidemiology of dracunculiasis and its socio-economic impact in a village in south-west Nigeria. *West African Journal of Medicine* **10**, 208–215.

Belcher, D.W., Wurapa, F.K., Ward, W.B. and Lourie, I.M. (1975). Guinea worm in southern Ghana: its epidemiology and impact on agricultural productivity. *American Journal of Tropical Medicine and Hygiene* **24**, 243–249.

Cairncross, S., Muller, R. and Zagaria, N. (2002). Dracunculiasis (Guinea worm disease) and the eradication initiative. *Clinical Microbiology Reviews* **15**, 223–246.

Centers for Disease Control and Prevention. (1995). Implementation of health initiatives during a cease-fire – Sudan, 1995. *Morbidity and Mortality Weekly Report* **44**, 433–436.

Centers for Disease Control and Prevention. (2004). Progress towards global eradication of dracunculiasis, 2002–2003. *Morbidity and Mortality Weekly Report* **53**, 871–872.

Chippaux, J.P., Benzou, A. and Agbede, K. (1992). Social and economic impact of dracunculiasis: a longitudinal study carried out in two villages in Benin. *Bulletin of the World Health Organization* **70**, 73–78.

Eberhard, M.L. (1990). Chemoprophylactic drug trials of dracunculiasis using the *Dracunculus insignis* – ferret model. *Journal of Helminthology* **2**, 79–86.

Edungbola, L.D. (1983). Babana parasitic disease project II. Prevalence and impact of dracontiasis in Babana District, Kwara State, Nigeria. *Transactions of the Royal Society of Tropical Medicine and Hygiene* **77**, 310–315.

Fedchenko, A.P. (1870). Concerning the structure and reproduction of the guinea worm (*Filaria medinensis* L.) *Proceedings of the Imperial Society of the Friends of Natural Sciences, Anthropology, and Ethnography*, Vol. 8 (in Russian). Reprinted in *American Journal of Tropical Medicine and Hygiene* (1971) **20**, 511–523.

Greenaway, C. (2004). Dracunculiasis (guinea worm disease). *Canadian Medical Association Journal* **170**(4), 495–500.

Hopkins, D.R. (1990). *Report on IDWSSD Impact on Dracunculiasis.* Report prepared for the Steering Committee for Cooperative Action, International Drinking Water Supply and Sanitation Decade, pp. 1–16.

Hopkins, D.R. and Foege, W.H. (1981). Guinea worm disease. *Science* **212**, 495.

Hopkins, D.R. and Hopkins, E. (1992). Guinea worm: the end is in sight. *Encyclopedia Britannica Medical Health Annual 1992*. Chicago: Encyclopaedia Britannica, Inc., pp. 10–26.

Hopkins, D.R. and Ruiz-Tiben, E. (1991). Strategies for dracunculiasis eradication. *Bulletin of the World Health Organization* **69**, 533–540.

Hopkins, D.R., Ruiz-Tiben, E., Diallo, N., Withers, P.C. and Maguire, J.H. (2002). Dracunculiasis eradication: and now Sudan. *American Journal of Tropical Medicine and Hygiene* **67**, 415–422.

Hopkins, D.R. and Withers, P.C. (2002). Sudan's war and eradication of dracunculiasis. *Lancet* **360** (supplement), S21–S22.

Ilegbodu, V.A., Ilegbodu, A.E., Wise, R.A., Christensen, B.L. and Kale, O.O. (1991). Clinical manifestations, disability, and use of folk medicine in dracunculiasis in Nigeria. *Journal of Tropical Medicine and Hygiene* **94**, 35–41.

Kale, O.O. (1977). The clinico-epidemiological profile of Guinea worm in the Ibadan District of Nigeria. *American Journal of Tropical Medicine and Hygiene* **26**, 208–214.

Kappus, K., Hopkins, D.R. and Ruiz-Tiben, E. (1991). A strategy to speed the eradication of dracunculiasis. *World Health Forum* **2**, 220–225.

Khan, H.D., Aminuddin, M. and Shah, C.H. (1986). Epidemiology and socio-economic implications of dracunculiasis in eleven rural communities of District Bannu (Pakistan). *Journal of the Pakistani Medical Association* **36**, 233–239.

Kim, A., Tandon, A. and Ruiz-Tiben, E. (1997). *Cost–Benefit Analysis of the Global Dracunculiasis Eradication Campaign.* Washington: World Bank, Africa Human Development Department, Policy Research Working Paper 1835, pp. 1–16.

Litvinov, S.K. and Lysenko, A. (1982). Dracunculiasis: its history and eradication in the USSR. *Workshop on Opportunities for Control of Dracunculiasis*, pp. 97–100.

Muller, R. (1971). *Dracunculus* and dracunculiasis. *Advances in Parasitology* **6**, 73–151.

Nwosu, A.B.C., Ifeluze, E.O. and Anya, A.O. (1982). Endemic dracontiasis in Anambra State of Nigeria. Geographic distribution, clinical features, and socio-economic impact. *Annals of Tropical Medicine and Parasitology* **76**, 187–200.

Rhode, J.E., Sharma, B.L., Patton, H., Deegan, C. and Sherry, J.M. (1993). Surgical extraction of Guinea worm: disability reduction and contribution to disease control. *American Journal of Tropical Medicine and Hygiene* **48**, 71–76.

Smith, G.S., Blum, D. and Huttley, S.R.A. (1989). Disability from dracunculiasis: effect on mobility. *Annals of Tropical Medicine and Parasitology* **83**, 151–158.

Suleiman, M.M. and Abdullahi, K. (1990). Guinea worm infection in Kiri-Manai village, Sokoto. *Nigerian Journal of Parasitology* **9–11**, 13–16.

Tayeh, A., Cairncross, S. and Maude, G.H. (1993). Water sources and other determinants of dracunculiasis prevalence in the Northern Region of Ghana. *Journal of Helminthology* **67**, 213–225.

Watts, S.J. (1987). Dracunculiasis in Africa: its geographical extent, incidence, and at-risk population. *American Journal of Tropical Medicine and Hygiene* **37**, 121–127.

Watts, S.J., Brieger, W.R. and Yacoob, M. (1989). Guinea worm: an in depth study of what happens to mothers, families, and communities. *Social Science Medicine* **29**, 1043–1049.

World Health Organization (2004). Global surveillance summary, 2003. *Weekly Epidemiologic Report*, No. 19, 181–189.

Intervention for the Control of Soil-Transmitted Helminthiasis in the Community

Marco Albonico[1], Antonio Montresor[2], D.W.T. Crompton[3] and Lorenzo Savioli[4]

[1]*Ivo de Carneri Foundation, Torino, Italy*
[2]*World Health Organization, Hanoi, Viet Nam*
[3]*Institute of Biomedical and Life Sciences, University of Glasgow, UK*
[4]*World Health Organization, Geneva, Switzerland*

ADVANCES IN PARASITOLOGY VOL 61
ISSN: 0065-308X
DOI: 10.1016/S0065-308X(05)61008-1

ABSTRACT

The global strategy for the control of soil-transmitted helminthiasis, based on regular anthelminthic treatment, health education and improved sanitation standards, is reviewed. The reasons for the development of a control strategy based on population intervention rather than on individual treatment are explained. The evidence and experience from control programmes that created the basis for (i) the definition of the intervention package, (ii) the identification of the groups at risk, (iii) the standardization of the community diagnosis and (iv) the selection of the appropriate intervention for each category in the community are discussed. How to best deliver the appropriate intervention, the impact of the control measures on morbidity and on indicators such as school attendance, cognitive development and productivity are presented. The factors influencing the cost–benefits of helminth control are also considered. The recent progress on the control of soil-transmitted helminth infections is illustrated. Research needs are analysed in relation to the most recent perceptions from private–public partnerships involved in helminth control. The way forward for the control of soil-transmitted helminth infections is described as a multi-disease approach that goes beyond deworming and fosters a pro-poor strategy that supports the aims of the Millennium Development Goals.

1. POPULATION-BASED INTERVENTIONS TO CONTROL SOIL-TRANSMITTED HELMINTHIASIS

Ascaris lumbricoides, *Ancylostoma duodenale*, *Necator americanus* and *Trichuris trichiura* constitute the major soil-transmitted helminth (STH) infections. Disease due to these infections is now recognized as a serious public health problem wherever suitable environmental conditions co-exist with inadequate sanitation and poor hygiene. In such conditions, STH infections are normally highly prevalent with 2 billion people infected worldwide and several million suffering from the chronic debilitating morbidity (Crompton, 1999, 2000; de Silva *et al.*, 2003).

The World Health Organization (WHO) promotes the combined control of soil-transmitted helminthiasis and schistosomiasis where both these infections are endemic (WHO, 2002a). Schistosomiasis and soil-transmitted helminthiasis present some similarities in terms of geographical distribution, epidemiology, groups at high risk and control interventions. Although this article focuses on the control of soil-transmitted helminthiasis, it should be noted that where the two infections are often co-endemic, combined control greatly increases impact and cost-effectiveness, and is strongly recommended where appropriate.

The WHO has identified the population-based approach as the main strategy for the control of mortality and morbidity due to STH infections, for the following reasons:

- The clinical appearance of STH infection often lacks specific symptoms and may not be recognized by the infected person, even when causing significant health damage. When control measures are limited to curative services, only a small fraction of the infected population receives appropriate treatment.
- Individual diagnosis is relatively expensive requiring the availability of microscopes, laboratory material and trained personnel. The cost of establishing and maintaining an efficient STH diagnosis facility at peripheral level is much more expensive than the cost of treatment, now available for a few US cents per dose (WHO, 2002a).
- Identifying risk is usually based on parasitological data that classify communities according to the risk of developing morbidity. To overcome the paucity of epidemiological information, environmental information can be used to predict the large-scale distribution of infection (Brooker *et al.*, 2002a). Epidemiological assessments can be undertaken in a limited number of communities in order to collect reliable data for risk identification and then select and monitor the appropriate intervention (Brooker *et al.*, 2002b; Montresor *et al.*, 2002).

- Drugs used in population-based interventions for the control of STH have a secure safety record. The drugs are given orally and, because they are usually poorly absorbed, they reach and kill the parasites in the digestive tract causing negligible side effects. Two WHO Informal Consultations have recommended treatment with anthelminthics of pregnant women after the first trimester (WHO, 1996) and of children over 1 year of age (WHO, 2002b) to improve the health and development of these two high-risk groups in endemic countries.
- Delivering population-based interventions for the control of STH requires minimal infrastructure. Owing to the safety profile of WHO-recommended anthelminthics, non-medically trained personnel can safely and effectively distribute the drugs after instruction (WHO, 2002a; Urbani and Albonico, 2003). Distribution by school-teachers is particularly well accepted by the community (Nwaorgu *et al.*, 1998; Partnership For Child Development, 2001).
- The morbidity caused by STH is directly related to the number of worms (intensity of infection) and the duration of infection. Infections of moderate to heavy intensity are mainly responsible for the morbidity due to STH. Regular treatment reduces the number of worms in each individual and keeps the worm burden permanently low throughout the year. Regular treatment, despite re-infection, is able to control morbidity in high-transmission areas (Savioli *et al.*, 2002) because, even if prevalence of infection remains high, moderate to heavy infections (responsible for morbidity) decline over time (Figure 1).

The use of anthelminthic treatment is no longer limited to the clinical domain; it has become the intervention for large-scale prevention and reduction of morbidity in endemic communities.

2. INTERVENTION PACKAGE

Three interventions are recommended by WHO to control morbidity due to STH infections: (i) regular drug treatment of high risk groups, aimed at reduction of the worm burden over time; (ii) health education to increase population health awareness; (iii) sanitation

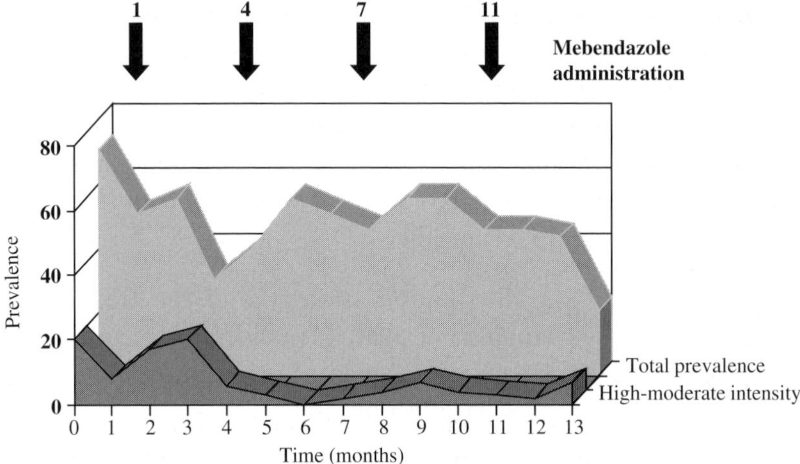

Figure 1 Effects of periodical treatment with mebendazole on total prevalence and prevalence of moderate–heavy *T. trichiura* infections. (Montresor *et al.*, unpublished data from the control programme in Zanzibar, United Republic of Tanzania.)

supported by personal hygiene aimed at reducing soil contamination with infected human faeces and the likelihood of re-infection (WHO, 2002a).

An appropriate combination of these three measures should be applied according to different epidemiological situations and to the availability of resources.

2.1. Regular Anthelminthic Treatment

Regular drug treatment represents the main measure in areas where infections are intensely transmitted, where resources for disease control are limited, and where funding for sanitation is insufficient.

Drug treatment can be administered in the community using different strategies:

- *Universal treatment.* Treatment is offered to the entire community, irrespective of age, sex, infection status and any other social characteristics.

- *Targeted treatment.* Treatment is targeted at population groups, which may be defined by age, sex or other social characteristics, irrespective of the infection status.
- *Selective treatment.* Individual-level application of anthelminthic drug administration, where selection is based on diagnosis to detect the most heavily infected people who will be most at risk of serious morbidity and mortality.

The selection of the distribution strategy and the frequency of treatment is based on analysis of available epidemiological data.

Recommended drugs (WHO, 2004a) for use in public health interventions to control STH infection are:

- Albendazole (400 mg) tablets given in single dose, reduced to 200 mg for children between 12 and 24 months.
- Levamisole (40 mg) tablets given in single dose by weight (2.5 mg/ kg). Levamisole at a dose of 80 mg has been successfully used in primary school-age children (Albonico *et al.*, 2003).
- Mebendazole (500 mg) tablets given in single dose.
- Pyrantel pamoate (250 mg) tablets given in single dose by weight (10 mg/kg). A combined preparation of pyrantel–oxantel has been proved more effective than pyrantel alone in treating *T. trichiura* infection (Albonico *et al.*, 2002).

These drugs are have undergone extensive safety testing and have been given to millions of individuals with only minimal adverse events (Horton, 2000; Urbani and Albonico, 2003). Anthelminthics can now be safely used in children as young as 12 months (Montresor *et al.*, 2003; WHO, 2002b). Drugs that do not need dosage according to weight, such as albendazole, mebendazole and levamisole (in school-age children) are considered easier to use for population-based interventions (de Silva *et al.*, 1997). All these drugs produce excellent egg reduction rates for *A. lumbricoides* (>95%) and for hookworms (>80%), but are less effective against *T. trichiura* (WHO, 1999; Bennet and Guyatt, 2000). The efficacy of single-dose anthelminthics is summarized in Table 1.

The patents of the anthelminthic drugs recommended by WHO have expired and therefore the drugs can be produced at very low

Table 1 Recommended drugs for the treatment of soil-transmitted nematode infections in public health

Substance	Therapeutic activity		Dosage	Use in pregnancy and in children
Albendazole (tablet 200 and 400 mg, suspension 100 mg/ 5 ml)	*A. lumbricoides*	+ + +	400 mg single dose	Not recommended in the first trimester of pregnancy. In children between 12 and 24 months use 200 mg
	T. trichiura	+ +	400 mg single dose	
	Hookworm infections	+ + +	400 mg single dose	
Levamisole (tablet 40 mg, syrup 40 mg/5 ml)	*A. lumbricoides*	+ + +	2.5 mg/kg single dose (80 mg single dose in school-age children)	No evidence of teratogenicity
	T. trichiura	+	2.5 mg/kg single dose (80 mg single dose in school-age children)	
	Hookworms	+ +	2.5 mg/kg single dose (80 mg single dose in school-age children)	
			For heavy necatoriasis repeat after 7 days	
Mebendazole (tablet 100 and 500 mg, suspension 100 mg/ 5 ml)	*A. lumbricoides*	+ + +	500 mg single dose	Not recommended in the first trimester of pregnancy and in children under 1 year
	T. trichiura	+ +	500 mg single dose	
	Hookworms	+ + +	500 mg single dose	
Pyrantel (tablet 250 mg, suspension 50 mg/ml)	*A. lumbricoides*	+ + +	10 mg/kg single dose	Not recommended in the first trimester of pregnancy
	T. trichiura	—	10 mg/kg single dose	
	Hookworms	+ +	10 mg/kg single dose. For heavy necatoriasis repeat for 3 days	

price by generic manufacturers. The price in the international market for mebendazole (500 mg), produced under Good Manufacturing Practice conditions is approximately US\$ 0.02 per tablet (Management Science for Health, 2004). The price is further reduced in case of local production, but in this case special attention should be given to assuring the good quality of the product. WHO, with a network of quality control laboratories, may facilitate the quality control exercise (Montresor *et al.*, 2002).

2.2. Health Education

Health education aims to increase health and hygiene awareness and to change health behaviour in the population. Health awareness is usually increased when communication strategies of proven efficacy are adopted (Kinzie, 2005). Marketing techniques and tools imported from the private sector are increasingly being advocated for their potential value in crafting and disseminating health messages (Bull *et al.*, 2001), but this technology should be appropriately transferred to reconcile differences between commercial marketing and public health (Walsh *et al.*, 1993). Education materials (posters, leaflets, radio and video messages) have been traditionally used to transmit and disseminate health messages. The expansion of commercial advertising in developing countries, however, calls for upgraded skills in designing such tools in order to compete for attention (Bull *et al.*, 2001; Whitelaw and Watson, 2005).

The adoption of safe behaviour is more difficult to obtain since it is not simply a direct consequence of the health awareness. Especially for diseases related to poverty such as STH infections, the suggested solution might not be available or too expensive to adopt. Although deprived communities understand the importance of the safe disposal of faecal matter and of wearing shoes, poverty often hinders the construction of latrines and the purchase of shoes.

For STH infections, the aims are: (i) to reduce the faecal contamination of the soil, by recommending the use of latrines, (ii) to develop self-protection from re-infection, through personal/family hygiene measures such as washing hands and proper food preparation, and (iii) to avoid spraying night soil on vegetables in communities where this habit is common.

Frequently, in STH endemic areas, latrines are not available or not in sufficient number for the population needs (Cairncross, 2003), therefore the knowledge and motivation for behavioural change must be sustained with the availability of proper facilities for excreta disposal.

Providing information on the disease and the possible adoption of preventive measures frequently results in increase of knowledge but not necessarily in behavioural change (O'Cathain *et al.*, 2002). Informed choice in the context of health care, competence (of patients to understand the problem) and the possibility of making a decision (availability of an alternative choice) are also necessary (Reeves, 2002).

Promotion of latrine maintenance and use, washing of hands and proper food handling have benefits that go beyond the control of STH infections. From this perspective, it is reasonable to include health education in all STH control programmes when the health education message can be provided in a simple and inexpensive way. Health education messages can be delivered by teachers in schools thereby fostering changes in health behaviour in children, which in turn involve their parents and guardians. On the other hand, intensive and sophisticated campaigns can represent the main cost for an STH control programme and impair significantly the cost-effectiveness of the control effort (Mascie-Taylor *et al.*, 1999). The effectiveness of health education campaigns in increasing health awareness and changing defecation habits varies according to different reports (Guanghan *et al.*, 2000; Lansdown *et al.*, 2002).

2.3. Sanitation

Sanitation is composed of two elements, which are complementary: "hardware" such as toilets, latrines and sewage treatments, and "software" such as personal hygiene and legislation. Sanitation in the context of economic development is the only definitive intervention that eliminates STH infections. STH infections are never a public health problem where hygiene and sanitation standards are appropriate. Improvement of the sanitation standard always has a repercussion on infection and re-infection levels. Studies from the West Indies showed that prevalence of STH infections were significantly lower in areas with improved sanitary conditions as was re-infection. Crowding and the type of excreta-disposal facility were the only significant predictors of re-infection (Henry, 1988). Similar results were obtained in urban slums of Bangladesh (Henry *et al.*, 1993) and in the plantation sector of Sri Lanka (Sorensen *et al.*, 1994).

Sanitation, however, does not become effective until it covers a high percentage of the population (Esrey *et al.*, 1991). In Zimbabwe, despite the marked increase in the number of latrines, no relationship was found between hookworm re-infection intensities and the availability of latrines on individual farms (Bradley *et al.*, 1993). The effect of improved sanitation on helminth transmission is slow to develop and may take decades to achieve a measurable impact. Often, the high costs involved, prevent the provision of sanitation to the communities most in need (Asaolu and Ofoezie, 2003).

In addition, latrine coverage is not a solution, unless the latrine is used and maintained. Studies in Senegal (Sow *et al.*, 2004) demonstrated that, despite high latrine coverage, the majority of the children in a village, interviewed with a questionnaire, claimed to defecate elsewhere. Experience in Mozambique demonstrated that in areas with low latrine coverage, even in houses where a well-maintained latrine existed, the soil in the house-yard was contaminated (Muller *et al.*, 1989).

On the other hand, an alternative model, which offers a market-based approach considers the rural poor as customers and not beneficiaries, and may accelerate access to sanitation, enhance sustainability and deliver services more efficiently. An international NGO recently launched a project to stimulate the acquisition and use of sanitation in rural areas of Viet Nam. A range of options that were appealing and affordable to potential customers was developed, the community's willingness to pay was assessed and the perception of benefits of sanitation was promoted through media channels and tailored messages. Within a year coverage of sanitation access has increased by 100% compared with the pre-project access rate. This success indicated that the population's willingness to pay for sanitation is often underestimated, provided that quality product and services are offered with effective information (Mukherjee, 2005).

3. GROUPS AT RISK

3.1. Preschool Children

Children between 1 and 5 years of age are particularly vulnerable to disease caused by STH infections (Carrera *et al.*, 1984; Oberhelman *et al.*, 1998; Crompton and Nesheim, 2002). Though they are less likely to harbour heavy infections, such young children, whose worm burdens are housed in smaller bodies, are at higher risk of anaemia and wasting malnutrition (Awasthi and Pande, 2001).

The negative effect of STH infection on iron status and nutrition in non-immune children with light infections may be linked to an inflammatory-triggered cytokine response in "naive" children, and a consequent suppression of protein metabolism, appetite and erythropoiesis, and not only to iron and micronutrient loss (Stoltzfus *et al.*, 2004).

3.2. School-Age Children

Children of primary school age (6–14 years) should be a major target for regular treatment, because they are the group that usually has the heaviest worm burdens for *A. lumbricoides* and *T. trichiura*, and are steadily acquiring hookworm infections. In addition, they are in a period of intense physical and intellectual growth and benefit most from deworming in terms of growth and school performance (Bundy *et al.*, 1992; Crompton and Nesheim, 2002). Schoolchildren are the most accessible group to reach in countries where school enrolment rates are good (Partnership For Child Development, 1999) and even non-enrolled siblings could be effectively outreached by promoting advocacy through the schools (Montresor *et al.*, 2001).

3.3. Women of Childbearing Age

Women between 15 and 49 years of age are susceptible to iron deficiency anaemia because of iron loss during menstruation and because of increased nutritional needs during pregnancy (Torlesse and Hodges, 2001; Nurdia *et al.*, 2001). The problem is aggravated if they have diets low in bioavailable iron and if they suffer from hookworm infection. Hookworms feed on blood and iron deficiency is often the consequence of this activity. Hookworm infection invariably reaches peak intensity in this age group (Bundy *et al.*, 1995a). Antenatal anthelminthic treatment in hookworm endemic areas is recommended for the control of maternal anaemia (WHO, 1996). The benefits of deworming after the first trimester far outweigh the health risks and result in improvements in maternal iron status, birth weight and perinatal survival (Christian *et al.*, 2004).

4. FREQUENCY OF TREATMENT

Frequency of regular treatment should vary according to the intensity of transmission and rates of re-infection. These factors must be considered in relation to the resources available and the cost involved in drug purchase and distribution. When there are budgetary constraints it is more efficient to treat a greater proportion of the population less frequently than to treat a smaller proportion of the population more often (Evans and Guyatt, 1995). For *A. lumbricoides* infections, the most cost-effective option is to treat infrequently (every 2 years) when effectiveness is assessed in terms of reduced mean worm burden and reduction in disease prevalence, both in low- and high-transmission areas. In contrast, when prevalence reduction is used as the measure of effectiveness (prevalence recovers more rapidly than intensity), the most cost-effective option is to treat every 4 months in high-transmission areas and every year in low-transmission areas (Guyatt *et al.*, 1993).

- Treatment frequency of twice or three times a year is effective in reducing morbidity in areas of intense transmission (prevalence

>70% and more than 10% of infections of moderate or heavy intensity) such as in Zanzibar (Albonico *et al.*, 1999b), Nepal (Khanal and Walgate, 2002) and Myanmar (Thein-Hlaing, 1989).
- In areas with a lower intensity of transmission (prevalence between 40% and 60% and less than 10% of infections of moderate and heavy intensity), for example in Oman (Idris *et al.*, 2001), India (Chhotray and Ranjit, 1990) and Brazil (Machado *et al.*, 1996), once-yearly intervention was found to be sufficient to reduce morbidity.

Based on these experiences and on logistic limitations, endemic communities are classified into three categories according to the levels of cumulative STH prevalence and intensity estimated in the population (Table 2). An indication of the epidemiological situation of the community can be estimated from the data collected in school-age children (Guyatt *et al.*, 1999) and guidelines on how to conduct school surveys have been proposed by WHO (Montresor *et al.*, 2002).

Each STH infection can be classified as being of light, moderate or heavy intensity according to the thresholds established by a WHO Expert Committee (WHO, 2002a) based on the number of STH eggs per gram of faeces (Table 2). Helminths in different areas of the world have different levels of egg output (Hall and Holland, 2000), so the thresholds proposed by WHO are not rigid and should be adjusted for the local situation. The appropriate population-based treatment strategies recommended for each category is illustrated in Table 3 (WHO, 2002a).

5. TARGETS

The World Health Assembly in 2001 endorsed a strategy for the prevention and control of schistosomiasis and soil-transmitted helminthiasis in high-transmission areas (WHO, 2001). In the short term, morbidity will be reduced by:

- access to drugs (praziquantel and broad-spectrum anthelminthics) and good case management in all health services;

Table 2 Community classification for soil-transmitted helminth infections

Community category	Results of school survey	
	Prevalence of any soil-transmitted helminthiasis	Percent of moderate-to-heavy infections
I High prevalence or high intensity	≥70%	≥10%
II Moderate prevalence and low intensity	≥50% but <70%	<10%
III Low prevalence and low intensity	<50%	<10%

Note: Each community can be classified according to prevalence and (if available) intensity of infection. Intensity of infections are classified as below:

Ascaris lumbricoides: Light 1–4999 epg; Moderate 5000–49 999 epg; Heavy >50 000 epg

Trichuris trichiura: Light 1–999 epg; Moderate 1000–9999 epg; Heavy >10 000 epg

Hookworms: Light 1–1999 epg; Moderate 2000–3999 epg; Heavy >4000 epg

Source: WHO (2002a).

Table 3 Recommended treatment strategies for soil-transmitted helminth infections

Community category	Intervention in schools (enrolled and non-enrolled children)	Community-based intervention
I	Targeted treatment of school-age children, 2–3 times/year	Systematic treatment of preschool children and women of childbearing age in mother and child health programmes
II	Targeted treatment of school-age children, once per year	Systematic treatment of preschool children and women of childbearing age in mother and child health programmes
III	Selective treatment	Selective treatment

Note: These treatment strategies always need to be accompanied by efforts to improve water supply, sanitation, information, education and communication.

Source: WHO (2002a).

- regular treatment of at least 75% of school-age children by 2010;
- targeting other high-risk groups (young children, women of childbearing age and occupational groups) through existing public health programmes and channels.

For long-term sustainability, environmental health will be required including:

- improving access to safe water and sanitation;
- improved hygiene behaviour through health education.

Field experience has shown that 75% coverage is an attainable target even in areas where school enrolment rates are low (Montresor *et al.*, 2001) and that a significant reduction in morbidity can be achieved in situations of intense transmission (Albonico *et al.*, 1999a). Cambodia is the first country to have reached this target ahead of schedule and other countries such as Brazil, Equador, Nepal, Tanzania, Uganda and Viet Nam are on track to succeed.

6. DELIVERING THE INTERVENTION

Implementation of any helminth control programme at country level requires strong links with existing interventions that already target women and children. Deworming can readily be added to ongoing public health programmes.

6.1. Helminth Control through Schools

Helminth control in schools is reckoned to be a most cost-effective public health intervention in low-income countries (World Bank, 1993). Schools represent an ideal setting to reach children. Trained teachers can distribute and administer the drug and give health education messages to the pupils (Montresor *et al.*, 2002). Schools can be used to reach non-enrolled school-age children with a simple child-to-child approach (Montresor *et al.*, 2001). Deworming of school-age children requires minimal financial input (Partnership For Child Development, 1999) and gives notable nutritional and cognitive benefits. In addition, enrolment figures and school attendance normally increase after such interventions (Miguel and Kremer, 2001).

School feeding programmes help to break the interrelated cycles of hunger, illiteracy, poverty and disease, and serve as a platform for deworming and other interventions (World Food Programme, 2004).

Thirty countries worldwide now report active deworming combined with school feeding programmes. Almost 2 million children were reached in 2002, nearly 3 million in 2003, and over 7 million in 2004 (WHO, 2003a). STH control programmes rely strongly on volunteer personnel who are not remunerated but need basic training for distributing the drug. The safety profile of drugs distributed without the supervision of medical personnel must be explained. In case of any adverse events the child should be referred to the nearest health centre. Close collaboration between the Ministry of Education and Ministry of Health at all levels is mandatory for the success of deworming and other control measures such as health education through the school system.

6.2. Helminth Control through Community-Based Intervention

Recent experience demonstrates that many preschool children can be reached by adding deworming to vitamin A distribution or immunization campaigns. Worms and vitamin A deficiency thrive in impoverished communities where the two problems often co-exist. The advantage of adding deworming to vitamin A supplementation is the coverage opportunity: over 167 million children are reached yearly by vitamin A supplementation programmes worldwide and more than 50 countries report more than 70% coverage (UNICEF, 2005). Deworming has been found to increase the vitamin A supplementation coverage and worm-free children have a better vitamin A status than infected children (Curtale *et al.*, 1995). Delivering deworming by using the vitamin A distribution infrastructure reduces costs and takes advantage of the access to remote communities that is already in place.

Nepal is successfully pioneering this approach. Deworming is now offered to children under 5 by using existing resources and the success of vitamin A distribution campaigns is being reinforced (Khanal and Walgate, 2002). Deworming is also being delivered during the National Child Health Days, a way of reaching children with a package of health measures including immunization and vitamin A supplementation. A similar intervention is proving to be successful in Angola, Republic of Korea, Tanzania and Uganda (WHO, 2004b, 2005a). In Cambodia, the Ministry of Health uses monthly outreach services to deliver a minimum package of activities through health centres including immunization, antenatal care, health education, family planning, tuberculosis, leprosy care, vitamin A supplements and deworming (WHO, 2004b, 2005a).

Mother and Child Health (MCH) services offer opportunities to provide regular deworming for childbearing women and children over the age of 1 year (Savioli *et al.*, 2003). The inclusion of routine deworming now reaches 75% of pregnant women in Sri Lanka (N.R. de Silva, personal communication). STH control measures can also be added to other public health initiatives including Integrated Management of Childhood Illness (IMCI), School Health Programmes, Roll Back Malaria, Micronutrient Initiatives and Reproductive Health—Making Pregnancy Safer.

7. IMPACT ON MORBIDITY

7.1. Preschool Children

Children under 5 experience the detrimental consequences of acute and chronic STH infections. Recent data from East Africa indicate that hookworms are an important cause of anaemia in preschool children (Brooker *et al.*, 1999) and that regular distribution of anthelminthics has a positive effect on motor and language development in this age group (Stoltzfus *et al.*, 2001). After 12 months of quarterly mebendazole treatment in Zanzibari children, mild wasting malnutrition was reduced by 62% in children <30 months, moderate anaemia (Hb $<9\,\mathrm{g/dl}$) was reduced by 59% in children <24 months, and appetite was improved by 48% in all 460 children (Stoltzfus *et al.*, 2004). In India, Awasthi *et al.* (2000) found that when children aged between 1.5 and 3.5 years received vitamin A and albendazole every 6 months they gained 3.5 kg in 2 years, compared with 2.5 kg gained by children given vitamin A only. In Nepal, twice-yearly distribution of vitamin A and albendazole to 2 million children under 5 reduced anaemia by 77% in 1 year (Mathema *et al.*, 2004).

7.2. School-Age Children

Deworming school-age children has a considerable benefit on their nutritional status (Stoltzfus *et al.*, 1996; Curtale *et al.*, 1995), physical fitness, appetite, growth (Stephenson *et al.*, 1993) and intellectual development (Partnership For Child Development, 2002). Although re-infection is inevitable where sanitation is lacking (Albonico *et al.*, 1995), treatment three times a year with a single dose of 500 mg mebendazole prevented 1208 cases of moderate–severe anaemia and 276 cases of severe anaemia in the schoolchildren study population ($n = 30\,000$) in Zanzibar (Stoltzfus *et al.*, 1998).

Studies in low-income countries of Africa (Kvalsvig *et al.*, 1991) and the Caribbean (Nokes *et al.*, 1992) have shown that children with intense STH infections perform poorly in learning ability tests, cognitive function and educational achievement. Differences in test performance equivalent to a 6-month delay in development can be attributed to moderate/heavy *T. trichiura* infections (Nokes and Bundy, 1994). Deworming schoolchildren assists their ability to learn. Tests have shown that a child's short-term memory, long-term memory, executive function, language, problem solving and attention respond positively to deworming (Watkins and Pollit, 1997). Interestingly, girls display greater improvements than boys. For the most heavily infected children, their educational performance shows an improvement after treatment. For the less heavily infected, deworming may allow them to catch up with uninfected peers over the longer term (Nokes *et al.*, 1992).

Deworming is usually followed by a significant reduction in school absenteeism. For example, Jamaican children enduring intense infections with *T. trichiura* miss twice as many school days as their infection-free peers (Nokes and Bundy, 1993). A randomized trial in Kenya indicated that school-based targeted treatment with deworming drugs reduced school absenteeism in treated schools by 25%. (Miguel and Kremer, 2001.)

7.3. Pregnant Women

Despite understandable concerns about the risk to the unborn child of offering deworming drugs to pregnant women, significant benefits follow for mother and infant when hookworm infections are reduced.

A study in Sierra Leone demonstrated that a single dose of albendazole given to pregnant women after the first trimester helped to prevent the decrease in haemoglobin concentrations that continued to occur in the untreated group (Torlesse and Hodges, 2001). An analysis of over 7000 pregnancies in Sri Lanka reported that mebendazole therapy during pregnancy is associated with a significant improvement in birth weights, fewer stillbirths and perinatal deaths, and that there was no increase of birth defect rates compared to the untreated women (de Silva *et al.*, 1999).

A controlled study in rural Nepal, where the prevalences of hookworm and *Ascaris* infection were roughly 70% and 50%, respectively, demonstrated that deworming greatly improves the health of pregnant women and the birth weight and survival of their infants. After albendazole treatment in the second trimester there was a significant decrease in the prevalence of severe anaemia in pregnant women, the birth weight of babies from mothers given two doses of albendazole rose on average by 59 g, and the infant mortality rate at 6 months had fallen by 41% (Christian *et al.*, 2004). This work confirms that deworming should be considered as part of routine antenatal care in areas where hookworm infections are endemic. The *Essential Care Practice Guide for Pregnancy and Childbirth* (WHO, 2003b), which provides support to the Integrated Management of Pregnancy and Childbirth (IMPAC), recommends anthelminthic treatment for all pregnant women in the second and third trimester attending clinics if they did not receive such treatment in the last 6 months, and also treatment for all postpartum women.

Women in the first trimester of pregnancy are precautionally excluded from any treatment (including anthelminthic). In developing countries, this principle presents some problem of application because some women in the first trimester of pregnancy may not be aware of their pregnancies. Also the performance of pregnancy testing in all women of childbearing age before administering anthelminthic treatment is not usually affordable. Adolescent girls who may be in early pregnancy while still at school and when the school is in a deworming scheme are a concern. Results from studies that have evaluated inadvertent deworming during the first trimester, however, have indicated that the risk of extra birth defects is negligible and that benefits in treating hookworm-induced iron deficiency anaemia both for the mother and the newborn far outweigh the risk of taking anthelminthic tablets in early pregnancy (de Silva *et al.*, 1999; Torlesse and Hodges, 2001; Diav-Citrin *et al.*, 2003; Christian *et al.*, 2004).

7.4. Adults

Adult populations are also vulnerable to high-intensity hookworm infections. Studies conducted in rural China, Brazil and elsewhere reveal that the elderly often suffer from high intensity of hookworm infection and clinical hookworm disease with impairment of work productivity (Gandhi *et al.*, 2001; Bethony *et al.*, 2002). The relationship between STH infections and labour productivity has been studied in various settings, such as tea-picking communities in Asia (Gardner *et al.*, 1977; Gilgen *et al.*, 2001), road workers in Africa (Brooks *et al.*, 1979; Wolgemuth *et al.*, 1982) and rural communities in Latin America (Viteri and Torun, 1974). Iron deficiency anaemia, the hallmark of hookworm infection, is the major cause of weakness and fatigue in adults in endemic countries (Crompton and Nesheim, 2002). Not only do the infections significantly reduce the ability to sustain even moderate levels of labour, they also reduce the pace and time spent at work. STH control would increase country productivity and aid economic development (Guyatt, 2000).

8. COST OF THE INTERVENTION

The cost–benefits of the control measures for morbidity due to STH infection is influenced by the ecological and environmental situation, by the availability of local anthelminthic drug production, and by the presence of infrastructures and facilities that can be used to reach the high-risk groups.

8.1. Regular Chemotherapy

Calculations indicate that a bundle of diseases, including schistosomiasis, soil-transmitted helminthiasis, onchocerciasis, lymphatic filariasis, trachoma and vitamin A deficiency, can be controlled at costs for drug and nutrients ranging from about US$ 1 to 2.50 per patient (Molyneux and Nantulya, 2004). Fenwick *et al.* (2005) estimated that a package of interventions could be provided at a cost of US$ 0.40 per person per year. The infrastructure for the delivery of such a package of health care to millions of poor people already exists in many endemic areas through primary health care provision, public and private schools, faith-based organizations and social institutions. In deprived communities, where sanitation is practically non-existent and the prevalence and intensity of infection are high, a suitable infrastructure (such as the school system or a national immunization day) should be used to distribute at least regular treatment to the groups at risk. The cost of adding this intervention is normally marginal.

Over 1.3 million preschool children were dewormed during the 2002 vitamin A distribution campaign in Nepal. The yearly cost of the vitamin A intervention is estimated at US$ 1.7 million (Fiedler, 2000). An additional expenditure of US$ 80 000 (about 4% of the cost of the vitamin A distribution) covered the cost of adding biannual deworming to the vitamin A campaign (Mathema *et al.*, 2004).

Since 1998, the World Food Programme (WFP) has incorporated deworming in the School Feeding Programme (SFP) in Nepal and, in light of the nutritional consequences, decided to include deworming (including schistosomiasis control) in all the countries where SFPs are conducted (Bordignon and Shakya, 2003). Thirty countries now conduct combined deworming and school feeding programmes. The average cost per child per year is 70 US cents: 4 cents for mebendazole, 25 cents for praziquantel, 30 cents for training, monitoring and educational materials; and the remaining 11 cents for delivering both drugs (WHO, 2003a).

In Ghana with over 80 000 school-age children treated and Tanzania with over 100 000 school-age children treated, the estimated costs for school-based delivery of albendazole was US\$ 0.04 and US\$ 0.03, respectively (Partnership for Child Development, 1999).

In Cambodian schools, deworming is promoted by means of a school kit, which contains deworming tablets, health education posters and pamphlets for teachers, games and attractive pictures giving simple messages on how to prevent infection. The coverage of primary school-age children was 84% in 2003, and the biannual deworming campaign from 2004 onward is estimated to cost US\$ 0.04 per child treated (Sinoun *et al.*, 2005).

The advantage of regular deworming lies in its simplicity (one tablet per child), cheap delivery (by teachers through schools), and safety record (the benefits of treatment far outweigh the risk of minor side effects). Many organizations, including NGOs, could include an STH control package in their routine activities and, even with limited budgets, relieve the burden of STH in the population covered.

8.2. Health Education

The contribution of health education towards the control of STH infections and morbidity varies according to different reports. A randomized trial in 25 schools in Viet Nam did not find that intensive health education had any effect on the intensity of re-infection 6 months after treatment (Partnership For Child Development, unpublished results). Other authors observed increased levels of knowledge and improved health behaviour in the population (Lansdown *et al.*, 2002), and measured a decrease in re-infection rates (Guanghan *et al.*, 2000). Cost analysis of work in Bangladesh indicates that regular mass treatment with albendazole is the most cost-effective control strategy and strategies involving health education were the least cost-effective (Mascie-Taylor *et al.*, 1999).

The importance of health education, however, should not be measured merely by cost-effectiveness alone. Health education, in community health, has the same role as the medical information and counselling given by the physician to the patient in clinical medicine.

The effects of establishing a good relationship between the health system and the community is not always directly measurable with regard to the success of the control measures. The effect of health education in community health includes improvement in loyalty and trust between the educators and the community. When such a relationship is established, the community is no longer a simple recipient of the medical intervention but becomes one of the partners in the health process.

8.3. Sanitation

The investment needed to provide access to adequate sanitation is beyond the resources of low-income countries. In addition, although improved water and sanitation contribute to reduce incidence of infection (Esrey *et al.*, 1991), morbidity due to infection may persist (Asaolu *et al.*, 2002). The coverage of properly built, used and maintained sanitation has to be higher than 90% to have any effects on worm transmission and critically depends on the general socioeconomic status of the community (Asaolu and Ofoezie, 2003).

A recent experience from STH control in Viet Nam, based on regular deworming, latrine construction and health education, has shown that the cost per child for each latrine has been estimated at US$ 7.9 (an amount equal to receiving over 200 doses of regular deworming). The building of new latrines was considered important as a good example for the schoolchildren and a way for providing essential sanitation at least in school. This intervention, however, increased the latrine coverage in each community of less than 1%. To have a significative impact (e.g. 20%) in the latrine coverage, an investment of US$ 50 000 is considered necessary in each community, and a total of over US$ 9 million for an entire province (Montresor, personal communication).

The magnitude of the problem of providing sewerage is a big challenge in large urban centres in developing countries. In Lagos, Nigeria, according to population projections, there may be an additional 1240 tons of human stool being deposited daily in the areas where the poor people live. The installation costs of modern sewerage similar to the type found in developed countries for the poor population of Lagos could amount to a billion US dollars or more. Progress has been made in developing a variety of latrines for rural communities, but these may not be appropriate for slums and squatter settlements with a shortage of land for dwellings and at sea level (Crompton and Savioli, 1993).

The resources needed to improve hygienic standards can be huge, but the collaboration of different initiatives dealing with hygiene and prevention of diseases related to poor hygiene will help create the synergy needed to reduce both disease and poverty. A reliable evaluation of the advantage of investments in sanitation must include the consequences for other health services and for economic development. An efficient sanitation infrastructure removes the underlying cause of most poverty-related communicable diseases and so supports the economic development of a country.

9. NEW TECHNOLOGY FOR SUSTAINING DEWORMING

Regular chemotherapy with single-dose anthelminthic drugs will be the mainstay for control of morbidity due to helminth infection in endemic countries for several years. No new drugs have been recently developed, tested and registered and it is essential to make the best use of existing products. This is particularly important in the light of increasing drug resistance of nematodes of livestock to veterinary versions of anthelminthic products also used in human (Geerts and Gryseels, 2001). Recent evidence suggests reduced efficacy of benzimidazoles against hookworm infections in humans after 15 rounds of treatment (Albonico *et al.*, 2003). Reduced efficacy after drug exposure and treatment failures are signs that drug resistance may emerge. Assessment and monitoring of efficacy of anthelminthic drugs in areas where they are commonly used should be performed in a standard way so as to warn of possible treatment failures and stimulate further investigations. In addition to the available measurement of reduction in faecal egg count following treatment, tests such as the Egg Hatch Assay have been developed to monitor benzimidazole efficacy against human hookworms (Albonico *et al.*,

2005). The development of molecular probes with PCR techniques offers a more sensitive technique for drug efficacy monitoring (Roos *et al.*, 1995). Research studies to identify sensitive and resistant genes in worm populations are still at an early stage in humans (Albonico *et al.*, 2004).

The creation of a global network for monitoring anthelminthic drug efficacy and resistance, coordinating research efforts, and translating operational research outcome into health policy is a much-needed response to this emerging threat. Such a network will depend on action by different partners and dedicated funding. A successful example is the concerted action on the use of praziquantel for the treatment of schistosomiasis in Africa, which is funded by the European Union and involves a forum of scientists and public health planners (Hagan *et al.*, 2004).

Combined treatment with two drugs with different modes of action or their alternate use are among the strategies used to safeguard efficacy and to delay the possible emergence of drug resistance. Combined treatment with mebendazole and levamisole has been proved safe and more effective than either drug alone (Albonico *et al.*, 2003). A pyrantel–oxantel combination is more effective than benzimidazole drugs in curing *T. trichiura* infections (Albonico *et al.*, 2002). Ivermectin and albendazole are effectively and safely given in combination in some countries as mass treatment to eliminate lymphatic filariasis and have ancillary benefits in controlling other helminthiases including strongyloidiasis (Belizario *et al.*, 2003). Co-administration of praziquantel and albendazole is recommended where schistosomiasis and intestinal helminthiasis are endemic (Olds *et al.*, 1999).

In addition to chemotherapy, a new hookworm vaccine against *N. americanus* infection is being developed and tested by the Human Hookworm Vaccine Initiative (Hotez *et al.*, 2003). It is proposed that chemotherapy would be given first to treat existing cases and then a vaccine would be administered to prevent or to delay further re-infection. It is unlikely that a hookworm vaccine will interrupt transmission due to the heterogenicity in hookworm transmission and the need for a vaccine to provide protection for at least two-thirds of an individual's lifetime (Anderson, 1982). The vaccine would decrease

the number of L3 larvae invading the gastrointestinal tract, prevent
their development into adult worms (larvicidal effect), and it would
also reduce the sexual development of female worms (antifecundity
effect). The major benefit will be directly reducing individuals' worm
burden. A first generation product known as *Na*-ASP-2 hookworm
vaccine against *N. americanus* has been developed and comprises a
larval hookworm recombinant protein engineered and purified from
yeast. Proof-of-concept for the efficacy of the *Na*-ASP-2 vaccine to
reduce hookworm burden and intestinal blood loss will be evaluated in
a Phase 2b clinical trial in Minas Gerais State, Brazil. An uncertainty is
how much such a vaccine costs to manufacture. Finding an innovative
financing mechanism and a cost-efficient delivery mechanism represent
the major challenges for the successful deployment of hookworm vaccines (Bundy *et al.*, 1995b; Brooker *et al.*, 2005).

10. SCALING UP DEWORMING FOR SCHOOL-AGE CHILDREN

Following the 2001 WHA resolution, WHO was requested to set up a
system to monitor each endemic country's progress towards the 2010
target. A global databank has been established at WHO (http://
www.who.int/wormcontrol) to track the number of people who are
treated each year for soil-transmitted helminthiasis and schistosomiasis, and epidemiological data describing the distribution of
infections are regularly collected and displayed using the geographical
information system technology. Country profiles, including information on coverage data, plans of action, anthelminthic drugs on the
Essential Drug List and their cost, are collected through questionnaires and extensive liaison with other partners, regional colleagues
and national programme managers. Global progress in coverage in
school-age children from 1999 to 2004 is reported from 73 out of 104
endemic countries. Although data is awaited from 26 countries in the
Pan American Health Organization and from India and China, there
is a steady increase of coverage over time. Thirty of the 73 countries
are known to be expanding control activities (Figure 2, which is Plate
8.2 in the separate colour plate section) (WHO, 2005b).

The Schistosomiasis Control Initiative (SCI) is assisting Uganda, Burkina Faso, Mali, Niger, Tanzania (including Zanzibar) and Zambia to scale up schistosomiasis and helminthiasis control to a national level. SCI has promoted integration of other deworming programmes at the country level, the synergistic deworming in collaboration with the Programme to Eliminate Lymphatic Filariasis (PELF) being an example. SCI, with funds from the Bill and Melinda Gates Foundation, has facilitated registration of drug products in each country, promoted local production by national pharmaceutical companies and strengthened procurement agencies at country level according to local needs (Fenwick, in press). In addition to these countries Cambodia, Nepal, Ecuador, Brazil, and Viet Nam, are also examples of good progress in helminth control.

WHO and other partners are building regional and country capacity to strengthen implementation of control programmes. WHO has provided evidence as to how deworming helps to meet some Millennium Development Goals and progress towards achieving them should be further documented (Lancet, 2004). In order to meet the target of reaching about 650 million children by 2010, deworming should become part of a multi-disease control approach, by maximizing links with chemotherapy-based control of lymphatic filariasis, onchocerciasis, trachoma and other diseases of poverty, thereby building a pro-poor strategy for sustainable development (Lancet, 2004; Molyneux and Nantulya, 2004; Molyneux *et al.*, 2005).

11. QUESTIONS NEEDING ANSWERS

Partners for Parasites Control recently gathered to discuss the best way forward in helminth control; the following research needs and priorities emerged (WHO, 2005b).

- Advocacy for sustaining the effort to control helminthiasis requires the latest and best information. The compelling evidence for detrimental effects of helminth infections and the benefits from deworming should be sustained with further knowledge and updated data. The disease burden should be regularly revised and expressed in terms of the most reliable DALYs available.

- There is emerging evidence that concurrent worm infections may have synergistic effects on the severity of malaria, on progression of HIV/AIDS, and on the development and effects of anaemia (Fincham *et al.*, 2003; Spiegel *et al.*, 2003). These interactions and potentially important consequences merit more extensive investigation.

- Impressive benefits of deworming on education, poverty reduction and contribution towards the Millennium Development Goals have been put forward, though they need further quantification and wider dissemination.

- Further research on the possible use of "packaging" deworming with other programmes is needed to sustain science-based synergy and integration with lymphatic filariasis and onchoceriasis elimination programmes, vitamin A distribution campaigns, Child Health Days, malaria, expanded programme of immunization.

- There is inconsistency between WHO recommendations and drug producers' prescribing information about the use of anthelminthic drugs during pregnancy. The WHO recommendations are based on toxicological evidence presented to experts in two Informal Consultations (WHO, 1996, 2002b). The full-scale toxicological review and the extensive process required by regulatory bodies should be undertaken by the pharmaceutical industry. A pressing issue to be addressed is the need to set up a reliable system for pharmacovigilance in community deworming campaigns.

- Sensitive molecular tools to monitor anthelminthic drug efficacy need to be developed. Waiting for drug resistance to occur before seeking funds for research on drug efficacy monitoring might be too late a response to this potential problem.

- The possibility of development of new anthelminthic drugs and the efficacy and safety of available drugs administered in combination should be evaluated.

- Availability of efficient vaccines would make a difference in helminth control. Trials for the development of vaccines against schistosomiasis and hookworms should be supported, and collaboration between research and control should be encouraged.

REFERENCES

Albonico, M., Bickle, Q., Haji, H.J., Ramsan, M., Khatib, J.K., Savioli, L. and Taylor, M. (2002). Evaluation of the efficacy of pyrantel-oxantel for the treatment of soil-transmitted nematode infections. *Transactions of the Royal Society of Tropical Medicine and Hygiene* **96**, 685–690.

Albonico, M., Bickle, Q., Ramsan, M., Montresor, A., Savioli, L. and Taylor, M. (2003). Efficacy of mebendazole and levamisole alone or in combination against intestinal nematode infections after repeated targeted mebendazole treatment in Zanzibar. *Bulletin of the World Health Organization* **81**, 343–352.

Albonico, M., Crompton, D.W.T. and Savioli, L. (1999a). Control strategies for human intestinal nematode infections. *Advances in Parasitology* **42**, 277–341.

Albonico, M., Smith, P.G., Ercole, E., Hall, A., Chwaya, H.M., Alawi, K.S. and Savioli, L. (1995). Rate of re-infection with intestinal nematodes after treatment of children with mebendazole or albendazole in a highly endemic area. *Transactions of the Royal Society of Tropical Medicine and Hygiene* **89**, 538–541.

Albonico, M., Stoltzfus, R.J., Savioli, L., Chwaya, H.M., d'Harcourt, E. and Tielsch, J.M. (1999b). A controlled evaluation of two school-based anthelminthic chemotherapy regimens on intensity of intestinal helminth infections. *International Journal of Epidemiology* **28**, 591–596.

Albonico, M., Wright, V. and Bickle, Q. (2004). Molecular analysis of the β-tubulin gene of human hookworms as a basis for possible benzimidazole resistance on Pemba Island. *Molecular and Biochemical Parasitology* **134**, 281–284.

Albonico, M., Wright, V., Ramsan, M., Haji, H.J., Taylor, M., Savioli, L. and Bickle, Q. (2005). Development of the Egg Hatch Assay for detection of anthelminthic resistance by human hookworms. *International Journal for Parasitology* **35**, 803–811.

Anderson, R.M. (1982). The population dynamics and control of hookworm and roundworm infection. In: *Population Dynamics of Infectious Diseases: Theory and Applications* (R.M. Anderson, ed.), pp. 67–109. London: Chapman & Hall.

Asaolu, S.O. and Ofoezie, I.E. (2003). The role of health education and sanitation in the control of helminth infections. *Acta Tropica* **86**, 283–294.

Asaolu, S.O., Ofoezie, I.E., Odumuyiwa, P.A., Sowemimo, O.A. and Ogunniyi, T.A. (2002). Effect of water supply and sanitation on the prevalence and intensity of *Ascaris lumbricoides* among pre-school-age children in Ajebandele and Ifewara, Osun State, Nigeria. *Transactions of the Royal Society of Tropical Medicine and Hygiene* **96**, 600–604.

Awasthi, S. and Pande, V.K. (2001). Six monthly de-worming in infants to study effects on growth. *Indian Journal of Pediatrics* **68**, 823–827.

Awasthi, S., Pande, V.K. and Fletcher, R.H. (2000). Effectiveness and cost-effectiveness of albendazole in improving nutritional status of preschool children in urban slums. *Indian Journal of Pediatrics* **37**, 19–29.

Belizario, V.Y., De Leon, W.U., Amarillo, M.E., De Los Reyes, A.E., Bugayong, M.G. and Macatangay, B.J.C. (2003). A comparison of the efficacy of single doses of albendazole, ivermectin, and diethylcarbamazine alone or in combinations against *Ascaris* and *Trichuris* spp. *Bulletin of the World Health Organization* **81**, 35–42.

Bennet, A. and Guyatt, H. (2000). Reducing intestinal nematodes infection: efficacy of albendazole and mebendazole. *Parasitology Today* **2**, 71–74.

Bethony, J., Chen, J.Z., Lin, S.X., Xiao, S.H., Zhan, B., Li, S.W., Xue, H.C., Xing, F.Y., Humphries, D., Wang, Y., Chen, G., Foster, V., Hawdon, J.M. and Hotez, P.J. (2002). Emerging patterns of hookworm infection: influence of aging on the intensity of *Necator* infection in Hainan Province, People's Republic of China. *Clinical Infectious Diseases* **35**, 1336–1344.

Bordignon, G.P. and Shakya, D.R. (2003). A deworming programme in Nepal supported by the World Food Programme. In: *Controlling Disease due to Helminth Infections* (D.W.T. Crompton, A. Montresor, M.C. Nesheim and L. Savioli, eds), pp. 87–92. Geneva: World Health Organization.

Bradley, M., Chandiwana, S.K. and Bundy, D.A.P. (1993). The epidemiology and control of hookworm infection in the Burma Valley area of Zimbabwe. *Transactions of the Royal Society of Tropical Medicine and Hygiene* **87**, 145–147.

Brooker, S., Beasley, N.M.R., Ndinaromtan, M., Madjiouroum, E.M., Baboguel, M., Djenguinabe, E., Hay, S.I. and Bundy, D.A. (2002a). Use of remote sensing and a geographical information system in a national helminth control programme in Chad. *Bulletin of the World Health Organization* **80**, 783–789.

Brooker, S., Bethony, J.M., Rodrigues, L.C., Alexander, N., Geiger, S. and Hotez, P. (2005). Epidemiologic, immunologic and practical considerations in developing, and evaluating a human hookworm vaccine. *Expert Review Vaccines* **4**, 1–16.

Brooker, S., Hay, S.I., Tchuem Tchuenté, L.A. and Ratard, R. (2002b). Using NOAA-AVHRR data to model helminth distributions for planning disease control in Cameroon, West Africa. *Photogrammetric Engineering and Remote Sensing* **68**, 175–179.

Brooker, S., Peshu, N., Warn, P.A., Mosobo, M., Guyatt, H.L., Marsh, K. and Snow, R.W. (1999). The epidemiology of hookworm infection and its contribution to anaemia among preschool children on the coast of Kenya. *Transactions of the Royal Society of Tropical Medicine and Hygiene* **93**, 240–246.

Brooks, R.M., Latham, M.C. and Crompton, D.W.T. (1979). The relationship of nutrition and health to worker productivity in Kenya. *East African Medical Journal* **56**, 413–421.

Bull, F.C., Holt, C.L., Kreuter, M.W., Clark, E.M. and Scharff, D. (2001). Understanding the effects of printed health education materials: which features lead to which outcomes? *Journal of Health Communication* **6**, 265–279.

Bundy, D.A., Chan, M.S. and Savioli, L. (1995a). Hookworm infection in pregnancy. *Transactions of the Royal Society of Tropical Medicine and Hygiene* **89**, 521–522.

Bundy, D.A.P., Chan, M.S. and Guyatt, H.L. (1995b). The practicality and sustainability of vaccination as an approach to parasite control. *Parasitology* **110**, S51–S58.

Bundy, D.A., Hall, A., Medley, G.F. and Savioli, L. (1992). Evaluating measures to control intestinal parasitic infections. *World Health Statistics Quarterly* **45**, 168–179.

Cairncross, S. (2003). Sanitation in the developing world: current status and future solutions. *International Journal of Environmental Health Research* **13** (supplement 1), S123–S131.

Carrera, E., Nesheim, M.C. and Crompton, D.W.T. (1984). Lactose maldigestion in *Ascaris* infected preschool children. *American Journal of Clinical Nutrition* **39**, 255–264.

Chhotray, G.P. and Ranjit, M.R. (1990). Effect of drug treatment on the prevalence of intestinal parasites amongst school children in a sub-urban community. *Indian Journal of Medical Research* **91**, 266–269.

Christian, P., Kathry, K.S. and West, K.P., Jr (2004). Antenatal anthelminthic treatment, birthweight, and infant survival in rural Nepal. *Lancet* **364**, 981–983.

Crompton, D.W.T. (1999). How much helminthiasis is there is in the world? *Journal of Parasitology* **85**, 397–403.

Crompton, D.W.T. (2000). *Ascaris* and ascariasis. *Advances in Parasitology* **48**, 285–375.

Crompton, D.W.T. and Nesheim, M.C. (2002). Nutritional impact of intestinal helminthasis during the human life cycle. *Annual Review of Nutrition* **22**, 35–59.

Crompton, D.W.T. and Savioli, L. (1993). Intestinal parasitic infections and urbanization. *Bulletin of the World Health Organization* **71**, 1–7.

Curtale, F., Pokhrel, R.P., Tilden, R.L. and Higashi, G. (1995). Intestinal helminths and xerophthalmia in Nepal. A case-control study. *Journal of Tropical Pediatrics* **41**, 334–337.

de Silva, N.R., Brooker, S., Hotez, P.J., Montresor, A., Engels, D. and Savioli, L. (2003). Soil-transmitted helminth infections: updating the global picture. *Trends in Parasitology* **19**, 547–551.

de Silva, N.R., Guyatt, H. and Bundy, D.A. (1997). Anthelminthics: a comparative review of their clinical pharmacology. *Drugs* **53**, 769–788.

de Silva, N.R., Sirisena, J.L.G.J., Gunasekera, D.P.S. and de Silva, H.J. (1999). Effect of mebendazole therapy during pregnancy on birth outcome. *Lancet* **353**, 1145–1149.

Diav-Citrin, O., Shechtman, S., Arnon, J., Lubart, I. and Ornoy, A. (2003). Pregnancy outcome after gestational exposure to mebendazole: a prospective controlled cohort study. *American Journal of Obstetrics and Gynecology* **188**, 282–285.

Esrey, S.A., Potash, J.B., Roberts, L. and Shiff, C. (1991). Effects of improved water supply and sanitation on ascariasis, diarrhoea, dracunculiasis, hookworm infection, schistosomiasis, and trachoma. *Bulletin of the World Health Organization* **69**, 609–621.

Evans, D.B. and Guyatt, H.L. (1995). The cost effectiveness of mass drug therapy for intestinal helminths. *Pharmacoeconomics* **8**, 14–22.

Fenwick, A. (in press). New initiatives against Africa's worms. *Transactions of the Royal Society of Tropical Medicine and Hygiene.*

Fenwick, A., Molyneux, D.H. and Nautulya, V. (2005). Achieving the millenium development goals. *Lancet* **365**, 1029–1030.

Fiedler, J.L. (2000). The Nepal National Vitamin A Program: prototype to emulate or donor enclave? *Health Policy and Planning* **15**, 145–156.

Fincham, J.E., Markus, M.B. and Adams, V.J. (2003). Could control of soil-transmitted helminthic infections influence the HIV/AIDS pandemic? *Acta Tropica* **86**, 315–333.

Gandhi, N.S., Chen, J.Z., Khoshnood, K., Xing, F.Y., Li, S.W., Liu, Y.R., Zhan, B., Xue, H.C., Tong, C.G., Wang, Y., Wang, W.S., He, D.X., Chen, C., Xiao, S.H., Hawdon, J.M. and Hotez, P.J. (2001). Epidemiology of *Necator americanus* hookworm infections in Xiulongkan Village, Hainan Province, China: high prevalence and intensity among middle-aged and elderly residents. *Journal of Parasitology* **87**, 739–743.

Gardner, G.W., Edgerton, V.R., Senewiratne, B., Barnard, R.J. and Ohira, Y. (1977). Physical work capacity and metabolic stress in subjects with iron deficiency anaemia. *American Journal of Clinical Nutrition* **30**, 910–917.

Geerts, S. and Gryseels, B. (2001). Anthelminthic resistance in human helminths: a review. *Tropical Medicine and International Health* **6**, 915–921.

Gilgen, D., Mascie-Taylor, C.G.N. and Rosetta, L. (2001). Intestinal helminth infections, anaemia and labour productivity of female tea pluckers in Bangladesh. *Tropical Medicine and International Health* **6**, 449–457.

Guanghan, H., Dandan, L., Shaoji, Z., Xiaojun, Z., Zenghua, K. and Guojun, C. (2000). The role of health education for schistosomiasis control in heavy endemic area of Poyang Lake region, People's Republic of

China. *Southeast Asian Journal of Tropical Medicine and Public Health* **31**, 467–472.

Guyatt, H.L. (2000). Do intestinal nematodes affect productivity in adulthood? *Parasitology Today* **16**, 153–158.

Guyatt, H., Brooker, S. and Donnelly, C.A. (1999). Can prevalence of infection in school-aged children be used as an index for assessing community prevalence? *Parasitology* **118**, 257–268.

Guyatt, H.L., Bundy, D.A.P. and Evans, D. (1993). A population dynamic approach to the cost-effectiveness analysis of mass anthelminthic treatment: effects of treatment frequency on *Ascaris* infection. *Transactions of the Royal Society of Tropical Medicine and Hygiene* **87**, 570–575.

Hagan, P., Appleton, C.C., Coles, G.C., Kusel, J.R. and Tchuem-Tchuenté. (2004). Schistosomiasis control: keep taking the tablets. *Trends in Parasitology* **20**, 92–97.

Hall, A. and Holland, C. (2000). Geographical variation in *Ascaris lumbricoides* fecundity and its implications for helminth control. *Parasitology Today* **16**, 540–544.

Henry, F.J. (1988). Re-infection with *Ascaris lumbricoides* after chemotherapy: a comparative study in three villages with varying sanitation. *Transactions of the Royal Society of Tropical Medicine and Hygiene* **82**, 460–464.

Henry, F.J., Huttly, S.R., Ahmed, M.U. and Alam, A. (1993). Effect of chemotherapy in slums and villages in Bangladesh. *Southeast Asian Journal of Tropical Medicine and Public Health* **24**, 307–312.

Horton, J. (2000). Albendazole: a review of anthelmintic efficacy and safety in humans. *Parasitology* **121**, S113–S132.

Hotez, P.J., Zhan, B., Bethony, J.M., Loukas, A., Williamson, A., Goud, G.N., Hawdon, J.M., Dobardzic, A., Dobardzic, R., Ghosh, K., Bottazzi, M.E., Mendez, S., Zook, B., Wang, Y., Liu, S., Essiet-Gibson, I., Chung-Debose, S., Xiao, S.H., Knox, D., Meagher, M., Inan, M., Correa-Oliveira, R., Vilk, P., Shepherd, H.R., Brandt, W. and Russell, P.K. (2003). Progress in the development of a recombinant vaccine for human hookworm disease: the human hookworm vaccine initiative. *International Journal for Parasitology* **33**, 1245–1258.

Idris, M.A., Shaban, M.A. and Fatahallah, M. (2001). Effective control of hookworm infection in school children from Dhofar, Sultanate of Oman: a four-year experience with albendazole mass chemotherapy. *Acta Tropica* **80**, 139–143.

Khanal, P. and Walgate, R. (2002). Nepal deworming programme ready to go worldwide. *Bulletin of the World Health Organization* **80**, 423–424.

Kinzie, M.B. (2005). Instructional design strategies for health behaviour change. *Patient Education and Counseling* **56**, 3–15.

Kvalsvig, J.D., Cooppan, R.M. and Connolly, K.J. (1991). The effects of parasite infections on cognitive processes in children. *Annals of Tropical Medicine and Parasitology* **85**, 551–568.

Lancet (2004). Thinking beyond deworming. *Lancet* **364**, 1993–1994.

Lansdown, R., Ledward, A., Hall, A., Issae, W., Yona, E., Matulu, J., Mweta, M., Kihamia, C., Nyandindi, U. and Bundy, D. (2002). Schistosomiasis, helminth infection and health education in Tanzania: achieving behaviour change in primary schools. *Health Education Research* **17**, 425–433.

Machado, M.T., Machado, T.M., Yoshikae, R.M., Schmidt, A.L., Faria, R.de C., Paschoalotti, M.A., Barata, R.de C. and Chieffi, P.P. (1996). Ascariasis in the subdistrict of Cavacos, municipality of alterosa (MG), Brazil: effect of mass treatment with albendazole on the intensity of infection. *Revista do Instituto de Medicina Tropical de São Paulo* **8**, 265–271.

Management Science for Health (2004). *Electronic Resource Center. International Drug Price Indicator* http://erc.msh.org/dmpguide

Mascie-Taylor, C.G., Alam, M., Montanari, R.M., Karim, R., Ahmed, T., Karim, E. and Akhtar, S. (1999). A study of the cost effectiveness of selective health interventions for the control of intestinal parasites in rural Bangladesh. *Journal of Parasitology* **85**, 6–11.

Mathema, P., Pandey, S. and Blomquist, P.O. (2004). Deworming impact evaluation of preschool children deworming programme in Nepal. Abstract from *International Nutritional Anaemia Consultative Group*, November 2004, Lima, Peru.

Miguel, E. and Kremer, M. (2001). *Worms: Education and Health Externalities in Kenya*. Working Paper no. w8481. Cambridge, MA: National Bureau of Economic Research http://www.nber.org/papers/W8481

Molyneux, D.H., Hotez, P.J. and Fenwick, A. (2005). Rapid impact interventions: How a policy of integrated control for Africa's neglected tropical diseases could benefit the poor. *PLOS Medicine* **2**, e 336.

Molyneux, D.H. and Nantulya, V.M. (2004). Linking disease control programmes in rural Africa: a pro-poor strategy to reach Abuja targets and millennium development goals. *British Medical Journal* **328**, 1129–1132.

Montresor, A., Awashti, S. and Crompton, D.W.T. (2003). Use of benzimidazoles in children younger than 24 months for the treatment of soil-transmitted helminthiasis. *Acta Tropica* **86**, 223–232.

Montresor, A., Crompton, D.W.T., Gyorkos, T.W. and Savioli, L. (2002). *Helminth Control in School Age Children*. Geneva: WHO.

Montresor, A., Ramsan, M., Chwaya, H.M., Ameir, H., Foum, A., Albonico, M., Gyorkos, T.W. and Savioli, L. (2001). Extending anthelminthic coverage to non-enrolled school-age children using a simple and low-cost method. *Tropical Medicine and International Health* **6**, 535–537.

Mukherjee, J.F.N. (2005). *Harnessing Market Power for Rural Sanitation.* WSP Field Notes, February 2005, Water and Sanitation Program, Jakarta, Indonesia.

Muller, M., Sanchez, R.M. and Suswillo, R.R. (1989). Evaluation of a sanitation programme using eggs of *Ascaris lumbricoides* in household yard soils as indicators. *Journal of Tropical Medicine and Hygiene* **92**, 10–16.

Nokes, C. and Bundy, D.A. (1993). Compliance and absenteeism in school children: implications for helminth control. *Transactions of the Royal Society of Tropical Medicine and Hygiene* **87**, 148–152.

Nokes, C. and Bundy, D.A. (1994). Does helminth infection affect mental processing and educational achievement? *Parasitology Today* **10**, 14–18.

Nokes, C., Grantham-McGregor, S.M., Sawyer, A.W., Cooper, E.S., Robinson, B.A. and Bundy, D.A. (1992). Moderate to heavy infections of *Trichuris trichiura* affect cognitive function in Jamaican schoolchildren. *Parasitology* **104**, 539–547.

Nurdia, D.S., Sumarni, S., Suyoko Hakim, M. and Winkvist, A. (2001). Impact of intestinal helminth infection on anemia and iron status during pregnancy: a community based study in Indonesia. *Southeast Asian Journal of Tropical Medicine and Public Health* **32**, 14–22.

Nwaorgu, O.C., Okeibunor, J., Madu, E., Amazigo, U., Onyegegbu, N. and Evans, D. (1998). A school-based schistosomiasis and intestinal helminthiasis control programme in Nigeria: acceptability to community members. *Tropical Medicine and International Health* **3**, 842–849.

Oberhelman, R.A., Guerrero, E.S., Fernandez, M.L., Silio, M., Mercado, D., Comiskey, N., Ihenacho, G. and Mera, R. (1998). Correlations between intestinal parasitosis, physical growth, and psychomotor development among infants and children from rural Nicaragua. *American Journal of Tropical Medicine and Hygiene* **58**, 470–475.

O'Cathain, A., Walters, S.J., Nicholl, J.P., Thomas, K.J. and Kirkham, M. (2002). Use of evidence based leaflets to promote informed choice in maternity care: randomised controlled trial in everyday practice. *British Medical Journal* **324**, 643.

Olds, G.R., King, C., Hewlett, J., Olveda, R., Wu, G., Ouma, J., Peters, P., McGarvey, S., Odhiambo, O., Koech, D., Liu, C.Y., Aligui, G., Gachihi, G., Kombe, Y., Parraga, I., Ramirez, B., Whalen, C., Horton, R.J. and Reeve, P. (1999). Double-blind placebo-controlled study of concurrent administration of albendazole and praziquantel in schoolchildren with schistosomiasis and geohelminths. *Journal of Infectious Diseases* **179**, 996–1003.

Partnership for Child Development (1999). The cost of large-scale school health programmes which deliver anthelminthics to children in Ghana and Tanzania. *Acta Tropica* **73**, 183–204.

Partnership for Child Development (2001). Community perception of school-based delivery of anthelmintics in Ghana and Tanzania. *Tropical Medicine and International Health* **6**, 1075–1083.

Partnership for Child Development (2002). Heavy schistosomiasis associated with poor short-term memory and slower reaction times in Tanzanian schoolchildren. *Tropical Medicine and International Health* **7**, 104–117.

Reeves, D. (2002). Provision of information is only one component of informed choice. *British Medical Journal* **325**, 43.

Roos, H.M., Kwa, M.S.G. and Grant, W.N. (1995). New genetic and practical implications of selection for anthelmintic resistance in parasitic nematodes. *Parasitology Today* **11**, 148–150.

Savioli, L., Crompton, D.W.T. and Neira, M. (2003). Use of anthelminthic drugs during pregnancy. *American Journal of Obstetrics and Gynecology* **188**, 5–6.

Savioli, L., Stansfield, S., Bundy, D.A., Mitchell, A., Bathia, R., Engels, D., Montresor, A., Neira, M. and Shein, A.M. (2002). Schistosomiasis and soil-transmitted helminth infections: forging control efforts. *Transactions of the Royal Society of Tropical Medicine and Hygiene* **96**, 577–579.

Sinoun, M., Tsuyuoka, R., Socheat, D., Montresor, A. and Palmer, K. (2005). Financial costs of deworming children in all primary schools in Cambodia. *Transactions of the Royal Society of Tropical Medicine and Hygiene* **99**, 664–668.

Sorensen, E., Ismail, M., Amarasinghe, D.K.C., Hettiarachchi, I. and Dassenaieke, de C.T.S. (1994). The effect of the availability of latrines on soil-transmitted nematode infections in the plantation sector in Sri Lanka. *American Journal of Tropical Medicine and Hygiene* **51**, 36–39.

Sow, S., de Vlas, S.J., Polman, K. and Gryseels, B. (2004). [Hygiene practices and contamination risks of surface waters by schistosome eggs: the case of an infested village in Northern Senegal] (in French). *Bulletin de la Société de Pathologie Exotique* **97**, 12–14.

Spiegel, A., Tall, A., Raphenon, G., Trape, J.F. and Druilhe, P. (2003). Increased frequency of malaria attacks in subjects co-infected by intestinal worms and *Plasmodium falciparum* malaria. *Transactions of the Royal Society of Tropical Medicine and Hygiene* **97**, 198–199.

Stephenson, L.S., Latham, M.C., Adams, E.J., Kinoti, S.N. and Pertet, A. (1993). Physical fitness, growth and appetite of Kenyan school boys with hookworm, *Trichuris trichiura* and *Ascaris lumbricoides* infections are improved four months after a single dose of albendazole. *Journal of Nutrition* **123**, 1036–1046.

Stoltzfus, R.J., Albonico, M., Chwaya, H.M., Savioli, L., Tielsch, J., Schulze, K. and Yip, R. (1996). Hemoquant determination of hookworm-related blood loss and its role in iron deficiency in African children. *American Journal of Tropical Medicine and Hygiene* **55**, 399–404.

Stoltzfus, R.J., Albonico, M., Chwaya, H.M., Tielsch, J.M., Schulze, K.J. and Savioli, L. (1998). Effects of the Zanzibar school-based deworming program on iron status of children. *American Journal of Clinical Nutrition* **68**, 179–186.

Stoltzfus, R.J., Chwaya, H.M., Montresor, A., Tielsch, J.M., Jape, J.K., Albonico, M. and Savioli, L. (2004). Low dose daily iron supplementation improves iron status and appetite but not anemia, whereas quarterly anthelminthic treatment improves growth, appetite and anemia in Zanzibari preschool children. *Journal of Nutrition* **134**, 348–356.

Stoltzfus, R.J., Kvalsvig, K.J., Chwaya, H.M., Montresor, A., Albonico, M., Tielsch, J.M., Savioli, L. and Pollitt, E. (2001). Effects of iron supplementation and anthelminthic treatment on motor and language development of Zanzibari preschool children. *British Medical Journal* **323**, 1384–1396.

Thein-Hlaing (1989). Burma. In: *Ascariasis and its Prevention and Control* (D.W.T. Crompton, M.C. Nesheim and Z.S. Pawlowski, eds), pp. 133–168. London: Taylor & Francis.

Torlesse, H. and Hodges, M. (2001). Albendazole therapy and reduced decline in haemoglobin concentration during pregnancy (Sierra Leone). *Transactions of the Royal Society of Tropical Medicine and Hygiene* **95**, 195–201.

UNICEF (2005). *The State of the World's Children 2005*. New York: United Nation Children Fund.

Urbani, C. and Albonico, M. (2003). Anthelminthic drug safety and drug administration in the control of soil-transmitted helminthiasis in community campaigns. *Acta Tropica* **86**, 215–221.

Viteri, F.E. and Torun, B. (1974). Anaemia and physical work capacity. *Clinical Haematology* **3**, 609–626.

Walsh, D.C., Rudd, R.E., Moeykens, B.A. and Moloney, T.W. (1993). Social marketing for public health. *Health Affairs (Bethesda MD)* **12**, 104–119.

Watkins, W.E. and Pollit, E. (1997). "Stupidity of worms": do intestinal worms impair mental performance? *Psychological Bulletin* **121**, 171–191.

Whitelaw, S. and Watson, J. (2005). Whither health promotion events? A judicial approach to evidence. *Health Education Research* **20**, 214–225.

Wolgemuth, J.C., Latham, M.C., Hall, A., Chesher, A. and Crompton, D.W.T. (1982). Worker productivity and the nutritional status of Kenyan road construction labourers. *American Journal of Clinical Nutrition* **36**, 68–78.

World Bank (1993). *World Development Report 1993: Investing in Health*. London: Oxford University Press.

World Food Programme (2004). *WFP Annual Report 2004*. Rome: WFP, pp. 36–38.

World Health Organization (1996). *Report of the WHO Informal Consultation on Hookworm Infection and Anaemia in Girls and Women*. Geneva: WHO, WHO/CTD/SIP/96.1.

World Health Organization (1999). *Report of the WHO Informal Consultation on Monitoring Drug Efficacy in the Control of Schistosomiasis and Intestinal Nematodes*. Geneva: WHO, WHO/CDS/CPC/SIP 99.1.

World Health Organization (2001). *Report of the 54th World Health Assembly. Control of Schistosomiasis and Soil-Transmitted Helminth Infections*. Geneva: WHO.

World Health Organization (2002a). *Prevention and Control of Schistosomiasis and Soil Transmitted Helminthiasis. Report of a WHO Expert Committee* Geneva: WHO, Technical Report Series 912.

World Health Organization. (2002b). *Report of the WHO Informal Consultation on the Use of Praziquantel during Pregnancy and Lactation and Albendazole/Mebendazole in Children under 24 Months*. Geneva: WHO, WHO/CPE/PVC 2002.4.

World Health Organization (2003a). *Action Against Worms*. Newsletter issue number 2: http://www.who.int/wormcontrol/newsletter/en/

World Health Organization (2003b). *Integrated Management of Pregnancy and Childbirth. Essential Care Practice Guide for Pregnancy and Childbirth*. Geneva: WHO Essential Care Series, WHO/RHR/2003.

World Health Organization (2004a). *WHO Model Formulary. Based on the 13th Model List of Essential Medicines 2003*. Geneva: WHO, pp. 82–85.

World Health Organization (2004b). *How to Add Deworming to Vitamin A Distribution*. Geneva: WHO, WHO/CDS/CPE/PVC/2004.1.

World Health Organization (2005a). *Action Against Worms*. Newsletter issue number 6: http://www.who.int/wormcontrol/newsletter/en (in production).

World Health Organization (2005b). *Deworming for Health and Development. Report of the Third Global Meeting of the Partners for Parasites Control*. Geneva: WHO, WHO/CDS/CPE/PVC/2005.14.

Control of Onchocerciasis

Boakye A. Boatin[1] and Frank O. Richards, Jr[2]

[1]*TDR, World Health Organization, CH-1211 Geneva 27, Switzerland*
[2]*The Carter Center, One Copenhill, Atlanta, GA 30307, USA*

ADVANCES IN PARASITOLOGY VOL 61
ISSN: 0065-308X
DOI: 10.1016/S0065-308X(05)61009-3

ABSTRACT

Onchocerciasis is a filarial infection which causes blindness and debilitating skin lesions. The disease occurs in 37 countries, of which 30 are found in Africa (the most affected in terms of the distribution and the severity of the clinical manifestations of the disease), six in the Americas and one in the Arabian Peninsula. The latest WHO Expert Committee on Onchocerciasis estimated that in 1995 around 17.7 million persons were infected, about 270 000 of whom were blind and another 500 000 severely visually impaired. The disease is responsible for 1 million DALYs. Eye disease from onchocerciasis accounts for 40% of DALYs annually although severe skin disease is also recognized as of public health significance. Great progress has been made in the last thirty years in the control of onchocerciasis, both in Africa and the Americas, and this progress has been due largely to international public–private partnerships, sustained funding regional programmes, and new tools and technology. Landmarks in the global control of river blindness include the significant success of the Onchocerciasis Control Programme of West Africa (1975–2002), and the donation of ivermectin (Mectizan®) by Merck & Co. Inc., in 1988, a medicine that is distributed to millions free of charge each year. Future major technical challenges of onchocerciasis control include ivermectin mass administration in areas co-endemic for the parasite *Loa loa* in the light of possible severe adverse reactions, ivermectin treatment in hypoendemic areas hitherto excluded from African control programmes, sustainability of ivermectin distribution, post-control surveillance for recrudescence detection, surveillance for emergence of resistance, and decisions of when to stop mass ivermectin treatments. There is the need to develop the appropriate information systems and diagnostic tools to help in accomplishing many of these tasks. A search for a second-line treatment or as an additional drug to ivermectin as well as a search for a macrofilaricide are issues that need to be addressed in the future.

1. INTRODUCTION

Onchocerciasis, also known as river blindness, is caused by a nematode filarial worm that causes blindness and debilitating skin lesions. The disease occurs in 37 countries, of which 30 are in Africa, six in the Americas and one in the Arabian Peninsula. Africa is by far the most affected continent both in terms of the extent of the distribution and the severity of the clinical manifestations of the disease. Onchocerciasis remains a major parasitic endemic disease especially in Central and East Africa. The latest World Health Organization (WHO) Expert Committee on Onchocerciasis estimated that in 1995 around 17.7 million persons were infected, about 270 000 of whom were blind and another 500 000 severely visually impaired (WHO, 1995a). Over 99% of the estimated 17.7 million persons infected with this filarial parasite live in Africa, while about 140 000 people in the Americas are infected with the worm. The disease is responsible for 1 million DALYs annually. Worldwide, onchocerciasis is one of the most important infectious causes of blindness, being second only to trachoma in number of persons affected (Thylefors *et al.*, 1995; Lewalen and Courtright, 2001). Eye disease from onchocerciasis therefore represents the main public health challenge accounting for 40% of the attributable DALYs although severe skin disease is also recognized as of major public health significance (Hagan, 1998). Great progress has been made in the last three decades to control onchocerciasis, both in Africa and the Americas, and this progress has been due largely to international public–private partnerships, regional programmes, sustained financing and the development of new tools and technology. Landmarks in the global control of river blindness include the significant success of the Onchocerciasis Control Programme (OCP) of West Africa (1975–2002), which is held as one of the great triumphs of tropical public health, and the donation of ivermectin (Mectizan®) by Merck & Co. Inc., in 1988, a medicine that is distributed to millions free of charge each year.

2. THE PARASITE LIFE CYCLE AND HUMAN DISEASE

2.1. *Onchocerca volvulus*

2.1.1. Life Cycle and Transmission

The parasite, *Onchocerca volvulus*, is transmitted by small blackflies of the genus *Simulium*, which breed in fast-flowing, highly oxygenated rivers and streams (Blacklock, 1926). An infected blackfly deposits one or more *O. volvulus* larvae into the human host when it takes a bloodmeal. These larvae develop into mature adult worms in about a year. They commonly aggregate into fibrous nodules that lie under the skin usually over bony prominences. The adult female has a mean life span of 12–15 years with a reproductive life span of about nine to 11 years (Habbema *et al.*, 1992). When fertilized by a male worm, she is viviparous, releasing millions of embryos called microfilariae (mfs), which themselves live for about two years. The mfs that are released by the adult worm migrate from the nodules to swarm in the dermal layers throughout the body where they can be taken up by blackflies during a blood meal. The mfs develop into infective larvae in the blackfly from which they can be deposited in another human being with a subsequent bite, thus completing the life cycle of the parasite and the transmission for the infection. *O. volvulus* develops only in man and has no animal reservoir. Two different types of *O. volvulus* are found in West Africa; the savanna and the forest types, each associated with the different species of the *Simulium damnosum* s.l. complex (Crosskey, 1990).

2.2. The Vector

S. damnosum s.l. which has a wide distribution in Africa and Yemen is the most important vector of the disease. The *S. damnosum* complex of species distributed in forest and savanna habitats have variables capacities to transmit *O. volvulus*. In East Africa, transmission of onchocerciasis also occurs by *S. neavei*. Several vectors transmit *O. volvulus* in Latin America; the most important vectors are *S. ochraceum* in Mexico and Guatemala, *S. metallicum* in Venezuela, *S. exiguum* in Ecuador, and *S. oyapockense* in Brazil (Zea Flores, 1990; Shelley, 1988). As a general rule, blackfly species are best adapted to transmit corresponding *O. volvulus* parasites from their original region (Duke *et al.*, 1991), and blackfly vectors in the Americas are less efficient in transmitting the parasite than those in Africa.

2.3. The Disease

2.3.1. Clinical Manifestations

Clinical manifestations of onchocerciasis occur one to three years after infection, when the adult worms begin producing mfs. Dead mfs provoke host inflammatory reactions in the tissue that presents as intense skin irritation and lesions of acute papular oncho dermatitis (APOD) and chronic papular oncho dermatitis (CPOD). Severe pruritus ("troublesome itching") is one of the most important symptoms of onchocerciasis (Brieger *et al.*, 1998; WHO, 1995b). Mfs can migrate from the skin to enter the eyes and cause ocular morbidity (Hall and Pearlman, 1999; Pearlman and Hall, 2000). Visual loss from acute and chronic ocular disease of both the anterior (sclerosing keratitis, irido-cyclitis) and posterior segments (optic atrophy, choroido-retinitis) occur. In the most severe cases, blindness in one or both eyes occurs. Recent evidence suggests *Wolbachia* endobacteria (symbionts of arthropods and filarial nematodes) contain lipopolysaccharides that are released with the death of mfs and contribute to the inflammatory pathology associated with the disease (Taylor and Hoerauf, 1999; Saint André *et al.*, 2002; Taylor *et al.*, 2005).

3. GEOGRAPHICAL DISTRIBUTION AND EPIDEMIOLOGICAL PATTERNS

3.1. Distribution in Africa

Onchocerciasis is widely distributed in Africa between latitudes 15°N and 14°S, extending from Senegal in the west to Ethiopia in the east and from Mali in the north to Malawi in the south. Outside Africa, onchocerciasis occurs in a highly focal manner in Latin American countries (Brazil, Colombia, Ecuador Guatemala, Mexico, and Venezuela) and in Yemen in the Arabian Peninsula (Figure 1).

In Africa, there are two broad clinical-epidemiological patterns of the disease; blinding (savanna) and the non-blinding (forest). In general, the primary manifestations of onchocerciasis in the forest belts are of severe skin disease. In West Africa, blindness rates are significantly higher in savanna communities with mf prevalence of greater than 60% (hyperendemic) compared to communities with similar prevalence in the rain forest (Anderson *et al.*, 1976; Dadzie *et al.*, 1989, 1990). In the most hyperendemic villages in the savanna over 10% of the population may be blind due to onchocerciasis. Without intervention more than 50% of the total village population may become ultimately blind. In Central Africa the pattern is less clear, with severe blinding as well as less-blinding onchocerciasis being found in both savanna and forest belts. Onchocercal skin disease is most prevalent in East Africa, where blindness is rare (Brieger *et al.*, 1998; WHO, 1995b). Skin disease and severe pruritus ("troublesome itching") has recently been recognized as affecting more than 50% of the population in some communities in the rain forest belt where the prevalence of blindness due to onchocerciasis is relatively low (Kale, 1998). "Troublesome itching" now accounts for 60% of DALYs attributable to onchocerciasis (Figure 2, which is Plate 9.2 in the separate colour plate section).

3.2. Distribution in the Americas

In the Americas, onchocerciasis occurs in 13 discrete foci in six countries: Brazil, Colombia, Ecuador, Guatemala, Mexico, and Venezuela

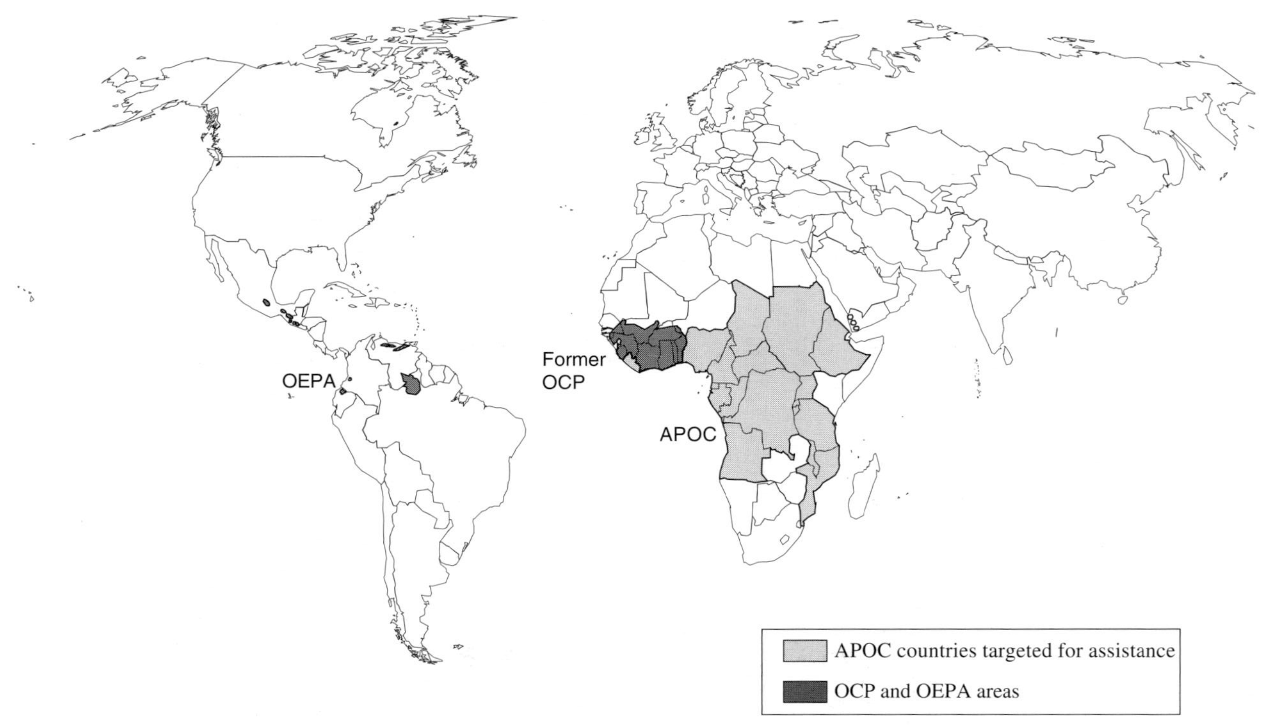

Figure 1 Geographic coverage of current regional Onchocerciasis Programmes.

(Figure 3, which is Plate 9.3 in the separate colour plate section). The disease was introduced into the region by the slave trade, and molecular studies indicate that it was the savanna blinding strain that was established in the Americas. In fact, the linkage between ocular disease and *O. volvulus* infection was not recognized initially in Africa, but in Guatemala by Rodolfo Robles near the turn of the last century. Ocular pathology attributable to onchocerciasis still occurs in many of the American foci, especially southern Venezuela and Brazil (Botto, 1997), but blindness is now rare to nonexistent. Skin disease and pruritus are the major clinical manifestations in the region. In the Yemen, the disease manifests as a pruritic and discolouring skin condition (Sowda), an apparent hyperreactive immune response to the infection.

4. DIAGNOSIS AND TREATMENT

4.1. Diagnosis

Diagnosis of onchocercal infection is required to determine individuals who need treatment, or, with mass treatment programmes, where treatment should be delivered. Diagnostics are also important to ascertain the impact an intervention is having on the infection and whether or not there is reappearance of the infection or renewed transmission in a given area. Diagnostics are important for validating model predictions, and in the future for helping to determine when and where mass-treatment activities can be stopped.

4.1.1. Parasitological Diagnosis

The skin snip biopsy, which affords both a parasitological diagnosis and allows the determination of intensity of infection, is the gold standard for the diagnosis of onchocerciasis. This method is very specific but insensitive when mf counts are low or absent, and so is inadequate for detecting early, low-intensity or pre-patent infections. Additionally, given that ivermectin treatment has a prolonged clearing effect on skin mf, this renders the skin snip method of diagnosis less sensitive in areas where mass ivermectin treatment is being delivered (Boatin *et al.*, 1998). As ivermectin is currently distributed in virtually all accessible onchocerciasis endemic areas (as well as in some lymphatic filariasis endemic areas that either overlap or are close to onchocerciasis zones), there is an urgent need for diagnostic tests which are sensitive enough to detect light infections or "amicrofiladermic" infections. Such tests should be biased towards specificity for *O. volvulus* (rather than sensitivity) to avoid long-lasting decisions made on false-positive results. The ideal test would be practical for field use, noninvasive, inexpensive, and acceptable to the community for large epidemiological assessments. Various tests have been developed in an effort to replace the skin biopsy (immunodiagnostics, DNA probes, and the DEC skin patch test), none of which have had the required characteristics to replace the skin biopsy. Antibody detection tests are not able to distinguish between past and current infections and so have not been useful in following up individuals after chemotherapy (Nutman *et al.*, 1994). For the purpose of ascertaining complete elimination of onchocerciasis in a community it would be profoundly useful to have a test which can detect *Onchocerca* antigens rather than antibodies.

4.1.2. Immunodiagnosis

The main challenge in the development of antibody detection tests for onchocerciasis is to produce an antigen, which would be sufficiently specific and sensitive. Earlier attempts with recombinant antigens showed that individually they were specific but adequately highly sensitive, or had variable sensitivity in different geographic areas. In an attempt to improve sensitivity, a combination of antigens ("the tricocktail" of OV-7, OV-11, and OV-16) was developed, which had an epidemiological sensitivity of 70–80% compared to the PCR (standard of 100%) depending on the locality. The specificity of this tricocktail was high (96–100%), but the test is not in common operational use.

Another test based on one of the tricocktail antigens, OV-16, was placed in a rapid-format card test that could detect IgG4 antibodies in 10 minutes (Weil *et al.*, 2000). The advantage of this test was that it could be performed in the communities and provide immediate results. The test was never placed into production and is no longer available in a rapid format. However, OV-16 testing in ELISA is still being used in sero-surveys in areas where transmission is thought to be interrupted in the Onchocerciasis Elimination Programme for the Americas (OEPA).

4.1.3. DNA Probes

Molecular techniques to detect the repetitive DNA sequence 0–150 (found in only *O. volvulus*) applied in entomological monitoring (see Section 6.1) have also been used to detect parasite DNA in skin snips, with epidemiological specificities of 100% (Zimmerman *et al.*, 1994). A major disadvantage of the PCR assay for routine use is its relative high cost and the need to perform the relatively invasive and often unpopular skin biopsy. At present, DNA probes for monitoring human disease is not generally used for the detection of *O. volvulus* infection.

4.1.4. The DEC Patch Test

The skin patch test is performed by the exposure of a small area of skin to a patch containing topical 10% DEC in Nivea cream for 48 hours. A positive test is the finding of a local "Mazzotti" reaction (Mazzotti, 1948) (most commonly a papular rash) under the patch, resulting from localized killing of dermal mfs. Noninvasive compared to the skin biopsy, the patch test was evaluated in OCP areas to assess its value in detecting infection in children born after the intervention started. The test has shown about 80% sensitivity when compared to the skin biopsy, with a specificity of 97%. Standardization of the test, and sensitivity issues, remain to be resolved before the test can be assimilated into routine epidemiological monitoring activities (Stingl *et al.*, 1984; Newland *et al.*, 1987).

5. TREATMENT

5.1. Suramin and Diethylcarbamazine

Until the 1980s only two drugs, suramin and diethylcarbamazine (DEC) were available for the treatment of onchocerciasis (WHO, 1987).

Suramin is macrofilaricidal (Ashburn *et al.*, 1949), and has been used successfully in limited mass treatment (Dawood, 1978; Rougemont *et al.*, 1980, 1984), but its toxicity (damage to the kidneys) and the difficulties associated with its mode of administration (repeated injections for several weeks) have limited its usefulness for both individual and large-scale treatment (Awadzi *et al.*, 1995). The piperazine derivative diethylcarbamazine (DEC) has only microfilaricidal action, has to be given over several days, and frequently produces severe adverse reactions such as fever, headache, rash, and oedema (the "Mazzotti" reaction), especially in those heavily infected (Awadzi and Gilles, 1980). DEC can also rapidly advance onchocercal eye disease leading to irreversible ocular damage. Accordingly, neither drug is recommended for routine onchocerciasis treatment or community control activities (WHO, 1995a, 2001). Given the lack of an appropriate drug, which was suitable for mass treatment or field use in the 1980s, most of those infected could not be treated, and ran the risk of developing eye lesions and subsequently blindness and/or skin manifestations from the infection.

5.2. Ivermectin

Ivermectin (Mectizan[®], Merck & Co.) is a semisynthetic macrocyclic lactone derived from *Streptomyces avermitilis*, which was registered for the treatment of human onchocerciasis in October 1987 in France. Ivermectin was the first microfilaricide suitable for large-scale onchocerciasis treatment (Awadzi *et al.*, 1985; De Sole *et al.*, 1989; Remme *et al.*, 1989; Prod'hon *et al.*, 1991; Whitworth *et al.*, 1991; Collins *et al.*, 1992). Donated free by Merck & Co. Inc. for as long as needed, the oral medication is safe and effective when given at the standard dose of 150 µg kg body weight^{-1}. Relative to DEC, its adverse effects are mild and non-ocular (Brown and Neu, 1990). One important characteristic is that despite its short half-life a single dose provides long-lasting suppression of microfilaridermia (Greene *et al.*, 1985), which makes it particularly suitable for community-based distribution in developing countries.

Since the early 1990s, ivermectin has not only become the drug of choice for the treatment and control of onchocerciasis, but the donation of the medicine by Merck & Co. Inc. has also opened up the avenue for mass presumptive treatment for all those living in hyper- and meso-endemic areas. A practical and easier method where the treatment is given on the basis of height, a good surrogate for the weight of an individual (Alexander *et al.*, 1993), has replaced the need to weigh individuals before treatment. This easy method has opened the way for the distribution of ivermectin to be undertaken by communities themselves through an approach known as Community Directed Treatment with Ivermectin (CDTI). CDTI embodies the philosophy of primary health care in that communities are encouraged to take responsibility for organizing their own distribution of ivermectin which is provided to the community free of charge. Distribution is undertaken according to a community's own chosen methods—door to door or at a central point. Ivermectin is always available in the communities to be given at a later time to those who might have been absent, sick, or unavailable during the chosen period. Cost of delivery is therefore reduced considerably.

5.2.1. Impact of Ivermectin on Adult O. volvulus Parasites

Ivermectin is largely a microfilaricide although there is evidence that there is an irreversible decline in female adult worm microfilaria production of approximately 30% per treatment (Plaisier *et al.*, 1995). This finding suggests that repeated treatment may ultimately sterilize the adult worms, although in a situation where transmission is not interrupted new infections continue to take the place of the older worms and so elimination of the parasite population would not be possible (Cupp *et al.*, 2004).

Gardon *et al.* (2002) conducted a three-year study in a hyperendemic focus in Cameroon comparing annual treatments ($150\,\mu g\,kg^{-1}\,year^{-1}$ and $400\,\mu g^{-1}\,year^{-1}$) with four times per year treatment using the same doses. They found significantly more female worms died from the three-monthly treatment regimens; the findings were not so striking as to suggest that four times per year treatments be generally recommended as an efficacious macrofilaricidal therapy. In addition, there are real concerns as to whether programmes can find resources to provide treatments four times per year, achieve sufficient coverage, or whether populations would accept such frequent treatment (Duke, 2005).

5.3. Doxycycline and *Wolbachia*

Wolbachia endobacteria (symbionts of arthropods and filarial nematodes) are now being considered as targets for the treatment of onchocerciasis. *Wolbachia* seem to be essential for fertility of *O. volvulus*, and perhaps for its survival. Treatment of *O. volvulus* infected Ghanaian individuals with doxycycline at $100\,\mathrm{mg\,day^{-1}}$ for six weeks resulted in an almost complete depletion of *Wolbachia* by 11 months and the inhibition of embryogenesis in female *O. volvulus* resulting in an apparently permanent elimination of skin microfilaria (Hoerauf *et al.*, 2000, 2001). Future clinical treatment of individuals with onchocerciasis might include prolonged doxycycline therapy, but the duration of the treatment is too long for any large-scale treatment. Studies are being undertaken to explore the use of shorter courses of doxycycline or other antibiotics in eliminating *Wolbachia* from *O. volvulus*.

5.4. Moxidectin

Moxidectin is a milbemycin compound, similar in structure to the avermectins (ivermectin). Moxidectin does not appear to be immediately macrofilaricidal, but nonetheless has been shown to induce sustained abrogation of embryogenesis in filarial animal models (Trees *et al.*, 2000). It has also been suggested that moxidectin given as a single dose, as in the case of ivermectin treatment, may have a similar but a longer duration of action than ivermectin, and so be effective (unlike ivermectin) in interrupting transmission when given yearly. There are attempts to develop this compound for use in humans. Given that the structure of moxidectin is similar to that of the avermectins if resistance were to develop, the possibility of cross-resistance between ivermectin and moxidectin may not be ruled out. de C. Bronsvoort *et al.* (2005) have investigated and studied the efficacy of high and prolonged doses of ivermectin and a related avermectin, doramectin, in cattle infected with *O. ochengi* and concluded that repeated high does may sterilize *O. volvulus* female worms for prolonged periods but is unlikely to kill them.

6. VECTOR CONTROL APPROACHES TO ONCHOCERCIASIS

Early attempts to control onchocerciasis utilized environmental management as a strategy for vector control of *Simulium*. The effort came soon after Blacklock had demonstrated that human onchocerciasis was transmitted by *Simulium* (Blacklock, 1926). In the Chiapas focus in Mexico, this involved clearing vegetation and applying plant extracts, Paris green, and creosote to the vector breeding sites. This attempt was unsuccessful. In Africa, S. *neavei* and onchocerciasis were successfully eradicated from a very small focus, the Riana focus, in Kenya by simply clearing riverine forest. Wide availability of DDT ushered in new campaigns against blackflies that succeeded in eradicating S. *neavei* from the Kodera valley in Kenya.

The interest in controlling onchocerciasis in West Africa was evident well before the OCP was formally launched in 1974. Ghana started vector control on a small-scale beginning in the Upper East region of the country in the Black Volta valley and later in the Lower Volta valley in the south, the latter to protect the workers at the Akosombo hydroelectric dam construction site (Davies, 1994).

Other early control efforts took place on the Comoé river in Burkina Faso and the Farako area of southeast Mali. During the 1960s, the Institut français de Recherche scientifique pour le Développement en Coopération (IRD), previously Office de Recherche scientifique et technique Outre-Mer (ORSTOM), and the Organisation de Coordination et de Coopération pour la Lutte contre les Grandes Endémies (OCCGE) carried out a series of vector control studies in Ivory Coast, Burkina Faso, and Mali.

6.1. The Onchocerciasis Control Programme in West Africa

The most comprehensive approach to the control of onchocerciasis and its elimination as a disease of public health importance in West

Africa began with the Preparatory Assistance Mission to the Governments of Dahomey (Benin), Ghana, Côte d'Ivoire, Mali, Niger, Togo, and Upper Volta (now Burkina Faso) in the early 1970s, which called for a vector control programme centered on aerial larviciding over a large area (the OCP area) to be carried out for a period of 20 years.

The Onchocerciasis Control Programme in West Africa (OCP) was launched in 1974 and during the early stages of the programme until ivermectin became available OCP was a purely vector control programme. The objective of vector control was to interrupt transmission of the parasite, *O. volvulus*, for a sufficiently long period of time to allow the human reservoir of the parasite to die out. The strategy was based on weekly aerial larviciding (where feasible ground larviciding), of *Simulium*-breeding sites. The OCP initially used Temephos (AgrEvo, France), which is a cheap and efficient organophosphorous insecticide with insignificant impact on non-target fauna. Following the use of Temephos, the OCP judiciously used seven environmentally friendly larvicides (organophosphates, carbamates pyrethroids, and biological *Bacillus thuringiensis* serotype H14–B.t.H14) in rotation to restrict emergence of insecticide resistance in vectors, to minimize adverse impact on non-target organisms and to have a cost-effective approach to the activity (Hougard *et al.*, 1993). The development of these insecticides to meet the requirements of the Programme was achieved through operational research which in many instances was done in partnership with industry. Larviciding was to be applied for 20 years. The duration of larviciding was informed by the then estimated life span of the adult worm. Later the period for larviciding was reduced to 14 years and then to 12 years when larviciding was combined with ivermectin treatment, in the light of new information from model predictions.

Parasitological surveys based on the skin biopsies of 1–2 mg skin were carried out in selected indicator villages at the start of the Onchocerciasis Control Programme in West Africa (OCP) in 1974. These surveys showed that the majority of these villages had hyperendemic *O. volvulus* infection, with more than 60% of residents having mfs in skin. The mean intensity of infection expressed as the Community Microfilaria Load (CMFL) was 30 mfs per biopsy in many villages.

Blindness rates as a result of onchocerciasis exceeded 3% in many villages and reached 10% in some of the worst affected villages. The entomological parameter, the annual transmission potential (ATP), which estimates number of *O. volvulus* larvae an individual is exposed to in a year, was over 800 in more than half of the monitoring points when the programme began.

In the original OCP area which comprises seven West African countries (Benin, Burkina Faso, Cote d'Ivoire, Ghana, Mali, Niger, and Togo) vector control has achieved the interruption of transmission in virtually all of the savanna areas (Molyneux, 1995; Boatin *et al.*, 1997) (Figure 4) except in a few pockets in Benin, Ghana, and Togo. Incidence of infection in children as measured by the skin snip biopsy has thus been reduced by 100% in almost all the areas that were under vector control. Infection in children has not occurred except in a small restricted area in the Mouhoun (Black Volta) basin in Burkina Faso where there was a recrudescence of infection (OCP, 1994). Annual transmission potentials are virtually zero in all these areas and have continued to be so after cessation of 12–14 years of weekly larviciding. In the other countries (Guinea Bissau, parts of Guinea Conakry, western of Mali, Senegal, and Sierra Leone) where no vector control was undertaken, known as the OCP "extension areas", the prevalence of infection has continued to decline through the repeated mass community treatment with ivermectin. Although

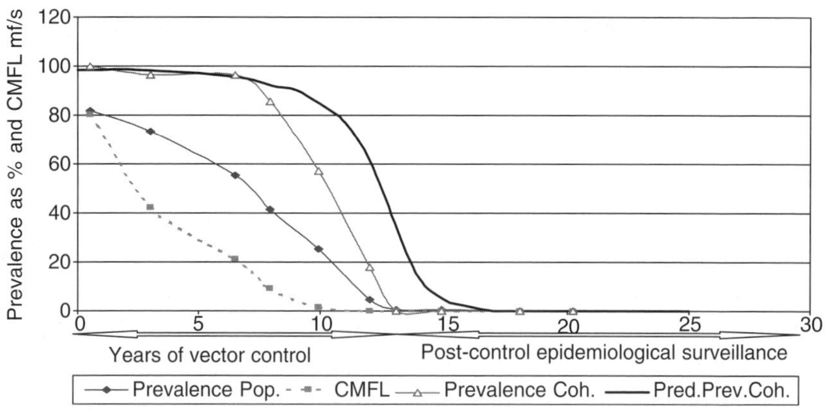

Figure 4 Epidemiological trends in the village of Niarba (White Volta, Burkina Faso).

transmission is only slowly on the decline in some areas, it seems to have been interrupted in Senegal where ivermectin treatment has been given on a twice-yearly basis for the last 12–15 years. Studies to obtain entomologic data to confirm or refute the impact of ivermectin treatment on transmission in this area are being undertaken. In the areas where there has been combined vector control and ivermectin treatment, prevalence of infection is low and incidence of infection is nil except in some areas in the north of Togo, in the Asubende focus in Ghana and small areas in Guinea Conakry. In Sierra Leone where control activities (large-scale ivermectin treatment) were completely halted for more than five years due to civil unrest the epidemiological situation has been static with no decline in the prevalence rates.

6.2. Vector Elimination/Eradication

Vector control has been particularly effective where *S. neavei* is the vector. *S. neavei* vector eradication has been possible particularly where the focus is small with simple river systems. In addition to ivermectin treatment, the African Programme for Onchocerciasis Control (APOC), is undertaking vector elimination and eventually eradication activities against other vectors through targeted larviciding of short duration in selected and isolated areas—the Tukuyu focus (Tanzania), Bioko island (Equatorial Guinea), and against *S. neavei* in Itwara and Mpamba-Nkusi (Uganda)—where it is believed that two to three years of larviciding will accomplish long-lasting impact. In all these foci, the hydrological and climatic conditions, river size, and flow speed, as well as the ecological conditions favour possible vector elimination. A post-elimination/eradication entomological evaluation over two to three years will be required following larviciding. An earlier study in Kabarole district, Uganda which began in 1996 showed that after the intervention programme was implemented (annual community-based treatment of the population with ivermectin (Mectizan) tablets and vector control measures using the organophosphorous larvicide temephos, flies were absent and no infested crabs (the biological (phoretic) substrate of *S. neavei* larvae) were detected at the last monitoring survey in 2000 (Garms and Kipp, 2001).

7. CONTROL THROUGH IVERMECTIN ADMINISTRATION

7.1. The Scale of Ivermectin Treatment

In 1987, Merck and Co. Inc. made the decision to launch the Mectizan® Donation Program (MDP) and provide ivermectin free of charge, in recognising that the medicine would need to be provided for many decades, if not indefinitely. Shortly thereafter, in 1988, an independent group of experts, the Mectizan® Expert Committee (MEC) was created to oversee the technical aspects of the donation. Among the many important initial partners in the distribution efforts that ensued were OCP and non-governmental development organizations (NGDOs), which, in collaboration with Ministries of Health of several endemic countries, established some of the first large-scale efforts to distribute ivermectin. In 1990, the River Blindness Foundation (RBF) was established by a private philanthropist to broaden the distribution of ivermectin, and provided millions of dollars in funding to aid in establishing treatment programmes in onchocerciasis endemic countries. The NGDO Coordination Group for Onchocerciasis Control was established at the WHO Prevention of Blindness Programme (PBL) in a combined effort to help promote distribution activities in non-OCP areas. All partners worked to develop guidelines and strategies for best practice through field experience, operations research, technical assistance and monitoring, and evaluation (Drameh *et al.*, 2002). TDR-sponsored studies (Ngoumou *et al.*, 1994) developed the methodology of Rapid Epidemiological Mapping of Onchocerciasis (REMO) and later CDTI followed by the launching of the APOC in 1995, and the funding by donors of the World Bank APOC trust fund, were landmark events in the continued growth of distribution of ivermectin in other parts of Africa. In the Americas, the 1991 Directing Council of PAHO passed Resolution XIV where ministers agreed to eliminate onchocerciasis morbidity, and wherever possible transmission from the Americas, and OEPA was launched in 1992. The donation of Mectizan has become a model of how industry, international organizations, donors, national Ministries of Health (MOHs), and affected communities can successfully work together toward solving a major health problem

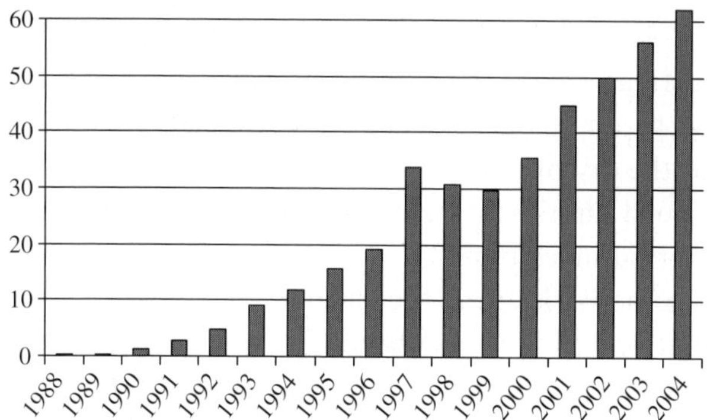

Figure 5   Treatments (in millions) approved and shipped by the Mectizan Donation Program 1988—2004. *Source:* Mectizan Program Notes No. 33, 2004 and http://www.mectizan.org/AH/AHeng.pdf (August 2005).

(Thylefors, 2004). Indeed, with the exception of the few areas where larviciding is undertaken by APOC to achieve vector eradication, large-scale ivermectin distribution is the only current tool being actively used to control or eliminate onchocerciasis.

The global initiative has now grown to one in which an estimated 62 million ivermectin treatments are provided per year, with over 400 million treatments enabled since the MDP began (Figure 5) (Mectizan Programme Notes, 2004). Roughly 8 million treatments are given annually in former OCP countries, 900 000 in the Americas, and the remainder in APOC countries. The ultimate treatment goal (UTG), which is the total number of people known or estimated to require and be eligible for ivermectin treatment, is currently estimated to be between 90 and 100 million; so much remains to be done, primarily in APOC countries or areas where conflict and insecurity limit the ability to distribute the medicine (Homeida *et al.*, 1999).

7.2. APOC and OEPA

The two regional programmes based primarily on ivermectin treatment are the APOC and the OEPA.

The objective of APOC is similar to that of the OCP: the control of onchocerciasis to a point where it is no longer a disease of public health importance through establishment of sustainable delivery mechanisms. In the 19 APOC countries, ivermectin is distributed annually in areas where the nodule prevalence exceeds 20% (which corresponds to an mf prevalence of between 35% and 40%). The approach to the distribution of ivermectin is to achieve sustainability. It was assumed that treatment must continue indefinitely without ongoing external investment. Key to the evaluations of APOC is the integration of activities into the primary health care system to support distribution, as well as the continued political will and local financing for onchocerciasis control activities. The impact of the control effort is also measured in changes in the prevalence and incidence of ocular onchocerciasis and reactive onchocercal dermatitis, as well as troublesome itching.

The objective of the OEPA programme is the regional elimination of onchocerciasis, with the assumption that at some point in time ivermectin distribution will cease. WHO estimate 140 000 persons to be infected and 4.7 million to be at risk in 1995, but most at risk population estimates are much lower now, at 500 000 persons. Over 95% of those at risk reside in Mexico, Guatemala, and Venezuela. Studies in the Americas in the late 1980s and early 1990s using twice yearly mass treatment with ivermectin demonstrated that transmission could be interrupted in Guatemala and Ecuador. These findings helped promote a Pan American Health Organization resolution in 1991 for a coordinated regional strategy based on intensive mass ivermectin treatment in all endemic areas (including hypoendemic areas) with the objectives of elimination not only of all disease manifestations but, wherever possible, transmission (Blanks *et al.*, 1998). Key to this decision were the entomological and epidemiological characteristics of onchocerciasis in the region. Many of the American *Simulium* vector species are inefficient vectors and sustained transmission requires high vector densities and heavy mf skin densities in infected populations. In most areas, health systems are sufficiently strong to be capable of delivering twice yearly treatments so that mf skin loads could be maintained at a level low enough to stop transmission.

Both APOC and OEPA programmes use baseline and post-treatment epidemiological, entomological, and ophthalmological data from sentinel areas to measure the impact of the effort.

7.3. Targeting of Distribution

The targeting of ivermectin distribution (as the frequency) depends on the strategy behind its use. In all instances, the aim is to find the optimum method of getting the drug to as many of the people who need it as possible. In original OCP areas, ivermectin distribution was guided by surveillance to provide treatment to pockets of residual transmission. In the extension areas of the OCP, however, ivermectin was used (a) in combination with larviciding in circumscribed areas and (b) in hyperendemic areas that did not have vector control. In the 19 APOC countries populations in hyperendemic areas who are at risk of developing ocular or skin manifestations of the diseases needed to be covered with ivermectin as a priority over those at less risk. The decision of where to initiate mass drug administration is through a well-planned, country by country, large-scale procedure called REMO (Ngoumou *et al.*, 1993). REMO used geographic attributes to determine areas likely to be permissive for *Simulium* breeding. This approach is rooted in the fact that the vectors for onchocerciasis have highly specific breeding site requirements and therefore it is possible solely with the aid of topographical maps to make a choice of representative villages most likely to be seriously affected by onchocerciasis. The REMO is followed by the Rapid Epidemiological Assessment (REA), a field evaluation of nodule rates in sample of 30–50 males aged 20 years and over in the communities drawn from those permissive areas. As a result of this mapping, it is now apparent that the 1995 WHO estimate of 17.7 million infected is likely to be revised upwards given that more countries than before have now undertaken more detailed mapping of onchocerciasis discovering foci hitherto not recorded. In the OEPA programme, all communities where there is the potential for transmission, regardless of endemicity, are targeted for treatment (Richards et al, 2001).

7.4. Coverage

Large-scale ivermectin distribution in APOC is monitored by the geographical and therapeutic coverage for each annual treatment round, aiming for 100% geographical coverage of all villages/communities demarcated through epidemiological mapping in the REMO exercise. For therapeutic coverage, the objective is to obtain at least 85% coverage for the eligible population (which excludes pregnant women, the very ill, and children under five years of age) and/or at least 65% coverage for the total population (all persons in the community). The UTG is a synthesis of the maximum geographic and eligible population coverage, and is the estimation of the number of people who would be treated if all persons eligible in all targeted communities were reached. Coverage is expressed as percentages calculated by dividing numbers of communities or persons treated by the various denominators (e.g., total communities, eligible population, total population) mentioned above. Since the OEPA goal is to provide ivermectin treatment twice a year in the target areas, treatment coverage is calculated as the number of treatments delivered during the year divided by twice the UTG value (termed the UTG (2)). The six American programmes have obtained at least 85% coverage of regional UTG (2) since 2002 (WHO, 2004).

7.5. Passive Distribution

Passive treatment strategies are based on having ivermectin delivered to health centres, clinics, and other health out-reach systems to support individual treatments in APOC areas where onchocerciasis is hypoendemic and therefore do not qualify for large-scale distribution. Passive treatments have not been well studied by the APOC or MDP programmes but are thought to account for a small percentage of the total number of people being treated. The use of "passive treatment coverage" as is calculated for large-scale distribution may not be justified nor useful given that the total or eligible population may not be known.

7.6. Challenges of Community-Directed Treatment with Ivermectin

7.6.1. CDTI

Distribution strategies for large-scale distribution in Africa have evolved from the use of relatively expensive mobile teams (called community-based distribution (CBD)) (Miri, 1998), in the early 1990s, to the current method of choice of CDTI. Distribution methods used in OEPA are selected at the discretion of the national programmes, and do not follow the strict guidelines of African CDTI.

The CDTI strategy has been successful over the years and through it millions in the affected communities who now receive ivermectin annually otherwise may not have received treatment early enough to save their sight. Like all novel strategies the implementation of CDTI has its own managerial challenges such as, for example, timely delivery of ivermectin in the community, reordering of medicines, management of mild adverse reactions, support (cash or in kind) for distributors, and record keeping. Investment in the programme, in support of local CDTI action, is required by local and state government if the process is to be sustained over many years; such support is often not forthcoming. Technical challenges include attaining the optimum coverage in the face of non-compliance for various reasons, the treatment of excluded pregnant women soon after parturition, integration of drug distributors with other health programmes, and the use of traditional African social structures such as kinship groups and socio-political challenges in terms of increasing the cultural appropriateness of the community distributors among others (Katabarwa *et al.*, 2000; Amazigo *et al.*, 2002; Burnham and Mebrahtu, 2004; Maduka *et al.*, 2004).

7.6.2. Impact of Ivermectin on the Eye and Skin Lesions

The impact of ivermectin on ocular onchocerciasis is seen in the reduction in and subsequent disappearance of ocular microfilaria from the anterior chamber of the eye, reduction in the prevalence of anterior segment lesions (punctuate keratitis, iridocyclitis, and sclerosing keratitis), and a beneficial effect on onchocercal optic nerve diseases, visual field loss, and visual acuity (Abiose, 1998; Emukah *et al.*, 2004). Impact of ivermectin treatment on posterior segment lesions appears minimal.

Results from a double-blind, placebo-controlled trial of different ivermectin regimens on onchocercal skin disease and severe itching showed that treatment results in a 40–50% decline in prevalence of severe itching relative to placebo, which is sustained for up to 12 months and that treatment results in a small, but significant decline in the prevalence of reactive skin lesions relative to placebo. Treating more frequently than once per year offered no significant advantage (Brieger *et al.*, 1998; WHO, 1997–1998). The overall impact of the millions of doses of ivermectin being distributed is difficult to measure in absolute terms but the direct and indirect benefits (not to mention the effect ivermectin has against intestinal worms and ecto-parasites; Heukelbach *et al.*, 2004; Heukelbach and Feldmeier, 2004) have had profound impact on the survival and quality of life for many millions of persons living in the onchocerciasis endemic areas (Tielsch and Beeche, 2004).

7.6.3. Impact on Transmission

A variety of studies conducted in several countries have all shown the unique effect of ivermectin on skin microfilaria. Although transmission is reduced, in some cases by as much as 65–85%, after an annual dose of ivermectin, the return of skin microfilaria six to nine months post-treatment reduces the potential for ivermectin to completely interrupt transmission when used in this way (Remme *et al.*, 1989). More frequent dosing of ivermectin (twice or four times per year) has been shown in some circumstances to interrupt transmission. In one river system in Ecuador, seven years of six-monthly mass treatment at 80% coverage of the eligible population resulted in an interruption of transmission. Twice per year treatment is also thought to have eliminated transmission in four communities in Guatemala, a focus in Mexico, and the single endemic focus in Colombia (Cupp *et al.*, 1989, 1992; Collins *et al.*, 1992; Guderian *et al.*, 1997; WHO, 2002). High treatment coverage is a key factor in stopping transmission.

In endemic areas in West Africa as for example Senegal, Guinea Bissau, and Sierra Leone where large-scale ivermectin treatment has been the only means to control onchocerciasis, complete interruption of transmission has not been proven (Dadzie *et al.*, 2003). However, in one focus where large-scale ivermectin treatment has been applied twice annually for close to 13 years, parasitological results suggest that ivermectin treatment may have interrupted transmission (Borsboom *et al.*, 2003). The implications of these findings, if confirmed by more detailed entomological studies, suggest the feasibility of elimination of onchocerciasis transmission in Africa by ivermectin treatment alone will need further consideration.

7.6.4. Duration of Treatment with Ivermectin

Although ivermectin treatment is very effective against onchocerciasis morbidity, the return of mf into the skin several months after treatment would mean that possibilities of transmission still exist in programmes based on annual therapy, and evidently that the treatment programme would need to be carried out indefinitely. The duration of treatment with ivermectin in those situations where transmission is interrupted continues to be a topic of intense discussion, and depends essentially on the reproductive life span of *O. volvulus* in the face of repeated ivermectin treatment. In non-endemic areas with no transmission, the conservative recommendation is to provide once a year treatment for up to 14 years to stride over the estimated life span of the adult worm determined in the OCP, in the absence of any ivermectin effect on the adult worms (WHO Certification, 2001). Simulations from the ONCHOSIM model (Plaisier, 1996) have suggested that the time required to eliminate infection depends on the coverage of treatment, frequency of treatment, habitual refusal to comply with treatment by infected persons, pre-control level of endemicity, and vector characteristics. At least 25 years of annual treatment at 65% total population coverage would be necessary to eliminate infection in areas of medium to high levels of infection, and more dire model predictions suggested that durations exceeding 35 years would be required if there were heterogeneity in exposure to *S. damnosum* vector bites (Winnen *et al.*, 2002). Modeling of the American situation using SIMON have given much more sanguine predictions (Davies, 1993). Validation of model predictions has been difficult because of inadequacy or paucity of real field data (Borsboom *et al.*, 2003).

8. IVERMECTIN "RESISTANCE"

The predictions that annual ivermectin treatments will need to be given for anything from 14–35 years or more have lead to a concern that resistance to ivermectin in *O. volvulus* will eventually emerge. Some authorities argue that resistance is unlikely (Taylor and Green, 1989) given the ineffective transmission of resistance through a vector-dependent life cycle of *O. volvulus*. Others note that no drug resistance has emerged in over 50 years of mass DEC use for lymphatic filariasis, or after years of intensive veterinary usage of ivermectin against dog heartworm (*Dirofilaria immitis*). A recent report from Ghana, however, of persistent microfilaridermias in several subjects despite multiple treatments with ivermectin led to concern that resistance of ivermectin had emerged. The observation was attributed to the 'non-response' of the adult female worms and not to inadequate drug exposure (Awadzi *et al.*, 2004).

9. SURVEILLANCE

The objective of the African onchocerciasis control programmes (OCP and APOC) is to eliminate onchocerciasis as a disease of public health importance. Given that regional elimination of the infection was not the goal of OCP, it is particularly important in onchocerciasis-freed zones where transmission has been eliminated, that a system of post-control surveillance is put in place to detect outbreaks of new infections before they reach the level where halting transmission becomes either difficult or impossible to overcome. The objective of the OEPA programme is the regional elimination of transmission, with the assumption that at some point in time ivermectin distribution will cease. Post ivermectin distribution surveillance will be required for a two-year period after the treatment programmes are discontinued, after which time surveillance may cease (WHO, 2001).

9.1. Entomological Surveillance

A surveillance system has been established in the onchocerciasis-freed zones (zones that benefited from the full 14 years of exclusive larviciding in the OCP area) based on molecular detection of *O.*

volvulus infection in blackflies. The system uses polymerase chain reaction (PCR) technology to detect the repetitive DNA sequence 0–150 (Meredith *et al.*, 1989) in pools of blackflies collected from monitoring sites. The PCR results are analysed using the Pool Screen method (Katholi *et al.*, 1995; Yameogo *et al.*, 1999). PCR analysis of blackflies collected from around the former OCP is carried out at a central point at the Molecular Biology Laboratory at the Multidisease Surveillance Centre in Ouagadougou, Burkina Faso. This process will gradually be decentralized initially to satellite laboratories in the areas in West Africa that have the capacity to undertake this procedure and later, at the opportune time, to the countries involved themselves.

Areas that are monitored were confirmed to be transmission-free through post-control entomological evaluation for a period of at least two years after larviciding ceased. The collection of flies, without any specific distinction for their ages, from designated zones every three years is carried out by community members with minimum supervision from the national health teams. PCR analysis is carried out to determine an infectivity index (number of infectious female flies among 1000 females captured). Three levels of the infectivity index are used to guide decisions: (i) If less than 0.5/1000 the three-yearly cycle of monitoring in the area concerned is maintained. (ii) An index of 0.5/1000 requires annual monitoring. (iii) An index greater than 0.5/1000 calls for immediate epidemiological surveys in the communities surrounding the capture points.

In the OCP areas that benefited from full-scale larviciding for a period of 14 years, interruption of transmission of infection was successfully achieved and the reservoir of infection has practically died out. Now that larviciding has stopped, reinvasion by *S. damnosum* has occurred and a permissive environment for resumption of transmission exits should reintroduction of *O. volvulus* take place. The participating countries have mounted a surveillance system (entomological and epidemiological) geared to detecting recrudescence of infection and to taking appropriate measures to control it should it occur. This is not only a long-term endeavour but it is also an important challenge for the countries to finance the surveillance system and sustain its efficiency. The development of a suitably sensitive, specific, rapid, and field-friendly diagnostic tool for the purposes of detecting recrudescence is a technical challenge that has not been addressed by the research community with the urgency it deserves. The OEPA programme needs a similar diagnostic test as it approaches a transmission interruption situation that requires at least two years of surveillance post-ivermectin stoppage prior to declaration of onchocerciasis elimination (WHO, 2001). Unfortunately, the largest and best-funded active onchocerciasis programme, APOC, utilizes a strategy that is unlikely to require deployment of a post-control monitor tool since transmission may not be interrupted (Richards *et al.*, 2000).

9.2. Epidemiological Surveillance

Post-control epidemiological surveillance in the former OCP areas is set up to detect the presence of new infections in humans in an area. The results are used to help determine if further control measures need to be undertaken. New infections suggest ongoing transmission, and in this instance it is defined as infection in children (as determined by skin snip until a better or equally specific method is found) born after transmission control was introduced. In the OCP situation, this defining point is when the programme of larviciding began. New infections may also be determined in adults who have been known to be parasitologically negative on two consecutive occasions separated by at least two years. This type of surveillance system will only be valid for areas that have had vector control or other means of control that has completely interrupted transmission and where there is no further intervention in progress.

ONCHOSIM, a micro-simulation mathematical model of the dynamics of *S. damnosum* onchocerciasis transmission, was used to investigate the risk and dynamics of onchocerciasis recrudescence after stopping vector control, in order to provide guidelines for operational decision-making in the OCP in West Africa. In the absence of immigration of infected humans or invasion by infected flies, the model predicted that 14 years of full-scale vector control would be required to reduce the risk of recrudescence to less than 1% (Plaisier *et al.*, 1990).

The model also suggests that if recrudescence is detected before it exceeds 1.0–1.5% annual infection incidence, then annual ivermectin distribution with at least 65% population coverage for 15 or more years should lead to suppression of the transmission and prevent nascent parasite populations from re-establishing (Plaisier *et al.*, 1991). Given the narrow window of 1–1.5% annual incidence of infection within which to decide whether or not to launch a long haul of ivermectin distribution, it is essential that any pronouncement of recrudescence is well verified through wide and detailed epidemiological investigation, in itself an expensive undertaking. On the other hand, any delays in taking the right decision could jeopardize the gains made in the onchocerciasis-freed zones. The entomological surveillance therefore complements the epidemiological surveillance activities. A challenge for the surveillance activity is how to detect infection (e.g., which diagnostic method to use) in the light of widespread use and distribution of ivermectin, not necessarily for onchocerciasis but for lymphatic filariasis as well, whose distribution overlaps that of the onchocerciasis-freed zones. If the distribution of ivermectin is efficient and the entomological surveillance network is optimum, the first indication of failure of the distribution may be detected through the presence of infected blackflies in the area concerned.

10. COST OF THE DISEASE AND COSTS OF THE PROGRAMMES

10.1. Social and Economic Costs of the Disease

The socio-economic impact of the disease is most marked in the rural hyperendemic areas where the vectors of the disease are predominant. Visual impairment and blindness which are recognized as telling consequences of the disease often result in families' inability to support themselves. Furthermore, the fear of blindness was a major reason for the depopulation of the fertile river valleys which made the disease an important obstacle to socioeconomic development in West African savannah regions.

Reactive skin lesions have severe social repercussions while onchocercal skin disease (OSD) diminishes income-generating capacity. It also contributes to the school drop-out rate that has been found to be twice as high among children from households whose head has OSD (WHO, 1995b). The consequences of onchocercal skin lesions, the stigmatization and psychosocial effect associated with the disease, are well known by the affected community. Skin diseases have been a major source of social stigma, whether they are infectious or not. It has been suggested that incessant itching and severe onchocerciasis lesions could be important predictors of failure of women to breast-feed for longer periods in rain-forest areas of Nigeria (Amazigo, 1994). Apart from blindness, those with skin-related symptoms and OSD have higher health-related expenditures and have diminished income-generating capacity compared with the uninfected (Benton, 1998).

10.2. Costs of the Programmes

Attempts to calculate the cost of treatment per person for the three strategies for large-scale distribution have been made. In Mali, the costs of treatment through CDTI were found to be US$0.06 compared with US$0.5 per person treated through the mobile teams (WHO, 1994), while a study in Nike and Achi in Nigeria estimated treatment costs which include direct financial costs, opportunity costs, advocacy, mobilizing the community, training, and distribution to be US$0.17 and US$0.13 per dose in these villages, respectively (Onwujekwe *et al.*, 2002; Waters *et al.*, 2004).

About US$560 million, provided by more than 22 non-African donor states, agencies, and the 11 African countries, was invested in the OCP for the period 1974–2002, excluding the cost of ivermectin which was generously donated free of cost by Merck and Co. The programme has been regarded by some commentators as having been expensive, however, the results have been equally impressive; 600 000 cases of blindness have been prevented, and 25 million hectares of formerly abandoned arable lands have been made safe for settlement and agriculture. These lands have the potential to feed an additional

17 million people. The African Programme APOC is supported entirely from voluntary contributions (75% from donors and 25% from NGDOs and African countries) and has a working budget of US$160 million to which could be added the cost of ivermectin tablets to treat over 50 million people. In West Africa, the OCP has achieved a 20% economic rate of return (Kim and Benton, 1995). Elsewhere in Africa, operations began in 1996 and achieved a 17% economic rate of return while preventing blindness, and eliminating disabling itching and stigmatizing skin disease. The cost of the OEPA Programme is estimated to be US$20 million so far, with over 50% of this contributed by the endemic countries.

11. FUTURE CHALLENGES

The principal goal common to all the onchocerciasis programmes is to ensure that onchocerciasis is permanently eliminated as an important public health problem throughout the world. The challenges vary with the three regional programmes (OCP, ivermectin, OEPA, APOC), based on their individual strategies for the use of the major control tool available (Dadzie, 1998; Richards *et al.*, 2000).

The OCP largely achieved its objective of eliminating onchocerciasis as a disease of public health importance and as an obstacle to socio-economic development. Before the programme terminated at the end of 2002, the participating countries were in a position to detect and control any recrudescence of infection. However, the disease itself was not eliminated, and certain foci have to continue with ivermectin distribution for the foreseeable future. Ongoing treatment in these residual foci, as well as surveillance for recrudescence, depends on the sustainability of the distribution process and how well this is integrated in the national health system and funded by national governments (Hopkins *et al.*, 2005). WHO authorities need to maintain their advocacy for these activities with ministries of health in the OCP area.

Future major technical challenges of onchocerciasis control include ivermectin mass administration in areas co-endemic for the parasite *L. loa*, ivermectin treatment in hypoendemic areas, sustainability, post-control surveillance for recrudescence detection, surveillance for emergence of resistance, and decisions of when to stop mass ivermectin treatments. There is the need to develop the appropriate information systems and diagnostic tools to help in accomplishing many of these tasks. A search for a second-line treatment or an alternative drug to ivermectin as well as a search for a macrofilaricide are issues that need to be addressed in the future.

11.1. Ivermectin Treatment of Onchocerciasis in Areas that are Co-Endemic for *Loa loa*

Human loiasis is caused by a filarial parasite transmitted by a deer fly vector (*Chrysops silacea* and *C. dimidiata*). The vector breeds in the high canopy forested areas of central Africa. The precise distribution of *L. loa* is unknown, but the most heavily infected populations are found in Angola, Benin, Cameroon, the Central African Republic, Congo, the DRC, Equatorial Guinea, Gabon, Nigeria, and Sudan.

Loa has been largely neglected because it does not in itself cause severe disease. Many persons are asymptomatic, and the most common clinical manifestations are periodic angioedematous swellings (known as "Calabar swellings") and/or passage of the adult *Loa* worms under the conjunctiva of the eye (*L. loa* also is known as the "eye worm"). *Loa* mf, which circulate diurnally in the peripheral blood, can occur in spectacular concentrations, reaching over 50 000 mf/ml of blood.

Central nervous system (CNS) dysfunction and coma from *L. loa*, associated temporally with microfilaricidal treatment, has been known for many years and was first described with the use of DEC. CNS-related adverse reactions have been reported during the first rounds of mass ivermectin treatment in areas where high-density *Loa* infections occur (Boussinesq *et al.*, 1998). These events generally occur in otherwise healthy persons who have high-density *Loa* microfilaremia ($>30\,000$ mf/ml of blood) (Gardon *et al.*, 1997) The pathogenesis leading to encephalopathy is unclear, but it appears related to rapid killing or immune unmasking of mf after the ingestion of DEC or ivermectin, leading to blockage of the microcirculation and ischaemia of vital organs, including the brain. Evidence suggests that promptly instituted basic supportive care (hydration, feeding, and nursing care) will result in complete patient recovery in most cases. The MDP, which is responsible for the release of ivermectin to both onchocerciasis and lymphatic filariasis programmes, has worked with APOC to develop strategies for ivermectin mass treatment in areas co-endemic for onchocerciasis and loiasis. MDP and APOC have jointly recommended that, in *L. loa* endemic areas, programmes must educate the population about possible complications of such treatment, intensify surveillance for severe adverse effects so that cases can be promptly referred, and assure the availability of trained healthcare personnel in well supplied referral units during and immediately following MDA. Thomson *et al.* (2000, 2004) created a spatial model of *L. loa* prevalence to identify areas where high endemicity may be associated with the occurrence of such reactions. The model results have been mapped and the areas of overlap between high *L. loa* prevalence and planned ivermectin distribution for onchocerciasis control may be identified. The RAPLOA (Rapid Assessment Procedure for Loiasis) is a rapid assessment method for quickly identifying (based on prevalence of the history of eye worm) potential risk of *L. loa* post-ivermectin treatment encephalopathy (Wanji *et al.*, 2005), so that the joint MDP/APOC recommendations can be put in place prior to launching mass treatment.

11.2. Ivermectin Distribution in Hypoendemic Areas

Ivermectin distribution in most of the remaining intervention areas in the former OCP is provided in hypoendemic areas and some endemic communities under treatment in the Americas are likewise considered hypoendemic. In contrast, the REMO exercise undertaken under APOC was designed to map out only those areas of greatest risk for onchocerciasis morbidity, where nodule rates were assumed to be at or above 20%. Whether or not there is a need for treatment in APOC to be expanded to hypoendemic zones in the APOC countries is an issue that needs to be addressed. The question that will continue to be posed is how much threat such untreated areas pose to neighbouring treated areas. The expense and benefit of treating hypoendemic areas with ivermectin needs to be studied well before APOC ends in 2010. Ivermectin distribution is envisaged in lymphatic filariasis areas which in most cases overlap the onchocerciasis endemic zones and go beyond into the hypoendemic zones of onchocerciasis which have not been eligible for treatment (Abiose *et al.*, 2000; Richards *et al.*, 2000). The wider distribution of ivermectin for lymphatic filariasis would cover such areas providing added value to the strategy for lymphatic filariasis elimination strategy.

11.3. Sustainability

The current approach to the distribution of ivermectin (CDTI) was developed with the condition of sustainability in mind. It was assumed that external investment in ivermectin distribution would be limited, but that such distribution would need to continue indefinitely. CDTI has been successful in getting ivermectin to a huge number of persons, but it is yet to be proven that the excellent geographic and therapeutic coverage now achieved can be sustained over an indefinite period without external investment. As external funding is withdrawn, there must be continued political will and the financing for onchocerciasis activities to continue to benefit from the considerable investments already made to generate the global momentum the programmes are currently riding on (Hopkins *et al.*, 2005). There are also examples of "population fatigue" at the community level, with opinions expressed of being tired of having to take the drug for years on end, especially given that the disease manifestations are no longer evident (Emukah *et al.*, 2004). Many have heard the health education message that only 15 years of treatment is needed to affect a "cure". Since ivermectin has been distributed in many areas since 1988, this understanding could affect coverage rates unless it is corrected.

11.4. Detection of Ivermectin Resistance

Although not yet identified to exist, emergence of resistance to ivermectin in *O. volvulus* is a potential threat to the great progress and considerable investment made so far to combat this disease. Surveillance mechanisms to detect the emergence of ivermectin resistance may be particularly important in APOC areas, where the number of parasites exposed to treatment is greatest and low levels of transmission seems to be ongoing and there is no vector control. DNA probes have been developed that could be used for such surveillance, based on sites of ivermectin resistance identified in intestinal trichostrongylid nematodes of sheep, goats, and cattle. If resistance is detected, many experts are of the opinion that the area should be intensely treated with replacement drugs, such as doxycycline or moxidectin, to prevent its spread to other areas.

11.5. Cessation of Ivermectin Distribution

The duration of treatment with ivermectin where transmission can be interrupted continues to be a topic of intense discussion, and depends essentially on the reproductive life span of *O. volvulus* in the face of repeated ivermectin treatment. The conservative recommendation, based on OCP observational data of reproductive life span of worms in the presence of complete vector control, is 14 years, further reduced to 12 years in the face of ivermectin treatment and vector control. The OEPA programme uses 12 years from the point of transmission interruption (WHO, 2001). The period of time required to cessation of ivermectin distribution would be further reduced if ivermectin has a permanent effect on female worm fecundity, male worm survival, or overall mortality (Cupp *et al.*, 2004). When once per year treatment is provided, transmission continues at low levels, new worms enter the system, and the ONCHOSIM model suggests that it would take at least 25 years to eliminate the infection if ivermectin were given at a minimum population coverage of 65%. All cessation considerations also need to consider the initial endemicity level and the vectorial capacity of the particular *Simulium* sp. concerned. To include the decision to stop treatment, there is need for new tools that could diagnose the presence of viable adult *O. volvulus* worms.

11.6. Macrofilaricides and Other Drugs

Even before the introduction of ivermectin it was recognized that the ideal drug for onchocerciasis should kill the adult worms (a "macrofilaricide") or permanently sterilize the adult females worms of *O. volvulus* without causing adverse reaction in the human host. The ideal drug would be safe under normal conditions of use, suitable for large-scale use orally, of low cost and effective in small number of doses. Macrofilaricides have a substantially higher potential for achieving onchocerciasis elimination than ivermectin, but high coverage levels will be key. When these drugs become available, onchocerciasis elimination strategies should be reconsidered in Africa (Alley *et al.*, 2001; Dadzie *et al.*, 2003). To date, the only known macrofilaricide for onchocerciasis is suramin. However, in several studies repeated treatments with ivermectin suggest increased mortality in adult worms examined after nodulectomy (Cupp *et al.*, 2002).

There is need to develop safe and easily administered drugs that can kill the adult *O. volvulus* parasite to reduce the time needed for the programme to eliminate adult worms from an endemic area. If such a drug became available cheaply, it could change the approach to onchocerciasis control in Africa. Research to develop a second microfilaricide (such as moxidectin, which has also a prolonged effect on the mfs) is also important, as a back-up to ivermectin.

12. MANAGERIAL CHALLENGES

Critical to all three onchocerciasis regional programmes is a functional central and peripheral health care system that can provide health education, training, supervision, and monitoring of the mass treatment programme. In Africa, it has been learned that CDTI does not function in a vacuum; government health systems must support the community and its decisions pertaining to ivermectin distribution, ideally through an integrated approach. Drug reporting, ordering, and supply are the most critical government function that must be strengthened and sustained. Communities must have an uninterrupted supply of ivermectin, when they need it, if the concept of community directed treatment is to flourish. Financial support emanating from the OCP/APOC Programmes and partner NGDOs so far has resulted in the success of the CDTI approach. The immediate challenge is to maintain this performance, with an indefinite horizon. This sustained approach is the strength of CDTI: it calls for integration with other ongoing management systems that must be permanently maintained, such as vaccination programmes, maternal child health, oral rehydration, and malaria treatment.

By the nature of its operations, the OCP from its inception operated mainly as a vertical public health and development programme. The programme, however, planned early on with the participating countries that residual activities be transferred with closure of the programme to national control, in particular the ivermectin distribution initiative. Other post-OCP managerial challenges include surveillance for recrudescence, and response/investigation when such surveillance gives a signal that action is required.

OEPA's challenge in the Americas is to reach and maintain the highest possible ivermectin treatment coverage, twice per year, to first interrupt transmission, and then maintain programme performance and coverage for the duration of the life span of the adult worms. This accomplished, the infection would be eliminated from a given endemic focus and treatment could be withdrawn with subsequent monitoring for recrudescence for a period of at least two years.

REFERENCES

Abiose, A. (1998). Onchocercal eye disease and the impact of Mectizan treatment. *Annals of Tropical Medicine and Parasitology* **92** (supplement 1), S11–S22.

Abiose, A., Homeida, M., Liese, B., Molyneux, D. and Remme, H. (2000). Onchocerciasis control strategies. *Lancet* **356**, 1523–1524.

Alexander, N.D., Cousens, S.N., Yahaya, H., Abiose, A. and Jones, B.R. (1993). Ivermectin dose assessment without weighing scales. *Bulletin of the World Health Organization* **71**, 361–366.

Alley, W.S., Oortmarssen, G.J., Boatin, B.A., Nagelkerke, N.J.D., Plaisier, A.P., Remme, J.H.F., Lazdins, J., Borsboom, G.J.J.M. and Habbema, J.D.F. (2001). Macrofilaricides and onchocerciasis control, mathematical modelling of the prospects for elimination. *BMC Public Health* **1**, 12.

Amazigo, U.O. (1994). Detrimental effects of onchocerciasis on marriage age and breast-feeding. *Tropical and Geographic Medicine* **46**, 322–325.

Amazigo, U.V., Brieger, W.R., Katabarwa, M., Akogun, O., Ntep, M., Boatin, B., N'doyo, J., Noma, M. and Sékétéli, A. (2002). The challenges of community-directed treatment with ivermectin (CDTI) within the African Programme for Onchocerciasis Control (APOC). *Annals of Tropical Medicine and Parasitology* **96** (supplement 1), S41–S58.

Anderson, J., Fuglsang, H. and Marshall, T.F. de C. (1976). Studies on onchocerciasis in the United Cameroon Republic III. A four year follow up of six forest and six savanna villages. The incidence of ocular lesions. *Transaction of Tropical Medicine and Hygiene* **79**, 362–373.

Ashburn, L.L., Burch, T.A. and Brady, F.J. (1949). Pathologic effects of Suramin, hetrazan and arsenamide on adult *Onchocerca volvulus*. *Boletin de la Oficina Sanitaria Panamericana* **28**, 1107–1117.

Awadzi, K., Boakye, D.A., Edwards, G., Opoku, N.O., Attah, S.K., Osei-Atweneboana, M.Y., Lazdins-Helds, J.K., Ardrey, A.E., Addy, E.T., Quartey, B.T., Ahmed, K., Boatin, B.A. and Soumbey-Alley, E.W. (2004). An investigation of persistent microfilaridermias despite multiple treatments with ivermectin, in two onchocerciasis-endemic foci in Ghana. *Annals of Tropical Medicine and Parasitology* **98**, 231–249(19).

Awadzi, K., Dadzie, K.Y., Schulz-Key, H. and Haddock, D.R.W. (1985). The chemotherapy of onchocerciasis. X. Assessment of four single dose treatment regimes of MK-933 (ivermectin) in human onchocerciasis. *Annals of Tropical Medicine and Parasitology* **79**, 63–78.

Awadzi, K. and Gilles, H.M. (1980). The chemotherapy of onchocerciasis. III. A comparative study of DEC and Metrifonate. *Annals of Tropical Medicine and Parasitology* **79**, 199–210.

Awadzi, K., Hero, M., Opoku, N.O., Addy, E.T., Büttner, D.W. and Ginger, C.D. (1995). The chemotherapy of onchocerciasis. XVIII. Aspects of treatment with suramin. *Tropical Medicine and Parasitology* **46**, 19–26.

Benton, B. (1998). Economic impact of onchocerciasis control through the African Programme for Onchocerciasis Control: an overview. *Annals of Tropical Medicine and Parasitology* **92** (supplement 1), S33–S39.

Blacklock, B.D. (1926). The development of *Onchocerca volvulus* in *Simulium damnosum*. *Annals of Tropical Medicine and Parasitology* **20**, 1–48.

Blanks, J., Richards, F., Beltran, F., Collins, R., Alvarez, E., Zea Flores, G., Bauler, B., Cedillos, R., Heisler, M., Brandling-Bennett, D., Baldwin, W., Bayona, M., Klein, R. and Jacox, M. (1998). The Onchocerciasis Elimination Program of the Americas: a history of partnership. *Pan American Journal of Public Health* **3**, 367–374.

Boatin, B., Molyneux, D.H., Hougard, J.-M., Christensen, O.W., Alley, E.S., Yaméogo, L., Sékétéli, A. and Dadzie, K.Y. (1997). Patterns of epidemiology and control of onchocerciasis in West Africa. *Journal of Helminthology* **71**, 91–101.

Boatin, B.A., Toé, L., Alley, E.S., Dembélé, N., Weis, N. and Dadzie, K.Y. (1998). Diagnostics in onchocerciasis: future challenges. *Annals of Tropical Medicine and Parasitology* **92** (supplement 1), S41–S45.

Borsboom, G., Boatin, B., Nagelkerke, N., Agoua, H., Akpoboua, K., Soumbey-Alley, W., Bissan, Y., Renz, A., Yameogo, L., Remme, J. and Habbema, D. (2003). Impact of ivermectin on onchocerciasis transmission: assessing the empirical evidence that repeated ivermectin mass treatments may lead to elimination/eradication in West Africa. *Filaria Journal* **2**, 8.

Botto, C. (1997). Onchocerciasis hyperendemic in the Unturan mountains— an extension of the endemic region in southern Venezuela. *Transactions of the Royal Society of Tropical Medicine and Hygiene* **91**, 150–152.

Boussinesq, M., Gardon, J., Gardon-Wendel, N., Kamgno, J., Ngoumou, P. and Chippaux, J.P. (1998). Three probable cases of *Loa loa* encephalopathy following ivermectin treatment for onchocerciasis. *American Journal of Tropical Medicine and Hygiene* **58**, 461–469.

Brieger, W.R., Awedoba, A.K., Eneanya, C.I., Hagan, M., Ogbuagu, K.F. and Okello, D.O. (1998). The effects of ivermectin on onchocercal skin disease and severe itching: results of a multicentre trial. *Tropical Medicine and International Health* **3**, 951–961.

Brown, K.R. and Neu, D.C. (1990). Ivermectin—clinical trials and treatment schedules in onchocerciasis. *Acta Leidensia* **59**, 169–175.

Burnham, G. and Mebrahtu, T. (2004). Review: the delivery of ivermectin (Mectizan®). *Tropical Medicine and International Health* **9** (supplement 4), A26–A44.

Collins, R.C., Gonzales-Peralta, C., Castro, J., Zea-Flores, G., Cupp, M.S., Richards, F.O., Jr. and Cupp, E.W. (1992). Ivermectin: reduction in prevalence and infection intensity of *Onchocerca volvulus* following bi-annual treatment in five Guatemalan communities. *American Journal of Tropical Medicine and Hygiene* **47**, 156–169.

Crosskey, R.W. (1990). *The Natural History of Blackflies*. Chichester, UK: Wiley.

Cupp, E., Ochoa, A., Collins, R.C., Ramberg, F.R. and Zea-Flores, G. (1989). The effect of multiple ivermectin treatments on infection of *Simulium ochraceum* with *Onchocerca volvulus*. *American Journal of Tropical Medicine and Hygiene* **40**, 501–506.

Cupp, E.W., Duke, B.O., Mackenzie, C.D., Guzman, J.R., Vieira, J.C., Mendez-Galvan, J., Castro, J., Richards, F., Sauerbrey, M., Dominguez, A.J., Eversole, R.R. and Cupp, M.S. (2004). The effects of long-term community level treatment with Ivermectin (Mectizan®) on adult *Onchocerca volvulus* in Latin America. *Journal of Tropical Medicine and Hygiene* **71**, 602–607.

Cupp, E.W., Ochoa, O., Collins, R.C., Cupp, M.S., Gonzales-Peralta, C., Castro, J. and Zea-Flores, G. (1992). The effects of repetitive community-wide ivermectin treatment on transmission of *Onchocerca volvulus* in

Guatemala. *American Journal of Tropical Medicine and Hygiene* **43**, 170–179.

Dadzie, K.Y. (1998). Control of onchocerciasis: challenges for the future. *Annals of Tropical Medicine & Parasitology* **29** (supplement 1), S65–S67.

Dadzie, K.Y., Remme, J., Baker, R.H.A., Rolland, A. and Thylefors, B. (1990). Ocular onchocerciasis and intensity of infection in the community III. West African rain-forest foci of the vector *Simulium sanctipauli*. *Tropical Medicine and Parasitology* **41**, 376–382.

Dadzie, K.Y., Remme, J., Rolland, A. and Thylefors, B. (1989). Ocular onchocerciasis an intensity of infection in the community: II. West African rain-forest foci of the vector *Simulium yahense*. *Tropical Medicine and Parasitology* **40**, 348–354.

Dadzie, Y., Neira, M. and Hopkins, D. (2003). Final report of the conference on the eradicability of onchocerciasis. *Filarial Journal* **2**, 2.

Davies, J.B. (1993). Description of a computer model of forest onchocerciasis transmission and its application to field scenarios of vector control and chemotherapy. *Annals of Tropical Medicine and Parasitology* **87**, 41–63.

Davies, J.B. (1994). Sixty years of onchocerciasis vector control: a chronological summary with comments on eradication, reinvasion and insecticide resistance. *Annual Review of Entomology* **39**, 23–45.

Dawood, M.S. (1978). *Field Treatment of Onchocerciasis in the Sudan with Suramin Preparations and Banocide*. Alexandra: World Health Organization.

de C. Bronsvoort, B.M., Renz, A., Tchakouté, V., Tanya, V.N., Ekale, D. and Trees, A.J. (2005). Repeated high doses of avermectins cause prolonged sterilisation, but do not kill, *Onchocerca ochengi* adult worms in African cattle. *Filaria Journal* **4**, 8.

De Sole, G., Remme, J., Awadzi, K., Accorsi, S., Alley, E., Ba, O., Dadzie, K., Giese, J., Karam, M. and Keita, F. (1989). Adverse reactions after mass treatment of onchocerciasis with ivermectin. Combined results from eight community trials. *Bulletin of the World Health Organization* **67**, 707–719.

Drameh, P., Richards, F., Derstine, P. and Cross, C. (2002). Ten years of NGO efforts in controlling onchocerciasis. *Trends in Parasitology* **18**, 378–380.

Duke, B.O.L. (2005). Evidence for macrofilaricidal activity of ivermectin against female *Onchocerca volvulus*: further analysis of a clinical trial in the Republic of Cameroon indicating two distinct killing mechanisms. *Parasitology* **130**, 447–458.

Duke, B.O.L., Zea-Flores, G., Castro, J., Cupp, E.W. and Munoz, B. (1991). Comparison of the effects of a single dose and four monthly doses of ivermectin on *Onchocerca volvulus*. *American Journal of Tropical Medicine and Hygiene* **45**, 132–137.

Emukah, E.C., Osuoha, E., Miri, E.S., Onyenama, J., Amazigo, U., Obijuru, C., Osuji, N., Ekeanyanwu, J., Amadiegwu, S., Korve, K. and Richards, F. (2004). A longitudinal study of impact of repeated mass ivermectin treatment on clinical manifestations of onchocerciasis in Imo State, Nigeria. *American Journal of Tropical Medicine and Hygiene* **70**, 556–561.

Gardon, J., Gardon-Wendel, N., Demanga-Ngangue, Kamgno, J., Chippaux, J.P. and Boussinesq, M. (1997). Serious reactions after mass treatment of onchocerciasis with ivermectin in an area endemic for *Loa loa* infection. *Lancet* **350**, 18–22.

Garms, R. and Kipp, W. (2001). Onchocerciasis control in a highly endemic onchocerciasis focus in Kabarole District, Uganda. *129th Annual Meeting of the American Public Health Association.*

Greene, B.M., Taylor, H.R., Cupp, E.W., Murphy, R.P., White, A.T., Schulz-key, H., D'Anna, S.A., Newland, H.S., Goldsmith, L.P., Auer, C., Hanson, A.P., Freeman, S.V., Reber, E.W. and Williams, P.N. (1985). Comparison of ivermectin and diethylcarbamazine in the treatment of onchocerciasis. *New England Journal of Medicine* **313**, 133–138.

Guderian, R.H., Anselmi, M., Espinel, M., Mancero, T., Rivadeneira, G., Proano, R., Calvopina, H.M., Vieira, J.C. and Cooper, P.J. (1997). Successful control of onchocerciasis with community-based ivermectin distribution in the Rio Santiago focus in Ecuador. *Tropical Medicine and International Health* **2**, 982–988.

Habbema, J.D.F., Alley, E.S., Plaisier, A.P., van Oortmarssen, G.J. and Remme, J.H.F. (1992). Epidemiological modeling for onchocerciasis control. *Parasitology Today* **8**, 99–103.

Hagan, M. (1998). Onchocercal dermatitis: clinical impact. *Annals of Tropical Medicine and Parasitology* **92** (supplement 1), S85–S96.

Hall, L.R. and Pearlman, E. (1999). Pathogenesis of onchocercal keratitis (river blindness). *Clinical Microbiological Review* **12**, 445–453.

Heukelbach, J. and Feldmeier, H. (2004). Ectoparasites—the underestimated realm. *Lancet* **363**, 889–891.

Heukelbach, J.B., Wilcke, T., Muehlen, M., Albrecht, S., Sales de Oliveira, F.A., Kerr-Pontes, L.R.S., Liesenfeld, O. and Feldmeier, H. (2004). Selective mass treatment with ivermectin to control intestinal helminthiases and parasitic skin diseases in a severely affected population. *Bulletin of the World Health Organization* **82**, 563–571.

Hoerauf, A., Mand, S., Adjei, O., Fleischer, B. and Büttner, D.W. (2001). Depletion of *Wolbachia* endobacteria in *Onchocerca volvulus* by doxycycline and microfilaridermia after ivermectin treatment. *Lancet* **357**, 1415–1416.

Hoerauf, A., Volkman, L., Hamelmann, C., Hamelmann, C., Adjei, O., Autenrieth, I.B., Fleischer, B. and Büttner, D.W. (2000). Endosymbiotic bacteria in worms as targets for a novel chemotherapy in filariasis. *Lancet* **355**, 1242–1243.

Homeida, M.M., Goepp, I., Ali, M., Hilyer, E. and Mackenzie, C.D. (1999). Medical achievements under civil war conditions. *Lancet* **354**, 601.

Hopkins, D.R., Richards, F. and Katabarwa, M. (2005). Whither onchocerciasis control in Africa? *American Journal of Tropical Medicine and Hygiene* **72**, 1–2.

Hougard, J.-M., Poudiougo, P., Guillet, P., Back, C., Akpoboua, L.K.B. and Quillévéré, D. (1993). Criteria for the selection of larvicides by the Onchocerciasis Control Programme in West Africa. *Annals of Tropical Medicine and Parasitology* **87**, 435–442.

Kale, O.O. (1998). Onchocerciasis: the burden of disease. *Annals of Tropical Medicine and Parasitology* **92** (supplement 1), S101–S115.

Katabarwa, M.N., Richards, F.R. and Ndyomugyenyi, R. (2000). In rural Ugandan communities the traditional kinship/clan system is vital to the success and sustainment of the African Programme for Onchocerciasis Control. *Annals of Tropical Medicine and Parasitology* **94**, 485–495.

Katholi, C.R., Toé, L., Merriweather, A. and Unnasch, T.R. (1995). Determining the prevalence of *Onchocerca volvulus* infection in vector populations by PCR screening of black flies. *Journal of Infectious Diseases* **172**, 1414–1417.

Kim, A. and Benton, B. (1995). *Cost–Benefit Analysis of the Onchocerciasis Control Program (OCP)*. Washington, DC: World Bank.

Lewalen, S. and Courtright, P. (2001). Blindness in Africa: present situation and future needs. *British Journal of Ophthalmology* **85**, 897–903.

Maduka, E.C., Nweke, L.N., Miri, E.S., Amazigo, U. and Richards, F. (2004). Missed treatment opportunities in onchocerciasis mass treatment programs for pregnant and breast-feeding women in southeast Nigeria. *Annals of Tropical Medicine and Parasitology* **98**, 697–702.

Mazzotti, L. (1948). Posibilidad de utilizar como medio diagnostico auxiliar en la onchocercosis, las reacciones alérgicas consecutivas a la administración del 'Hetrazan'. *Revista de Instituto de Salubridad y Enfermedadas Tropicales* **38**, 235–237.

Meredith, S.E.O., Unnasch, T.R., Karam, M., Piessen, W. and Wirth, D.F. (1989). Cloning and characterization of an *Onchocerca volvulus* specific DNA sequence. *Molecular Biochemical Parasitology* **36**, 1–10.

Miri, E.S. (1998). Problems and perspectives of managing an onchocerciasis control programme. *Annals of Tropical Medicine and Parasitology* **92** (supplement 1), S121–S128.

Molyneux, D.H. (1995). Onchocerciasis control in West Africa: current status and future of the onchocerciasis control programme. *Parasitology Today* **11**, 399–402.

Newland, H.S., Kaiser, A. and Taylor, H.R. (1987). The use of diethylcarbamazine cream in the diagnosis of onchocerciasis. *Tropical Medicine and Parasitology* **38**, 143–144.

Ngoumou, P., Walsh, J.F. and Mace, J.M. (1994). A rapid mapping technique for the prevalence and distribution of onchocerciasis: a Cameroon case study. *Annals of Tropical Medicine and Parasitology* **88**, 463–474.

Nutman, T.B., Zimmerman, P.A., Kubofcik, J. and Kostyu, D.D. (1994). A universally applicable diagnostic approach to filarial and other infections. *Parasitology Today* **9**, 76–79.

Onwujekwe, O., Chima, R., Shu, E. and Okwonko, P. (2002). Community directed treatment with ivermectin in two Nigerian communities: an analysis of first year start-up process, costs and consequences. *Health Policy* **62**, 31–51.

Pearlman, E. and Hall, L.R. (2000). Immune mechanisms in *Onchocerca volvulus*—mediated corneal disease (river blindness). *Parasite Immunology* **22**, 625–631.

Plaisier, A.P. (1996). *Modeling onchocerciasis transmission and control*. Ph.D Thesis, Erasmus University, Rotterdam.

Plaisier, A.P., Alley, E.S., Boatin, B.A., Van Oortmarssen, G.J., Remme, H., De Vlas, S.J., Bonneux, L. and Habbema, J.D. (1995). Irreversible effects of ivermectin on adult parasites in onchocerciasis patients in the Onchocerciasis Control Programme in West Africa. *Journal of Infectious Diseases* **172**, 204–210.

Plaisier, A.P., van Oortmarssen, G.J., Habbema, J.D., Remme, J. and Alley, E.S. (1990). ONCHOSIM: a model and computer simulation program for the transmission and control of onchocerciasis. *Computer Methods and Programs in Biomedicine* **31**, 43–50.

Plaisier, A.P., van Oortmarssen, G.J., Remme, J., Alley, E.S. and Habbema, J.D. (1991). The risk and dynamics of onchocerciasis recrudescence after cessation of vector control. *Bulletin of the World Health Organization* **9**, 169–178.

Prod'hon, J., Boussinesq, M., Fobi, G., Prod'hum, J.M., Enyong, P., Lafluer, C. and Quillévéré, D. (1991). Lutte contre onchocercose par ivermectin; résultats d'une campagne de masse au Nord-Cameroun. *Bulletin of the World Health Organization* **69**, 443–450.

Remme, J., Baker, R.H.A., De Sole, G., Dadzie, K.Y., Adams, M.A., Alley, E.S., Avissey, H.S.K. and Walsh, J.F. (1989). A community trial of ivermectin in the onchocerciasis focus of Asubende, Ghana. I. Effect on the microfilarial reservoir and the transmission of *Onchocerca volvulus*. *Tropical Medicine and Parasitology* **40**, 367–374.

Richards, F., Boatin, B., Sauerbrey, M. and Sékétéli, A. (2001). Control of onchocerciasis today: status and challenges. *Trends in Parasitology* **17**, 558–563.

Richards, F., Hopkins, D. and Cupp, E. (2000). Commentary: varying programmatic goals and approaches to river blindness. *Lancet* **255**, 1663–1664.

Rougemont, A., Hien, M., Thylefors, B., Prost, A. and Rolland, A. (1984). Traitement de l'onchocercose par la suramin à faibles doses progressive dans les collectivités hyperendémiques d'Afrique occidentale. 2. Résultats cliniques, parasitologiques et opthalmologique en de transmission contrôlée. *Bulletin of the World Health Organization* **62**, 261–269.

Rougemont, A., Thylefors, B., Duncan, M., Prost, A. and Ranque, P.H. (1980). Traitement de l'onchocercose par la Suramin à faibles doses progressive dans les collectivités hyperendémiques d'Afrique occidentale. 1. Résultats parasitologique et surveillance opthalmologique en zone de transmission non interrompue. *Bulletin of the World Health Organization* **58**, 917–922.

Saint André, A., Blackwell, N.M., Hall, L.R., Hoerauf, A., Brattig, N.W., Volkmann, L., Taylor, M.J., Ford, L., Hise, A.G., Jonathan, H., Lass, J.H., Diaconu, E. and Pearlman, E. (2002). The role of endosymbiotic *Wolbachia* bacteria in the pathogenesis of river blindness. *Science* **295**, 1892–1895.

Shelley, A.J. (1988). Vector aspects of the epidemiology of onchocerciasis in Latin America. *Annual Review of Entomology* **33**, 337–366.

Stingl, P., Ross, M., Gibson, D.W., Ribas, J. and Connor, D.H. (1984). A diagnostic patch test for onchocerciasis using topical diethylcarbamazine. *Transactions of the Royal Society of Tropical Medicine and Hygiene* **78**, 254–258.

Taylor, H.R. and Green, B.M. (1989). The status of ivermectin in the treatment of human onchocerciasis. *American Journal of Tropical Medicine and Hygiene* **41**, 460–466.

Taylor, M.J., Bandi, C. and Hoerauf, A. (2005). *Wolbachia* bacterial endosymbionts of filarial nematodes. *Advances in Parasitology* **60**, 247–286.

Taylor, M.J. and Hoerauf, A. (1999). *Wolbachia* bacteria of filarial nematodes. *Parasitology Today* **15**, 437–442.

Thomson, M.C., Obsomer, V., Dunne, M., Connor, S.J. and Molyneux, D.H. (2000). Satellite mapping of *Loa loa* prevalence in relation to ivermectin use in west and central Africa. *Lancet* **356**, 1077–1078.

Thomson, M.C., Obsomer, V., Kamgno, J., Gardon, J., Samuel Wanji, S., Takougang, I., Enyong, P., Remme, J.H., Molyneux, D.H. and Boussinesq, M. (2004). Mapping the distribution of *Loa loa* in Cameroon in support of the African Programme for Onchocerciasis Control. *Filaria Journal* **3**, 7.

Thylefors, B. (2004). Eliminating onchocerciasis as a public health problem. *Tropical Medicine and International Health* **9** (supplement 4), A1–A3.

Thylefors, B., Negrel, A.D., Pararajasegaram, R. and Dadzie, K.Y. (1995). Global data on blindness. *Bulletin of the World Health Organization* **73**, 115–121.

Tielsch, J.M. and Beeche, A. (2004). Impact of ivermectin on illness and disability associated with onchocerciasis. *Tropical Medicine and International Health* **9** (supplement), A45–A56.

Trees, A.J., Graham, S.P., Renz, A., Bianco, A.E. and Tanya, V. (2000). *Onchocerca ochengi* infections in cattle as a model for human onchocerciasis: recent developments. *Parasitology* **120** (supplement), S133–S134.

Wanji, S., Tendongfor, N., Esum, M., Siker, S.J., Yundze, S.S.J., Taylor, M.J. and Enyong, P. (2005). Combined utilisation of rapid assessment procedures for loiasis (RAPLOA) and onchocerciasis (REA) in rain forest villages of Cameroon. *Filaria Journal* **4**, 2.

Waters, H.R., Rehwinkel, J.A. and Burnham, G. (2004). Economic evaluation of Mectizan distribution. *Tropical Medicine and International Health* **9** (supplement), A16–A25.

Weil, J., Steel, C., Liftis, F., Li, B.W., Mearns, G., Lobos, E. and Nutman, T.B. (2000). A rapid-format antibody card test for diagnosis of onchocerciasis. *Journal of Infectious Diseases* **182**, 1796–1799.

Whitworth, J.A.G., Gilbert, C.E., Mabey, D.M., Maude, G.H., Morgan, D. and Taylor, D.W. (1991). Effects of repeated doses of ivermectin on ocular onchocerciasis: community-based trial I, Sierra Leone. *Lancet* **ii**, 1100–1120.

Winnen, M., Plaisier, A.P., Alley, E.S., Nagelkerke, N.J.D., van Oortmarssen, G., Boatin, B.A. and Habbema, J.D.F. (2002). Can ivermectin mass treatments eliminate onchocerciasis in Africa? *Bulletin of the World Health Organization* **80**, 384–390.

World Health Organization (1987). *WHO expert committee on onchocerciasis: third report.* Technical Report Series No. 752. Geneva: WHO.

World Health Organization (1995a). *Expert committee on onchocerciasis control.* Technical Report Series No. 852. Geneva: WHO.

World Health Organization (1995b). *The importance of onchocercal skin disease: report of the Pan-African Study Group on onchocercal skin disease.* Document TDR/AFR/RP/95. Geneva: WHO.

World Health Organization (1997–1998). *The importance of onchocercal skin disease; report of the Pan-African Study Group on onchocercal skin disease.* Document TDR/AFR/RP/95.1 18. Geneva: WHO.

World Health Organization (2001). *Criteria for certification of interruption of transmission/elimination of human onchocerciasis.* Document WHO/CDS/CEE/2001.18a. Geneva: WHO.

World Health Organization (2002). River Blindness. *Weekly Epidemiological Bulletin* **77**, 249–256.

World Health Organization (2004). Onchocerciasis (river blindness). Report from the thirteenth InterAmerican Conference on Onchocerciasis, Cartagena de Indias, Colombia. *Weekly Epidemiological Record* **79**, 310–312.

Yaméogo, L., Toe, L., Hougard, J.M., Boatin, B.A. and Unnasch, T.R. (1999). Pool screen polymerase chain reaction for estimating the prevalence of *Onchocerca volvulus* infection in *Simulium damnosum sensu lato*: results of a field trial in an area subject to successful vector control. *American Journal of Tropical Medicine and Hygiene* **60**, 124–128.

Zea Flores, G. (1990). Situation of onchocerciasis in the Americas. *Acta Leidensia* **59**, 59–60.

Zimmerman, P.A., Guderian, R.H., Aruajo, E., Eslon, L., Kubofcik, J. and Nutman, T.B. (1994). Polymerase chain reaction-based diagnosis of *Onchocerca volvulus* infection: improved detection of patients with onchocerciasis. *Journal of Infectious Diseases* **169**, 686–689.

Lymphatic Filariasis: Treatment, Control and Elimination

Eric A. Ottesen

Lymphatic Filariasis Support Centre, The Task Force for Child Survival and Development, 750 Commerce Drive Decatur, GA 30030, USA

ABSTRACT

Lymphatic filariasis (LF) is a disease not just treatable or controllable; it is a disease that can be eliminated. Indeed, LF is currently the target of a major global initiative to do just that; a few visionaries of the past 50 years did hypothesize that LF elimination was feasible. However, for most of the scientific and global health

ADVANCES IN PARASITOLOGY VOL 61
ISSN: 0065-308X
DOI: 10.1016/S0065-308X(05)61010-X

"

communities, the elimination of such a broadly disseminated, mosquito-borne disease has seemed highly unlikely. During the past decade, however, both the treatment strategies and the control strategies for LF have undergone profound paradigm shifts—all because of a rapid increase in knowledge and understanding of LF that derived directly from a series of remarkable achievements by the scientific and medical research communities. As a result, a public health dimension with a focus on affected populations, now supplements the earlier, predominantly patient-oriented clinical approach to LF. The early uncertainties, then the essential steps leading to this change in outlook are outlined below, followed by descriptions of the new strategy for LF elimination, the Global Programme created to attain this goal and the successes achieved to date.

1. SETTING THE STAGE FOR THE ELIMINATION OF LYMPHATIC FILARIASIS

1.1. Recognizing the Barriers/Challenges to LF Elimination

1.1.1. Biological Barriers Imposed by the Parasite

(a) *Scope of the infection.* The term lymphatic filariasis (LF) denotes infection with any of three different species of filarial parasites—*Wuchereria bancrofti, Brugia malayi and B. timori.* The mere scope and distribution of LF infection provides an enormous challenge to its elimination. Over 120 million people in at least 80 countries throughout the tropics and sub-tropics (Figure 1) are affected by LF, and more than 1 billion people live in areas where they are at risk of acquiring infection (Ottesen *et al.*, 1997). Of these infections 90% are caused by *W. bancrofti*; most of the remaining, by *B. malayi.*

(b) *Vectors.* Mosquito vectors are essential for the life cycle of LF parasites (Figure 2) and the diversity of the vector species provides an additional challenge for efforts to eliminate LF. The major vectors for *W. bancrofti* are culicine mosquitoes in most urban and

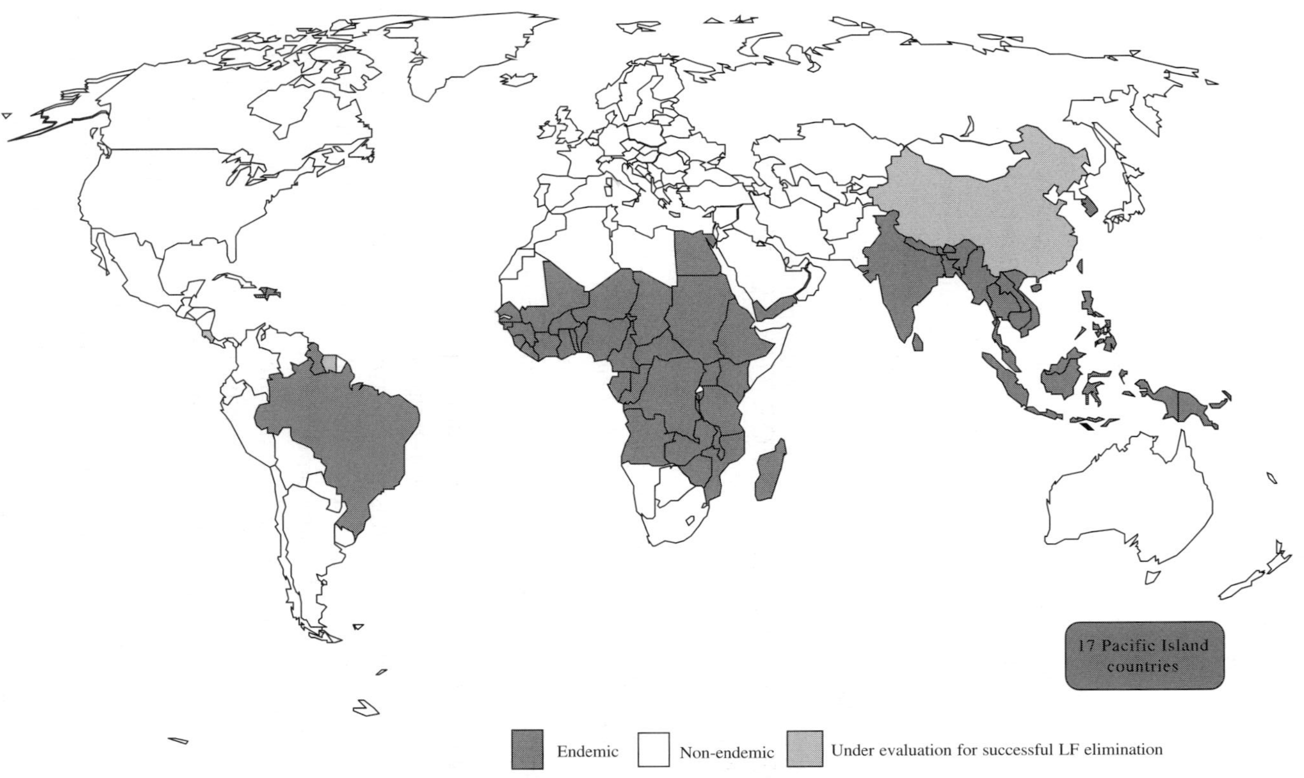

Figure 1 Lymphatic filariasis endemic countries (http://www.filariasis.org).

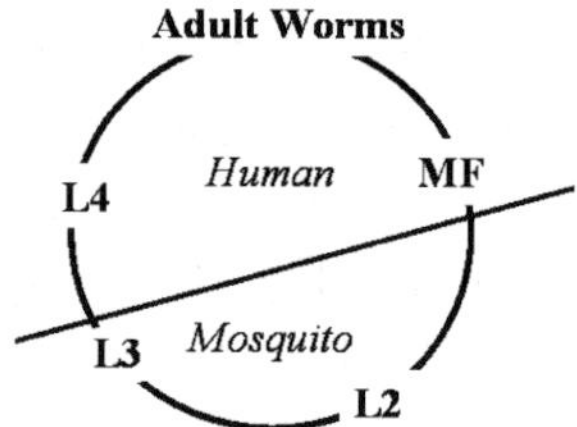

Figure 2 Life cycle of lymphatic filarial parasites. Developmental stages in the vector last approximately 2–4 weeks (depending on environmental conditions). After humans are infected by the mosquito-borne 3rd stage larvae, development through two molts to the fecund adult stage lasts approximately 6–12 months. The life span of the adult is estimated at 4–6 years during which millions of microfilariae (MF) are produced, each with a life span of an estimated 12 months (Sasa, 1976).

semi-urban areas, anopheline mosquitoes in the more rural areas of Africa and elsewhere, and *Aedes* species in many of the endemic Pacific islands (Sasa, 1976). For the *Brugia* parasites, *Mansonia* species serve as the major vectors, but in some areas anopheline mosquitoes are responsible for transmitting infection as well (Sasa, 1976). The fact that so many different species of mosquitoes (each with its distinctive biological behaviour) are responsible for transmitting LF makes very much greater the challenge of developing effective vector-control strategies to eliminate the spread of these infections.

(c) *Parasite life span.* The fecund life span of the parasite's adult stage is generally estimated at 4–8 years (Michael *et al.*, 2004). Since this is the stage producing the microfilariae (MF) responsible for transmission, its longevity provides another significant challenge to LF elimination. In addition, since the duration of the developmental phase from infective larva to mature adult is estimated at 6–12 months, there is necessarily a long 'diagnostic lag' between the time one is infected and the time when the infection can be detected, either parasitologically or by detecting circulating filarial antigen.

(d) *Microfilaraemia.* Microfilaraemia, which is obviously essential for the transmission of LF (Figure 2), has its own biological peculiarities that provide special challenges to LF elimination. First, not all infected individuals are microfilaraemic; many have active infection with living adult parasites, but with no MF circulating in the blood (Beaver, 1970); such individuals provide a significant challenge for diagnosing LF. Second, there is the problem of microfilarial 'periodicity'. Nocturnal periodicity (MF circulating in the blood only during the few hours on either side of midnight) is a feature of LF infection essentially everywhere in the world except for some regions of the Pacific and South Asia, where sub-periodic infections (MF present in the blood for most of the day, often peaking in late afternoon) are found (Sasa, 1976). Such microfilarial periodicity has, in the past, been an enormous practical barrier both to diagnosing the infection and to understanding its distribution.

1.1.2. Social and Political Barriers to LF Elimination

The very lack of attention paid to LF has in the past been a significant barrier to efforts to control or eliminate this infection. Three principal reasons account for this lack of attention:

(1) *The true impact of the infection/disease is not well understood.* One important reason for this lack of understanding is that LF has been understudied, largely because the available diagnostic and investigative tools were so poor, but also because the disease itself is hidden from view—as a disease of poor, isolated populations and as a disease whose principal clinical manifestations [elephantiasis and genital disease (hydrocele)] are 'covered up' because of the personal shame and stigma they engender (Krishna *et al.*, 2005). Not only has this 'hiddenness' prevented full appreciation of both the scope and impact of the infection in adults, but it has also inhibited the recognition that in many individuals, and perhaps especially in children (Witt and Ottesen, 2001), LF is a progressive sub-clinical disease [see Section 1.2.3(a)]. Even more challenging has been establishing links between this "hidden" infection and the economic and social burden it exacts on affected communities (Ramaiah *et al.*, 2000).

(2) *Those affected are the poorest of society and, therefore, politically voiceless.* The weakness or complete lack of any political constituency, except for a few notable exceptions, has led either to a total neglect of LF by national health authorities or, at the least, to its being ranked inappropriately low among national health problems.

(3) *The disease is generally not fatal.* Thus, there is decreased awareness of the degree of its endemicity and of the impact that chronic debilitation from LF [the second leading cause of permanent, long-term disability worldwide (World Health Organization, 1995)] has on endemic communities.

1.2. Reasons for Optimism about the Feasibility of Eliminating LF

The barriers or challenges to LF elimination are formidable, but there are many factors favouring potential success as well. While there is no single attribute or feature of an infectious disease that determines whether or not it is 'eliminatable' (Ottesen *et al.*, 1998), and while technical considerations actually play a more significant role than the biological ones (see below), for LF both are highly favourable (Centres for Disease Control, 1993).

1.2.1. Biological Features of LF that Favour its Elimination

(a) The single most important biological attribute favouring successful elimination of any infectious disease is that humans are essential for the organism's 'life cycle', i.e., the organism does not multiply freely in the environment and has no significant non-human vertebrate host serving as a reservoir of infection (Ottesen *et al.*, 1998). For Bancroftian filariasis (accounting for 90% of LF infections) there is no non-human host. Even for *Brugia* infections, where a number of other animal species (particularly felines and monkeys) may also harbour the less-common, sub-periodic parasite strains of *B. malayi*, it is not clear that there is any significant epidemiologic overlap between the cycles of *Brugia* infection in human and non-human hosts.

(b) The fact that the life cycle of LF parasites requires a vector mosquito gives a second potential target (in addition to the infection in humans) for interventions to interrupt LF transmission. Since transmission obviously requires host–vector contact, efforts to decrease this contact through vector control may well be very helpful for LF elimination (Sasa, 1976), and perhaps in some cases, even essential (Burkot and Ichimori, 2002).

(c) Other biological attributes of LF parasites also promote their 'eliminatability' by decreasing their "force of infection". These include the fact that the adult worms do not multiply in the human host (i.e., infections only expand through acquisition of additional new infection), nor does the infection amplify itself within the vector (in contrast, e.g., to schistosomiasis, malaria and others). Also, for whatever reason, people do not appear to acquire LF infection after a single (or even multiple) mosquito bites; rather, epidemiological observations suggest that a minimum of 3–6 months of exposure (Wartman, 1947) and many vector mosquito bites (Gubler and Bhattacharya, 1974) are required before infection actually develops.

1.2.2. Social (Historical) Considerations

Possibly, the most significant reason for optimism about the feasibility of eliminating LF is the fact that such elimination has already been achieved in a number of different settings and with a number of different strategies! (Laigret *et al.*, 1966). Active programmes based on mass and/or targeted chemotherapy with diethylcarbamazine (DEC) have eliminated Bancroftian filariasis from Japan (Sasa, 1976), Trinidad (Rawlins *et al.*, 2004), most areas of Brazil (Schlemper *et al.*, 2000) and essentially all of China (The Editorial Board of Control of Lymphatic Filariasis in China, 2003). In addition, vector control alone (through targeting the anophelines in an effort to control malaria) actually eliminated Bancroftian filariasis from the Solomon Islands, since transmission of LF there was maintained by the same anophelines vectors (Webber, 1975). Finally, numerous instances are also recorded where social, civic and environmental development (with improved sanitation and consequent decrease in vector exposure) has resulted in the concomitant disappearance of LF from previously endemic areas [e.g., in the Southeastern United States (Chernin, 1987), in Northeastern Australia (Sprent, 1986) and elsewhere].

1.2.3. Technical Considerations: The Availability of Effective Tools (for Treatment, for Diagnosis)

What most clearly distinguishes eliminatable from non-eliminatable diseases is not so much a particular biological property of the infection itself but, rather, having the appropriate tools both to treat it effectively and to detect (diagnose) any incidence of infection or re-infection (Ottesen *et al.*, 1998). Indeed, it was the development of such tools for effective treatment and diagnosis of LF that has spurred all of the activity of the past decade towards creating a global initiative to eliminate LF.

(a) *Treatment tools.* To interrupt transmission of LF it is necessary either to eliminate (or reduce to very low levels) the microfilaraemia in humans or to achieve effective control of the mosquito vector (Figure 2). Since efforts at vector control have proven expensive, difficult to sustain and often ineffective in the past, and since drugs for very effective control of microfilaraemia are now available (Gyapong *et al.*, 2005), the focus of efforts to interrupt transmission has shifted from the earlier attempts at vector control, now to treating infections in humans.

Two dramatic advances in the understanding of how best to use the available antifilarial drugs changed the entire approach to controlling LF (Gyapong *et al.*, 2005). The first was the recognition that single doses of any of the three antifilarial drugs were very effective at reducing microfilaraemias for extended periods (up to 12 months for DEC, ivermectin and albendazole; Figure 3). The second was the discovery that single administrations of a combination of any two of these drugs given together were significantly more effective for the long-term reduction of microfilaraemia than any of the drugs given alone. All three drugs have different modes of action and while none is completely effective in killing adult worms or inhibiting MF production by them, still microfilaraemia can be reduced for very long periods (1 year or more) by these single-dose, two-drug treatment regimens (Figure 4).

For the disease manifestations of affected individuals new therapeutic tools and management techniques have also been developed in recent years—largely as a result of the increased understanding of

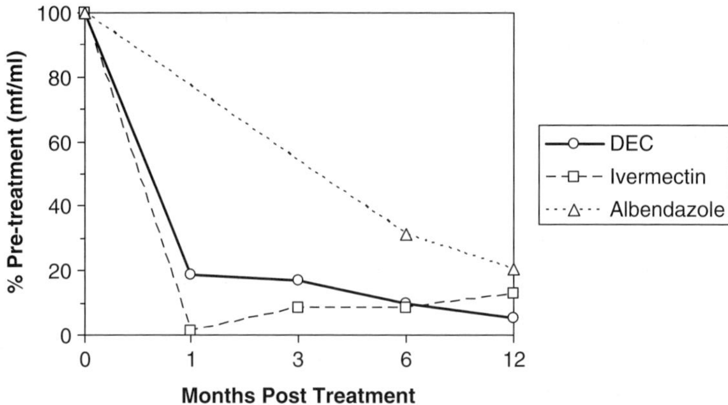

Figure 3 Effect of single doses of DEC (6 mg/kg; circles), ivermectin (200 μg/kg; squares) and albendazole (400 mg; triangles) in decreasing levels of microfilaraemia in *W. bancrofti* infections. (Redrawn from Gyapong *et al.*, 2005.)

LF's pathogenesis. Use of lymphoscintigraphy and ultrasonography techniques confirmed that sub-clinical, asymptomatic dilation and progressive functional incompetence of the lymphatics were induced by adult LF parasites (reviewed by Ottesen, 1994). However, since it is the recurrent inflammatory episodes (earlier termed 'filarial fevers') that are principally responsible for determining the progression of patients from an asymptomatic state to clinically manifesting lymph-oedema and then elephantiasis (Dreyer *et al.*, 2000), when the cause of the inflammatory responses was recognized to be principally bac-terial superinfection of these tissues with compromised lymphatic function (Olszewski *et al.*, 1997; Dreyer *et al.*, 2000), it became clear that the use of antibiotics to treat (and sometimes to prevent) these episodes was essential, as were aggressive washing and other hygiene management techniques. Such approaches to lymphoedema manage-ment have yielded excellent results (Olszewski *et al.*, 1997; Dreyer *et al.*, 2002). For hydrocele, the principal management tool remains surgery; but when the scrotal skin is involved with lymphoedema, the same management principles as those used for lymphoedema of the arms or legs also apply (Dreyer *et al.*, 2002).

(b) *Diagnostic tools.* Developing a sensitive, specific and user-friendly diagnostic for active infections has been a *sine qua non* for

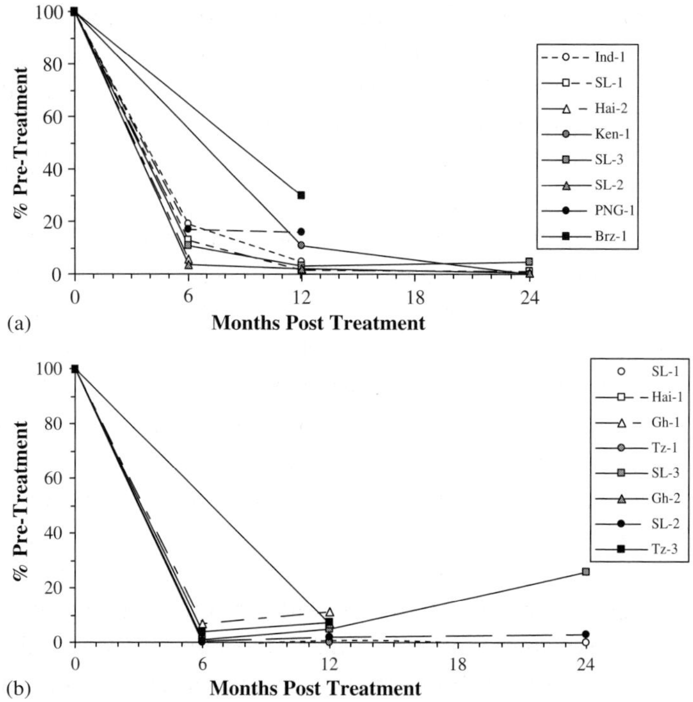

Figure 4 (a) Effect of a single dose of co-administered albendazole (400 mg) and DEC (6 mg/kg) on levels of microfilaraemia in *W. bancrofti* infections at eight study sites (*n* = 13–86 patients per group; median = 22) (Gyapong *et al.*, 2005). (b) Effect of a single dose of co-administered albendazole (400 mg) and ivermectin (200 µg/kg) on levels of microfilaraemia in *W. bancrofti* infections at eight study sites (*n* = 12–148 patients per group; median = 36) (Gyapong *et al.*, 2005).

creating the Global Programme to Eliminate LF (GPELF). Until the very effective antigen-detection techniques were devised (Weil *et al.*, 1997), LF diagnosis required laborious microscopic detection of MF in blood specimens; and to make matters still more cumbersome, the blood had to be collected at a time (generally around midnight) to allow for the parasite's microfilarial periodicity [see Section 1.1.1(d)]. With such a tool, it was difficult to diagnose even individual cases of LF, much less to consider the assessment of whole populations that might be at risk. However, the development of antigen detection assays [with their later refinement into a field-friendly card format requiring only a finger-prick specimen of blood taken at any time of day (Weil *et al.*, 1997)] changed all that. LF went from having one of the poorest, most cumbersome diagnostics for any parasite infection to having perhaps the best. Indeed, the antigen-detection test's only 'drawback' is its specificity—detecting only Bancroftian filarial infections (90% of all LF infections), but not those caused by *Brugia* species. For these latter infections (as well as for identifying any LF infection in mosquitoes) techniques for DNA detection by PCR are available (Zhong *et al.*, 1996; Williams *et al.*, 2002), though they have not yet been utilized on a public health scale in the field. Similarly, an IgG4-based antibody assay for detecting active *Brugia* infections is under evaluation (Rahmah *et al.*, 2003), again because there is still no antigen detection assay for these infections.

Another diagnostic tool, now increasingly needed for the assessment of long-term programme effectiveness, is an assay not just detecting active infection (as antigen and PCR assays do) but one looking to detect even exposure to infection and that can be used for monitoring and surveillance of areas thought to be freed of LF transmission. IgG4 antibody assays utilizing highly specific recombinant antigens have been recently developed for this purpose and are currently being tested for their practical usefulness to meet such a need (Lammie *et al.*, 2004).

Though not yet having a ready use in field settings, one of the most significant advances in diagnostic techniques for LF has been the use of ultrasound to detect living adult worms in both patent (MF-producing) and non-patent infections (Amaral *et al.*, 1994). Not only has this tool been important in improving our understanding of the pathogenesis of the lymphatic damage in LF, it has also allowed direct observation of therapeutic drug effects on adult worms (Dreyer *et al.*, 1995), a capability essential for the further development or optimization of LF treatment regimens.

1.2.4. A Promising Strategy to Eliminate LF

Because of the new intervention and diagnostic tools available and the new understandings of disease pathogenesis, a new strategy for

LF elimination could be formulated (Ottesen *et al.*, 1997). The strategy has two essential components: first, stopping the spread of infection (i.e., interrupting transmission); second, alleviating the suffering of affected individuals (i.e., controlling morbidity).

(a) *Interrupting LF transmission.* As already indicated, current efforts towards interrupting transmission (Figure 2) are focused on MF reduction in the human host. Two different single-dose, two-drug treatment regimens have been shown to be extremely effective in reducing blood microfilarial levels by more than 90% for periods up to 1 year and beyond (Gyapong *et al.*, 2005) (Figure 4). These are:

- Albendazole (400 mg) plus DEC (6 mg/kg)
- Albendazole (400 mg) plus ivermectin (200 μg/kg).

Extensive safety and pharmacokinetic studies have shown that these drugs at these dosages are safe and essentially without side effects when administered alone or together to individuals who are not microfilaraemic (Horton *et al.*, 2000). In patients with LF microfilaraemia, side reactions do occur as a result of rapid MF killing by the microfilaricidal action of either DEC or ivermectin, but the side reactions are essentially identical to those described previously in the treatment of LF with these single drugs alone (Ottesen, 1987; Horton *et al.*, 2000); they are most prominent in the most heavily infected individuals, but can be safely managed in both clinic and field situations. The addition of albendazole, whose action is principally on adult-stage parasites, to either DEC or ivermectin does not increase the frequency or severity of adverse reactions seen in microfilaraemic individuals (Horton *et al.*, 2000).

Because, DEC can induce severe, unacceptable reactions in patients with onchocerciasis, LF-endemic communities where onchocerciasis may be co-endemic are treated only with the albendazole-plus-ivermectin regimen. Outside of the onchocerciasis-endemic areas, the recommended two-drug treatment regimen is albendazole-plus-DEC (Ottesen, 2000).

To interrupt transmission in an endemic community, the 'community microfilarial load' must be reduced below that necessary to sustain transmission and for a period long enough to exceed the effective fecund (i.e., MF-producing) life span of the adult parasites. Unfortunately, the precise value of neither of these figures is known for certain, but it has been estimated that a period of 4–6 years during which MF are absent or at very low levels in a community will be sufficient to break transmission. Mathematical modelling generally supports such estimates (Stolk *et al.*, 2003), but only if population 'compliance' in taking the MF-reducing drug regimens approximates 80% and if the 'non-compliers' are randomly distributed. It is also clear from these models that greater efficacy of the drug combinations, higher drug 'coverage' in the treated populations and lower initial prevalences of LF, all will lead to fewer rounds of mass drug administration (MDA) required to interrupt transmission (Stolk *et al.*, 2003; Michael *et al.*, 2004).

Based on all these considerations, the strategy formulated to interrupt LF transmission through microfilarial reduction by this intermittent drug treatment calls for use of either of the two drug regimens (albendazole + DEC or albendazole + ivermectin) once yearly to achieve 4–6 rounds of high-coverage MDA to all endemic and at-risk communities.

An alternative (and already proven effective) MDA strategy for reducing MF to interrupt transmission is to substitute regular table/ cooking salt with DEC-fortified salt (Houston, 2000). Though used widely in China's national Filariasis Elimination Programme (The Editorial Board of Control of Lymphatic Filariasis in China, 2003), elsewhere it has been employed principally in demonstration projects, where its effectiveness, based on treatment for periods ranging from 18 days to 1 year, has been documented (Houston, 2000). Current WHO guidelines suggest that the DEC-fortified salt strategy can be used to interrupt transmission if applied to endemic communities for a period of 1–2 years (World Health Organization, 2000). This approach is currently being selected by very few countries, and its most valuable role might eventually prove to be as an adjunct or supplement for treating residual microfilaraemia in MDA programmes using DEC (tablets)-plus albendazole after the yearly two-drug MDAs have finished.

Vector reduction, too, remains a potentially valuable strategic adjunct for interrupting transmission, especially when used in conjunction with two-drug MDA programmes (Reuben *et al.*, 2001). Though a strategic plan for employing vector control routinely in LF elimination programmes has not yet been formulated, research studies have clearly demonstrated the remarkable value of bednets (insecticide treated and not treated) (Bockarie *et al.*, 2002; Pedersen and Mukoko, 2002), residual spraying (Webber, 1975) and use of polystyrene beads (Curtis *et al.*, 2002) for source reduction, depending on the different mosquito species involved. Because there is no specific agreed strategy for the use of vector control to interrupt the transmission of LF, current recommendations call only for the use of such techniques to supplement the MDA activities whenever feasible and affordable (World Health Organization, 2000).

(b) *Alleviating the suffering caused by LF disease.* While all of the clinical manifestations of LF (including chyluria, nephropathy, tropical pulmonary eosinophilia and others) cause suffering that needs to be alleviated (Ottesen, 2004), the public health strategies for addressing the problems of LF disease focus on its three principal clinical manifestations—lymphoedema/elephantiasis, acute inflammatory episodes and hydrocele.

Lymphoedema/elephantiasis. Care of lymphoedema in filariasis endemic areas is, as it should be, very similar to the care of lymphoedema elsewhere. Because avoidance of secondary bacterial infection is essential to prevent worsening lymphoedema or its progression to elephantiasis, the cornerstone of all lymphoedema management should be a strong focus on hygiene, skin care [with detection, treatment and prevention of 'entry lesions' (McPherson *et al.*, 2006)], appropriate footwear and elevation of the affected limb; prophylactic antibiotics may be indicated for some patients (Dreyer *et al.*, 2002). These measures may be augmented by others (e.g., compressive bandages or garments and physical lymphatic drainage techniques in countries with more highly developed health care options), but the most important elements of lymphoedema management can be carried out very appropriately even in resource-constrained environments and, particularly importantly, by the affected individual or by minimally trained, 'informal caregivers'

(Vaqas and Ryan, 2003; Addiss and Brady, 2005). Thus, the goal of lymphoedema management on a public health scale is home-based self-care. To achieve this goal requires means for (1) identifying and bringing patients to treatment, (2) educating patients and family members on the principles and practice of lymphoedema self-care, (3) encouraging and supporting sustainable self-care and (4) providing referral networks for acutely infected or complicated patients (Addiss and Brady, 2005).

Acute inflammatory episodes: acute dermatolymphangioadenitis (ADLA). The majority of acute inflammatory reactions seen in LF patients are induced by secondary bacterial infections in skin whose underlying lymphatic function is compromised and which frequently is lymphoedematous; only a small percentage of such reactions are induced by immune responses to dying adult worms in lymph nodes and lymphatic vessels (Dreyer *et al.*, 2000). The management of these ADLA episodes (which usually last 4–8 days) is, therefore, similar to that for erysipelas in parts of the world not endemic for LF; namely, rest, cooling the affected area to relieve pain, analgesics, antipyretics, elevation of the affected limb and systemic antibiotics (Dreyer *et al.*, 2002). Since prevention of such episodes is the goal, their management on a public health scale should rely not primarily on active involvement of the formal health-delivery system but (as for lymphoedema management) on self-care or on informal caregivers from the community, except for those severe cases where further referral will be necessary (Addiss and Brady, 2005).

Hydrocele. The treatment for hydrocele is surgery, and if properly carried out, it is curative. Techniques such as recurrent aspiration of the hydrocele fluid or injection of sclerosing substances are not only less effective but also may have unacceptable side effects. Therefore, the public health strategy to alleviate the suffering from LF-associated hydrocele is to provide access to surgery to as many of those needing it as possible (World Health Organization, 2000).

To be sure, not all LF genital lesions termed 'hydrocele' are simply that (Addiss and Brady, 2005). Rupture of lymphatic vessels inside the scrotal cavity can introduce lymph and red blood cells into the otherwise 'transudate fluid' of a hydrocele. The pathogenic implications of this lymph-contaminated hydrocele fluids have not been fully delineated, but it has been speculated to cause more severe clinical consequences in patients, both with and without surgery. Since the public health approach to 'hydrocele' does require direct involvement of the formal health-delivery system (for its surgical expertise), effective triaging of patients is necessary to ensure appropriate management of simple hydrocele, complicated hydrocele, lymph–scrotum and other 'genital' conditions (including hernias) presenting as hydrocele. Such clinical distinctions will only be possible once the clinical definitions and therapeutic implications have been instilled in the health system personnel through education and training (Addiss and Brady, 2005).

2. TURNING POTENTIAL INTO REALITY: THE GLOBAL PROGRAMME TO ELIMINATE LF

The Global Programme to Eliminate LF came to life unexpectedly, almost spontaneously. Critical scientific advances were made one after another but generally independently, and then as these came together, a concept, goal and vision developed that subsequently attracted resources, partnerships of interested organizations and finally a political concern and determination that led to the birth of a Global Programme (Ottesen *et al.*, 1997; Ottesen, 2000).

2.1. 'Drivers' of the Programme

2.1.1. Scientific Underpinning

As indicated (Section 1.2), it was the scientific advance in diagnostics, therapeutics and strategic thinking, linked with a history of earlier successes in eliminating LF from a number of countries, which provided the science base for developing the Global Programme.

(a) *Diagnostics.* For filariasis control to become effective as a public health measure, microfilarial detection had to be replaced as the principal diagnostic. For Bancroftian filariasis two remarkably effective antigen detection tests were developed [immunochromatographic test

(ICT) and enzyme-linked immunosorbent assay (ELISA); Weil *et al.*, 1997] plus an effective parasite DNA-detection PCR assay (Zhong *et al.*, 1996) that could be used with human blood specimens collected on filter paper. Though each of these diagnostic tools is highly effective, in practice what has been utilized by the Global Programme almost exclusively to 'map' the distribution of LF by detecting infected populations has been the ICT. Its format as a card test using finger-prick blood and yielding answers within 10 minutes has made it the preferred diagnostic for LF mapping worldwide (e.g., Gyapong *et al.*, 2002; Eigege *et al.*, 2003) and, in some instances, for monitoring the effects of treatment as well (Fraser *et al.*, 2005).

For Brugian filariasis, the story has not been so straightforward. Many efforts at creating an antigen-detection test were unsuccessful, and the highly sensitive, specific PCR test to identify parasite DNA in finger-prick blood specimens that works so well in the laboratory (Lizotte *et al.*, 1994) has just never been broadly employed as a field diagnostic. Instead, efforts have been focused on utilizing an antibody assay based on detecting IgG4 antibodies, the sub-class of IgG responses that reflects chronic antigenic stimulation and therefore most likely to be associated with active infection. While one candidate IgG4 assay does show promise for use as a diagnostic to map Brugian infections, it is still being assessed for practical usefulness in the Global Programme (Rahmah *et al.*, 2003).

For both Brugian and Bancroftian filariasis, the new 'pathology diagnostics' based on ultrasound and lymphoscintigraphy have proven to be important adjuncts both in the clinical assessment of patient disease (Amaral *et al.*, 1994; Freedman *et al.*, 1994) and in the development and monitoring of patient management (e.g., Dreyer *et al.*, 1995, 2001).

(b) *Therapeutics.* Extensive studies (see Section 1.2.3) of the safety and effectiveness of the two-drug treatment regimens for decreasing microfilaraemia in both Brugian and Bancroftian infections led to the recommendations for their being administered to affected populations once yearly to interrupt LF transmission. Such a strategy of decreasing microfilaraemia in populations through mass drug treatment has proven successful elsewhere (Schlemper *et al.*, 2000; The Editorial Board of Control of Lymphatic Filariasis in China, 2003; Rawlins *et al.*, 2004), and predictions from mathematical models suggest that the current strategy can be successful if programmes can maintain adequate levels of population 'compliance' for a period of at least 4–6 years (Stolk *et al.*, 2003; Michael *et al.*, 2004). The two-drug regimen should be albendazole (400 mg) + ivermectin (200 µg/kg) in areas where onchocerciasis may be co-endemic with LF, and it should be albendazole (400 mg) + DEC (6 mg/kg) elsewhere in the world. The effectiveness of these regimens and this strategy is currently being documented in programmes from many parts of the world (see Section 2.2.2).

The approach to disease management described above (hygiene, antisepsis and physical measures for lymphoedema and elephantiasis; surgery for hydrocele) are based on an increased understanding of the pathogenesis of filarial disease (Dreyer *et al.*, 2000, 2002). The success achieved by such therapeutic measures is increasingly being documented both in programmes and in programmatic study settings where they have been employed (World Health Organization, 2004b).

2.1.2. Resources

A strong science base has been essential for developing the GPELF, but without resources no Programme could have been established. The most important (non-personnel) resources enabling the Programme have been the enormous drug donations and the essential implementation funds.

(a) *Pharmaceutical donations.* Just as the principal strategy of global immunization programmes relies on distribution of vaccines to at-risk populations, the principal strategy of the GPELF relies on the distribution of drugs to at-risk populations. The drug needs for the GPELF are enormous, given that all 1.2 billion people at risk of LF infection are expected to receive a regimen of two drugs once yearly for a period of at least 4–6 years (Ottesen, 2000). Albendazole is required for all of these at-risk individuals, ivermectin for approximately 1/3 of them (in the onchocerciasis-endemic countries of Africa and Yemen) and DEC in the remaining 2/3. Clearly, without availability of these drugs there would be no GPELF!

To meet these needs, two pharmaceutical companies, GlaxoSmith-Kline and Merck & Company, Inc., have pledged the most remarkable, largest drug donations ever made to help the developing world. In 1998, GlaxoSmithKline pledged to the World Health Organization a donation of as much albendazole as would be needed to achieve the goals of the Global Programme, as well as additional measures of support for the programme itself (Molyneux and Zagaria, 2002). That same year Merck & Company, Inc. agreed to expand its original donation of ivermectin (Mectizan) for onchocerciasis control to include all those countries (principally in Africa), where LF and onchocerciasis overlap (Colatrella, 2003). This expanded donation represents a 10-fold increase of their original 1987 donation of Mectizan for onchocerciasis. Together these unprecedented donations by GlaxoSmithKline and Merck & Company, Inc. hold the potential for extraordinary health benefits for an enormous number of people worldwide, among whom are the very poorest populations anywhere. The value of these donations must be calculated literally in billions of dollars.

(b) *Implementation funds*. It is necessary, but not sufficient to have the drugs and strategies needed to overcome LF in endemic populations; there must also be funds to help implement the programmes. While some endemic countries are able to fund programme implementation themselves, most must rely (particularly in the initial phases) on external support. At the Programme's inception one foundation (the Arab Fund for Economic and Social Development) and two national development agencies (from the United Kingdom and Japan) provided the funds necessary for programme initiation in selected countries. Soon thereafter a donation from the Bill and Melinda Gates Foundation became a main driver of programme implementation, along with other important support from a number of additional bilateral development agencies and non-governmental organizations [see (http://www.filariasis.org)].

2.1.3. Political Will and Partnership

The science and the resources are the 'things' essential for a Global Programme, but it is 'people' who must utilize these things wisely to establish an effective programme. Partnerships with agreed goals and defined roles must be formed, and political will to support and champion these national programmes must be established.

The most important fillip in transforming the Global Programme from simply a visionary concept to an acceptable political goal was the Resolution by the World Health Assembly in 1997 calling for member states to eliminate LF as a public health problem and for the Director General of the World Health Organization to facilitate efforts to achieve this goal (www.filariasis.org). The Resolution was formulated in response to the remarkable set of scientific advances that preceded it and to recognition of the extraordinary potential that such a Programme would have for improving the lives of so many people worldwide. Its acceptance by all member nations of the World Health Assembly meant that efforts towards developing the Global Programme could then shift to focus more on challenges of implementation than on the challenge of determining whether such national programmes should be established or not.

The development of a global health programme of such magnitude requires very large number of individuals and organizations to work together effectively. Extremely important in the development of the GPELF was the bringing together of organizations (NGOs, international agencies, scientific institutions, academic organizations) in advance of the Programme launch, in order to identify roles, responsibilities and contributions best suited for each organization. These commitments by the partner organizations were captured in an agreed strategic plan for the Global Programme that recognized the essentialness of building effective partnerships to ensure programmatic success (World Health Organization, 1999).

Just as important as the political will embodied in the World Health Assembly Resolution and the partnership of supporting organizations has been the engagement of the endemic country Ministries of Health (MOH) for actually undertaking national LF elimination programmes. Without question, MOH in all LF-endemic countries are greatly challenged by an enormous array of often competing needs and always insufficient resources. Given that LF is a non-fatal disease and that it is most prevalent in the poorest, most politically voiceless sectors of society, MOH decision-makers have frequently ascribed LF a priority lower than many other conditions. Once national programmes began, however, it became clear that for a very small investment, enormous good could be brought to very large segments of the population; furthermore, the donated medications (albendazole and ivermectin) proved to be extremely popular in these populations because of their immediate de-worming and other health benefits (Stephenson *et al.*, 2000). When programmes are popular with people, they become popular with politicians, and when they are popular with politicians, they are much more effectively implemented. Indeed, recent evaluation of the economic contributions of different partners has made it clear that the MOH (stimulated by programme effectiveness and popularity) voluntarily contribute very significantly to the costs of implementation of these national programmes (e.g., Ramzy *et al.*, 2005).

2.1.4. Management

As important as any other driver of GPELF success have been programme management and oversight. Establishing an appropriate framework proved to be particularly challenging for the GPELF, but finally a very effective Global Alliance of all partner organizations has been created as a means of generating support for the Global Programme, which is coordinated principally by WHO [see (www. filariasis.org)]. The *Programme's* principal functions are setting guidelines, supporting all aspects of implementation and assessing outcomes of the national programmes, while members of the *Global Alliance* contribute not only to programme implementation but also to problem solving, technical support and fundraising in support of the Global Programme. General guidelines for programme implementation are developed by WHO and its Technical Advisory Group, but then modified as appropriate by national programme managers who work together in regional coordinating bodies, the Regional Programme Review Groups. Data are compiled at the National, Regional and Global levels. This new management framework, in effect only since 2004 (www.filariasis.org), takes advantage of the contributions and comparative advantages of each of the partners to contribute to a Global Programme that is coordinated centrally but with principal oversight at the Regional and National levels.

2.2. Achievements of the Global Programme: 1999–2005

2.2.1. Scope of Programme Implementation

(a) *Mapping the distribution of LF worldwide* has been one of the great challenges and achievements of the Global Programme to date. It was the extraordinarily cumbersome nature of the only diagnostic test available (i.e., microscopic identification of MF in blood) prior to the development of the antigen detection assays that resulted in few health workers having sufficient motivation to undertake studies to define the geographic distribution of LF; consequently little was known about it. The GPELF, using the ICT antigen detection technique to assess populations at risk (i.e., those defined operationally as having an antigen prevalence $>1\%$), developed specific, population-based protocols for mapping the distribution of *W. bancrofti* LF and then trained and supported national mapping efforts (e.g., Gyapong *et al.*, 2002; Eigege *et al.*, 2003; Onapa *et al.*, 2005). The result has been a rapid, phased mapping strategy that should see the completion of mapping in 66 countries by the end of 2005 and in all 83 endemic countries 1 year later (www.filariasis.org). These maps are generally not prevalence maps, as the sampling techniques being used are designed only to determine whether or not areas (Implementation units [IUs]) have an antigen prevalence (detected by ICT card tests) of $>1\%$. The size of the IU varies by country, but generally is in the order of the size of a health district.

(b) *Implementation of MDAs.* Only after the mapping of a country is complete (or at least well underway) are the MDA programmes to interrupt transmission generally undertaken.

MDAs are enormously complex, with elements of social mobilization at all levels, logistical planning, training, drug distribution and monitoring and evaluation of the total effort, its effectiveness and its cost-effectiveness. Some countries have employed a strategy of focusing efforts on a single yearly 'Filaria Day' or 'Filaria Week(s)'.

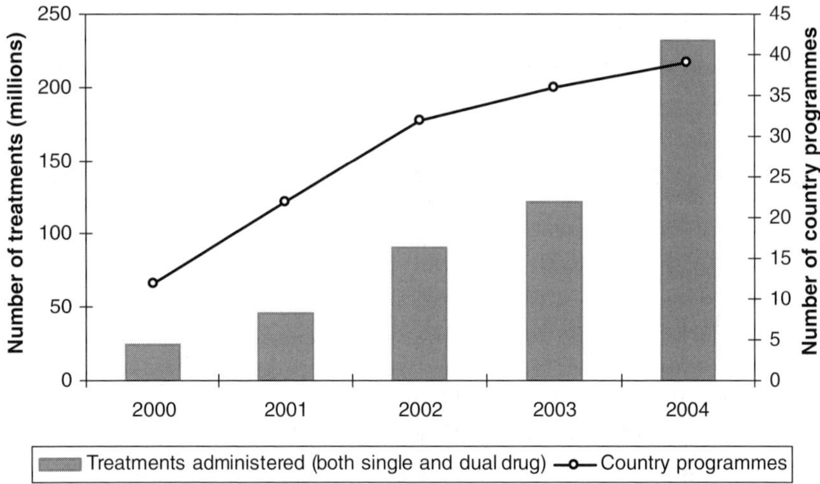

Figure 5 Progressive scaling-up of Global Programme to Eliminate LF. Line denotes number of countries with active LF elimination programmes and bars identify the number of treatments (one- and two-drug regimens) administered to at-risk populations.

Others have used the Community-Directed Treatment (COMDT) approach developed by the onchocerciasis control programmes (Katabarwa and Mutabazi, 2000), and still others have created locally appropriate variations on these themes. While there is no question but that MDAs utilizing Directly Observed Treatment are preferable to the alternatives, not all national programmes have been able to manage such approaches. Despite all this complexity, there has been progressive expansion of the number of countries initiating these MDAs, and by the end of 2004 there were 39 countries with active national programmes to eliminate LF (Figure 5).

Even more remarkable, however, is the number of people covered under these MDAs. Because India had earlier established an MDA programme using the single drug DEC alone, in 1999 there were already 12 million people being covered under antifilarial MDAs, but the expansion of this number over the next 5 years has been extraordinary. By the end of 2004, a total of 248 million people (Figure 5) were being reached through antifilarial MDAs [though 172 million of those still received only single-drug treatment with DEC, since India had not yet completely converted its MDA strategy to the more

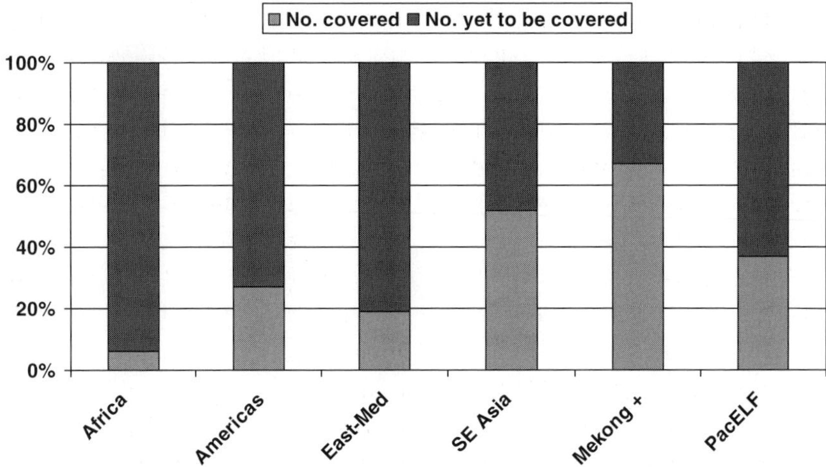

Figure 6   Proportion of at-risk populations reached by MDAs in each of the six regions of the GPELF.

effective two-drug regimen (World Health Organization, 2005a)]. Still, however, the up-scaling of these numbers has occurred at an extraordinary rate over the past 4 years—indeed, a rate unmatched by any other global health programme.

Despite the impressively broad scope of programme activities to date, it is still clear that 79% of the total 1.2 billion at-risk population remains unreached by any antifilarial MDAs (Figure 6), and only 6% are currently covered by two-drug-regimen MDAs (World Health Organization, 2005a). Unfortunately, further ramping up of programme activities is now constrained principally by insufficient financial resources (see Section 2.4), but the Programme's target still remains focused on reaching all of the at-risk populations by 2010.

2.2.2. Impact on LF Transmission and Disease

(a) *Transmission.* At the end stages of national programmes, transmission will be assessed by using antibody assays to determine potential LF exposure of children born after the MDAs began (Lammie *et al.*, 2004). Monitoring for effects on transmission during the MDA phase of the programme relies principally on assessing microfilaraemia in the at-risk population, though antigen detection by

ICT is also sometimes used. Operationally, the individuals tested are part of 'sentinel sites' (villages, blocks, etc. of about 500 persons each) evaluated at 2- or 3-year intervals during the course of MDA activities. One or more sites are monitored in each IU, and this information is correlated with information on programme coverage at that site, as determined by reports from drug distributors and by active coverage surveys (World Health Organization, 2005b).

Since the Global Programme really began only in 2000, few countries have had time to complete five or six rounds of MDA. Most of the available data, therefore, comes from progress being made in the 39 countries with active MDA programmes. Two types of datasets are available. The first includes all of the data reported to WHO by programme managers in each participating country, and the second is from a number of more intensively studied programmes, where multiple markers of potential transmission interruption (e.g., antigen levels or mosquito infection rates, in addition to MF prevalence) or more frequent time points of assessment are included. Figure 7a, showing the data from 102 sentinel sites in all programmes reporting to WHO, indicates that after only 2–3 rounds of MDA, 43% of sentinel sites had already reduced MF prevalence to zero, while 44% had lowered MF counts to less than half of what they had been pretreatment, and only 13% still had MF prevalence more than half of their pretreatment levels (World Health Organization, 2004a). Figure 7b shows the mean decrease in prevalence reported from these same sentinel sites in six different sub-regions reporting to WHO. Similar findings are seen in the data from the individual country programmes following this and other monitoring parameters (Figure 8), including infection in vector mosquitoes (Figure 9), more closely.

(b) *Morbidity Management.* Treatment strategies for managing the disease associated with LF infection have been well documented to be effective in individual patients (Dreyer *et al.*, 2002). The public health challenge now is to implement these strategies (home-based self-care of lymphoedema/elephantiasis through rigorous hygiene; surgery for hydrocele) on a population-wide scale and to assess their effectiveness for affected individuals when implemented in this fashion.

GPELF's success in implementing its morbidity management strategy can best be described as extending, at least in some measure, to all

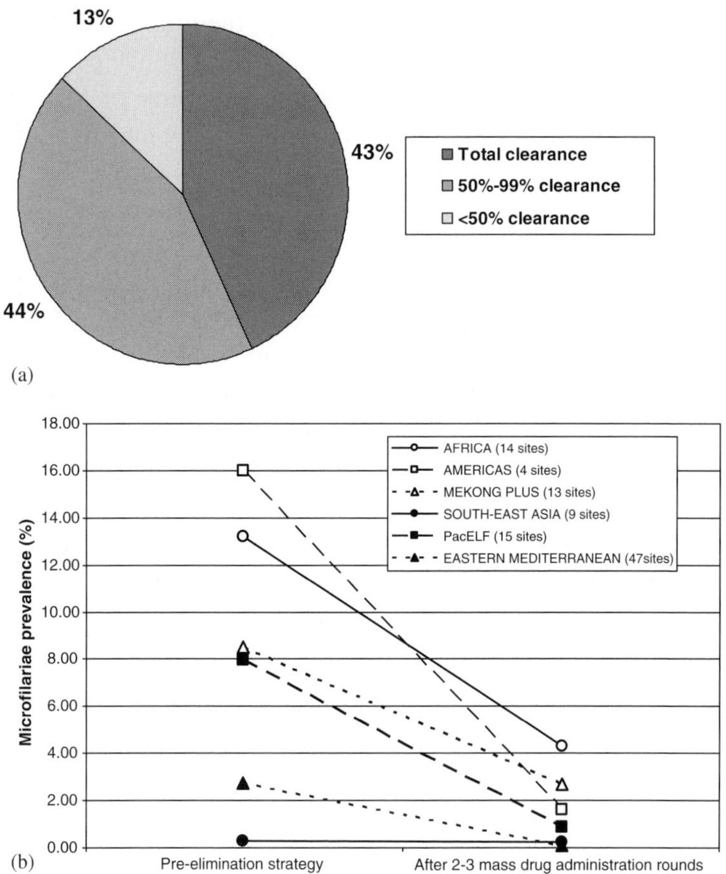

Figure 7 Impact of MDAs on microfilarial clearance (World Health Organization, 2004a). (a) Summary of results at all 102 sentinel sites (in 15 countries) reporting to WHO after two or three rounds of MDA using the two-drug treatment regimens. Forty three percent of sites showed total clearance of microfilaraemia, 44% showed 50–99% clearance, and 13% showed <50% clearance. (b) Same data from 102 sentinel sites but plotted to show reductions in mean microfilarial prevalence at sites in each of the six regions of the GPELF.

of the 39 active national LF elimination programmes. The reason is not just that 'alleviating the suffering of those affected' is the second pillar of the GPELF (Seim *et al.*, 1999); rather, it is because one really cannot carry out a programme simply focused on interrupting transmission (i.e., preventing LF) without attending to the needs and

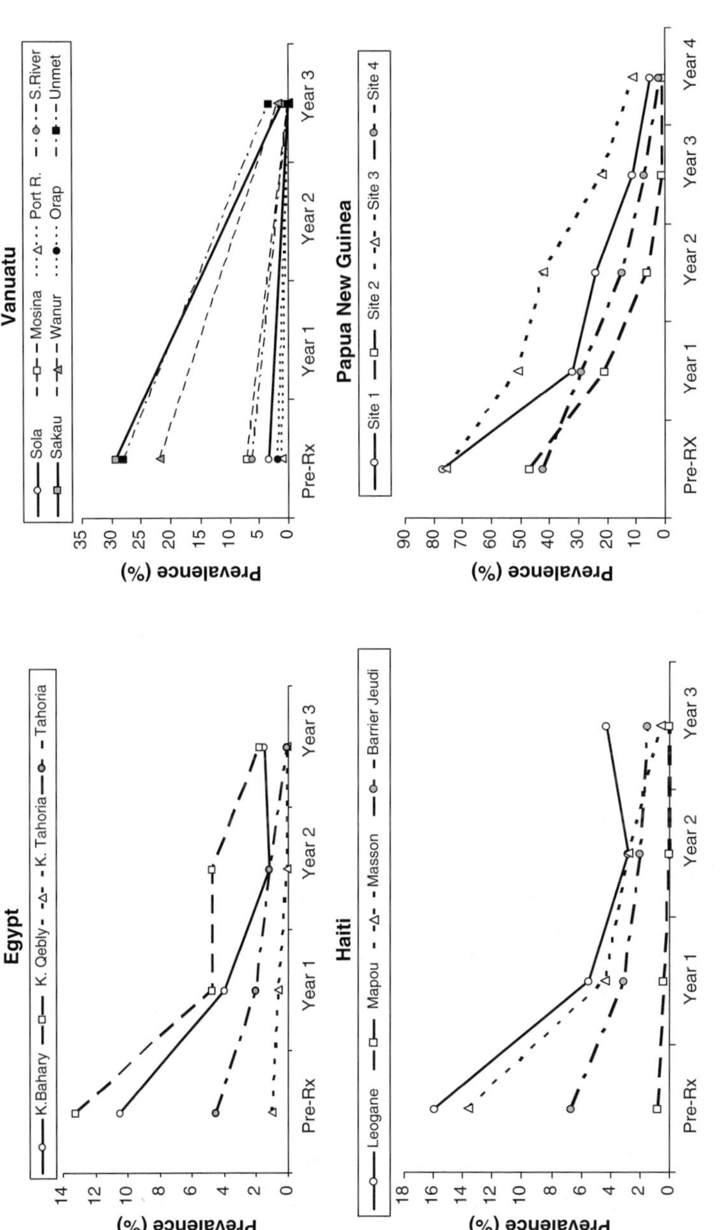

Figure 8 Microfilaria prevalence (*W. bancrofti*) decreases progressively with yearly MDA treatment. Each line represents a single sentinel site (~100–500 population) with data assessed 9–12 months after each MDA (albendazole + DEC) in national LF elimination programmes [Egypt (Ramzy *et al.*, 2006), Vanuatu (Fraser *et al.*, 2005), Haiti (Beau de Rochars *et al.*, 2005)] or in community-based research studies [PNG (Bockarie *et al.*, 2002)] where single-dose ivermectin + DEC (solid lines) or DEC alone (hatched lines) was used. Note different levels of initial MF prevalence in the populations and the more rapid approach to complete clearance at the sites with lower initial prevalence levels. Mean population coverage was 88%, 84%, 71% and 80% for Egypt, Vanuatu, Haiti and PNG, respectively.

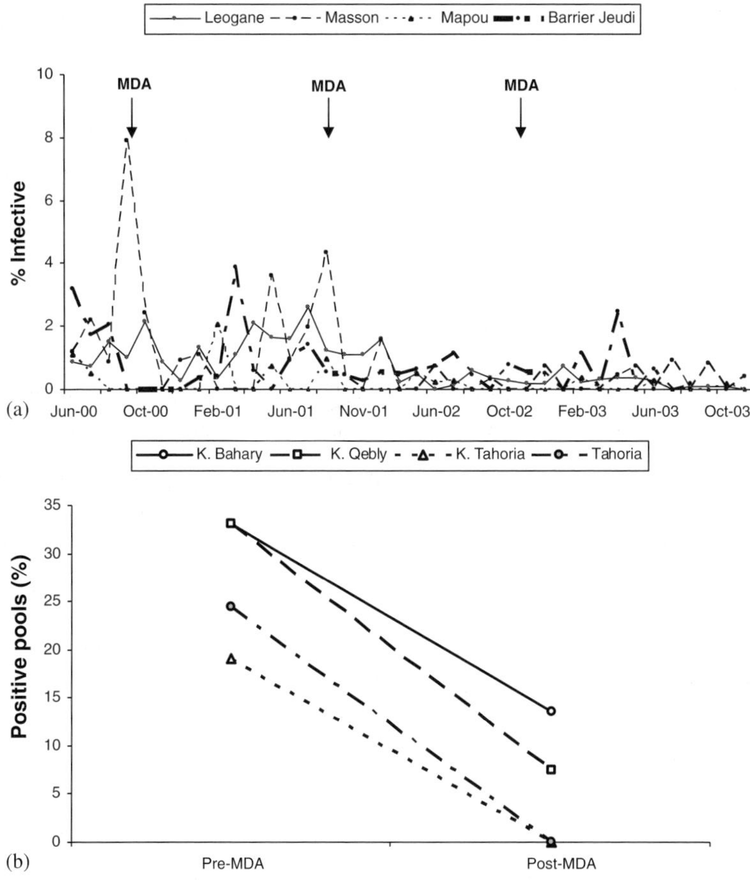

Figure 9   (a) Decline in mosquito infectivity (presence of L3 s) following MDA seen in monthly collections and dissections of mosquitoes at four sentinel sites in Haiti (Lammie, P., personal comm., 2005). (b) Decline in mosquito infection rates (assessed by PCR) 9 months after three cycles of MDA (albendazole + DEC) at four sentinel sites in Egypt (Ramzy *et al.*, 2006). Mean population coverage was 71% for Haiti and 88% for Egypt.

clinical conditions of affected individuals as well. Certainly, not all national programmes have equally developed morbidity management components, and, indeed, quantifying the extent of these programmes (which is necessary for assessing programme impact) does present a significant challenge.

For lymphoedema the principal programmatic activity is training, focused around both health-system clinics and home-based care.

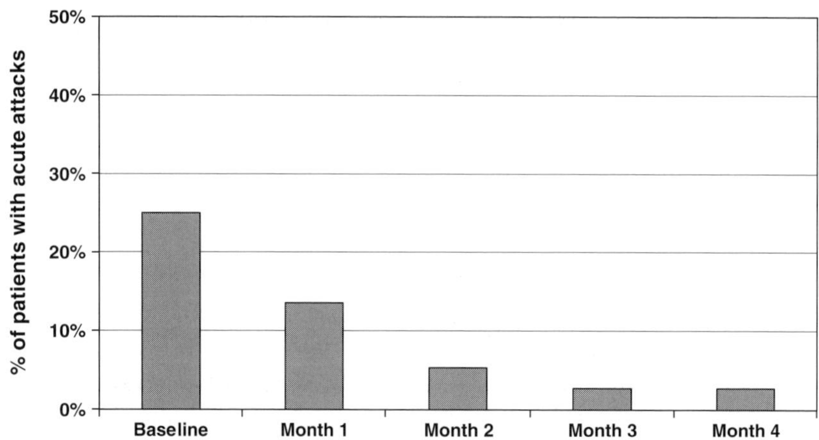

Figure 10   Decreasing occurrence of acute attacks in a cohort of patients followed monthly for 4 months after the introduction of a footcare hygiene regimen (World Health Organization, 2004).

Though the available estimates are likely to underestimate the real situation, already by 2003 almost 500 training workshops for morbidity management had been documented in countries with national LF elimination programmes and more than 24 000 people had been trained (World Health Organization, 2004b). Further, because the training strategy is a cascade of activities, many more individuals actually received training and retraining than documented by these figures. Indeed, when the early impact of such training and public health implementation of lymphoedema management principles has been examined, it is clear that these programmes can achieve excellent results towards their principal goal of decreasing acute inflammatory attacks in affected individuals (Figure 10; World Health Organization, 2004b).

For hydrocele, the number of surgical workshops and the number of surgeries performed are quantifiable measures of morbidity management programmes that allow the impact of GPELF efforts to be calculated. However, both because the national health systems are not always responsible for the surgeries performed for hydrocele and because mechanisms to track the number of such surgeries (or surgical workshops) have not yet been well developed, little of the essential basic information is currently available on a global scale to describe the impact of these approaches to LF genital morbidity.

2.2.3. Ancillary Health Benefits

One of the most extraordinary and valuable attributes of the GPELF is that two of the three drugs it relies on (albendazole and ivermectin) are also the most effective drugs available today for treating all intestinal helminth infections, especially including hookworm, and other conditions as well (Table 1). Therefore, at every MDA not only LF but all the intestinal helminth infections are being treated as well, and the effectiveness of this treatment has been well documented both in pilot studies on carefully followed individuals (Belizario *et al.*, 2003) and in actual LF programme settings and populations (Beau De Rochars *et al.*, 2004; Mani *et al.*, 2004).

As a result, all of the health and development benefits of treating intestinal helminth infections (e.g., Crompton, 2000; O'Lorcain and Holland, 2000; Stephenson *et al.*, 2000) must be added to those gained from treating LF infections when gauging the impact of the GPELF on the health of affected populations. For children, these benefits include very well-documented improvements in growth

Table 1 Broad antiparasitic effectiveness of single-dose albendazole or ivermectin when used alone

Parasite/Infection	Albendazole 400 mg[a] (%)	Ivermectin 200 µg/kg (%)
Hookworm	95	0–20
Ascaris	100	100
Trichuris	40–60	10–50
Strongyloides	45	95
Cutaneous larva migrans	80	100
Enterobius	85	85
Onchocerciasis	—	95[b]
Lice	—	100
Scabies	—	100

[a]Also effective against other parasitic infections (Cysticercosis, Echinococcus, Giardia, Trichomonads, Microsporidia and Crytosporidia) but requiring multiple doses.
[b]Killing effect against MF stage only.

(height and weight), school attendance, performance on cognitive tests, fitness, appetite and activity (Stephenson *et al.*, 2000). For women of child-bearing age, the reduction in hookworm infection contributes greatly to protecting these women from maternal anaemia, a major determinant of low-birth-weight babies and childhood growth failure (Crompton, 2000; Stephenson *et al.*, 2000). Quantifying the impact of all these ancillary health benefits (in terms of DALYS or some other measure) should certainly be feasible, but at the moment it still remains an incompletely met challenge.

The benefits of de-worming in children may extend even beyond the nutrition-related ones described above. Recent evidence that clearance of intestinal helminth infection improves responses to certain vaccines (Cooper *et al.*, 2000) and that the presence of intestinal helminths may exacerbate malaria or other infections (Nacher *et al.*, 2002; Shin *et al.*, 2004; Druilhe *et al.*, 2005) suggests that there might be important interactions (immunologic or otherwise) between these intestinal parasite infections and the host response to other infections or protective antigens. These latter might also be significantly improved through population-wide distribution of albendazole and ivermectin as part of the GPELF.

2.2.4. Integrated Management of Public Health Programmes

Many of the components and many of the needs of different public health programmes are really so similar that the concept of integrating programme activities or 'packaging' health initiatives is not only obvious but of very great practical significance (Molyneux and Nantulya, 2004). Importantly, the national programmes to eliminate LF have a number of unique (or at least, very special) characteristics that make them particularly effective partners for integrating with other health initiatives. Especially important is that their target in at-risk areas is the 'entire population', since all segments and age groups of the population are at risk and must be reached for the LF programmes to be successful. Thus, other programmes that focus on sub-sets of the population can link with national LF elimination programmes, as well as those which must reach the most remote, underserved populations (e.g., for the delivery of bednets for malaria prevention). In addition, as indicated above, the drugs used by the GPELF are the very ones used for intestinal helminth control programmes, so that coordinated programmatic linkages between these initiatives should be particularly straightforward. Finally, the fact that the donated drugs (albendazole, ivermectin) are not only free for the affected populations but also extremely popular with them (because of the very recognizable health benefits they bring to the individual), enhances the compliance of communities towards the LF elimination activities and towards any other health initiatives associated with it.

As a result of such great potential for linkages, the GPELF is now being 'packaged' in a number of different countries with a range of health initiatives that focus on control of intestinal parasites, schistosomiasis, onchocerciasis, trachoma, leprosy and malaria (Fenwick *et al.*, 2005). While the 'impact' of this new thrust towards integrated programme implementation and management has not yet been quantified, its potential for enhancing the effectiveness of all of these programmes appears to be very great. In addition, since most of these programmes are undertaken by the same health workers at the community, district and even national levels, the packaging of currently independent initiatives should prove to be of very great value to the efficient management, operation and strengthening of the health-delivery system itself. Though to date there is still minimal documentation, the anticipated benefits are appreciable.

2.3. Raising Awareness of Global Health Issues and their Solutions

One of the most important achievements of the GPELF has been awakening the global health community to the enormous burden currently saddling endemic populations as a consequence of lymphatic filarial infection. LF is much more widespread and affects many more of the world's most underserved communities than previously recognized. The GPELF, however, has not just raised awareness of this important global health problem; it has also raised awareness that the problem can be solved. Furthermore, its solution can be an essential and integral part of a larger global health implementation programme that is extremely cost-effective and has significant pro-poor benefits that will act effectively to reduce poverty and be fully in line with efforts to achieve the globally agreed Millennium Development Goals (Molyneux, 2004; Molyneux and Nantulya, 2004).

Public–private partnerships have been essential to the development of the GPELF and will unquestionably prove to be equally important for meeting the challenges of other global health concerns. The partnerships created between the GPELF and both GlaxoSmithKline and Merck & Company, Inc. (Molyneux and Zagaria, 2002) not only have helped to break down earlier barriers to effective coordination of LF and other global health efforts but also have facilitated the entry of additional pharmaceutical companies into similar partnering roles in other health initiatives. Indeed, the value to global health of increasing first the awareness and then the willingness of partners to deal with the extraordinarily debilitating effects of LF is matched in importance only by the demonstration of the value, power and feasibility of all facets of the healthcare framework coming together to share ideas, resources and best practices to overcome so many of the health problems inhibiting advancement of the developing world.

2.4. Principal Challenges Now Facing the Global Programme to Eliminate LF

The GPELF has done a remarkable job in rapidly translating critical scientific advances first into programme development, then to health policy and finally into programme implementation. The rapid scale-up achieved (almost 300 million people treated in 2004) is unprecedented and reflects both the Programme's popularity and its strategic feasibility. However, a number of challenges and uncertainties still facing the Programme must be addressed. The most important of these are:

(1) *Financial resources for programme implementation.* Despite the fact that LF elimination programmes (either 'stand-alone' or 'packaged') are extraordinarily inexpensive and cost-effective (Fenwick *et al.*, 2005), because LF and the other 'neglected diseases' with which it is

packaged are predominantly chronic, debilitating diseases of poverty and not ones associated with acute illness and death, it has been difficult for them to gain wide recognition and broad financial support. The low costs of successful implementation of a 'neglected diseases package' have been contrasted quite clearly with per-person costs of HIV/AIDS, tuberculosis, malaria and other international health programmes (Molyneux and Nantulya, 2004; Fenwick *et al.*, 2005), and there is a definite willingness of affected countries to strongly support the LF elimination programmes, both politically and economically (e.g., Ramzy *et al.*, 2005). Still, however, support from outside the developing world remains insufficient for the necessary expansion of MDA activities and for needed enhancement of morbidity management activities. Indeed, the financial resource shortfall for programme implementation is currently the major barrier to the success of this initiative, especially in Africa, and efforts to develop creative financing options provide a major challenge for GPELF activities.

(2) *Financial support for operational research.* The need for financial resources is not limited just to programme implementation. It is widely appreciated that a mark of all successful public health programmes is the continuing involvement of an active research community capable of providing solutions both to programme problems as they arise and to anticipated problems or barriers that might arise during programme activities. Operational research is necessary for continuing to improve the tools (diagnostic and therapeutic) and strategies on which the Programme rests (Ottesen and Weil, 2004). Particularly important for the GPELF now are the tools and strategies to define successful end-points to the LF MDA programs. These most likely will be antibody assays to detect evidence of exposure to infection in cohorts of children born after the LF elimination programme has begun. While potential tools and sampling strategies are available (Lammie *et al.*, 2004; World Health Organization, 2005b), operational research to define their diagnostic effectiveness for monitoring and surveillance is still necessary. Similarly, while the two-drug regimens for use in interrupting transmission are very good, there might be still more effective ways either of using the same drug combinations now employed or developing alternative drug regimens to interrupt transmission more rapidly and, thereby, help to protect

from any potential drug resistance that might otherwise compromise programme success (Bradley and Kumaraswami, 2004).

(3) *Strategies for utilizing vector control.* To interrupt transmission,the parasite can be attacked in both the vector and the human host (Figure 2), but essentially all current efforts of the GPELF are focused on chemotherapeutic targeting of the parasite in the human host. As there is, however, a large body of knowledge and understanding of the vector biology associated with LF, it is essential to develop a strategy that would effectively and cost-effectively utilize this knowledge to hasten the achievement of GPELF's goal of LF elimination (Burkot and Bockarie, 2004). Indeed, in some situations it has been hypothesized that without effective vector control it might prove impossible to eliminate infection using the current drug-based strategy alone (Burkot and Ichimori, 2002). In any case, the potential value of vector control efforts to support the chemotherapeutic ones is so great that the challenge of finding an appropriate strategy for utilizing vector control presents itself as an urgent unmet need whose solution should prove extraordinarily valuable for the success of GPELF.

(4) *Identifying programme impact.* That there is an enormous, cost-beneficial impact of the GPELF, both when implemented alone and especially when packaged with other disease control programmes, is already clear. However, in order for society to make the appropriate choices in allocating its resources, it is necessary for this impact to be as well defined and quantified as possible. Efforts to achieve such quantification are actively being pursued, but, still, meeting this public health challenge remains extremely important for the continued success of the Global Programme.

3. TREATING INDIVIDUALS WITH LF

3.1. Treating LF Infection in Individuals

In contrast to the therapeutic objective of the GPELF where the goal of treating infection in individuals in endemic populations is to prevent the spread of infection from that individual to others, the goal of treating the infection in individuals in the clinic is to prevent development of *disease* in that individual.

Most LF disease (lymphoedema and its consequence; hydrocele and its consequence) is induced by the adult-stage filarial worms. Therefore, the most appropriate therapeutic target to prevent disease is the adult worm. The understanding of how best to kill this stage of the parasite, however, remains remarkably limited. In part, this limitation results from the few tools available for assessing adult worm viability [e.g., ultrasound visualization of both brugian and bancroftian parasites; circulating antigen (derived from adult worms) detection for *W. bancrofti* infections only], and in part, it results from the lack of potent macrofilaricidal drugs.

The effectiveness of DEC in killing many but not all LF adult worms is well recognized (Ottesen, 1985; Noroes *et al.*, 1997) but not explained, and the finding that a single dose of DEC (6 mg/kg) is as effective in killing adult worms as is a multiple-week course (Figure 11; Noroes *et al.*, 1997) has not been challenged. For albendazole, a single dose (400 mg) does appear to affect adult worms (killing?, inhibiting MF production?; Gyapong *et al.*, 2005), but a 3-week course of 400 mg twice daily showed very much greater (perhaps 100%) killing of adult worms (Jayakody *et al.*, 1993). Ivermectin, on the other hand, appears not to kill adult-stage parasites at all (Dreyer

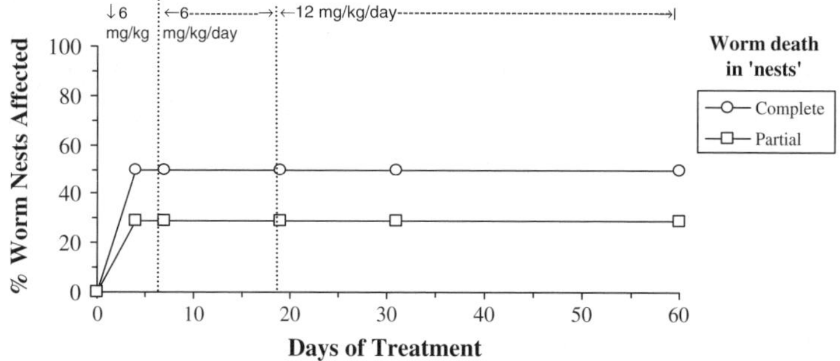

Figure 11 Macrofilaricidal effects of DEC on *W. bancrofti* parasites, assessed by ultrasonography, following a single dose of DEC (6 mg/kg) at Day 0, then 12 days of DEC (6 mg/kg/day) beginning at Day 7, followed by 42 days of high-dose DEC (12 mg/kg/day). Maximal effect was achieved after the first dose of DEC (Noroes *et al.*, 1997; Gyapong *et al.*, 2005).

et al., 1996). A recent study indicated that a single dose of albendazole + DEC was equally effective in killing adult worms as 7 days of this two-drug combination (El Setouhy *et al.*, 2004). Most recently another approach (i.e., targeting the worm's *Wolbachia* endosymbionts) showed that 8-week treatment with doxycycline resulted in macrofilaricidal effects in patients with *W. bancrofti* infection (Taylor *et al.*, 2005). However, for none of these antifilarial agents have there been recent formal clinical trials focused on optimizing treatment of the infection in individual patients, so that textbooks of medicine are still left with espousing the very old recommendations for treating LF patients with a 12-day course of DEC (6 mg/kg/day) for Bancroftian filariasis and a 6-day course for Brugian filariasis (Ottesen, 2004). Clearly, the more recent research observations demonstrating the equivalence of single- and multiple-dose DEC and the action of long-term albendazole or doxycycline treatment for killing adult worms have very effectively set the stage for additional clinical trials to revise these outdated treatment recommendations.

Though adult-stage parasites do cause most of the damage that one tries to prevent in treating individuals with LF infection, MF, too, can induce disease. Indeed, term 'asymptomatic microfilaraemia' belies the pathogenicity of this stage of the parasite. Most commonly associated with microfilaraemia is a nephropathy manifesting as microscopic or gross hematuria (Dreyer *et al.*, 1992). The frequency of such hematuria is high, but the long-term consequences of it have not been well explored. Since both DEC and ivermectin are very effective microfilaricides, and since the hematuria resolves after treatment, it is appropriate to use single doses of either of these drugs (DEC, 6 mg/kg; ivermectin, 200 µg/kg) to decrease microfilaraemia.

The tropical pulmonary eosinophilia syndrome, though caused by hyperresponsiveness to the microfilarial stage of the parasites, actually requires treatment with an adulticidal regimen of DEC [6 mg/kg/day × 3–4 weeks (Ottesen and Nutman, 1992)]. Interestingly the microfilaricidal drug ivermectin is not effective in treating this syndrome, probably because the DEC, through its macrofilaricidal activity, stops microfilarial production by the adult worms more effectively than ivermectin.

Neither DEC nor ivermectin, given separately or together at the doses necessary to treat microfilaraemic patients, has any significant drug toxicity in normal individuals or in amicrofilaraemic patients. However, in microfilaraemic individuals the rapid killing of MF by these drugs presumably releases so much antigen that the modulating effects of the host immune system appear to be overwhelmed and a variety of side reactions is induced (Ottesen, 1987). These occur in direct proportion to individuals' pre-treatment microfilarial loads and include headaches, fever, lymphoadenopathy and occasionally rash, itching and other symptoms. Although the most severely affected patients can also experience postural hypotension, generally these reactions are well managed through the use of antipyretics, antihistamines or, in the most severe instances, corticosteroids.

3.2. Treating the Disease in Individuals with LF

Although trying to cure the infection is important, it is managing the disease consequences of LF infection (i.e., lymphoedema/elephantiasis, genital pathology and acute inflammatory episodes) that is most often of greatest concern to the patient. Effective antifilarial chemotherapy will arrest further parasite-induced damage to lymphatics, but the already-damaged vessels continue to render the affected patients susceptible to secondary bacterial infections, likely for the rest of their lives. Since repeated episodes of such infections are the principal determinant to progression of the morbidity associated with LF, all infected individuals (even those manifesting only microfilaraemia) should be enrolled in programmes of hygiene and limb care that will effectively decrease the frequency of bacterial infections. As already described [Section 1.2.4(b)], this should include training on washing and care of the limbs, prompt recognition and treatment of minor injuries, wearing of shoes and other foot protection, limb elevation, exercise and judicious use of antibiotics [to treat acute inflammatory attacks and for prophylaxis when indicated (Dreyer *et al.*, 2002)].

For hydrocele and other even more complicated manifestations of genital pathology, surgery is indicated (DeVries, 2002).

Chyluria is best managed through dietary modification, especially replacement of fat-rich diets with high-protein, high-fluid diets supplemented where possible with medium-chain triglycerides (Dreyer *et al.*, 2002). Surgery or the sclerosing effects of lymphangiography have also been used when nutritional management has not been successful (Ottesen, 2004).

4. THE FUTURE

The recent history of LF has been one of rapid acceleration in our understanding and potential mastery over this parasite. First described 125 years ago, LF needed 75 years before the discovery of its first practical, effective drug treatment (DEC), but during the past 20 years there has been such rapid development of new, powerful diagnostics and drug regimens that a GPELF could actually be created, just over 5 years ago. Already during the short span of these 5 years more than 20% of the world's at-risk population has been reached in the effort to eliminate LF, and the Global Programme remains on target to reach its goal of LF elimination as a public health problem by the year 2020—provided that necessary resources continue to be made available.

While the principal goal of the GPELF remains LF elimination, it has become increasingly clear that this programme can, and indeed must, extend its benefits more broadly through integrating its own programmatic activities (both MDA and morbidity management) with those of other programmes utilizing similar strategies and tools. Such integration should be especially effective with those global health programmes focused on what have been termed 'rapid impact diseases' (World Health Organization, 2005c)—diseases for which technical solutions have already been defined but which today lack the public health resources to deliver these solutions to the poor, underserved populations burden by these 'neglected diseases'. Indeed, the argument has already been made quite forcefully (Fenwick *et al.*, 2005) that investment in a package of health initiatives directed at these neglected diseases is likely the best buy in Global Health today.

The achievements of the GPELF, founded on the scientific advances of an effective, determined research community and supported by an extraordinary partnership of public- and private-sector organizations, have already translated into health and productivity benefits for almost 300 million people living in LF-endemic regions worldwide, and the Programme is on target to reach all 1.2 billion people at risk during the next decade. A critical challenge, while undertaking this expansion, will be for the GPELF now to utilize its organizational and cost-effective implementation strategies for integrating with other global health initiatives to deliver even greater value towards improving health in the developing world and thereby exert strong impetus towards achieving the globally agreed Millennium Development Goals (Molyneux and Nantulya, 2004). Thus, the vision for the future of the GPELF today is not one focused solely and exclusively on eliminating LF; rather, the vision is nothing short of a global LF elimination programme fully integrated into national health care systems and serving as a strong vehicle and partner for delivering the goods and services necessary to make a broad, effective impact on the health and development of the world's neediest and most neglected populations.

REFERENCES

Addiss, D.G. and Brady, M.A. (2005). *Morbidity management in the Global Programme to Eliminate Lymphatic Filariasis—a review of the scientific literature.* Background paper. Special Programme for Research and Training in Tropial Diseases (TDR) Scientific Working Group Meeting on Lymphatic Filariasis, May 2005, Geneva.

Amaral, F., Dreyer, G., Figueredo-Silva, J., Noroes, J., Cavalcanti, A., Samico, S.C., Santos, A. and Coutinho, A. (1994). Live adult worms detected by ultrasonography in human Bancroftian filariasis. *American Journal of Tropical Medicine and Hygiene* **50**, 753–757.

Beau De Rochars, M.B., Direny, A.N., Roberts, J.M., Addiss, D.G., Radday, J., Beach, M.J., Streit, T.G., Dardith, D., Lafontant, J.G. and Lammie, P.J. (2004). Community-wide reduction in prevalence and intensity of intestinal helminths as a collateral benefit of lymphatic filariasis elimination programs. *American Journal of Tropical Medicine and Hygiene* **71**, 466–470.

Beaver, P.C. (1970). Filariasis without microfilaremia. *American Journal of Tropical Medicine and Hygiene* **19**, 181–189.

Belizario, V.Y., Amarillo, M.E., de Leon, W.U., de los Reyes, A.E., Bugayong, M.G. and Macatangay, B.J. (2003). A comparison of the efficacy of single doses of albendazole, ivermectin, and diethylcarbamazine alone or in combinations against *Ascaris* and *Trichuris* spp. *Bulletin of the World Health Organization* **81**, 35–42.

Bockarie, M.J., Tavul, L., Kastens, W., Michael, E. and Kazura, J.W. (2002). Impact of untreated bednets on prevalence of *Wuchereria bancrofti* transmitted by *Anopheles farauti* in Papua New Guinea. *Medical and Veterinary Entomology* **16**, 116–119.

Bradley, M.L. and Kumaraswami, V. (2004). Towards a strategic plan for research to support the Global Program to Eliminate Lymphatic Filariasis. 2. Reserach directly linked with GPELF activities (operational research). 2.2. Essential tools—drugs and clinical drug trials. *American Journal of Tropical Medicine and Hygiene* **71**, supplement, 7–11.

Burkot, T. and Bockarie, M.J. (2004). Towards a strategic plan for research to support the Global Program to eliminate lymphatic filariasis. 2. Research directly linked with GPELF activities (operational research). 2.7. Vectors. *American Journal of Tropical Medicine and Hygiene* **71**, supplement, 24–26.

Burkot, T. and Ichimori, K. (2002). The PacELF programme: will mass drug administration be enough? *Trends in Parasitology* **18**, 109–115.

Centers for Disease Control and Prevention (1993). Recommendations of the International Task Force for Disease Eradication. *Morbidity and Mortality Weekly Report* **42**, 1–38.

Chernin, E. (1987). The disappearance of Bancroftian filariasis from Charleston, South Carolina. *American Journal of Tropical Medicine and Hygiene* **37**, 111–114.

Colatrella, B. (2003). The Mectizan Donation Programme—successful collaboration between the public and private sectors. *Essential Drugs Monitor* **33**, 28–29.

Cooper, P.J., Chico, M.E., Losonsky, G., Sandoval, C., Espinel, I., Sridhara, R., Aguilar, M., Guevara, A., Guderian, R.H., Levine, M.M., Griffin, G.E. and Nutman, T.B. (2000). Albendazole treatment of children with ascariasis enhances the vibriocidal antibody response to the live attenuated oral cholera vaccine CVD 103-HgR. *Journal of Infectious Diseases* **182**, 1199–1206.

Crompton, D.W. (2000). The public health importance of hookworm disease. *Parasitology* **121**(supplement), S39–S50.

Curtis, C.F., Malecela-Lazaro, M., Reuben, R. and Maxwell, C.A. (2002). Use of floating layers of polystyrene beads to control populations of the filaria vector *Culex quinquefasciatus*. *Annals of Tropical Medicine and Parasitology* **96**(supplement 2), S97–S104.

DeVries, C.R. (2002). The role of the urologist in the treatment and elimination of lymphatic filariasis worldwide. *British Journal of Urology* **89**(supplement 1), 37–43.

Dreyer, G., Addiss, D., Dreyer, P. and Noroes, J. (2002). *Basic Lymphoedema Management: Treatment and Prevention of Problems Associated with Lymphatic Filariasis*, pp. 112. Hollis, New Hampshire: Hollis Publishing Company.

Dreyer, G., Addiss, D., Noroes, J., Amaral, F., Rocha, A. and Coutinho, A. (1996). Ultrasonographic assessment of the adulticidal efficacy of repeat high-dose ivermectin in Bancroftian filariasis. *Tropical Medicine and International Health* **1**, 427–432.

Dreyer, G., Amaral, F., Noroes, J., Medeiros, Z. and Addiss, D. (1995). A new tool to assess the adulticidal efficacy *in vivo* of antifilarial drugs for Bancroftian filariasis. *Transactions of the Royal Society of Tropical Medicine and Hygiene* **89**, 225–226.

Dreyer, G., Figueredo-Silva, J., Carvalho, K., Amaral, F. and Ottesen, E.A. (2001). Lymphatic filariasis in children: adenopathy and its evolution in two young girls. *American Journal of Tropical Medicine and Hygiene* **65**, 204–207.

Dreyer, G., Noroes, J., Figueredo-Silva, J. and Piessens, W.F. (2000). Pathogenesis of lymphatic disease in Bancroftian filariasis: a clinical perspective. *Parasitology Today* **16**, 544–548.

Dreyer, G., Ottesen, E.A., Galdino, E., Andrade, L., Rocha, A., Medeiros, Z., Moura, I., Casimiro, I., Beliz, F. and Coutinho, A. (1992). Renal abnormalities in microfilaremic patients with Bancroftian filariasis. *American Journal of Tropical Medicine and Hygiene* **46**, 745–751.

Druilhe, P., Tall, A. and Sokhna, C. (2005). Worms can worsen malaria: towards a new means to roll back malaria? *Trends in Parasitology* **21**, 359–362.

Eigege, A., Richards, F.O., Jr., Blaney, D.D., Miri, E.S., Gontor, I., Ogah, G., Umaru, J., Jinadu, M.Y., Mathai, W., Amadiegwu, S. and Hopkins, D.R. (2003). Rapid assessment for lymphatic filariasis in central Nigeria: a comparison of the immunochromatographic card test and hydrocele rates in an area of high endemicity. *American Journal of Tropical Medicine and Hygiene* **68**, 643–646.

El Setouhy, M., Ramzy, R., Ahmed, E., Kandil, A., Hussain, O., Farid, H., Helmy, H. and Weil, G. (2004). A randomized clinical trial comparing single-multi-dose combination therapy with diethylcarbamazine and albendazole for treatment of Bancroftian filariasis. *American Journal of Tropical Medicine and Hygiene* **70**, 191–196.

Fenwick, A., Molyneux, D. and Nantulya, V. (2005). Achieving the millennium development goals. *Lancet* **365**, 1029–1030.

Fraser, M., Taleo, G., James, Y., Amos, M., Babu, M. and Kalkoa, M. (2005). Evaluation of the Program to eliminate lymphatic filariasis in

Vanuatu following two years of mass drug administration implementation: results and methodological approach. *American Journal of Tropical Medicine and Hygiene* **73**, 753–758.

Freedman, D.O., de Almeida Filho, P.J., Besh, S., Maia e Silva, M.C., Braga, C. and Maciel, A. (1994). Lymphoscintigraphic analysis of lymphatic abnormalities in symptomatic and asymptomatic human filariasis. *Journal of Infectious Diseases* **170**, 927–933.

Gubler, D.J. and Bhattacharya, N.C. (1974). A quantitative approach to the study of Bancroftian filariasis. *American Journal of Tropical Medicine and Hygiene* **23**, 1027–1036.

Gyapong, J.O., Kumaraswami, V., Biswas, G. and Ottesen, E.A. (2005). Treatment strategies underpinning the global programme to eliminate lymphatic filariasis. *Expert Opinion on Pharmacotherapy* **6**, 179–200.

Gyapong, J.O., Kyelem, D., Kleinschmidt, I., Agbo, K., Ahouandogbo, F., Gaba, J., Owusu-Banahene, G., Sanou, S., Sodahlon, Y.K., Biswas, G., Kale, O.O., Molyneux, D.H., Roungou, J.B., Thomson, M.C. and Remme, J. (2002). The use of spatial analysis in mapping the distribution of Bancroftian filariasis in four West African countries. *Annals of Tropical Medicine and Parasitology* **96**, 695–705.

Horton, J., Witt, C., Ottesen, E.A., Lazdins, J.K., Addiss, D.G., Awadzi, K., Beach, M.J., Belizario, V.Y., Dunyo, S.K., Espinel, M., Gyapong, J.O., Hossain, M., Ismail, M.M., Jayakody, R.L., Lammie, P.J., Makunde, W., Richard-Lenoble, D., Selve, B., Shenoy, R.K., Simonsen, P.E., Wamae, C.N. and Weerasooriya, M.V. (2000). An analysis of the safety of the single dose, two drug regimens used in programmes to eliminate lymphatic filariasis. *Parasitology* **121**(supplement), S147–S160.

Houston, R. (2000). Salt fortified with diethylcarbamazine (DEC) as an effective intervention for lymphatic filariasis, with lessons learned from salt iodization programmes. *Parasitology* **121**(supplement), S161–S173.

Jayakody, R.L., De Silva, C.S. and Weerasinghe, W.M. (1993). Treatment of Bancroftian filariasis with albendazole: evaluation of efficacy and adverse reactions. *Tropical Biomedicine* **10**, 19–24.

Katabarwa, N.M. and Mutabazi, D. (2000). Controlling onchocerciasis by community-directed, ivermectin-treatment programmes in Uganda: why do some communities succeed and others fail? *Annals of Tropical Medicine and Parasitology* **94**, 343–352.

Krishna, K., Harichandrakumar, K., Das, L. and Krishnamoorthy, K. (2005). Physical and psychosocial burden due to lymphatic filariasis as perceived by patients and medical experts. *Tropical Medicine and International Health* **10**(June), 567–573.

Laigret, J., Kessel, J.F., Bambridge, B. and Adams, H. (1996). 11 years of chemoprophylaxis of non-periodic lymphatic filariasis with diethylcarbamazine in Tahiti. *Bulletin of the World Health Organization* **34**, 925–938.

Lammie, P.J., Weil, G., Noordin, R., Kaliraj, P., Steel, C., Goodman, D., Lakshmikanthan, V.B. and Ottesen, E. (2004). Recombinant antigen-based antibody assays for the diagnosis and surveillance of lymphatic filariasis—a multicenter trial. *Filaria Journal* **3**, 9.

Lizotte, M.R., Supali, T., Partono, F. and Williams, S.A. (1994). A polymerase chain reaction assay for the detection of *Brugia malayi* in blood. *American Journal of Tropical Medicine and Hygiene* **51**, 314–321.

Mani, T.R., Rajendran, R., Sunish, I.P., Munirathinam, A., Arunachalam, N., Satyanarayana, K. and Dash, A.P. (2004). Effectiveness of two annual, single-dose mass drug administrations of diethylcarbamazine alone or in combination with albendazole on soil-transmitted helminthiasis in filariasis elimination programme. *Tropical Medicine and International Health* **9**, 1030–1035.

McPherson, T., Persaud, S., Singh, S., Fay, M. P., Addiss, D., Nutman, T.B. and Hay, R. (2006). Interdigital lesions and acute dermatolymphangioadenitis in lymphatic filariasis. *British Journal of Dermatology*, in press.

Michael, E., Malecela-Lazaro, M.N., Simonsen, P.E., Pedersen, E.M., Barker, G., Kumar, A. and Kazura, J.W. (2004). Mathematical modelling and the control of lymphatic filariasis. *Lancet Infectious Diseases* **4**, 223–234.

Molyneux, D.H. (2004). "Neglected" diseases but unrecognised successes—challenges and opportunities for infectious disease control. *Lancet* **364**, 380–383.

Molyneux, D.H. and Nantulya, V.M. (2004). Linking disease control programmes in rural Africa: a pro-poor strategy to reach Abuja targets and millennium development goals. *British Medical Journal* **328**, 1129–1132.

Molyneux, D.H. and Zagaria, N. (2002). Lymphatic filariasis elimination: progress in global programme development. *Annals of Tropical Medicine and Parasitology* **96**(supplement 2), S15–S40.

Nacher, M., Singhasivanon, P., Yimsamran, S., Manibunyong, W., Thanyavanich, N., Wuthisen, R. and Looareesuwan, S. (2002). Intestinal helminth infections are associated with increased incidence of *Plasmodium falciparum* malaria in Thailand. *Journal of Parasitology* **88**, 55–58.

Noroes, J., Dreyer, G., Santos, A., Mendes, V.G., Medeiros, Z. and Addiss, D. (1997). Assessment of the efficacy of diethylcarbamazine on adult *Wuchereria bancrofti in vivo*. *Transactions of the Royal Society of Tropical Medicine and Hygiene* **91**, 78–81.

O'Lorcain, P. and Holland, C.V. (2000). The public health importance of *Ascaris lumbricoides*. *Parasitology* **121**(supplement), S51–S71.

Olszewski, W., Jamal, S., Manokaran, G., Pani, S., Kumaraswami, V., Kubicka, U., Lukomska, B., Dworczynski, A., Dworczynski, A., Swoboda, E. and Meisel-Mikolajczyk, F. (1997). Bacteriologic studies of skin, tissue fluid, lymph, and lymph nodes in patient with filarial lymphedema. *American Journal of Tropical Medicine and Hygiene* **57**, 7–15.

Onapa, A.W., Simonsen, P.E., Baehr, I. and Pedersen, E.M. (2005). Rapid assessment of the geographical distribution of lymphatic filariasis in Uganda, by screening of schoolchildren for circulating filarial antigens. *Annals of Tropical Medicine and Parasitology* **99**, 141–153.

Ottesen, E.A. (1985). Efficacy of diethylcarbamazine in eradicating infection with lymphatic-dwelling filariae in humans. *Reviews of Infectious Diseases* **7**, 341–356.

Ottesen, E.A. (1987). Description, mechanisms and control of reactions to treatment in the human filariases. *Ciba Foundation Symposium* **127**, 265–283.

Ottesen, E.A. (1994). The human filariases: new understandings, new therapeutic strategies. *Current Opinion in Infectious Diseases*, 550–558.

Ottesen, E.A. (2000). The global programme to eliminate lymphatic filariasis. *Tropical Medicine and International Health* **5**, 591–594.

Ottesen, E.A. (2004). Filariasis. In: *Infectious Diseases* (J. Cohen and W. Powderly, eds), pp. 1607–1613. London: Elsevier.

Ottesen, E.A., Dowdle, W., Fenner, F., Habermehl, K., John, T., Koch, M., Medley, G., Muller, A., Ostroff, S. and Zeichhardt, H. (1998). How is eradication to be defined and what are the biological criteria? In: *The Eradication of Infectious Diseases* (W. Dowdle and D. Hopkins, eds). Wiley. Chickester, UK.

Ottesen, E.A., Duke, B.O., Karam, M. and Behbehani, K. (1997). Strategies and tools for the control/elimination of lymphatic filariasis. *Bulletin of the World Health Organization* **75**, 491–503.

Ottesen, E.A. and Nutman, T.B. (1992). Tropical pulmonary eosinophilia. *Annual Review of Medicine* **43**, 417–424.

Ottesen, E.A. and Weil, G. (2004). Towards a strategic plan for research to support the Global Programme to Eliminate Lymphatic Filariasis— introduction. *American Journal of Tropical Medicine and Hygiene* **71** (supplement), 1–2.

Pedersen, E.M. and Mukoko, D.A. (2002). Impact of insecticide-treated materials on filaria transmission by the various species of vector mosquito in Africa. *Annals of Tropical Medicine and Parasitology* **96**(supplement 2), S91–S95.

Rahmah, N., Shenoy, R.K., Nutman, T.B., Weiss, N., Gilmour, K., Maizels, R.M., Yazdanbakhsh, M. and Sartono, E. (2003). Multicentre laboratory evaluation of Brugia rapid dipstick test for detection of brugian filariasis. *Tropical Medicine and International Health* **8**, 895–900.

Ramaiah, K.D., Das, P.K., Michael, E. and Guyatt, H. (2000). The economic burden of lymphatic filariasis in India. *Parasitology Today* **16**, 251–253.

Ramzy, R., El Setouhy, M., Helmy, H., Ahmed, E., Abdel Aziz, K., Farid, H. and Weil, G. (2006). Comprehensive monitoring of the impact of mass drug administration with diethylcarbamazine and albendazole on Bancroftian filariasis in Egypt. *Lancet*.

Ramzy, R., Goldman, A. and Kamal, H. (2005). Defining the cost of the Egyptian lymphatic filariasis elimination program. *Filaria Journal* **4**, 7.

Rawlins, S.C., Siung-Chang, A., Baboolal, S. and Chadee, D.D. (2004). Evidence for the interruption of transmission of lymphatic filariasis among school children in Trinidad and Tobago. *Transactions of the Royal Society of Tropical Medicine and Hygiene* **98**, 473–477.

Reuben, R., Rajendran, R., Sunish, I.P., Mani, T.R., Tewari, S.C., Hiriyan, J. and Gajanana, A. (2001). Annual single-dose diethylcarbamazine plus ivermectin for control of Bancroftian filariasis: comparative efficacy with and without vector control. *Annual Tropical Medicine Parasitology* **95**, 361–378.

Sasa, M. (1976). *Human Filariasis. A Global Survey of Epidemiology and Control*, pp. 819. Tokyo: University Park Press.

Schlemper, B.R.J., Steindel, M., Grisard, E.C., Carvalho-Pinto, C.J., Bernardini, O.J., de Castilho, C.V., Rosa, G., Kilian, S., Guarneri, A.A., Rocha, A., Medeiros, Z. and Ferreira Neto, J.A. (2000). Elimination of Bancroftian filariasis (*Wuchereria bancrofti*) in Santa Catarina State, Brazil. *Tropical Medicine and International Health* **5**, 848–854.

Seim, A.R., Dreyer, G. and Addiss, D.G. (1999). Controlling morbidity and interrupting transmission: twin pillars of lymphatic filariasis elimination. *Revista de Sociedade Brasileira de Medicina Tropical* **32**, 325–328.

Shin, J.L., Gardiner, G.W., Deitel, W. and Kandel, G. (2004). Does whipworm increase the pathogenicity of *Campylobacter jejuni*? A clinical correlate of an experimental observation. *Canadian Journal of Gastroenterology* **18**, 175–177.

Sprent, J.F. (1986). Parasitology in Brisbane. *International Journal of Parasitology* **16**, 281–285.

Stephenson, L.S., Latham, M.C. and Ottesen, E.A. (2000). Malnutrition and parasitic helminth infections. *Parasitology* **121**(supplement), S23–S38.

Stolk, W.A., Swaminathan, S., van Oortmarssen, G.J., Das, P.K. and Habbema, J.D. (2003). Prospects for elimination of Bancroftian filariasis by mass drug treatment in Pondicherry, India: a simulation study. *Journal of Infectious Diseases* **188**, 1371–1381.

Taylor, M.J., Makunde, W.H., McGarry, H.F., Turner, J.D., Mand, S. and Hoerauf, A. (2005). Macrofilaricidal activity after doxycycline treatment of *Wuchereria bancrofti*: a double-blind, randomised placebo-controlled trial. *Lancet* **365**, 2116–2121.

The Editorial Board of Control of Lymphatic Filariasis in China. (2003). *Control of Lymphatic Filariasis in China*, 230pp. World Health Organization Regional Office for the Western Pacific, Manila.

Vaqas, B. and Ryan, T.J. (2003). Lymphoedema: pathophysiology and management in resource-poor settings—relevance for lymphatic filariasis control programmes. *Filaria Journal* **2**, 4.

Wartman, W.B. (1947). Filariasis in American armed forces in World War II. *Medicine* **26**, 27–38.

Webber, R.H. (1975). Vector control of filariasis in the Solomon Islands. *Southeast Asian Journal of Tropical Medical Public Health* **6**, 430–434.

Weil, G.J., Lammie, P.J. and Weiss, N. (1997). The ICT filariasis test: a rapid-format antigen test for diagnosis of Bancroftian filariasis. *Parasitology Today* **13**, 401–404.

Williams, S.A., Laney, S.J., Bierwert, L.A., Saunders, L.J., Boakye, D.A., Fischer, P., Goodman, D., Helmy, H., Hoti, S.L., Vasuki, V., Lammie, P.J., Plichart, C., Ramzy, R.M.R. and Ottesen, E.A. (2002). Development and standardization of a rapid, PCR-based method for the detection of *Wuchereria bancrofti* in mosquitoes, for xenomonitoring the human prevalence of Bancroftian filariasis. *Annual Tropical Medicine Parasitology* **96**, S41–S46.

Witt, C. and Ottesen, E.A. (2001). Lymphatic filariasis: an infection of childhood. *Tropical Medicine and International Health* **6**, 582–606.

World Health Organization (1995). *World Health Report*, 118pp. Geneva, Switzerland: World Health Organization.

World Health Organization (1999). *Building Partnerships for Lymphatic Filariasis Strategic Plan* (September 1999), 64pp. WHO/FIL 99.1998. Geneva, Switzerland: World Health Organization.

World Health Organization (2000). *Preparing and Implementing a National Plan to Eliminate Lymphatic Filariasis*, Geneva, Switzerland: World Health Organization 65pp. WHO/CDC/CPE/CEE/200.15.

World Health Organization (2004a). Report on the mid-term assessment of microfilaraemia reduction in sentinel sites of 13 countries of the GPELF. *Weekly Epidemiological Record* **79**, 358–365.

World Health Organization (2004b). Lymphatic filariasis: progress of disability prevention activities. *Weekly Epidemiological Record* **79**, 417–424.

World Health Organization (2005a). Global Programme to Eliminate Lymphatic Filariasis: progress report for 2004. *Weekly Epidemiological Record* **80**, 202–212.

World Health Organization (2005b). Monitoring and Epidemiological Assessment of the Programme to Eliminate Lymphatic Filariasis at Implementation Unit Level. Geneva, Switzerland: World Health Organization, WHO/CDS/CPE/CEE 2005.50.

World Health Organization (2005c). Strategic and Technical Meeting on Intensified Control of Tropical Diseases. http://www.who.int/neglected diseases/rationale, (accessed August 2005).

Zhong, M., McCarthy, J., Bierwert, L., Lizotte-Waniewski, M., Chanteau, S., Nutman, T.B., Ottesen, E.A. and Williams, S.A. (1996). A polymerase chain reaction assay for detection of the parasite *Wuchereria bancrofti* in human blood samples. *American Journal of Tropical Medicine and Hygiene* **54**, 357–363.

Control of Cystic Echinococcosis/ Hydatidosis: 1863–2002

P.S. Craig[1] and E. Larrieu[2]

[1]*Cestode Zoonoses Research Group, Biomedical Sciences Institute & School of Environment and Life Sciences, University of Salford, Salford, Greater Manchester M5 4WT, UK*
[2]*Veterinary Faculty, University of La Pampa, General Pico, Calle 5y116, (6360), La Pampa Province, Argentina*

ADVANCES IN PARASITOLOGY VOL 61
ISSN: 0065-308X
DOI: 10.1016/S0065-308X(05)61011-1

ABSTRACT

Echinococcosis/hydatidosis, caused by *Echinococcus granulosus*, is a chronic and debilitating zoonotic larval cestode infection in humans, which is principally transmitted between dogs and domestic livestock, particularly sheep. Human hydatid disease occurs in almost all pastoral communities and rangeland areas of the underdeveloped and developed world. Control programmes against hydatidosis have been implemented in several endemic countries, states, provinces, districts or regions to reduce or eliminate cystic echinococcosis (CE) as a public health problem. This review assesses the impact of 13 of the hydatid control programmes implemented, since the first was introduced in Iceland in 1863. Five island-based control programmes (Iceland, New Zealand, Tasmania, Falklands and Cyprus) resulted, over various intervention periods (from <15 to >50 years), in successful control of transmission as evidenced by major reduction in incidence rates of human CE, and prevalence levels in sheep and dogs. By 2002, two countries, Iceland and New Zealand, and one island-state, Tasmania, had already declared that hydatid disease had been eliminated from their territories. Other hydatid programmes implemented in South America (Argentina, Chile, Uruguay), in Europe (mid-Wales, Sardinia) and in East Africa (northwest Kenya), showed varying degrees of success, but some were considered as having failed. Reasons for the eventual success of certain hydatid control programmes and the problems encountered in others are analysed and discussed, and recommendations for likely optimal approaches considered. The application of new control tools, including use of a hydatid vaccine, are also considered.

1. INTRODUCTION

The history of control programmes against cystic hydatidosis or cystic echinococcosis (CE) due to infection with *Echinococcus granulosus* is an under-recognized success story of 20th century parasitology. Cystic hydatidosis is a classic zoonosis in which most transmission depends on domestic animal reservoir hosts, livestock husbandry and dog management practices as well as human behaviour (Nelson, 1972). Hydatid disease is one of the few examples where elimination of transmission of a parasitic zoonosis from a defined region has been achieved as a result of purposeful control campaigns. Currently, however, the parasite still remains endemic on all continents except Antarctica, and also appears to have emerged or re-emerged in several regions including parts of Central Asia, China, Europe, East Africa and South America (Craig and Pawlowski, 2002; Torgerson and Budke, 2004). This review aims to describe and assess all the successful hydatid control programmes, to consider failed campaigns and to discuss control options and modern surveillance tools.

Human CE is a chronic, potentially life-threatening infection with the larval cystic stage (hydatid) of the dog taeniid tapeworm *E. granulosus* (Batsch, 1786). It was recognized as a human infection by Hippocrates (379 BC), but its animal (parasitic) origin was not identified until the work of Redi in 17th-century Italy. Batsch named the cystic parasite as *Hydatigera granulosa* in 1786, and in 1808 Rudolphi introduced the name *Echinococcus* (spiny berry) probably to describe the hooked protoscoleces found in hydatid cysts. It took another 50 years or so, however, before the life cycle of *E. granulosus* was determined in the decade 1850–1860 by the work of von Siebold, Naunyn and Krabbe following their independent experiments to infect dogs with hydatid cyst material (Grove, 1990). Subsequently, Krabbe in Iceland in 1863 successfully infected sheep with eggs from adult *E. granulosus* tapeworms, and the life cycle of the hydatid-forming tapeworm was thus confirmed. In 1854, Kuchenmeister in Germany published some of the '*Principles of hydatid control*' including prevention of dogs being fed livestock offal (Grove, 1990). By 1863, Krabbe used this new life cycle knowledge to recommend implementation of the the world's first national programme to control a parasite, that is, hydatid disease in Iceland (see Section 2.1).

1.1. Life Cycle Biology of *Echinococcus. granulosus*

The adult tapeworm is small, being only 2–7 mm in length comprising 2–6 segments, with a scolex that bares two rows of hooks and four suckers. The pre-patent period in the dog's small intestine is around 6 weeks, but may vary according to genotype of the parasite as well as breed of the dog so that the range may be 34–58 days (Thompson, 1995). Gravid proglottids are shed approximately every 7–14 days, each proglottis containing around 500–600 eggs. A dog may harbour <10–>25000 worms in the intestine, but the mean number is probably more like 200–300. Most worms are attached between the villi in the first third of the small intestine. Worm longevity in the dog is estimated to be about 1 year (probable range 6–20 months) (Gemmell *et al.*, 1986; Torgerson and Heath, 2003). (Plate 11.1.A and E in colour plate section) The mature eggs of *E. granulosus* are typical of taeniid cestodes, 30–40 μm in size with a thick embryophore that protects an enclosed, fully developed six-hooked oncosphere (hexacanth). Eggs of *E. granulosus* cannot be distinguished under light microscopy from eggs of other *Echinococcus* or *Taenia* species, but may be specifically identified using monoclonal antibodies or by PCR amplification of DNA (Craig and Nelson, 1986; Cabrera *et al.*, 2002a). The eggs may contaminate not only the perianal area of a dog but also the snout, flanks and paws (Torgerson and Heath, 2003). *Echinococcus* eggs in the environment may remain viable for months and withstand temperatures of approximately −30°C to +30°C, but desiccate when relative humidity is 25% or lower and at temperatures >45°C (Eckert *et al.*, 2001). Viable eggs may be mechanically transported on or within the gut of dipteran flies or other arthropods (Lawson and Gemmell, 1990), but the majority contaminate the immediate environment of the infected dog around its home area and on pastures where dog defaecation may occur (Gemmell *et al.*, 1986; Craig *et al.*, 1988).

Following ingestion by a suitable intermediate host, e.g. sheep or human, the egg hatches in the upper small intestine to release an activated oncosphere, which penetrates the gut epithelium with the aid of hook movements and proteolytic secretions. Penetration may occur within minutes, and the oncosphere usually enters a capillary so that the venous flow ensures that the majority will pass directly to the liver and/ or the lungs. Oncospheres that fail to penetrate within about 1 hour usually die and are digested (Lethbridge, 1980). Within hours of penetration and site location, the oncosphere begins to vesiculate in tissues, and by 3–8 days a clearly laminated layer is visible in the small hydatid cyst (<1 mm diameter) (Holcman and Heath, 1997). The invasive oncosphere and early post-oncosphere metacestode stages are vulnerable to antibody-dependent, complement-mediated immune damage and may be killed in the first few days of infection before the formation of the protective laminated layer. Pre-encystment immunity can also be artificially stimulated using native extracts, or recombinant oncosphere antigens, which form the basis of the highly effective EG95 *E. granulosus* vaccine (Lightowlers *et al.*, 1996). Once the unique acellular mucin-rich laminated layer is secreted from the thin cellular germinal layer, the fluid-filled unilocular hydatid cyst grows relatively slowly at the rate of about 0.5 cm to several centimetres per year. In sheep older than 5 years, hydatid cysts may reach 5–7 cm. (see Plate 11.1 A in colour plate section) In other more long-lived livestock species (e.g. camels, cattle and horses) and in humans, hydatid cysts may be significantly larger. In untreated humans, CE annual hydatid cyst growth ranged from 0 to 160 mm, but average growth was 7–29 mm (Romig *et al.*, 1986; Frider *et al.*, 1999). Humans become infected with CE only through accidental ingestion of the infective egg(s) and normally are a dead-end host and take no part in the transmission cycle, though a human–dog cycle may theoretically be possible (Macpherson, 1983) Plate 11.1 in the separate colour plate section).

Within 4 to 12 months post-infection of a susceptible animal or human host, brood capsules bud from the inner germinal layer of the hydatid cyst and asexual protoscolex production occurs within each brood capsule. A 10 cm human hydatid cyst contained 87 920 brood capsules within which a total of approximately 1.3 million protoscoleces were counted (Wen and Ding 2000). After ingestion of a fertile hydatid cyst by a suitable definitive host, e.g. the dog, each protoscolex can transform into an adult tapeworm to complete its life cycle. Protoscoleces may, however, also vesiculate in their own right and develop in the cystic direction, for example, when a cyst is damaged, and results in formation of daughter cysts in human CE, termed secondary echinococcosis.

1.2. Medical Importance

Human CE is characterized by a variable asymptomatic period during hydatid cyst growth, which is affected by patient age, site of cyst development and whether infection is with a single or multiple cysts. Approximately 70–80% of hydatid cysts in human CE develop in the liver, 10–20% in the lungs and around 5% in any other site in the body (WHO/OIE, 2001). Hydatid cysts may remain asymptomatic for life especially if they remain small. Symptoms are usually associated with pressure effects of the cyst on adjacent tissues/organs, but traumatic hydatid cyst rupture may result in a fatal anaphylaxis. Human CE may be fatal in around 5% of primary cases, and >10–20% of secondary echinococcosis cases. The burden of disease associated with echinococcosis is significant in highly endemic regions, for example regions of China and South America (Budke *et al.*, 2004a; 2004b; Carabin *et al.*, 2005). Surgical cyst removal or drainage is the main form of treatment and therefore human CE represents a serious and costly public health challenge in endemic areas (Larrieu *et al.*, 2000a; Torgerson *et al.*, 2000). Approximately 5–27% of hydatid patients experience a recurrence following surgery, which then usually results in higher morbidity and mortality rates (WHO/OIE, 2001). Use of benzimidazole drugs, such as albendazole and percutaneous cyst aspiration, provide useful additional approaches for treatment of complicated CE and simple hepatic CE, respectively (WHO/OIE, 2001; Larrieu *et al.*, 2004).

1.3. Epidemiology of *E. granulosus* Transmission

Transmission of *E. granulosus* between domestic livestock and canids is predominantly a feature of pastoral communities in temperate or semi-arid rangeland areas of the world. The dominant strain, sub-species or genotype of *E. granulosus* is the sheep–dog form or G1 genotype (McManus and Thompson, 2003). The sheep–dog strain is cosmopolitan, with high endemicity in the Mediterranean Basin (including North Africa), the Near and Middle East, Central Asia, western China, Russia, East Africa and large regions of South America (central Andes, south Brazil and Uruguay, to southern Patagonia), and this strain is responsible for >95% of all human hydatid cysts that have been DNA typed after surgical removal or biopsy (WHO/OIE, 2001; McManus and Thompson, 2003). In addition to the G1 genotype, up to nine other genotypes have been described using mitochondrial gene analysis, including horse, bovid, camel, pig and cervid forms, and all except the horse strain show evidence of zoonotic potential, albeit only identified in relatively small numbers of human hydatid cases (Kamenetzky *et al.*, 2002; McManus and Thompson, 2003). Phenotypic differences between strains of *E. granulosus* may be important for transmission dynamics, for example the pre-patent period in the sheep–dog strain is approximately 45 days, in contrast to the cattle–dog strain which is quite short at 33–35 days. (WHO/OIE, 2001)

From our experience in South America, East Africa and China, it appears that, in general, when ovine CE and canine echinococcosis prevalence rates are 10–20% or greater, the parasite will potentially cause human incidence rates >5 cases per 100 000 per year and human hepatic CE prevalence (by ultrasound mass screens) of >1–2%. Such CE disease rates in humans, though low compared to other helminthic infections such as schistosomiasis, may nevertheless be significant in terms of the public health impact due to the high morbidity and the complicated nature of treatments for human CE (Craig *et al.*, 1996; Budke *et al.*, 2004a). Recent estimates for average cost for surgical treatment of CE was >US$10 000 in UK (Torgerson and Dowling, 2001), >US$4000–6700 in Argentina and Uruguay (Larrieu *et al.*, 2000a; Torgerson *et al.*, 2000) and at least US$700 in China (Craig, 2004). In addition to public health impacts, economic losses due to condemnation of sheep and bovid offal may be significant, and for example were estimated to be US$10–15 million annually in Tunisia (Carabin *et al.*, 2005).

Adults >20 years of age are usually at greater risk of CE but many probably contract the disease as children. Children may however be symptomatic and require treatment. One study in the Xinjiang Region of northwest China showed that 36.4% of 21 560 CE patients treated in hospital over an extended period were under the age of 14 years (Xu, 1995; Ito *et al.*, 2003). Other risk factors for human CE from case control and community mass screening surveys appear to be livestock ownership (especially sheep), occupation in pastoralism/ rangeland, ethnicity (e.g. Turkana in Kenya, and Tibetans and Kazahks in China), gender (females often at higher risk), dog ownership (number of dogs, years owned and caregiver), feeding uncooked viscera to dogs, source of drinking water, knowledge about CE and poor hygienic practices (Dowling *et al.*, 2000; Larrieu *et al.*, 2002; Craig, 2004).

2. HYDATID CONTROL PROGRAMMES LEADING TO ELIMINATION OR NEAR ELIMINATION OF *E. GRANULOSUS*

Five 'island-based' hydatid control programmes, i.e. Iceland, New Zealand, Tasmania, Falkland Islands and Cyprus, have been successful in the eventual elimination of CE as a public health problem, and even to the elimination of the parasite in dogs and sheep.

2.1. Iceland (1863–1960)

Cystic hydatid disease probably became established in Iceland by 1200 AD when livestock numbers on the island began to increase, and after the parasite was possibly imported with dogs brought via trading routes from north Germany. The first clear autopsy records that described human hydatid infection in Iceland appeared in the 1760s, and hydatid rates as high as 26–30% were recorded for autopsies performed at the beginning of the 20th century on persons born from the 1840s (Dungal, 1957). Of 7333 autopsies performed in the capital Reykjavik, from 1932 to 1966, hydatid cysts were detected in 190 (2.6%) of the deceased. However, very high post-mortem prevalence rates for CE of 15–62% occurred for persons born between the years

1860 and 1899 (Palsson, 1976). Probably the last confirmed case of human CE contracted in Iceland during the 20th century was diagnosed in 1960 in a 23-year-old female who died 6 months after surgery for a hydatid cyst of the ileum (Beard *et al.*, 2001). In the intervening 100 years a deliberate hydatid control campaign resulted in a remarkable reduction in human CE, and the disease was considered to have been 'eradicated' from Iceland by the 1960s (reported by the National Hydatids Council of New Zealand, 1965).

The Iceland hydatid campaign must be one of the earliest control programmes specifically directed against any parasite. It was instigated in 1863 by a Danish veterinarian, Harald Krabbe, which was in the same year that Bernard Naunyn, in Germany, succeeded in infecting dogs with *E. granulosus* worms after feeding them human hydatid cysts (Grove, 1990). Krabbe was Professor of Veterinary Science in Copenhagen, and became chief adviser to the Icelandic government on hydatid disease control from 1860 to 1890. In 1864, he wrote an 18-page general information booklet on hydatid disease that was distributed free of charge, which emphasized the life cycle of the parasite and the role of the dog as the key to prevention of hydatid disease. The prophylactic measures he recommended included the destruction of cyst-infested offal from livestock, a reduction in the number of dogs and avoidance of close contact with dogs (Krabbe, 1864). A similar pamphlet written by the chief medical officer for Iceland (J. Jonassen) was also distributed to all households in 1884 and 1891 (Palsson, 1976). During that period there were relatively few books, apart from the Bible and Icelandic Sagas, thus the hydatid pamphlets became one of the most widely read printed works by the poor but highly literate society whose population was only around 70 000 (Beard *et al.*, 2001). In 1890, a Hydatid law was passed by the government, which imposed a tax on every dog (payable by owners), and it also outlawed feeding of dogs offal from slaughtered sheep and cattle, and furthermore stated that livestock cysts should be buried or burnt. Significantly, this law also required that every dog was to be treated once a year with a vermifuge, which at that time was areca seed extract (later arecoline hydrobromide), and each community had to nominate a 'dog-cleaner'. In addition, a 'dog-cleaning house' was to be constructed in each village. Dogs were purged on wood shavings, that were then burnt, and each dog was then washed (Beard *et al.*, 2001). This Act was upgraded by parliament in the years 1924, 1953 and 1957. In the early part of the 20th century, slaughterhouses were built all over Iceland and it was made illegal to kill livestock outside them. Changes in sheep husbandry that occurred in Iceland in the early 20th century also reduced the risk of transmission from sheep to dogs. Lambs were slaughtered at 4–5 months of age replacing the previous reliance on 3–4 year old wethers (castrated male sheep) for meat, and also the milking of ewes was discouraged.

Krabbe was far-sighted and had correctly considered that it would take a generation before any public health effects of the educational campaign would be seen. By the decade 1890–1900, new cases of human CE had virtually disappeared, and only two cases in the under 40 years age group were detected between 1930 and 1950, the re-maining cases ($n = 70$) were >51 years of age (Dungal, 1957). In 1883, Krabbe found 28% of 100 dogs at necropsy infected with *E. granulosus* worms, and a much later necropsy survey, in the decade 1950–1960, failed to find the parasite in 200 dogs, though the non-pathogenic tapeworm *Taenia hydatigena* (syn. *T. marginata*, which is also transmitted by offal from sheep to dogs) persisted at low (5.5%) prevalence (Palsson, 1976). There are no reliable records of ovine CE in the early decades of the campaign, but during the period 1948–1953 the prevalence in sheep was around 0.0008%; the last sheep confirmed infected with hydatids were 21 aged ewes identified between the years 1953 and 1973 on the east of the island (Dungal, 1957; Beard *et al.*, 2001) (Table 1).

Thus the Icelandic hydatid campaign was astonishingly successful, even though it was based solely on an educational campaign for the first 20 years, with subsequent enforcements after 1890 and the intro-duction of beneficial changes in sheep husbandry in the early 1900s. Continued strict controls on dog behaviour and slaughter practices for the next 50 years (to the 1960s and currently) as a 'maintenance of eradication' phase, have ensured control of transmission and probable elimination of *E. granulosus* from the Island. The Iceland experience served to demonstrate for the first time that total control and even elimination of hydatid disease was possible, albeit over a very long period in an island state with a small rural though literate population.

Table 1 Island control programmes for cystic echinococcosis (CE) that lead to elimination or near elimination of human CE and transmission of *E. granulosus*

Region (control period)	Pre-control	Intermediate impact (i)	Intermediate impact (ii)	Post-control impact
Iceland (1860–1960)	1861–1870	1924–1935	1946–1957	1967–1973
Dogs (%)	28		0	
Sheep (%)		12.4 (1924)	0.0008	19 ewes
Humans autopsy (%)	22	5.9	1.5	0
New Zealand (1959–1997)	1947–1955	1959–1963	1975–1982	1993–2002
Dogs (%)	10	37	<5%	0
Sheep (%)	80	48–58	0.43–15.6	<1 in 10^6
Human incidence per 100 000 pa	4.5	3.2	0.7	Last old cases
Tasmania (1965–1996)	1953–1967	1971–1975	1981–1985	1996–2000
Dogs (%)	12.7	0.8	0.06	
Sheep (%)	52.2	8.7	0.6	0.0002
Human incidence per 100 000 pa	537 cases 15	28 cases	0 cases	
Falklands (1965–1997)	1965–1969	1977–1983	1991–1993	2000–
Dogs (%)			1.7%[a]	
Sheep (%)	59	1.8	0.11–0.47	
Human incidence per 100 000	55	18 seropositves		Last old cases
Cyprus (1971–1985)	1972	1982–1984	1993–1998	2000–
Dogs (%)	6.8	<0.02	0.17 (3%[a], 1995)	(2.6%[a], 1997–2000)
Sheep (%)	66	0.9	0.014	
Humans per 100 000 pa	12.9		0<20 years 3.5–8 (NC)	25 cases (NC)

[a]Coproantigen test; NC, Northern Cyprus.

Interestingly and possibly uniquely, the health education message alone was successful, as evidenced by the autopsy data, which indicated that the risk to humans fell dramatically within 30 years of the distribution in 1864 of Krabbe's hydatid booklet. The success in Iceland encouraged the initiation of other hydatid control programmes on the islands of New Zealand, Tasmania, Cyprus and the Falklands, which to varying degrees, have been highly effective. New Zealand and Tasmania both declared their islands provisionally free of hydatids by 2002.

2.2. New Zealand (1938–2002)

The population of New Zealand in 1955, four years prior to formal control, was around 3 million people, while the number of sheep was more than 39 million, owned by 37000 sheep ranchers (Schwabe, 1979). Of a sample of 25 991 sheep from both North and South Islands, 48.4% were infected with hepatic hydatidosis, and >80% of the farms surveyed were affected (Gemmell, 1961). There were approximately 200 000 dogs in New Zealand, and arecoline surveys for canine echinococcosis indicated a prevalence range of 10% to >37% in some regions (Gemmell, 1990). Human hydatidosis was recognized in the country since 1862, but unlike Iceland, control was not seriously considered prior to 1938 (Pharo, 2002). Between 1946 and 1956, hydatid disease was indicated as the cause of death in 142 persons. The autopsy rate was about 1%, and a national surgical incidence rate of 4.5 per 100000 per year was calculated for the period 1941–950, with higher rates (11.8 per 100000) in rural areas (Gemmell, 1990; Heath *et al.*, 1999).

From 1938 to 1958, prior to the start of the formal hydatid control campaign, a 'voluntary educational campaign' was instigated (eventually using voluntary committees) that gave advice on safe ways to feed dogs and dispose of offal, and it also provided enough arecoline hydrobromide for owners who registered their dogs, to enable dosing four times per year (Gemmell, 1990). The Meat Act 1940 also made it illegal to feed raw offal to dogs. However, unlike the situation described above for Iceland, little or no change occurred in neither human CE rates nor the prevalence of ovine hydatidosis in New Zealand over the 20-year period of the initial 'educational campaign' (Gemmell, 1990).

In 1959, an independent National Hydatids Council was formed by the Hydatids Act of parliament, which worked through local county councils and municipalities and was funded by a mandatory dog licence fee (about 400 000 rural and urban dogs were registered). This local management and dedicated funding stream were an operational advantage for the Hydatids Council, but later it became apparent that transformation from the arecoline testing/anthelmintic dosing 'attack' phase, to a 'consolidation' phase based on livestock quarantine, was problematic without legislative powers for proper surveillance and quarantine of infected farms. Arecoline is a purgative, so infected dogs could be identified and quarantined after macroscopic then microscopic examination of the purge, and their owners given more intensive education. Dog testing in New Zealand was done in a semi-automated central testing laboratory that could process 1 million faecal samples per year, rather than by a mobile arecoline field unit (as adopted more successfully in the shorter duration Tasmanian hydatid programme— see Section 2.3). In 1972, arecoline screening was replaced by a more costly 6 weekly anthelmintic dog-dosing programme involving 400 technicians who were employed by the Hydatids Council of New Zealand. Initially the anthelmintic niclosamide was used, then after 1978 it was replaced by the more effective drug praziquantel (PZQ) (Gemmell, 1990; Economides *et al.*, 1998).

Thus the first part of the 'attack' phase in New Zealand from 1959 to 1972 (13 years) was based on arecoline surveillance of dogs (up to four testings per year) under the direction of the National Hydatids Council, followed by 19 years of 6 weekly anthelmintic dosing (1972–1991).

In 1967, it was recommended that the control programme be transferred to the Ministry of Agriculture in order to reduce costs and use the government-trained veterinary workforce. This proposal was however rejected at the time and transfer to full Government control did not take place until 1991, when the 6 weekly dosing programme ceased and the National Hydatids Council was disbanded. In 1990, movement control of livestock was introduced by the Ministry of Agriculture, and slaughterhouse surveillance with trace back to infected farms became the core of the 'consolidation' phase over the next 11 years (1991–2002).

It is probable that hydatid control in New Zealand could have been more rapid in the 'attack' phase (total 32 years) and transferred earlier to a 'consolidation' phase (termed 'maintenance of eradication phase' at the time, which depended on quarantine of farms with infected animals) if the Ministry of Agriculture had managed the programme earlier. This is because the Ministry of Agriculture already had a large pool of salaried skilled technical staff employed in farm outreach (e.g. for tuberculosis and brucellosis control). Also because it possessed the necessary quarantine authority and measures, which could not be applied under the authority of a National Hydatids Council (Gemmell, 1994; M.A. Gemmell, personal communication).

Despite the lengthy 32-year 'attack' phase of the New Zealand hydatid control programme, evidence of a rapid decline and even cessation in transmission to humans, under 19 years of age, occurred within 12 years (1959–1971) of the start of the 'attack' phase (Gemmell, 1990, 1994). Over the same period, prevalence in sheep had declined from >50% to 25%, and 10 years later (in 1981) the national prevalence of ovine hydatidosis was only 0.43% (National Hydatids Council of New Zealand, 1980). Prevalence in dogs had declined from >30% to <5% over the period 1959–1972, and in 1980 only five dogs in the country were confirmed by purgation to be infected with *E. granulosus*. After 1987, all cysts detected at meat inspection were submitted for histological diagnosis (Heath *et al.*, 1999). From 1991, the parasite was rarely seen in sheep at slaughter, and the last true outbreak occurred in 1995 when fertile hydatid cysts were found in an aged ewe from an isolated property. This property was subsequently quarantined by the Ministry of Agriculture and a 6 weekly dog-dosing regime enforced (Heath *et al.*, 1999). After 1996, no confirmed hydatid lesions or cysts have been recorded in the >25 million sheep slaughtered annually in New Zealand. In 2002, the country declared itself provisionally free from hydatids, 43 years after the start of the control programme (Pharo, 2002) (Table 1).

2.3. Tasmania (1964–1996)

In 1953, Harold Dew, an Australian surgeon and world authority on the clinical pathology of cystic hydatidosis, had estimated the annual incidence of human CE for the island of Tasmania (a State of Australia, population about 402 000 in 1964) to be 9.3 per 100 000 in the decade 1941–1950, but with an incidence of 27.4 per 100 000 in the rural population (Dew, 1953). In the following decade, 1953–1962, there were 537 new cases of human hydatid disease in Tasmania, or an average of one case per week (McConnell and Green, 1979). In the early 1960s, about 50% of sheep >3 years old were infected with hydatids, and at least 12% of dogs carried the *Echinococcus* tapeworm (Bramble, 1974; McConnell and Green, 1979).

The Tasmanian hydatid control programme was largely conceived by Trevor Beard, an English physician who moved to the island in the 1950s, but soon began to see many paediatric and adult hydatid cases in his practice in Campbell Town. In 1962, a local Farmers and Stockowners Association, in consultation with the Department of Agriculture, produced a small booklet on hydatid control (reprinted in 1964), and the voluntary group formed the Tasmanian Hydatids Eradication Council. By that time the formal New Zealand hydatid campaign had been running for 3 years. Following a fact-finding visit to New Zealand in 1961–1962, Beard was able to help formulate an official hydatid control programme for the State of Tasmania with support from the Department of Agriculture and the Department of Primary Industry (Beard *et al.*, 2001).

The Tasmanian programme however would be different to the New Zealand programme in four important ways, which almost certainly resulted in a much shorter 'attack' phase (11 years in Tasmania compared to the 32 years of the New Zealand campaign) and thus earlier transformation to the less costly 'consolidation' phase. Firstly, the Tasmanian hydatid control programme was funded and managed by the State Department of Agriculture, rather than a Voluntary Hydatid Commission as was initially used in New Zealand (although dog registration in Tasmania remained under the control of the local authorities and community participation was kept active through an advisory committee). Secondly, mobile dog testing units (with 'dog testing strips' set up annually in each locality) were used in Tasmania rather than a central testing laboratory as employed in New Zealand, and the former approach also gave a greater educational impact to the sheep farmers themselves. Thirdly, dog testing/treatment, which in Tasmania became legally compulsory in 1965, was confined to rural dogs (approximately 20 000 dogs; city dogs were ignored as low risk after 1967). Fourthly, high-risk farms in Tasmania were identified initially by arecoline testing of dogs (1965–1974), then by trace back of infected sheep (from 1975–1997), and subsequently quarantined under very strict State government enforced legislation (Beard *et al.*, 2001).

As a direct result of the control programme transmission of hydatid disease to humans had ceased in Tasmania by 1974 within only 10 years after the start of the official campaign, and possibly even earlier, as there were no new cases in the <9 years of age group after that date. Furthermore, no human hydatid cases occurred in the under 20 years age group after 1976 (McConnell and Green, 1979; Gemmell, 1990). Abattoir inspection of sheep offal was introduced in 1967, and data from that year showed that 52% of sheep >3 years old were infected, reducing to 8.4% in 1972–1973 and to 3.4% in 1977–1978 (McConnell and Green, 1979). Prevalence of *E. granulosus* in dogs by arecoline purgation declined from 12.7% in 1965–1966 to 1.1% in 1972–1973, was 0.22% in 1977–1978, and by 1981–1985 prevalence in dogs was only 0.06% (McConnell and Green, 1979; Beard *et al.*, 2001).

The Tasmanian hydatid control programme was, and still is, considered one of the fastest, most successful and cost-effective hydatid programmes yet introduced anywhere in the world. It cost only 0.5% of the State health budget (McConnell and Green, 1979; Gemmell, 1990). In 1996, Tasmania was officially declared provisionally free from hydatidosis, 32 years after the start of the control programme (Jenkins, 2005). The Island then entered the so-called 'maintenance of eradication' phase, which depended on permanent annual notification of abattoir inspection records for both sheep and cattle. As a result of this legislation, two farms were quarantined in 1997 following detection of small hydatid cysts in a single sheep and a cow. Subsequent investigation identified an infected dog that had been brought in from mainland Australia within 18 months of the abattoir findings. This event led to the current legal requirement of a veterinary certification of PZQ treatment for all dogs within 14 days of entry to Tasmania (Economides *et al.*, 1998).

2.4. Falkland Islands (1965–1997)

These remote islands in the South Atlantic (permanent human population <2000) held a sheep population of about 700 000 in the early 1990s which were located on about 90 large farms, which also owned approximately 900 dogs (Reichel *et al.*, 1996). The first official record of ovine hydatidosis in the Falklands was reported in 1941 in one of 2000 sheep (Gibbs, 1946). By 1969, slaughter records, largely from Stanley abattoir, indicated that 59.3% of sheep were infected (Whitely, 1983). This dramatic increase in the prevalence of ovine hydatidosis paralleled the first reports of human cases from 1965, and 11 cases were confirmed by 1975 (Bleaney, 1984). This was equivalent to an annual incidence rate of at least 55 cases per 100 000. An official local government advisory committee on hydatidosis was established in 1965 to undertake education (including safe disposal of offal on farms), together with compulsory licencing and annual arecoline dosing of dogs. From 1970, anthelmintic dosing of dogs every 12 weeks with bunamidine was instigated, and from 1977 was replaced by 6 weekly dosing with PZQ (the drug paid for by owners); furthermore, quarantine was introduced for premises with infected livestock (Gemmell, 1999). By 1981, hydatid prevalence in sheep had declined to 1.8% (Whitely, 1983) and further to 0.16% in 1993 (Reichel *et al.*, 1996). The 1993 prevalence was, however, still more than double the ovine prevalence recorded in 1991. Almost all these residual hydatid infections originated from sheep farms on the more remote East Falkland Islands (Reichel *et al.*, 1996). During the period 1995–1996, slaughter surveillance records for the islands revealed only two infected sheep (Economides *et al.*, 1998). In 1988, no confirmed cases of human CE were detected, although 18 seropositve persons (by Arc 5 diffusion test) were identified. There appear to be no available reports of the prevalence of echinococcosis in dogs prior to the control programme; however, from 1992 to 1993 a serological and coproantigen survey was carried out on almost the entire dog population ($n = 908$) of the Islands, of which 2.1% were seropositve, and 1.7% of 464 dogs were coproantigen positive (Reichel *et al.*, 1996).

The Falkland Islands hydatid control programme thus spent about 32 years in the 'attack' phase (1965–1997), moving to a consolidation phase in 1997, which, like New Zealand and Tasmania, relied on strict abattoir and slaughterhouse surveillance with quarantine of infected properties. Dog owners also continued to be supplied with PZQ and assumed direct responsibility for dosing their own dogs; in addition, restriction on dog entry to the islands is currently enforced (Gemmell, 1994).

2.5. Cyprus (1971–1985)

The Mediterranean Basin has a long history of endemic CE with recognizable descriptions of hydatid cysts from ancient Greece (Grove, 1990). Recent overviews of the status of CE in this region indicate a continued significant problem that includes regions of *all* the countries on the Mediteranean littoral from Portugal to Lebanon, and from Israel to Morocco, including all the large Mediterranean islands (Ecca *et al.*, 2002; Seimenis, 2003). Only the island nation of Cyprus however has embarked on a national-level hydatid control programme, which was highly successful during the period 1971–1985 when the parasite was almost eliminated. However, transmission had re-emerged in several areas of the island by the early 1990s (Economides and Christofi, 2002).

In the late 1960s and early 1970s, human hydatidosis was a common disease in Cyprus whose population was 615 000 (with approximately the same number of sheep and goats) on an island about seven times smaller than Tasmania. There was on average two surgical cases per week for CE, and the annual surgical incidence was calculated at 12.9 per 100 000 in the late 1960s (Economides *et al.*, 1998). Prior to the control programme, ovine CE prevalences ranged from 25% to >80% in aged ewes, and cattle and pigs were also infected up to 60% and 30%, respectively. The dog population was probably around 50 000 many of which were stray/unwanted animals, and in 1972 overall prevalence at necropsy (or arecoline purge) was 6.8%, with 14% of farm dogs infected (Polydorou, 1976). In 1971, the Department of Veterinary Services, under the direction of Kristacos Polydorou, embarked on a national hydatid control campaign. The main thrust was a draconian euthanasia programme (by current standards) to reduce stray dog numbers, combined with obligatory registration of all owned dogs, and the spaying (sterilization) of large numbers of female dogs. In addition, arecoline purge testing of all registered dogs occurred every 3 months, with infected owned dogs being euthanized. A public health education programme was also initiated, as well as slaughter control and meat inspection (Economides *et al.*, 1998).

Between the years 1971 and 1985, more than 85 000 stray dogs were exterminated, and >13 000 female dogs sterilized. Arecoline purge data for owned dogs showed that prevalence of *E. granulosus* had dropped from 6.8–7.4% in 1972–1973 to 0.6–0.75% in 1977–1978; and by 1984–1985 no dogs were found infected from more than 36 000 that were arecoline tested (Economides, 1994). Over the control period, the prevalence of CE in sheep (>2 years old) dropped from 50% in 1971 to 13% in 1978, and was only 0.1% in 1985. The human CE surgical case numbers also reduced over the control period so that by 1993–1998 no new cases under 20 years of age were diagnosed in the Cyprus Government Controlled Area (GCA). Consequently, by 1985 it was considered that hydatid disease had been 'eradicated' from Cyprus and the programme was terminated (Polydorou, 1993). The partitioning of the island after 1974, however, meant that the hydatid control programme was effectively restricted to the GCA and could not be properly continued in the northern Turkish occupied territory or non-GCA (also referred to as Northern Cyprus). Initially after 1985, only sporadic cases of ovine CE were detected in abattoirs and it was assumed that these animals came from the non GCA. A survey in the main GCA zone of Cyprus between 1993 and 1996, however, revealed that 21% of villages harboured small numbers of infected livestock (sheep and cattle), and 0.7% of dogs tested arecoline purge positive. Furthermore, *Echinococcus* coproantigen ELISA surveys in 1995 and during 1997–2000, obtained positive results in 0.1% (1/700) and 2.8% (184/6551) of dogs, respectively, with 8.1% positivity for dogs from Northern Cyprus (non-GCA) (Economides *et al.*, 1998; Christofi *et al.*, 2002). No human CE cases <20 years old were treated in the GCA between 1990 and 1993, while three cases were identified in the northern non-GCA zone, and an incidence of human CE of eight per 100 000 in the non-GCA was calculated for the period 1997–1998 (Economides and Christofi, 2002).

In order to prevent a major recurrence of transmission in Cyprus, hydatid control measures were re-introduced in 1993 (in the GCA zone) by the Department of Veterinary Services. This was effectively a new 'consolidation' phase to replace that which had probably previously been prematurely stopped, and which had been disrupted as a result of a breakdown of control measures in Northern Cyprus. The new control measures included dog registration, treatment of imported dogs, safe destruction of livestock carcasses, a re-vitalized education programme and importantly abattoir surveillance of all livestock with active trace back of infected animals. Infection of livestock with the related dog–sheep cestode *T. hydatigena* (non-pathogenic to humans) was also used as a marker for farms with high-risk dog behaviour and/or unhygienic slaughter practices. Farms and villages with evidence of either *E. granulosus* or *T. hydatigena* transmission were subjected to additional control measures, i.e. treatment of all dogs with PZQ two to three times per year, strict control of stray dogs, movement control of both dogs and livestock, prosecution for illegal slaughtering and PZQ baits for stray dogs (and foxes). In addition, quarantined premises were not released from restrictions until there was no further evidence of infection with either *E. granulosus* or *T. hydatigena* in livestock for at least 3 years (Economides and Christofi, 2002). Thus, in Cyprus, an island-wide control programme changed effectively to a 'continental' style programme as a result of partitioning of the island in 1974, with resultant need to maintain a permanent or long-term 'consolidation' phase, which is still ongoing in the GCA (Economides *et al.*, 1998).

3. LESSONS LEARNED FROM ISLAND HYDATID CONTROL PROGRAMMES

By the late 1970s, it was clear that CE was a zoonotic disease that could be effectively controlled, by, quote, 'active implementation of a programme by a recognized authority on an instruction from the legislature to limit prevalence' (Gemmell and Roberts, 1998). This confidence was gained from the five island control programmes described above, all of which resulted in elimination or near elimination of transmission of *E. granulosus*, and the demise of CE as a public health problem. In the case of Iceland this took >100 years beginning from the 1860s, for New Zealand it took around 50 years (from 1938), but by contrast control measures were already effective within about 10 years in Tasmania (from 1964) and Cyprus (from 1971). It is therefore reasonable to ask two questions, firstly, 'why did some programmes work better and faster than others?' Secondly, 'can the island campaigns against cystic hydatidosis be applied successfully to continental control programmes?' (Table 1).

3.1. Slow-Track versus Fast-Track

The control approach in Iceland over more than 100 years, was considered, not illogically, as being 'slow-track', as was the New Zealand programme at least initially (Gemmell, 1990). Both, relied solely on specific health education (mainly concerning safe offal disposal and dog management), for Iceland from 1863 to 1890, and in New Zealand the educational phase ran from 1938 to 1958. The late Dr. Mike Gemmell categorized this kind of educational/development approach to control as a 'horizontal approach', in which emphasis was placed on health education, but also meat inspection and upgrading of abattoirs (Gemmell, 1986, 1999). In contrast, Gemmell considered that a 'vertical approach' involved the setting up of an appropriate structure to apply veterinary public health measures principally using an 'attack phase' targeted at testing and/or treating dogs, and this could be a 'fast-track' approach (Gemmell and Roberts, 1998). The 'education-only approach' had a historically significant and measurable effect on human CE rates in Iceland so that the disease had virtually disappeared in younger persons (<20 years old) within 30 years after 1890 (Dungal, 1957). However, in the 20th century, 20–30 years of specific health education aimed at sheep farmers in New Zealand failed to significantly reduce human or ovine CE rates over that period (Gemmell, 1990). Iceland is now considered to be a unique example of an education-based horizontal approach to hydatid control that was ultimately effective. The main reasons for success in Iceland were the highly literate population and the obligatory reading of Krabbe's hydatid control booklet (Krabbe, 1864), so that virtually the whole population became aware of the parasite life cycle and the basic control measures of offal disposal and avoidance of close contact with dogs. Furthermore, changes in Icelandic sheep husbandry in the early 20th century in favour of fat lambs, also reduced transmission potential.

Health education for prevention of hydatidosis, on its own, with the exception of Iceland, appears generally not to lead to significant reduction in transmission (Gemmell, 1990; Lloyd *et al.*, 1996; Buishi *et al.*, 2005). The biotic potential of *E. granulosus*, though lower than other taeniid species, is enough to ensure that despite applying basic horizontal measures, transmission may continue through pasture contamination by a relatively small number of dogs with high worm burdens (Gemmell *et al.*, 1986, 1987; Torgerson and Heath, 2003). Two advantages of health education, however, are (i) it is relatively cheap, (ii) it provides an important avenue to enable endemic rural communities to accept and participate in a 'fast-track' vertical hydatid control programme.

Both the New Zealand (from 1959) and the Tasmania (from 1964) 'attack' phases of their respective hydatid control programmes started around the same time, with Tasmania about 3 years behind New Zealand. The Tasmanians, from the start however, put the dog-centred control under the funding and implementation responsibilty of the State Department of Agriculture. In contrast, the New Zealand programme was funded by a specially created National Hydatids Council that derived its funding from dog registrations, and this non-government body also specifically hired and trained the hydatid technical workforce. The Tasmania government-based hydatid control authority was much more cost-effective, efficient and committed, and ultimately lead to an overall faster control of CE in the 'attack' phase with easier conversion to a less intensive surveillance-based 'consolidation' phase. Though both programmes used extensive arecoline purge testing of dogs, the Tasmanian option of mobile testing units making annual visits to localities contrasted to the centralized purge screening facility used in New Zealand. As a result, the Tasmanian approach had a greater educational impact at grass roots and resulted in more effective implementation of quarantine measures on hydatid positive farms. Even without the availability of the highly effective anthelmintic, PZQ, to treat dogs (which was introduced in New Zealand in 1978), the Tasmanian programme resulted in a cessation of transmission to humans within 10 years of the start of the 'attack' phase of their campaign (McConnell and Green, 1979). In New Zealand, the attack phase lasted a total of 32 years, moving from arecoline purgation to 6 weekly dosing with niclosamide, then 6 weekly with PZQ. The New Zealand Ministry of Agriculture only assumed responsibility for the programme when it was clear that the Hydatids Council did not have the legislative authority to undertake abattoir surveillance as the mainstay of the consolidation phase.

The Falkland islands hydatid programme (1965–1997) also lasted 32 years and has also been relatively effective, mainly because the following features applied; (i) a small number of registered dogs were treated regularly every 6–12 weeks with an anthelmintic (bunamidine, then PZQ from 1977), (ii) introduction of strict quarantine for infected sheep farms and (iii) hydatid control was under the responsibility of the Department of Agriculture. The parasite has not however been totally eliminated from the Falkland islands, and like Iceland in the early 20th century this was mainly due to difficulty of enforcing measures in several very remote sheep farms (Reichel *et al.*, 1996).

The 'fast-track' option of a massive reduction in dog numbers by extermination of strays and unregistered dogs was applied in Cyprus, and when coupled with 3 monthly obligatory arecoline testing also had a dramatic and rapid effect on reducing transmission of *E. granulosus* to the point of cessation of new human CE cases within 7–10 years. The Cyprus example also illustrates that when hydatid control measures were prevented (or ceased) in one area of a control zone (i.e. Northern Cyprus) this would lead to re-emergence of the parasite as a result of dog and livestock movement from the non-intervention to the intervention areas. That situation then required the re-introduction of hydatid control measures in 1993 to Cyprus in the form of a protracted consolidation phase based on long-term surveillance and trace back of livestock. Effectively, breakdown in hydatid control in Cyprus occurred when the island-wide programme essentially converted, after territorial partition, into a 'continental-type' control problem (Economides *et al.*, 1998).

3.2. Options and Phases for Control of Cystic Hydatidosis

A critical analysis of all the island-based hydatid control programmes lead Gemmell and colleagues to consider five options and four phases in any control programme for CE (Gemmell, 1986, 1990; Gemmell and Roberts, 1998; Gemmell *et al.*, 2001).

Option 1: Decision not to proceed. For example, because human CE is not a priority public health issue, such health data is not available, suitable control structure and funding are not available or there are unfavourable epidemiological features (e.g. an active wildlife cycle) or socio-economic features (e.g. underdeveloped region with dispersed population and no abattoirs). Decision may be temporary until the situation changes.

Option 2: Implementation of a long-term (slow-track) horizontal approach involving health education, upgrading of abattoirs and meat inspection, with reliance on owners to treat dogs (e.g. Iceland and New Zealand programmes required 30–100 years).

Option 3: Vertical slow-track approach incorporating at least annual arecoline purge testing of dogs with on-site education of owners and quarantine of positive dogs (e.g. Tasmania, 10–30 years).

Option 4: Vertical fast-track approach, but with elimination of stray dogs and euthanasia for arecoline test positive dogs (e.g. Cyprus, 10–15 years).

Option 5: Vertical fast-track approach with specified regular (usually 6-12 weeks) treatment of all registered dogs with PZQ (e.g. New Zealand after 1990, Falkland islands after 1977, 10–15 years).

Gemmell (1986, 1999), influenced by generic ideas of Yekutiel (1980), divided implementation of hydatid control into four phases, which have now generally been accepted as the most useful way to consider control of CE within any specific option or approach (WHO/OIE, 2001).

1. *Preparatory or planning phase*: Identify the control authority, its legislative powers and funding commitments (must be long term), quality of baseline data on human and livestock CE incidence and prevalence, public health impact and priority, consider

whether to designate CE as a notifiable disease, undertake a cost-benefit analysis for options (e.g. horizontal versus vertical approach), role of education, identify needs for staff (veterinary and technical staff, medical advisors, quantitative epidemiologists, etc.), cooperation with local/rural groups (e.g. 'voluntary farmers' unions), operational research needs, logistics and establish quality of surveillance potential. Also liaison avenues between the Control Authority, the Ministry of Agriculture/Dept of Veterinary Services, the Ministry of Health, the Municipalities and if appropriate specific research agencies ('planning' phase needs 1–2 years).

2. *Attack phase*: The control measures are applied, principally to involve dog registration, and then specified regular mass treatment (or testing) of the entire owned dog population (rural preferably) ideally by trained operatives, reduction in stray dog numbers (if possible), parallel health education at community and school levels. Set-up of abattoir surveillance for specified areas and preferably also a dog surveillance approach (arecoline and/or coproantigen testing). This is the most costly phase and therefore should be as short as possible. A reduction in livestock and dog infection prevalences should occur within 5–7 years and human CE rates within 10 years ('attack' phase usually requires 10–15 years).

3. *Consolidation phase*: Pro-active identification of infected food animals at abattoir meat inspection with trace back ability, use of enforced dog treatment and legislation to quarantine affected and neighbouring premises (with specified period free from CE and possibly also *T. hydatigena*) may involve provision of PZQ to dog owners at low cost. Prosecution for illegal slaughtering (if appropriate). This is a long-term phase after the 'attack' phase, but should require a reduction in field staff and cost of anthelmintics (phase needs >20 years and may need to be permanent).

4. *Maintenance of elimination phase*: Specific control activities have stopped. However, vigilance to be maintained through meat inspection, and measures applied to prevent entry of infected animals (easier on islands). Develop ability for trace back from abattoirs and control limited out-breaks on infected properties.

The definition of elimination of *E. granulosus* for a specified territory becomes an important issue. This is a permanent phase, but it may be required to re-adopt consolidation measures if re-emergence of transmission occurs (e.g. as occurred in Cyprus).

4. CONTINENTAL HYDATID CONTROL PROGRAMMES WITH VARIABLE SUCCESS—SOUTH AMERICA

With the growing and evident success of the island hydatid control programmes, several regions in South America opted to undertake or improve hydatid control because of the high incidence of the disease in rural populations in endemic areas. Two of these continental programmes (in Region XII in Chile, and in Rio Negro Province in Argentina) have been successful, and benefited from the knowledge gained in the island programmes and the ready availability of the anthelmintic PZQ. Other South American programmes have been less successful, but eventually had a significant impact, e.g. in Uruguay, or have had variable impact, e.g. in Neuquen Province, Argentina.

4.1. Epidemiology of Cystic Echinococcosis in South America

Cystic echinococcosis is one of the zoonotic diseases with significant public health impact in Argentina, Uruguay, Chile, Peru, Bolivia and Brazil. CE also causes significant economic losses for livestock due to confiscated viscera and losses in wool, milk and meat production (Larrieu *et al.*, 2000b; Torgerson *et al.*, 2000). For example, in the Province of Rio Negro, Argentina, with a human population of 500 000 inhabitants, the average cost of CE treatment has been estimated to be US$4511 (Larrieu *et al.*, 2000a). CE has been known along the Rio de la Plata from the last decades of the 18th century. After the Spanish Viceroyalty organized the fishing industry and whale-fleets by setting up factories along the coasts of Argentina and Uruguay, it is thought that dogs, transported as mascots in whaling ships, contaminated sheep and cattle spreading *E. granulosus* throughout the region.

Echinococcus granulosus is responsible for human hydatid cases in the region, although some cases of *E. vogeli* have been identified in Amazonian Venezuela, Brazil, Columbia and Peru (Rausch and D'Alessandro, 2002; Somocursio *et al.*, 2004). The presence of several strains/genotypes of *E. granulosus* have been described in South America, including the G1 sheep–dog strain (the most geographically widespread and significant for human health), the G2 Tasmanian ovine strain (identified in rural mountain areas in the Province of Tucumán, Argentina), the G5 cow strain, the G6 camel strain and the G7 porcine strain. All these strains possess variable pre-patency in the dog and can differ in their infectivity for humans (Eckert, 1997; Rosenzvit *et al.*, 1999; Kamenetzky *et al.*, 2002). As in other parts of the world, the domestic sheep–dog strain of *E. granulosus* persists due to indiscriminate home-slaughter and feeding hydatid infected offal to dogs. Additionally, slaughterhouses and butchers without appropriate facilities or veterinary inspection constitute important sources of infection for dogs in urban areas, a frequent situation in small urban populations in Argentina, Uruguay and Peru.

Before the application of control measures, prevalence of ovine CE reached 26% in southern Brazil, 26.7% in Peru, 80% in Chile Region XI and 60% in Region XII, 41% in Uruguay, and for Argentina 61% in the Province of Rio Negro and 52% in the Province of Tierra del Fuego (Ruiz *et al.*, 1994; Moro *et al.*, 1999). Canine prevalence with *E. granulosus* was recorded to be 28.3% in Brazil, 26–79% in Peru, 10.1% in Uruguay, 54% in Region XI of Chile, 71% in Region XII of Chile, 11% in Region VII of Chile, and in the pastoral Argentinian Provinces, 42% in Rio Negro, 28.2% in Neuquén and 40.2% in Cushamen (Chubut) (Ruiz *et al.*, 1994; Moro *et al.*, 1999; Lópera *et al.*, 2003).

Canine re-infection rates in the rural environment, may be rapid. In Uruguay, dogs from endemic areas treated with anthelmintics showed re-infection rates ranging from 5.2% at 60 days post-treatment up to 18.6% after 120 days. Similarly in Rio Negro (Argentina), dog re-infection rates were 6.7% and 21.3%, respectively (Larrieu *et al.*, 1999). Case control studies have allowed identification of the main risk factors for human CE in Argentina (Larrieu *et al.*, 2002). Risk factors of greater epidemiological importance detected using multivariate analysis included, slaughtering sheep at home (OR 3.2), ownership and contact with large numbers of dogs during the first years of life (OR 2.6), presence of CE cases in the family nucleus (OR 2.5) and quality of drinkable water (OR 0.1, protection factor). Contact with an infected dog presented an attributable risk of 0.77, and there was a statistically significant increase in risk in relation to owning a greater number of dogs during a persons lifetime ($p = 0.0003$), as well as the number of years spent in a rural endemic environment ($p = 0.033$) (Larrieu *et al.*, 2002).

More than 2000 new human CE cases were reported every year in South America in the 1990s, with annual incidence rates of 41 per 100 000 in the Patagonian region of south Argentina, 137 per 100 000 in General Carrera Province of Region XI, Chile and 100 per 100 000 in the Department of Flores, Uruguay (Ruiz *et al.*, 1994; Gemmell, 1997). More recent studies indicate a human CE incidence rate of 38.5 per 100 000 in Region XI (Aliaga and Oberg, 2000) and a human prevalence of 3.6% in the north of Argentina (Lopez, 2002). The advent of ultrasonographic screening with portable scanners applied to asymptomatic human populations have allowed more accurate evaluation of the true prevalence of the human CE in the diverse affected communities, and more recently have become a valuable surveillance screening tool for hydatid control programmes. Relatively high human CE prevalence rates by ultrasound have been reported in South America: 5.5% in Rio Negro (Argentina), 14.2% in Loncopué, Neuquén (Argentina), 1.6% in Tacuarembó (Uruguay), 1.6% in Florida (Uruguay), 3.6% in Durazno (Uruguay) and 5.1% in Vichaycocha (Peru) (Frider *et al.*, 1988; Carmona *et al.*, 1998; Cohen *et al.*, 1998; Moro *et al.*, 1999; Larrieu *et al.*, 2004) (Plate 11.1. B in colour plate section).

4.2. Hydatid Control Programmes in South America

The first structured hydatid control programmes were the Pilot Program to Study and Combat Hydatidosis developed by the Province of Neuquén in the Huiliches Department, Argentina from 1970 to 1985 (De Zavaleta *et al.*, 1986), and in 1973 the Pilot Program for

Hydatidosis Control developed in Flores Department, Uruguay. Both these pilot programmes were based on the regular 6 weekly testing of dogs with arecoline hydrobromide. Later, programmes based on the systematic dosing of dogs with PZQ were implemented in Uruguay, Chile and Argentina, with distinct organization models for the Control Authority. In Uruguay, they opted for a 'New Zealand-style' Hydatids Comission under the jurisdiction of the Ministry of Public Health. Chile opted for the Ministry of Agriculture (similar to Tasmania, Cyprus and the Falkland islands), and Argentina used the Ministry of Health as the control authority (Plate 11.1.C and D in colour plate section).

With minor local differences, current hydatid control activities (since late 1990s) have been based on registration and PZQ treatment of dogs at the dose of 5 mg/kg every 6 weeks; accompanying health education, slaughter control to prevent access of dogs to viscera; legislation for the regulation of dog populations, and recommendations for construction of basic infrastructure in cattle and sheep ranches/estancias comprising designated slaughter area and a pit for disposal of infected viscera. The Chilean control programme in Region XII was successful from the outset with evidence of reduction in transmision within the first 5 years (1979–1984), and the Neuquén Province (Argentina) pilot programme resulted in significant control and cessation of new human cases after 17 years (1970–1986). In contrast, the Uruguayan hydatid control programme had little effect on livestock or human CE rates over the first 20 years of the control campaign (1972–1992) (Gemmell, 1994). Similarly, the programme in Sierra Central Peru (1992–2002) made no impact (Table 2).

4.2.1. Hydatid Control in Chile, Regions XI (1982–1997) and XII (1979–1997)—Evidence of Success

CE has been highly endemic in Chile since Spanish colonization, especially in the rich pastoral areas of the south. In 1951, CE was made a notifiable disease in Chile and the national incidence of human CE was estimated to be 6.6–8.4 per 100 000. Human incidence of CE in the two southern areas i.e. Regions XI and XII was between 38 and 80 per 100 000 per year prior to intervention in the late 1970s. The Ministry of Agriculture (Ministerio de Agricultura y Servicio

Agricola y Ganadero—SAG) implemented two hydatid control programmes, one in 1979 (Region XII) and the other in 1982 (Region XI). Both were based on the 'fast-track' Option 5 (see above) involving 6 weekly dosing of dogs (eight times per year) in the 'attack' phase with parallel health education (Vidal, 1989; Gemmell and Roberts, 1998).

Region XII was more accessible with a population of 125 000, about 1700 farms/ranches and >2 million sheep. Region XI with a human population of 80 000, a total of 1400 farms and 300 000 sheep was less accessible due to harsh terrain and poor roads, and was less developed socio-economically. Each region had about 8000–9000 dogs (approximately four dogs per owner in Region XII and two per owner in Region XI) for which pre-control prevalence of *E. granulosus*, based on arecoline purge, was 71% in Region XII and 31–54% in Region XI. In 1979, for both Regions, between 60% and 80% of sheep were infected with CE at slaughter.

Within 5 years (1979–1984) of implementation of hydatid control, ovine CE prevalence in Region XII had declined to 25% in sheep and 1% in lambs, and canine echinococcosis rates were reduced dramatically to 1.6%; human CE incidence was also down to 19.6 per 100 000 by 1984, and reduced further to 11.8 per 100 000 in 1992 (Gemmell, 1994, 1997) (Table 2). In 1991, the prevalence in sheep was 7%, and the average prevalence in dogs for both regions was 5% (Vidal *et al.*, 1994; Ruiz *et al.*, 1994). The 'attack' phase in Region XII lasted a total of 18 years (1979–1997), but from 1987 dog dosing was reduced to twice annual treatments and owners were also instructed how to treat their dogs in order to save on costs and improve logistics. However, in 1991 the SAG authority (Ministry of Agriculture) re-introduced the eight treatments per year schedule (half by dog owners themselves) in Region XII in order to further reduce transmission to sheep which had plateaued at a prevalence of 5–7% after 1986 (Gemmell, 1997). This re-introduction of full dog treatment with increased cover (>90% dogs were treated) brought the prevalence of *E. granulosus* in dogs and lambs close to zero by 1994, that is within 3 years of the re-introduction of the enhanced counter-measures.

Hydatid control was initiated in Region XI of Chile in 1982. Due to difficulties in movement of veterinary/technical SAG staff between

Table 2 Impact of hydatid control programmes in South America

Region	Pre-control	Impact (i)	Impact (ii)
Brasil (Río Grande) (1983–2000)	1983	—	2000
Dog (%)	28.3		9
Sheep (%)	26		3
Human (per 100 000)	—		
Screening (%)	1.7		
Perú (Sierra Central) (1992–2002)	1992	—	2002
Dog (%)	26		51–79
Sheep (%)	26.7		38
Human (cases)	600		2000
Screening (%)	5.8(DD5)		5.1(US)
Uruguay (2nd program 1994–2002)	1991	1994	1997/8
Dog (%)	10.1	16.1	0.7
Sheep (%)	41	9	8.5
Human (per 100 000)	12.4		6.5
Screening (%)			0.04(ELISA[a])
Argentina (Rio Negro) (1980–1997)	1980	1998	2003
Dog (%)	41	2.9	2.5
Sheep (%)	61	18	
Human (per 100 000)	73	22	
Screening (%)	2 (DD5)/5(US[a])	1.6(US[a])	0.4(US[a])
Argentina (Tierra del Fuego) (1980–2001)	1980	1985	2001
Dog (%)	36	27	2.5
Sheep (%)	52	20	2.5
Human (per 100 000)			3.1
Screening (%)			0.2(US[a])
Chile (Región XI–XII) (1982–1997)	1979	1991	1997
Dog (%)	31–71	1.6–5	0.35–6.5
Sheep (%)	60–80	5–25	1.3–10.4
Human (per 100 000)	38–80	11.8	6–20

Notes: Dogs: surveys with arecoline hydrobromide or coproantigens; sheep: surveys in slaughter houses; human cases: based on hospital records; screening: population surveys with ultrasonography (US) or DD5 or ELISA.

[a]Studies in school populations.

sheep farms, PZQ treatment of dogs was carried out on dosing strips—similar to that used in Tasmania. As described above for Region XII, there was a dramatic reduction in the prevalence of canine echinococcosis (from 35% to <5%) within the first 3–4 years of introduction of 6 weekly dosing in Region XI, as was also the case for ovine CE (>80% in sheep in 1982 to about 25% in 1986). The dog-dosing frequency was subsequently though prematurely reduced after 1986. As a result, CE prevalence in adult sheep remained at around 25–30% after 1986, but importantly declined close to zero in lambs. Residual infections may be expected to last longer in older livestock even when transmission has nearly ceased to young food animals. Nevertheless, the SAG control authority re-introduced 6 weekly PZQ dosing in Region XI from 1992 (Vidal et al., 1994).

After 1997, both the Region XII and Region XI hydatid control programmes entered the consolidation phase based on abattoir surveillance of food animals. Continued success will depend on maintenance of a permanent consolidation phase. These two programmes, especially in Region XII, may be considered as exemplars for a 'modern' fast-track vertical approach to control of CE in a continental region. Success was achieved by the Ministry of Agriculture (SAG) using a small number of well-trained technical staff i.e. only seven veterinarians and 18 technicians for Region XII, with good starting baseline data and control impact evidence based on comprehensive abattoir records and dog arecoline surveys. Both sets of animal data (sheep post-mortem and dogs by arecoline purge) clearly showed a dramatic reduction in transmission of *E. granulosus* within 5 years of implementation of control in Region XII, as did human incidence which declined from >40 to 11.8 per 100 000 within 10 years, and indeed probably ceased to persons aged <15 years (Gemmell, 1997). Recent reports after 2000, however, suggest that prevalence in sheep has increased again in both regions, possibly associated with transfer of the control authority from the Ministry of Agriculture to the Ministry of Health (E. Larrieu, personal observations).

4.2.2. Hydatid Control in Argentina, Provinces of Neuquén (1970–1988) and Rio Negro (1980–1997)—Evidence of Success but Continued Transmission

In contrast to Chile, the federal government of Argentina devolves public health to its 23 Provinces, and hydatid control comes under the responsibility of the Provincial Council of Public Health rather than the Ministry of Agriculture. The Neuquen programme was effectively based on Option 3 (Section 3.2) as used in Tasmania with regular arecoline testing of dogs and health education. In contrast, the Rio Negro programme was able to use PZQ and implemented a 6 weekly dosing programme with accompanying health education, as used in Chile, i.e. a fast-track approach described in Option 5 (Section 3.2).

In Neuquen Province ($94\,000\,\mathrm{km}^2$) in 1970, prior to the pilot control programme, 71% of sheep and 90% of cattle had CE, 28% of dogs were infected with *E. granulosus* and the incidence of human CE was one of the highest in the world at 567 per 100 000 (Larrieu, 1994). Fifteen years later in 1985, two years before termination of the of the Neuquen pilot programme, parasite prevalences had dropped 95% in dogs to 1.2%, were down 76% in sheep to 2.1% and the human CE incidence had reduced 86% to 75 cases per 100 000 per year. Despite this significant reduction in parasite burden, transmission continued and human CE incidence remained high, by global standards, at 67 per 100 000 during 1988–1992 (Larrieu, 1994).

The hydatid control programme in the Province of Rio Negro ($203\,000\,\mathrm{km}^2$ with a population of 600 000 in 13 Departments) was the most successful in Argentina. It has been maintained to date, though it has not completely transfered from the 'attack' to the 'consolidation' phase. Under the authority of the Provincial Council of Public Health and the Department of Zoonoses, the hydatid control programme in Rio Negro Province was implemented in 1980 and employed nine veterinarians and 64 rural health/veterinary assistants. Just prior to start of control, the provincial human CE incidence rate was 73 per 100 000 with a rate of 50 per 10 000 in children < 10 years; ovine CE prevalence by abattoir inspection was 61%, and the prevalence of canine echinococcosis by arecoline purge testing was 41.5% (Larrieu *et al.*, 2000a). The control programme approach was similar to that implemented in Chile in 1979. After registration of all dogs, and a health education programme, intervention consisted of an 8 weekly dog dosing frequency using PZQ, which was provided free to dog owners. Surveillance of ovine CE was instigated in 10 abattoirs across the Province. In 1994, it became compulsory for owners to register all dogs and to comply with control measures.

The Rio Negro programme, however, incorporated additional sur-veillance methods for the human population that had not previously been applied in other hydatid control campaigns. These included sero-logical (initially the DD5 diffusion test, then from 1993 the ELISA) and abdominal ultrasound surveys for the 6–13 years age group (Frider *et al.*, 1986; Coltorti *et al.*, 1988). Within 5 years (1980–1985) of the start of the programme the canine infection rate had dropped to a prevalence of <5%, and the ovine CE prevalence down to 7%. It took 12 years for the CE incidence in children (<13 years) to drop below 20 per 100 000, while the total number of CE cases diagnosed was reduced from 1720 in the period 1980–1986 down to 275 for the period 1990–1996. Ultra-sound rates in children, which largely reflects asymptomatic hepatic CE, were reduced from 5.5% in 1984, to 4% in 1986 and to 1.1% by 1997; by 2003 overall human CE ultrasound prevalence was 0.4%, and canine prevalence down to 2.5% (Larrieu *et al.*, 2000a; Frider *et al.*, 2001). Table 2 up to the year 1997, the total cost of treating 12 000 dogs (with health education for owners) was US$440 000, for the child surveys the cost was US$17 000 and for treatment of human CE cases US$243 000. Thus, the whole programme (over 17 years) cost approximately US$41 000 per year to run, which must be highly cost-effective consid-ering the average cost of treatment for a single human CE case in Rio Negro was US$4500 (Larrieu *et al.*, 2000b).

In Rio Negro Province, epidemiological surveillance systems have continued to use arecoline purging of dogs and slaughterhouse sur-veys for ovine CE (Larrieu *et al.*, 2001). Surveillance in humans con-tinues by means of registration of operated CE cases, serological screening and in the last few years, ultrasonographic screening of high-risk groups (Coltorti *et al.*, 1988; Frider *et al.*, 1988). From the year 2003, in Argentina, farm surveillance also included use of co-proantigen techniques on ground-collected faecal samples (Guarnera *et al.*, 2000). In a first study in the Patagonian region, a total of 262 homesteads in 18 departments were surveyed, of which 5.4% of 813 faecal samples were positive for *Echinococcus* coproantigens (Cavag-ion *et al.*, 2004).

In the case of the Patagonian provinces in Argentina, including Tierra Del Fuego (Table 2), the difficulties of access to the rural communities and discontinuity in field actions due to budgetary limitations, have lead to an excessive number of years of the 'attack' phase so that a full consolidation phase has not been achieved. This has lead to the persistent occurrence of new cases of human CE albeit at much lower levels.

4.2.3. Hydatid Control in Uruguay (1965–2002)—Initial Failure followed by Evidence of Success

Uruguay, population 3.2 million, with 25 million sheep and approximately 160 000 dogs (in 1994), occupies 177 500 km^2 and is divided into 19 Departments. The national incidence of human CE in the decade 1962–1971 was 20 per 100 000 and exceeded 75 per 100 000 for some Departments (Purriel *et al.*, 1973; Bonifacino *et al.*, 1991). In 1965, a national hydatid control programme was initiated by Uruguayan law under administration of a National Commission against Hydatidosis (Comision Honoraria de Lucha Contra la Hidatidosis), which derived its funding from a dog tax. This was similar to the control structure in the first 32 years of the New Zealand hydatid control programme (Section 2.2); however, in Uruguay the owners were provided arecoline and were expected to treat their own dogs after appropriate education. During the period 1965–1972 no useful abattoir or dog surveillance data were collected, but from 1972 to 1985 ovine CE prevalence did not appear to alter significantly remaining at 40–65% each year, despite the fact that 30–50 000 dogs per year were registered between 1980 and 1986 (the military government in this period did however affect the programme) (Gemmell, 1994). In 1991–1992 the programme was re-invigorated with more funds as a result of a new law which made the police responsible for collection of the dog tax. About 10% of the dogs tested positive with arecoline by veterinary teams (Plate 11.1, C–E, see colour plates); however, sheep CE prevalence remained at around 40%, while human incidence was 12.4 per 100 000. From 1994, the Honorary Hydatid Commission was able to mount a programme of systematic PZQ treatment of 140 000 rural dogs, and by 1997 the prevalence rate in dogs dropped to 0.7%. In parallel, ovine CE rates declined to 12.5% (7.7% in lambs) in 1998 (Cabrera *et al.*, 1996, 2003), and were recorded at 3.8% in 2002 (D. Orlando, personal communication). Mass ultrasound surveys of the human population in Durazno Department, 1991–1992, obtained a prevalence of asymptomatic hepatic CE of 3.6% (Cohen *et al.*, 1999). By 1998, human incidence was down to 6.5 per 100 000, and 139 CE cases nationally were operated on in 2002 compared to 367 in 1992.

Uruguay currently is the only country in the world that has a national level hydatid control programme, and it now appears to have moved into a consolidation phase. As in Rio Negro Province (Argentina), however, human CE cases are still detected though transmission to children appears to have ceased. The hydatid programme in Uruguay did not work for 27 years (1965–1992), largely because of the following factors. Too much reliance was placed on large numbers of rural owners to dose their own dogs; the use of a purgative rather than a cestocidal drug; when arecoline dosing teams did operate the proportion of dogs tested and treated was probably less than 50%; the Honorary Commission (which came under the Ministry of Health) did not employ enough local municipality staff and did not raise sufficient funds from the dog tax; baseline data for sheep (and dogs) was neither collected nor livestock surveillance implemented to provide feedback to measure progress; political upheaval during the 1980s also caused inertia in the programme. Evidence of success was only achieved after 1994 through implementation of 6 weekly PZQ dosing and proper abattoir surveillance of livestock.

The Uruguay hydatid programme was in some ways a poor version of the New Zealand campaign. Both started with an Option 2 type approach using health education and owner-based treatment of dogs, which had little or no effect for 20–27 years. Then both the programmes converted to an Option 5 'fast-track' vertical approach based on 6 weekly supervised anthelmintic dosing of dogs, achieving cessation of transmission to humans within 12 years for New Zealand and probably also for Uruguay.

5. OTHER HYDATID CONTROL PROGRAMMES WITH NO OR LIMITED SUCCESS—WALES, KENYA, SARDINIA

The 'island' hydatid control programmes in Australasia, the Mediterranean and the Atlantic were all eventually successful, though the time taken varied from around 10–>100 years. The 'Continental' hydatid programmes of South America have also been a success, either from the outset (e.g. Option 5 approach in Region XII, Chile), or only after re-invigoration of a vertical approach to the programme following years of poor impact (e.g. Uruguay). It is however clear that in almost all these programmes when dog testing or anthelmintic treatment was efficient and well managed, the incidence rates of human CE disease began to fall within 5–10 years of strict implementation of those control measures.

On the other hand, there have been at least three other hydatid control programmes, all initiated or re-activated in the 1980s, which have failed for different reasons. Reasons for failure included: (i) the premature withdrawal of funding by the legislature of a well-organized programme (e.g. the mid-Wales programme), (ii) the control authority was too small, under-funded and there was difficulty in implementation/logistics (e.g. the Turkana pilot programme, Kenya), (iii) the control authority was ineffective and management of stray dogs was an issue (e.g. Sardinia) and (iv) presence of political upheaval, and/or security issues (e.g. Cyprus, Turkana-Kenya).

5.1. Mid-Wales, UK (1983–1989)

The South Powys hydatid control scheme was introduced in mid-Wales in 1983 after proper consideration and deliberation in the 'planning' phase. The control authority was the the UK Ministry of Agriculture (MAFF) and the State Veterinary Service with administrative and funding support from the Agriculture Department of the Welsh Office. In addition, a Local Liason Committee was established (as in the Australasian and Argentinian programmes). The programme adopted was Option 5, that is a 'fast-track' approach based on supervised 6 weekly PZQ dosing of rural dogs by MAFF veterinarian/ technical staff. There was also an educational component directed at sheep farmers and other dog owners through specific visits and use of printed leaflets. Education was directed at owners preventing their dogs gaining access to raw offal either by illegal home-slaughter or through scavenging sheep carcasses (Clarkson, 1978; Walters, 1984).

Various surveys before the mid-1980s in Powys and other areas of mid-Wales indicated prevalence of echinococcosis in farm dogs to be 4.6–25% (Williams, 1976a; Walters and Clarkson, 1980; Jones and Walters, 1992), 9–29% in hunting dogs, i.e. 'foxhounds' (Williams, 1976b; Walters, 1977) and around 7% in red foxes (*Vulpes vulpes*) (Hackett and Walters, 1980). Prevalence of CE in adult sheep in mid-Wales in the 1970s and early 1980s was 23–37% (Walters, 1978; Palmer *et al.*, 1996). Average annual incidence of human CE in Powys County between 1953 and 1983 was 3.7–3.9 cases per 100 000 (Palmer *et al.*, 1996). The Breconshire/Radnorshire areas of south Powys recorded the highest human incidence rates at 4.7–6.3 cases per 100 000 over the period 1981–1983 (Stallbaumer *et al.*, 1986).

Data from the main abattoir in the South Powys Hydatid Control Area within 5 years of application of control measures indicated a reduction in ovine CE prevalence from 23.5% in 1984–1986 to 10.5% in 1988–1989. A genus specific coproantigen ELISA test employed as a measure of canine echinococcosis prevalence in the south Powys control zone in 1993, recorded 0% coproantigen positive farm dogs compared to 2.4–9.2% in neighbouring non-intervention areas. Furthermore, human CE incidence in the intervention area, for the period 1984–1990, fell from 3.9 per 100 000 to 2.3 per 100 000 with no cases in the under 15 years of age group (Palmer *et al.*, 1996).

In 1989, only 6 years after implementation of the control programme, the major funding from the Welsh Office stopped and the supervised dog-dosing programme was replaced by a health education programme (directed by the Powys Health Promotion Unit funded by the Dyfed-Powys Health Authority) targeted to schoolchildren and sheep farmers. Sheep farmers were encouraged to purchase Droncit (PZQ) and dose their own dogs every 6–8 weeks. Essentially, this converted the 'attack' phase from a 'fast-track' Option 5 vertical approach to a slow-track education-only based Option 2 style approach.

Two post-control surveys (after 1989) for exposure of *E. granulosus* in sheep and dogs in the hydatid control zone in 1995–1996 and 2002, respectively, indicated the presence of active transmission. Therefore, the termination of the dog-dosing programme was premature, and the health education programme had largely failed to prevent re-emergence of transmission (Lloyd *et al.*, 1996; Buishi *et al.*, 2005). Specifically, in the main intervention area, 6% of sentinel lambs became infected with *E. granulosus* within 15 months of natural exposure (compared to 10% in the non-intervention area) (Lloyd *et al.*, 1996). In addition, 8.1% of dogs from the intervention area tested coproantigen positive (compared to 0–3.4% in 1993) (Buishi *et al.*, 2005). Highly significant risk factors for a coproantigen positive farm dog were owners who reported infrequent anthelmintic dosing (>4 month intervals) and allowing their dogs to roam free (Buishi *et al.*, 2005). There are no recent data on human CE incidence after 1990. In 2005, a health education programme continues in south Powys at schools and farmers' markets.

5.2. Northwest Turkana, Kenya (1983–2000)

The annual incidence of human CE in the Turkana District (70 000 km^2, population approximately 160 000) of Kenya in the 1970s was estimated to be 220 cases per 100 000, with a significant public health impact (French and Nelson, 1982; French *et al.*, 1982). In order to reduce the high incidence of CE in this remote region, a pilot hydatid control programme was initiated in 1983 in a 9000 km^2 region in the northwest of the District (bordering Uganda and Sudan) under the authority of the African Medical and Research Foundation (AMREF), a non-government organization (Macpherson *et al.*, 1984). The control zone had a population of around 12 000 Turkana tribespeople, 70% of whom were nomadic or semi-nomadic, and for whom the local incidence of CE was 198 per 100 000. This scattered population, in a control zone the size of Cyprus with few roads and towns, owned a total of about 120 000 sheep/goats, 45 000 cattle and 3500 camels (also 8000 donkeys). They also owned 6–8000 dogs of which 63.5% of population samples were infected with *E. granulosus* at necropsy (Macpherson *et al.*, 1985). Wild canids and several wild ungulate species though susceptible to infection with *E. granulosus* were not considered to be important in the epidemiology of CE in Turkana (Nelson, 1986; Macpherson and Craig, 1991). Prevalence in livestock in the 1970s was difficult to estimate because there was no slaughterhouse in the Control Zone and only one in the whole of Turkana District. Limited data from this latter abattoir (in Lodwar) showed a prevalence of 2–7% in sheep, goats and cattle, and approximately 60% in camels (Macpherson, 1981). A recent slaughterhouse survey in northern and central areas of Turkana, outside the Pilot Control Zone, also found relatively low CE prevalences of <1% in sheep and up to 10% in cattle, but 50–80% in camels (Njoroge *et al.*, 2002). The low prevalence in sheep and goats, but high prevalence in humans contributed to speculation about an active intermediate host role for humans (burial customs are uncommon in Turkana) (Macpherson, 1983). However, molecular analysis of >200 hydatid isolates from CE patients showed all but one to be infected with the common sheep strain (G1 form) of *E. granulosus* (Wachira *et al.*, 1993; Dinkel *et al.*, 2004). The camel strain of *E. granulosus* also occurs in Turkana and appears to infect goats and cattle as well as camels (Dinkel *et al.*, 2004).

From the outset control of CE in Turkana was considered to be difficult for the following reasons: there were virtually no educational, medical or veterinary facilities; there were poor communications and road network with few settlements; no abattoirs; a population of nomadic and largely illiterate indigenous people; occurrence of frequent droughts; inter-tribal livestock raiding and fighting was common; the Turkana tribe were a marginalized population with low contribution to the national GNP (Macpherson and Wachira, 1997). Despite these inherent problems, a vertical approach to control was adopted from 1983. It was essentially a combination of Option 4 (dog culling, sterilization and testing/dosing, with health education) and Option 5 (specified 6 weekly treatment of dogs with PZQ) (Section 3.2). The 'attack' phase lasted about 10 years (1983–1994), but difficulties in transport, manpower and under-funding meant that only about 30% of dogs were registered in the first 2 years, and of those only between 30% and 60% were followed up for anthelmintic treatment (Macpherson *et al.*, 1986; Macpherson and Wachira, 1997). The dog-dosing frequency was also reduced from 6 weeks to 12–15 weeks. Owing to the absence of livestock data, surveillance was uniquely placed on dog and human prevalence surveys using necropsy/arecoline testing and ultrasound scanning, respectively. Within 4 years of the start of hydatid control in northwest Turkana, human CE prevalence using ultrasound scanning had reduced from >7% to <4%, with very few cases in the under 5 years age group. Human prevalence then appeared to plateau around 3% after the mid-1990s (E. Zeyhle, personal communication). Prevalence in dogs by necropsy, reduced from 63% to around 45% within 5 years and was ~27% after 11 years (1983–1994) of control implementation (Macpherson and Wachira, 1997). In a recent *Echinococcus* coproantigen survey (2002) of owned dogs in the Control Zone, 31% (29/94) tested positive (I. Buishi, Ph.D. Thesis, University of Salford, 2005).

While the Turkana control effort made some impact on transmission and reduction in human morbidity, existence of relatively high infection rates in both dogs and humans after 10 years of intervention suggests that control was not as effective as anticipated in this nomadic population in a remote semi-arid region of Kenya. The AMREF supported programme could not enter a 'consolidation' phase because, like Uruguay, the 'attack' phase was not sufficiently comprehensive. The number of staff employed was probably also too small for the dispersed population (i.e. one physician, one veterinarian, six technical assistants, one educationalist and about 10 local health workers). From the late 1990s, the reduced resources of the Turkana control programme were re-focussed largely on appropriate health education and patient management. The ongoing extensive health education programme in northwest Turkana may eventually have an impact, as in the example of Iceland, but it is more likely that such an approach alone will have limited effect in these nomadic pastoralists. The concept of combining control of more than one zoonotic disease and of integrating both medical and veterinary outreach programmes for nomadic populations as has been advocated (Zinsstag and Weiss, 2001) and could be a future option for hydatid disease control in this semi-arid remote region of East Africa.

5.3. Sardinia (1960–1997)

Human CE is particularly endemic in southern Italy including the islands of Sicily and Sardinia. The population of Sardinia ($24\,000\,\mathrm{km}^2$) in the 1980s was about 1.6 million, with about 3.5 million sheep (predominently under transhumance husbandry). There were around 150 000 owned dogs and 80 000 stray dogs (Attanasio *et al.*, 1985). Prevalence of CE in sheep in 1981 was 85%, *E. granulosus* in farm dogs was 24% and 10–20% in stray dogs. For the period 1948–1970, human CE incidence in different provinces of Sardinia ranged from 13.4 to 22.2 per 100 000, with an average of 16 per 100 000 producing about 200 human CE cases per year, and with a mortality of 5% (Maggi, 1980; Attanasio *et al.*, 1985). The first programme to try and control transmission of *E. granulosus* in Sardinia was implemented from 1960 to 1967 in three of the most endemic provinces (Nuoro, Sassari and Cagliari), and was re-activated further in 1973 by enactment in Regional law. The initial approach was essentially one of intense health education (leaflets, posters, radio, TV, films, meetings, etc.) combined with annual or twice yearly arecoline testing of owned dogs, i.e. essentially equivalent to 'Option 3' described by Gemmell and Roberts (1998) (Section 3.2). After the mid-1970s, dog owners were encouraged to dose their own dogs with PZQ, and many of the numerous small, rural slaughter-houses were closed (about 500) or upgraded (about 109) (Conchedda *et al.*, 2002). Over the period 1969–1990, it became clear that the Sardinian hydatid control programme had little or no effect. Sheep prevalence was still very high at 87% in 1988–1989 and human incidence did not change significantly remaining between 13–14 cases per 100 000.

In 1987, an Action Plan for 'Eradication of Hydatidosis' was issued by the Sardinian Government who made a Research Agency (the Sardinian Experimental Institute for Zooprophylaxis) responsible for managing control, and provided 15 million euros for the programme. The plan was to register all owned dogs and dose them with PZQ at specified intervals, control the stray dog population, improve abattoir inspection and apply health education to rural populations especially regarding home-slaughter (Battelli *et al.*, 2002; Conchedda *et al.*, 2002). A law on strays was also approved in 1991, which forced communes to keep and treat indefinitely (privately or in pounds but not to euthanize) all stray dogs collected by municipalities. Ten years of formal control over the period 1987–1997, however, did not provide the expected decline in neither CE infection rates in sheep and humans nor the cost-benefit that had been carefully predicted/anticipated prior to implementation (Attanasio and Palmas, 1984). Canine prevalence, 5 years after the start of the 'new' programme, was still 25% for sheep–dogs and 11% in stray dogs (Conchedda *et al.*, 2002); for the period 1998–2003 ovine CE prevalence in Nuoro and Sassari Provinces was 75% (Scala *et al.*, 2005). Average human CE incidence for Sardinia appeared to have fallen only slightly to 9.8 per 100 000 by the mid-1990s (Gabriele *et al.*, 2004).

Reasons for failure of hydatid control in Sardinia are probably several, but the main factors may be the following. Not surprisingly the significant stray dog issue became difficult to manage both ethically, logistically and cost-wise; also problems arose for cooperation and appropriate funding between the various operational sectors. Crucially, the non-government Control Agency was not readily accepted in rural areas nor could its staff effectively provide outreach to remote farms, in contrast to the regional veterinary services. Thus in the Sardinian programme from 1997, the important dog-centred 'attack' phase was neither implemented effectively nor was it well managed. Finally, despite > 30 years of health education to sheep farming communities, there was still a major lack of awareness of the parasite and/or unwillingness to change entrenched cultural behaviour patterns (Conchedda *et al.*, 1997, 2002).

6. CURRENT OPTIONS AND TOOLS FOR HYDATID CONTROL

6.1. Epidemiological Modelling

A detailed knowledge of the life cycle of the parasite is important in relation to rational implementation of hydatid control programmes as evidenced as early as the mid-19th century in Iceland. In addition, an understanding of the transmission dynamics and development of a locally relevant transmission model is theoretically also an advantage to optimize a modern cost-effective control programme. A quantitative modelling approach though of great potential, has not been shown historically to be a necessity for eventual control. For example, from the mid-1860s to the year 2000 at least seven national or regional hydatid control programmes have been successfully implemented across the globe (in Iceland, New Zealand, Tasmania, Cyprus, Falkland islands, Chile and Argentina—see Sections 2 and 4) without the benefit of a detailed quantitative transmission modelling approach. On the other hand, at least four programmes have been only partially successful or unsuccessful (in Uruguay, Wales, Sardinia and Kenya—see Sections 4 and 5), and these may have benefited enormously from computerized simulations using locally relevant parameters such as age-related abundance of ovine and canine infections and relative cost-effectiveness of different dog-dosing frequencies and percentage cover for dosed dogs (Torgerson, 2003; Torgerson and Heath, 2003).

In the 1970s and 1980s, approximately 120 years after the discovery of the life cycle of *E. granulosus*, experimental determination of the transmission dynamics of the parasite led to the development of a quantitative epidemiological approach to model transmission (e.g. egg output in dogs, age-specific intensity rates in sheep, etc.), and to theoretically help determine the feasibility and economics of hydatid control (Gemmell and Johnstone, 1977; Gemmell *et al.*, 1986; Gemmell, 1990). These, and other related seminal studies from New Zealand, enabled the contribution of the parasite (biotic potential—adult, egg, oncosphere and metacestode stages), the hosts (e.g. aquired immunity in definitive and intermediate hosts) and the environment (egg survival and dispersal, socio-economic factors) to be measured, and the construction of a quantitative modelling approach. This allowed determination of the parasite's basic reproductive ratio or number (Ro), and thus quantitative definitions of extinction, endemic or hyperendemic steady states (Gemmell and Roberts, 1998). Estimates of Ro (i.e. the number of new infections in the next generation in the absence of density-dependent constraints chief of which is host aquired immunity) for *E. granulosus* were usually low. For example, an Ro of 1.3 was calculated retrospectively in New Zealand (prior to introduction of hydatid control measures), which manifested as theoretically 0.4 infections per year per sheep (Gemmell *et al.*, 1986). Similarly, exposure to low numbers of hydatid cyst infections per year for intermediate hosts (range 0.025–0.44) were also determined for endemic areas of China, Kazakhstan, Jordan, Tunisia, Peru and Uruguay (reviewed by Torgerson and Heath, 2003). These studies suggest that in most areas of the world *E. granulosus* transmission between dogs and sheep is in an 'endemic steady state' (i.e. appears as a linear increase in age-specific cyst intensity rates in sheep) rather than a 'hyperendemic state' (i.e. plateau of age-specific cyst intensity rates in sheep due to aquired immunity), and therefore in theory the former state will be more amenable to control intervention. Hyperendemic status for *E. granulosus* therefore appears unlikely in the sheep–dog domestic cycle; however, hyperendemic levels of exposure may occur in wildlife, e.g. within the deer–wolf, or the wallaby–dingo cycles, and perhaps in a wild ungulate–lion transmission cycle (Rausch, 2003; Jenkins and Macpherson, 2003; Torgerson and Heath, 2003).

Recent epidemiological data from necropsy and arecoline purge studies of dog populations in areas without hydatid control intervention, e.g. in Kazakhstan, China, Tunisia and Libya, now strongly indicates that immunity, in addition to acting against infection in livestock hosts, also occurs in the dog definitive host against the adult tapeworm stage of *E. granulosus*. Epidemiological studies suggest that resistance or immunity in dogs is manifested by significant higher worm burdens in young dogs compared to animals over 4 years old (Torgerson and Heath, 2003; Budke *et al.*, 2004a; Buishi *et al.*, 2005). In practical terms, this means that computer simulations based on transmission models that realistically take into account immunity in both the intermediate and final hosts, will be more likely to assist in planning and implementation of hydatid control, and for cost-benefit analysis (Torgerson, 2003). For example, such refined models can help determine the optimal frequency and cover of anthelmintic treatment of dogs, the best use of combined dosing of dogs and vaccination of sheep and the cost effectiveness of health education to reduce infection pressure to dogs (Torgerson and Heath, 2003).

6.2. Surveillance Tools

6.2.1. Ovine Hydatidosis

The gold standard approach for surveillance of the impact of control programmes for CE is the use of reliable specific meat (offal) inspection in designated abattoirs or slaughterhouses, primarily for sheep as the most important intermediate host. These data should be collected for three different age groups of sheep for more sensitive variation in prevalence rates. Care should also be taken to differentiate CE from other lesions e.g. caused by cysticercus tenuicollis (*T. hydatigena*) especially in lambs where cysts will be smaller and may therefore require histological confirmation (e.g. Cabrera *et al.*, 1995; Larrieu *et al.*, 2001). Annual CE prevalence figures in lambs, juveniles and adult sheep will enable the control authority to measure control impact and adjust dog-dosing regimens if necessary, for example as used in Chile Region XII (Vidal *et al.*, 1994). Specific training of abattoir inspectors and/or veterinarians may be required whether employed by the municipality, health services, veterinary services or a hydatid commission/research agency. Abattoir inspection of slaughtered sheep, and other livestock, is also critical for transfer from the 'attack' to the 'consolidation' phase of control. The latter relies on trace back of infected animals to identify infected farms/properties in order to impose restrictions on livestock and dog movement and treatment of dogs. The additional use of abattoir data for *T. hydatigena* infection can be important in identifying potential problem properties, as for example was effectively employed in Cyprus (Economides and Christofi, 2002).

Ante-mortem approaches for diagnosis or detection of ovine CE using modern serological methods or portable ultrasound scanning are as yet not sufficiently specific and sensitive to be of significant assistance in hydatid control programme surveillance of livestock CE (Craig *et al.*, 2003). However, such approaches may be useful to identify exposure in epidemiological studies, or be applied if slaughterhouse data is unavailable or difficult to collect, e.g. in northwest Turkana (Njoroge *et al.*, 2000).

Use of lambs as sentinel animals to detect natural exposure to *E. granulosus* has been quite successfully applied in control programmes in Wales and Uruguay. In Wales, 6% of sentinel lambs became infected within 15 months from exposure in an area subject to full control (PZQ and education) over the previous 5 years (compared to 10% in a neighbouring area where control was not implemented), indicating continued transmission from dogs to sheep (Lloyd *et al.*, 1998). In Uruguay, one study to determine optimal PZQ dosing frequency found that sentinel lambs were not infected when a 6 weekly dosing regimen was used, but in contrast, 4–18% of sentinel lambs became infected when the dosing interval was extended to 12 or 16 weeks (Cabrera *et al.*, 2002b).

6.2.2. Canine Echinococcosis

Post-mortem examination of the small intestines of dogs is the gold standard for detection of the adult tapeworm of *E. granulosus* (WHO/ OIE, 2001). However, such an approach cannot usually be applied for surveillance of owned dogs, and it is difficult to necropsy large numbers of unwanted or stray dogs even when humane culling is undertaken, for example by a municipality. Use of areca extracts, and later arecoline salts, as an ante-mortem purge for detection of *E. granulosus* in dogs has been applied in hydatid control programmes since the 1890s when it was first used in the Iceland campaign (Beard *et al.*, 2001). Arecoline is not an anthelmintic so it cannot be reliably used to treat dogs. Rather as a strong purgative it may eliminate a large proportion of resident tapeworms (including all main genera, *Echinococcus, Taenia, Spirometra, Dipylidium, Mesocestoides*, etc.), and in that regard should be viewed as an ante-mortem diagnostic test. The great advantage of arecoline is that it should be 100% specific and purgation also provided an important on-site educational tool for dog owners. Arecoline sensitivity however is normally around 70%, as small burdens of *E. granulosus* may not be completely voided with the purge, and up to 25% of dogs fail to purge; it may also be stressful for dogs (dehydration may occur), potentially biohazardous for operatives and logistically difficult and time consuming (Craig, 1997).

Despite these drawbacks until the mid-1990s, purgation was the only reliable and practical test for canine echinococcosis, and was used to great effect in several hydatid control programmes especially those carried out in Tasmania, New Zealand and Cyprus, where hundreds of thousands of dogs were screened (Section 2). Arecoline testing remains a very useful surveillance approach during the 'attack' phase and particularly the 'consolidation' phase of hydatid control. The advent of PZQ in the late 1970s and its widespread availability in the 1980s meant however that this anthelmintic could replace the reliance on arecoline purgation as the main tool of the 'attack' phase. Furthermore, the development in 1992 of a highly specific laboratory test, based on coproantigen ELISA, provided a potential alternative approach to ante-mortem diagnosis of canine echinococcosis (Allan *et al.*, 1992; Deplazes *et al.*, 1992). Coproantigen testing could be performed on faecal supernatants extracted from less than 1 gm of frozen or formalin-preserved samples, faecal samples could be collected per rectum or from the ground, the test could identify a proportion of dogs with low burdens (< 50 worms), was at least as sensitive as arecoline purgation, was able to detect pre-patent juvenile infections and dogs became copro-negative within 4–5 days post-treatment (Allan *et al.*, 1992; Craig *et al.*, 1995; Jenkins *et al.*, 2000). Comparison of the coproantigen ELISA with necropsy or purge indicated the following characteristics: specificity, 91–98% and sensitivity, 62–100% (Craig *et al.*, 1995; El-Shehabi *et al.*, 2000; Christofi *et al.*, 2002; Lopera *et al.*, 2003; Buishi *et al.*, 2005). The coproantigen approach was also shown to be superior to serological diagnosis, mainly due to the poor correlation of serum antibodies with current infection (Craig *et al.*, 1995).

Coproantigen ELISA has already been used for surveillance purposes in at least three formal hydatid control programmes, i.e. Wales, Falkland islands and Cyprus. In the Falkland islands, the test was used in the 'consolidation' phase to screen about 50% of the dog population in order to identify the remaining foci of infected sheep farms (Reichel *et al.*, 1996). Similarly, in Cyprus > 6500 owned dogs were screened (2.8% were copro-positive) using a commercial *Echinococcus* coproantigen test, in a low prevalence zone in the 'consolidation' phase of hydatid control, and positive dogs were treated with PZQ (Christofi *et al.*, 2002). Coproantigen testing of farm dogs in mid-Wales was used to assess the impact of the 'attack' phase of hydatid control and whether canine echinococcosis rates had changed after the termination of the control programme. Dosing of dogs had been effective in Wales as the coproantigen prevalence in farm dogs remained at 0% in the control zone 4 years after cessation of supervised dosing. However, after 13 years the coproantigen positive rate had increased to 8%, signalling a re-emergence of transmission (Palmer *et al.*, 1996; Buishi *et al.*, 2005).

The recent development of copro-PCR tests for *E. granulosus* shows great promise as a 100% specific confirmatory tool for dog infection (Abbasi *et al.*, 2003; Stefanic *et al.*, 2004). Such tests, which detect *Echinococcus* DNA, may be best applied in confirmation of coproantigen tests and will be invaluable in the 'consolidation' phase of control (Craig *et al.*, 2003).

6.2.3. Human Cystic Echinococcosis

Surveillance of human CE is critical in order to measure the public health impact of any hydatid control programme, and to inform the Control Authority and Public Health agencies about its efficacy and success. The gold standard has been and remains, the use of annual CE surgical/treatment incidence rate per 100 000 population within the control zone. Age-specific incidence rates for the under 15 or under 10 years age groups will in addition provide data on recent transmission, as opposed to old (pre-intervention) CE cases. Such data retrospectively indicated the positive impact of the Iceland education focussed and the Chile dog-dosing-based campaigns, or by contrast the failure of hydatid control in Sardinia (see Sections 2 and 5). Such hospital-derived data are, however, not always accurate and treatment access may be poor for underdeveloped regions, e.g. northwest Kenya (Schantz, 1997; Craig *et al.*, 2003).

Radiographic surveys using imaging techniques, especially portable ultrasound scanners at community level, provide a relatively new mass screening approach for human surveillance in hydatid control programmes. Advantages of ultrasound scanning over hospital data include the detection of asymptomatic cases and confirmation of clinical status of previous cases, early clinical information in respect of treatment options and natural history of disease, the true age-specific prevalence of abdominal CE, longitudinal data in follow-up and an educational effect for rural communities (Macpherson *et al.*, 2003). Ultrasound-based screening in endemic populations has been applied for surveillance in at least two hydatid control programmes i.e. Rio Negro (Argentina) and Turkana (Kenya). In the Rio Negro programme, the ultrasound prevalence of CE in children (aged under 13 years) was shown to reduce from 5.5% to 1.1% over a 13-year period of intervention, and furthermore that characteristic hydatid cyst pathology indicated that 65% of cysts were of the 'early growth' i.e. type CE 1 (Larrieu *et al.*, 2000a; Frider *et al.*, 2001). In the Turkana hydatid control programme, human US screening data were very important for surveillance on two counts. Firstly, because hospital-based incidence data was difficult to collect especially after a deliberate reduction in surgical provision (due to high recurrence rates) and more emphasis on albendazole outpatient therapy by AMREF. Secondly, the virtual absence of slaughterhouses in the region meant that ovine CE data could not easily be obtained (Macpherson and Wachira, 1997).

Serosurveys using sensitive and/or specific tests, such as Arc-5/DD5 agar tests, cyst fluid antigen or antigen B-ELISA or immunoblot tests, have not been employed extensively in surveillance of hydatid control programmes. Rather, use of hospital and/or ultrasound-based data sets were preferred because of their unequivocal diagnostic status. The DD5 test was however used to screen humans in the Falkland islands, and was applied in the Rio Negro programme (later replaced by ELISA) to identify exposure in children, but are now used primarily only in confirmation of ultrasound screening.

6.3. Vaccination against *Echinococcus granulosus*

An effective vaccine against CE in livestock or canine echinococcosis in dogs would have enormous potential for hydatid control. A dog vaccine is currently not available and assuming research occurs, probably would not be for the next 5–10 years. Livestock vaccination however is practical but would probably not replace dog dosing, rather act as an additional measure that would reduce the biomass of cysts developing especially in sheep and thus the infection pressure to dogs. It would therefore also reduce the frequency of anthelmintic dosing of dogs. As discussed above, several hydatid control programmes have failed or had poor impact, because of difficulties in maintaining the accepted standard of 6- or 12-week dog-dosing regimens for several years. Also because not high enough proportions of dogs were treated over the 'attack' phase (e.g. as occurred during control efforts in Uruguay, Chile Region XI, Falkland islands and Sardinia).

Extensive research on immune responses against larval cestodes was undertaken from the 1930s to 1980s using experimental animal cysticercosis due to *Taenia* spp. infection, and then from the 1960s to 1990s using experimental livestock infections with either *Taenia* spp. or *E. granulosus* (largely in New Zealand and Australia) (reviewed by Rickard and Williams, 1982; Lightowlers *et al.*, 2003). This research culminated in the development of the first defined subunit vaccine with high efficacy against any helminth. The first antimetacestode vaccine utilized a recombinant oncosphere peptide (45 W) against *T. ovis* infection in sheep (Johnson *et al.*, 1989), which quickly lead to the development of a similarly effective recombinant oncosphere vaccine (EG95) against ovine echinococcosis (Lightowlers *et al.*, 1996). Two subcutaneous injections in sheep of the EG95 vaccine with Quil A adjuvant lead to the production of complement fixing IgG antibodies lethal to *E. granulosus* oncospheres that resulted in 96–100% protection against *E. granulosus* egg challenge infections for up to 12 months; and furthermore for up to 3 months in lambs born to vaccinated ewes (Lightowlers, 2002; Heath *et al.*, 2003).

This development of an effective vaccine against ovine hydatidosis provides the potential for implementation of a more rapid and cost-effective 'attack' phase for ongoing or future hydatid control programmes. Though not yet formally included in any national or provincial hydatid control programme, two large-scale pilot trials of the vaccine in highly endemic areas in western China and one in southern Argentina, confirmed its high efficacy, optimal delivery and safety, against natural challenge with *E. granulosus* (Heath *et al.*, 2003). Trials indicate that one effective strategy would be to combine spring and autumn vaccination of lambs/sheep (two injections 1 month apart followed by a third at 6–12 months) with only twice yearly PZQ dosing of dogs. Furthermore, computer simulations of transmission in which control interventions were modelled (involving, anthelmintic treatment of dogs, vaccination of sheep and/or health education), indicated that vaccination of sheep alone can be highly effective if >90% are protected. Even more realistically a 75% vaccine cover of sheep, coupled with twice annual dog dosing would have an equal effect (Torgerson and Heath, 2003).

6.4. Options for Control of *Echinococcus multilocularis*

Human alveolar echinococcosis (AE), due to liver infection with the larval stage of *E. multilocularis*, is a much rarer though more pathogenic form of hydatidosis compared to human CE, furthermore AE disease has a significantly higher fatality rate in untreated cases (Craig, 2003; McManus *et al.*, 2003). *E. multilocularis* transmission is considered to be spreading and potentially emergent in rural and urban parts of Europe (Deplazes *et al.*, 2004). Transmission of *E. multilocularis* occurs only in the northern hemisphere, and is maintained principally within sylvatic (wildlife) cycles between fox definitive and rodent intermediate hosts, and therefore control is potentially much more difficult compared to interruption of the main domestic animal cycle of *E. granulosus*.

There has been one successful example of total control, in Reuben island (Japan) in the 1930s, where *E. multilocularis* was eliminated as a result of deliberate extermination of the red fox reservoir; however, the parasite is now endemic over the whole of the main island of Hokkaido (Ito *et al.*, 2003). In Alaska, an intense localized focus of transmission on St. Lawrence island was controlled in the 1980s by supervised PZQ dosing of sled dogs, which were responsible for the main zoonotic risk to the indigenous Inuit population, so that the risk of human disease also decreased (Rausch *et al.*, 1990). In two other regions (southern Germany and Hokkaido, Japan), PZQ baits, similar to rabies-vaccine baits, have been successfully used to reduce the prevalence of *E. multilocularis* in red fox populations over local to medium scales (90–3500 km^2) (Ito *et al.*, 2003). In the pilot control programmes in Germany, based on monthly or 6-week intervals for bait distribution, prevalence in fox populations declined from 32–64% to 4–15% over 14–18 months (Ito *et al.*, 2003). Direct dosing of domestic dogs, and use of PZQ baits for fox or stray dog populations, are thus able to reduce transmission and therefore also the public health risk of AE. However, sustained long-term dosing or baiting programmes will be required to maintain reduced levels of transmission, and therefore the potential for a long-acting vaccine against *E. multilocularis* in the canid host would be a major improvement.

7. CONCLUDING REMARKS

Several cystic hydatid control programmes to reduce or eliminate transmission of *E. granulosus* are likely to be planned in a number of countries or regions, where human CE cases continue to increase, and where CE has re-emerged or is newly emerged, or newly recognized as a public health problem (Eckert *et al.*, 2000; Craig and Pawlowski, 2002; Torgerson and Budke, 2004). Nearly 150 years of hydatid control programmes clearly show that human CE can be eliminated as a public health problem. The best results occurred when a well-managed control authority implemented a medium to long-term (>10 years) vertical campaign directed at the treatment of owned rural dogs with appropriate community education and surveillance in sheep, canid and human populations. Future CE programmes may be more efficient and cost-effective than those previously implemented if an integrated approach is used. Therefore, a new option for CE control i.e. Option 6, can now be considered, and would be based on a vertical fast-track approach with specified lower frequency of PZQ treatment (e.g. as low as two times per year) of registered dogs, combined with annual or twice annual vaccination of sheep against *E. granulosus* egg exposure.

Use of PZQ baits for fox populations can have a significant, albeit temporary, effect on transmission of *E. multilocularis*; however, long-term reduction in risk of human AE in endemic areas (e.g. Alaska and Tibet) will depend on the regular dosing of domestic dogs. Future research to develop effective dog and fox vaccines against *Echinococcus* spp. could lead to more effective control programmes.

ACKNOWLEDGEMENTS

We are grateful for the many insightful discussions with the late Dr. Michael Gemmell, to whom this review is dedicated. Thanks also to David Heath (Ag Research Limited, Wallaceville Animal Research Centre, Upper Hutt, New Zealand) and David Jenkins (Australian Hydatid Control and Epidemiology Program, Fyshwick, Australia) for provision of reports and papers relating to the New Zealand hydatid control programme. Research support in part from the NIH/ NSF Ecology of Infectious Diseases Program (TWO 1565) is gratefully acknowledged.

REFERENCES

Abbasi, I., Branzburg, A., Campos-Ponce, M., Abdel-Hafez, S.K., Raoul, F., Craig, P.S. and Hamburger, J. (2003). Coprodiagnosis of *Echinococcus granulosus* infection in dogs by amplification of a newly identified repeated DNA sequence. *American Journal of Tropical Medicine and Hygiene* **69**, 324–330.

Aliaga, F. and Oberg, C. (2000). Epidemiology of human hydatidosis in the IX Region of la Araucania, Chile 1991–1998. *Boletin Chileno Parasitologia* **55**, 54–58.

Allan, J.C., Craig, P.S., Garcia-Noval, J., Mencos, F., Liu, D., Wang, Y., Wen, H., Zhou, P., Stringer, R., Rogan, M.T. and Zeyhle, E. (1992). Coproantigen detection for immunodiagnosis of echinococcosis and taeniasis in dogs and humans. *Parasitology* **104**, 347–356.

Attanasio, E., Ferretti, G. and Palmas, C. (1985). Hydatidosis in Sardinia: review and recommendations. *Transactions of the Royal Society of Tropical Medicine and Hygiene* **79**, 154–158.

Attanasio, E. and Palmas, C. (1984). Cost-effectiveness analysis of echinococcosis-hydatidosis eradication project in Sardinia. *Social Science and Medicine* **19**, 1067–1072.

Battelli, G., Mantovani, A. and Seimenis, A. (2002). Cystic echinococcosis and the Mediterranean region: a long-lasting association. *Parassitologia* **44**, 43–57.

Beard, T.C., Bramble, A.J. and Middleton, M.J. (2001). *Eradication in Our Time. A Log Book of the Tasmanian Hydatid Control Programs, 1962–1996.* Hobart: University of Tasmania.

Bleaney, A. (1984). *Hydatid Disease in Humans in the Falkland islands 1984.* Port Stanley, 21st March.

Bonifacino, R., Malagor, R., Barbeito, R., Balleste, R., Rodriguez, M.J., Botto, C. and Klug, F. (1991). Seroprevalence of *Echinococcus granulosus* infection in a Uruguayan rural human population. *Transactions of the Royal Society of Tropical Medicine and Hygiene* **85**, 769–772.

Bramble, A.J. (1974). Hydatid disease control 1964–1974. A report of ten years of effort to control hydatid disease in Tasmania. *Tasmanian Journal of Agriculture* **45**, 225–232.

Budke, C.M., Qiu, J., Craig, P.S. and Torgerson, P.R. (2004a). Modelling the transmission of *Echinococcus granulosus* and *Echinococcus multilocularis* in dogs for a high endemic region of the Tibetan plateau. *International Journal for Parasitology* **35**, 163–170.

Budke, C.M., Qiu, J., Zinsstag, J., Wang, Q. and Torgerson, P.R. (2004b). Use of disability adjusted lifeyears in the estimation of the disease burden of echinococcosis for a high endemic region of the Tibetan Plateau. *American Journal of Tropical Medicine and Hygiene* **71**, 56–64.

Buishi, I., Walters, T., Guildea, Z., Craig, P.S. and Palmer, S. (2005). Re-emergence of canine *Echinococcus granulosus* infection, Wales. *Emerging Infectious Diseases*, Ph D. Thesis **11**, 568–571.

Cabrera, M., Canova, S., Rosenzvit, M. and Guarnera, E. (2002a). Identification of *Echinococcus granulosus* eggs. *Diagnostic Microbiology and Infectious Diseases* **44**, 29–34.

Cabrera, P.A., Haran, G., Benavidez, V., Valledor, S., Pererra, G., Lloyd, S., Gemmell, M.A., Barbaibar, M., Morana, A., Maissonave, J. and Carballo, M. (1995). Transmission dynamics of *Echinococcus granulosus, Taenia hydatigena and Taenia ovis* in sheep in Uruguay. *International Journal for Parasitology* **25**, 807–813.

Cabrera, P.A., Irabedra, P.M., Orlando, D., Rista, L., Haran, G., Vinals, G., Blanco, M.T., Alvarez, M., Elola, S., Morosoli, D., Morana, A., Bondad, M., Sambran, Y., Heinzen, T., Chans, L., Pineyro, L., Perez, D. and Pereyra, I. (2003). National prevalence of larval echinococcosis in sheep in slaughtering plants (*ovis aries*) as an indicator in control programmes in Uruguay. *Acta Tropica* **85**, 281–285.

Cabrera, P.A., Lloyd, S., Haran, G., Pineyro, L., Parietti, S., Gemmell, M.A., Correa, O., Morana, A. and Valledor, S. (2002b). Control of *Echinococcus granulosus* in Uruguay: evaluation of different treatment intervals for dogs. *Veterinary Parasitology* **103**, 333–340.

Cabrera, P.A., Parietti, S., Haran, G., Benavidez, V., Lloyd, S., Valledor, S., Pererra, G., Gemmell, M.A. and Botto, T. (1996). Rates of reinfection with *Echinococcus granulosus, Taenia hydatigena, Taenia ovis* and other cestodes in a rural dog population in Uruguay. *International Journal for Parasitology* **26**, 79–83.

Carabin, H., Budke, C.M., Cowan, L.D., Willingham, A.L. and Torgerson, P.R. (2005). Methods for assessing the burden of parasitic zoonoses: echinococcosis and cysticercosis. *Trends in Parasitology* **21**, 327–333.

Carmona, C., Perdomo, R., Carbo, A., Alvarez, C., Monti, J., Graubert, D., Stern, G., Perera, G., Lloyd, S., Bazini, R., Gemmell, M.A. and Yarzabal, L. (1998). Risk factors associated with human cystic echinoccoccosis in Florida, Uruguay: results of a mass screening study using ultrasound and serology. *American Journal of Tropical Medicine and Hygiene* **58**, 599–605.

Cavagion, L., Perez, A., Zanini, F., Jensen, O., Saldía, L., Diaz, M., Cantoni, G., Herrero, E., Costa, M., Volpe, M., Araya, D., Alvarez Rubianes, N.,

Aguado, C., Meglia, G., Santillan, G., Guarnera, E. and Larrieu, E. (2004). Diagnosis of cystic echinococcosis in cattle farms in the south of Argentina: areas with a control program. *Veterinary Parasitology* **128**, 73–81.

Christofi, G., Deplazes, P., Christofi, N., Tanner, I., Economides, P. and Eckert, J. (2002). Screening of dogs for *Echinococcus granulosus* copro-antigen in a low endemic situation in Cyprus. *Veterinary Parasitology* **104**, 299–306.

Clarkson, M.J. (1978). Hydatid disease in Wales: 2 Eradication. *Veterinary Record* **102**, 259–261.

Cohen, H., Paolillo, E., Bonifacino, R., Botta, B., Parada, L., Cabrera, P., Alfaro, H., Rogan, M. and Craig, P.S. (1998). Human cystic echino-coccosis in a Uruguayan community: a sonographic, serologic and epidemiologic study. *American Journal of Tropical Medicine and Hygiene* **59**, 620–627.

Coltorti, E.A., Fernandez, E., Guarnera, E., Lago, J. and Iriate, J. (1988). Field evaluation of an enzyme immunoassay for detection of asympto-matic patients in a hydatid control programme. *American Journal of Tropical Medicine and Hygiene* **38**, 603–607.

Conchedda, M., Ecca, A.R., Gabrielle, F., Bortoletti, G. and Palmas, C. (2002). In: *Cestode Zoonoses: Echinococcosis and Cysticercosis. An Emergent and Global Problem* (P.S. Craig and Z. Pawlowski, eds), pp. 343–354. Amsterdam: IOS Press, NATO Science Series.

Conchedda, M., Palmas, C., Bortoletti, F., Gabrielle, F. and Ecca, A.R. (1997). Hydatidosis: a comprehensive view of the Sardinian case. *Parassitologia* **39**, 359–366.

Craig, P.S. (1997). Immunodiagnosis of *Echinococcus granulosus* and a comparison of techniques for diagnosis of canine echinococcosis. In: *Compendium on Cystic Echinococcosis in Africa and in Middle Eastern Countries with special Reference to Morocco* (F.L. Andersen, H. Ouhelli and M. Kachani, eds), pp. 85–118. Provo: Brigham Young University Print Services.

Craig, P.S. (2003). *Echinococcus multilocularis. Current Opinion in Infectious Diseases* **16**, 437–444.

Craig, P.S. (2004). Epidemiology of echinococcosis in China. *Southeast Asian Journal of Tropical Medicine and Public Health* **35**, supplement 1, 158–169.

Craig, P.S., Gasser, R.B., Parada, L., Cabrera, P., Parietti, S., Borgues, C., Acuttis, A., Gulla, J., Snowden, K. and Paolillo, E. (1995). Diagnosis of canine echinococcosis: comparison of coproantigen and serum antibody tests with arecoline purgation in Uruguay. *Veterinary Parasitology* **56**, 293–301.

Craig, P.S., Macpherson, C.N.L., Watson-Jones, D.L. and Nelson, G.S. (1988). Immunodetection of *Echinococcus* eggs from naturally infected dogs and from environmental contamination sites in settlements in Turkana, Kenya. *Transactions of the Royal Society of Tropical Medicine and Hygiene* **82**, 268–274.

Craig, P.S. and Nelson, G.S. (1986). The identification of eggs of *Echinococcus* by immunofluorescence using a specific anti-oncospheral monoclonal antibody. *American Journal of Tropical Medicine and Hygiene* **35**, 152–158.

Craig, P.S. and Pawlowski, Z. (2002). *Cestode Zoonoses: Echinococcosis and Cysticercosis. An Emergent and Global Problem*. Amsterdam: IOS Press, NATO Science Series.

Craig, P.S., Rogan, M.T. and Allan, J.C. (1996). Detection, screening and community epidemiology of taeniid cestode zoonoses: cystic echinococcosis, alveolar echinococcosis and neurocysticercosis. *Advances in Parasitology* **38**, 169–250.

Craig, P.S., Rogan, M.T. and Campos-Ponce, M. (2003). Echinococcosis: disease, detection and transmission. *Parasitology* **127**, S5–S20.

Deplazes, P., Gottstein, B., Eckert, J., Jenkins, D.J., Ewald, D. and Jiminez-Palacios, S. (1992). Detection of *Echinococcus* coproantigens by enzyme-linked immunosorbent assay in dogs, dingoes and foxes. *Parasitology Research* **78**, 303–308.

Deplazes, P., Hegglin, D., Gloor, S. and Romig, T. (2004). Wilderness in the city: the urbanization of *Echinococcus multilocularis*. *Trends in Parasitology* **20**, 77–84.

Dew, H.R. (1953). Hydatid disease in Australia. *Archivos Internacionales de la Hidatidosis* **13**, 1319–1332.

De Zavaleta, O., Losada, C. and Galardi, M. (1986). Epidemiología y control de la hidatidosis en Neuquen 1970–1985. Subsecretaría de Salud de Neuquen.

Dinkel, A., Njoroge, E.M., Zimmermann, A., Walz, M., Zeyhle, E., Elmahdi, I.E., Mackenstedt, U. and Romig, T. (2004). A PCR system for detection of species and genotypes of the *Echinococcus granulosus*-complex, with reference to the epidemiological situation in eastern Africa. *International Journal for Parasitology* **34**, 645–653.

Dowling, P., Abo-Shehada, M. and Torgerson, P.R. (2000). Risk factors associated with human cystic echinococcosis in Jordan: results of a case control study. *Annals of Tropical Medicine and Parasitology* **94**, 69–75.

Dungal, N. (1957). Eradication of hydatid disease in Iceland. *New Zealand Medical Journal* **56**, 213–222.

Ecca, A.R., Conchedda, M., Gabrielle, F., Bortoletti, G. and Palmas, C. (2002). Cystic echinococcosis in the Mediterranean Basin. In: *Cestode Zoonoses: Echinococcosis and Cysticercosis. An Emergent and Global Problem* (P.S. Craig, and Z. Pawlowski, eds), pp. 41–55. Amsterdam: IOS Press, NATO Science Series.

Eckert, J. (1997). Epidemiology of *Echinococcus multilocularis* and *E granulosus* in Central Europe. *Parassitologia* **39**, 337–344.

Eckert, J., Conraths, F.J. and Tackmann, K. (2000). Echinococcosis: an emerging or re-emerging zoonosis? *International Journal for Parasitology* **30**, 1283–1294.

Eckert, J., Gottstein, B., Heath, D. and Liu, F-J. (2001). Prevention of echinococcosis in humans and safety precautions. In: *WHO/OIE Manual on Echinococcosis in Humans and Animals: A Public Health Problem of Global Concern* (J. Eckert, M.A. Gemmell, F.-X. Meslin and Z.S. Pawlowski, eds), pp. 238–247. Paris: World Health Organization for Animal Health.

Economides, P. (1994). Echinococcosis in Cyprus—10 years after the eradication campaign. In: *Mediterranean Zoonoses Control Programme (MZCP) Consultation on the Echinococcosis/Hydatidosis National Control Activities and Programmes in the MZCP countries*, 16–18 November, Valladolid, pp. 22–34. Athens: World Health Organization Mediterranean Zoonoses Control Centre.

Economides, P. and Christofi, G. (2002). Experience gained and evaluation of the echinococcosis/hydatidosis eradication programmes in Cyprus 1971–1999. In: *Cestode Zoonoses: Echinococcosis and Cysticercosis. An Emergent and Global Problem* (P.S. Craig and Z. Pawlowski, eds), pp. 367–379. Amsterdam: IOS Press, NATO Science Series.

Economides, P., Christofi, G. and Gemmell, M.A. (1998). Control of *Echinococcus granulosus* in Cyprus and comparison with other island models. *Veterinary Parasitology* **79**, 151–163.

El-Shehabi, F.S., Kamhawi, S.A., Schantz, P.M., Craig, P.S. and Abdel-Hafez, S.K. (2000). Diagnosis of canine echinococcosis: comparison of coproantigen detection with necropsy in stray dogs and red foxes from northern Jordan. *Parasite* **7**, 83–90.

French, C.M. and Nelson, G.S. (1982). Hydatid disease in the Turkana district of Kenya, II. A study in medical geography. *Annals of Tropical Medicine and Parasitology* **76**, 439–457.

French, C.M., Nelson, G.S. and Wood, M. (1982). Hydatid disease in the Turkana district of Kenya, I. The background to the problem with hypotheses to account for the remarkably high prevalence of the disease in man. *Annals of Tropical Medicine and Parasitology* **76**, 425–437.

Frider, B., Larrieu, E. and Aguero, A. (1986). Catastro ecografico de hidatidosis en un area endemica, studio comparative con DD5. *Revista Iberica Parasitologia* **46**, 257–266.

Frider, B., Losada, C., Larrieu, E. and De Zavaleta, O. (1988). Asymptomatic abdominal hydatidosis detected by ultrasonography. *Acta Radiologica* **29**, 431–434.

Frider, B., Larrieu, E. and Odriozola, M. (1999). Long-term outcome of asymptomatic liver hydatidosis. *Journal of Hepatology* **30**, 228–231.

Frider, B., Moguilensky, J., Salvitti, J., Odriozola, M., Cantoni, G. and Larrieu, E. (2001). Epidemiological surveillance of human hydatidosis by means of ultrasonography: its contributions to evaluation of control programs. *Acta Tropica* **79**, 219–223.

Gabriele, F., Bortoletti, G., Conchedda, M., Palmas, C. and Ecca, A.R. (2004). [Human cystic hydatidosis in Italy: a public health emergency? Past to present] [In Italian]. *Parassitologia* **46**, 39–43.

Gemmell, M.A. (1961). An analysis of the incidence of hydatid cysts (*Echinococcus granulosus*) in domestic food animals in New Zealand, 1958–1959. *The New Zealand Veterinary Journal* **9**, 29–41.

Gemmell, M.A. (1987). A critical approach to the concepts of control and eradication of echinococcosis/hydatidosis and taeniasis/cysticercosis. In: *Parasitology—Quo Vadis?* (M.J. Howell, ed.), pp. 465–472. Canberra: Australian Academy of Sciences.

Gemmell, M.A. (1990). Australasian contributions to an understanding of the epidemiology and control of hydatid disease caused by *Echinococcus granulosus*—past, present and future. *International Journal for Parasitology* **20**, 431–456.

Gemmell, M.A. (1994). Current progress in control of *Echinococcus granulosus*: a global summary. *Meeting of the Scientific Working Group on the Advances in Prevention, Control and Treatment of Hydatidosis*. Montevideo: Pan American Health Organization, 26–28 October.

Gemmell, M.A. (1997). Report on progress in control of hydatidosis caused by *Echinococcus granulosus* in the Republic of Chile (1979–1997). World Health Organization, Consultative Report.

Gemmell, M.A. (1999). Contributions of epidemiological research into island programmes for control of *E. granulosus* during the 20th century. XIX International Congress of Hydatidology San Carlos de Bariloche, Rio Negro, Argentina.

Gemmell, M.A. and Johnstone, P.D. (1977). Experimental epidemiology of hydatidosis and cysticercosis. *Advances in Parasitology* **15**, 311–369.

Gemmell, M.A., Lawson, J.R. and Roberts, M.A. (1986). Population dynamics in echinococcosis and cysticercosis: biological parameters of *Echinococcus granulosus* in dogs and sheep. *Parasitology* **92**, 599–620.

Gemmell, M.A., Lawson, J.R. and Roberts, M.A. (1987). Population dynamics in echinococcosis and cysticercosis: evaluation of the biological parameters of *Taenia hydatigena* and *T. ovis* and comparison with those of *Echinococcus granulosus*. *Parasitology* **94**, 161–180.

Gemmell, M.A. and Roberts, M.A. (1998). Cystic echinococcosis. In: *Zoonoses* (S.R. Palmer, E.J.L. Soulsby and D.I.H. Simpson, eds), pp. 665–716. Oxford: Oxford University Press.

Gemmell, M.A., Roberts, M.G., Beard, T.C., Campano Diaz, S., Lawson, J.R. and Nonnemaker, J.M. (2001). Control of echinococcosis. In: *WHO/OIE Manual on Echinococcosis in Humans and Animals: a Public*

Health Problem of Global Concern (J. Eckert, M.A. Gemmell, F.-X. Meslin and Z.S. Pawlowski, eds), pp. 195–204. Paris: World Health Organization for Animal Health.

Gibbs, J.G. (1946). Agricultural Department Report 1937–1946. The Secretariat, Port Stanley, Falkland islands.

Grove, D.I. (1990). *A History of Human Helminthology*. Wallingford, UK: CAB International.

Guarnera, E., Santillan, G., Botinelli, R. and Franco, A. (2000). Canine echinococcosis: an alternative for surveillance epidemiology. *Veterinary Parasitology* **88**, 131–134.

Hackett, F. and Walters, T.M.H. (1980). Helminths of the red fox in mid-Wales. *Veterinary Parasitology* **7**, 181–184.

Heath, D.D., Jensen, O. and Lightowlers, M.W. (2003). Progress in control of hydatidosis using vaccination—a review of formulation and delivery of the vaccine and recommendations for practical use in control programmes. *Acta Tropica* **85**, 133–143.

Heath, D.D., Pharo, H. and van der Loght, P. (1999). Hydatids close to eradication in New Zealand. *Archivos Internacionales de la Hidatidosis* XXXIII, 39–40.

Holcman, B. and Heath, D.D. (1997). The early stages of *Echinococcus granulosus* development. *Acta Tropica* **64**, 5–17.

Ito, A., Romig, T. and Takahashi, K. (2003). Perspective on control options for *Echinococcus multilocularis* with particular reference to Japan. *Parasitology* **127**, S159–S172.

Ito, A., Urbani, C., Qiu, J.M., Vuitton, D.A., Qiu, D.C., Heath, D.D., Craig, P.S., Feng, Z. and Schantz, P.M. (2003). Control of echinococcosis and cysticercosis: a public health challenge to international cooperation in China. *Acta Tropica* **86**, 3–17.

Jenkins, D.J. (2005). Hydatid control in Australia: where it began, what we have achieved and where to go from here. *International Journal of Parasitology* **35**, 733–740.

Jenkins, D.J., Fraser, A., Bradshaw, H. and Craig, P.S. (2000). Detection of *Echinococcus granulosus* coproantigens in Australian canids with natural or experimental infection. *Journal of Parasitology* **86**, 140–145.

Jenkins, D.J. and Macpherson, C.N.L. (2003). Transmission ecology of *Echinococcus* in wild-life in Australia and Africa. *Parasitology* **127**, S63–S72.

Johnson, K.S., Harrison, G.B., Lightowlers, M.W., O'Hoy, K.L., Cougle, W.G., Dempster, R.P., Lawrence, S.B., Vinton, J.G., Heath, D.D. and Rickard, M.D. (1989). Vaccination against ovine cysticercosis using a defined recombinant antigen. *Nature* **338**, 585–587.

Jones, A. and Walters, T.M.H. (1992). A survey of taeniid cestodes in farm dogs in mid Wales. *Annals of Tropical Medicine and Parasitology* **86**, 137–142.

Kamenetzky, I., Gutierrez, A., Canova, S., Haag, K., Guarnera, E., Parra, A., Garcia, G. and Rosenzvit, M. (2002). Several strains of *Echinococcus granulosus* infect livestock and humans in Argentina. *Infection Genetics and Evolution* **2**, 129–136.

Krabbe, H. (1864). Athugasemdir handa islendingum um sullaveikina og varnir moti henni. Copenhagen.

Larrieu, E. (1994). Hydatidosis situation in Argentina. *Meeting of the Scientific Working Group on the Advances in Prevention, Control and Treatment of Hydatidosis.* Montevideo: Pan American Health Organization, 26–28 October.

Larrieu, E., Costa, M., Cantoni, G., Alvarez, R., Cavagion, L., Labanchi, J., Bigatti, R., Araya, D., Herrero, E., Mancini, S. and Cabrera, P. (2001). Ovine *Echinococcus granulosus* transmission dynamics in the province of Rio Negro, Argentina, 1980–1999. *Veterinary Parasitology* **98**, 263–272.

Larrieu, E., Costa, M., Cantoni, G., Labanchi, J., Bigatti, R., Araya, D., Herrero, E., Iglesias, L., Mancini, S. and Thakur, A. (1999). Rate of infection and of reinfection by *Echinococcus granulosus* in rural dogs of the Province of Rio Negro. *Veterinary Parasitology* **87**, 281–286.

Larrieu, E., Costa, M., Cantoni, G., Labanchi, J., Bigatti, R., Perez, A., Araya, D., Mancini, S., Herrero, E., Talmon, G., Romeo, S. and Thakur, A. (2000a). Control program of hydatid disease in the Province of Rio Negro, Argentina, 1980–1997. *Boletin Chileno Parasitologia* **55**, 49–53.

Larrieu, E., Costa, M., Del Carpio, M., Moguillansky, S., Bianchi, G. and Yadon, Z.E. (2002). A case-control study of the risk factors among children of Rio Negro Province, Argentina. *Annals of Tropical Medicine and Parasitology* **96**, 43–52.

Larrieu, E., Del Carpio, M., Salvitti, J., Mercapide, C., Sustersic, J., Panomarenko, H., Costa, M., Bigatti, R., Labanchi, J., Herrero, E., Cantoni, G., Perez, A. and Odiozola, M. (2004). Ultrasonographic diagnosis and medical treatment of human cystic echinococcosis in asymptomatic school age carriers: 5 years of follow-up. *Acta Tropica* **91**, 5–13.

Larrieu, E., Mercapide, G., Del Carpio, M., Salvitti, J., Costa, M., Romeo, S., Cantoni, G., Perez, A. and Thakur, A. (2000b). Evaluation of the losses produced by hydatidosis and cost/benefit analysis of different interventions of control in the Province of Rio Negro, Argentina. *Boletin Chileno Parasitologia* **55**, 8–13.

Lawson, J.R. and Gemmell, M.A. (1990). Transmission of taeniid tapeworm eggs via blowflies to intermediate hosts. *Parasitology* **100**, 143–146.

Lethbridge, R.C. (1980). The biology of the oncosphere of cyclophyllidean cestodes. *Helminthological Abstracts Series A* **49**, 59–72.

Lightowlers, M.W. (2002). Vaccines for control of cysticercosis and hydatidosis. In: *Cestode Zoonoses: Echinococcosis and Cysticercosis. An*

Emergent and Global Problem (P.S. Craig and Z. Pawlowski, eds), pp. 381–391. Amsterdam: IOS Press, NATO Science Series.

Lightowlers, M.W., Colebrook, A.L., Gauci, C.G., Gauci, S.M., Kyngdon, C.T., Monkhouse, J.L., Vallejo Rodriquez, C., Read, A.J., Rolfe, R.A. and Sato, C. (2003). Vaccination against cestode parasites: anti-helminth vaccines that work and why. *Veterinary Parasitology* **115**, 83–123.

Lightowlers, M.W., Lawrence, S.B., Gauci, C.G., Young, J., Ralston, M.J., Maas, D. and Heath, D.D. (1996). Vaccination against hydatidosis using a defined recombinant antigen. *Parasite Immunology* **18**, 457–462.

Lloyd, S., Martin, S.C., Walters, T.M.H. and Soulsby, E.J.L. (1996). Use of sentinel lambs for early monitoring of the South Powys hydatidosis control scheme: prevalence of *Echinococcus granulosus* and some other helminths. *Veterinary Record* **129**, 73–76.

Lloyd, S., Walters, T.M.H. and Craig, P.S. (1998). Use of sentinel lambs to survey the effect of an education programme on control of transmission of *Echinococcus granulosus* in South Powys, Wales. *Bulletin of the World Health Organization* **76**, 469–473.

Lopera, L., Moro, P.L., Chavez, A., Montes, G., Gonzales, A. and Gilman, R.H. (2003). Field evaluation of a coproantigen enzyme-linked immunosorbent assay for diagnosis of canine echinococcosis in a rural Andean village in Peru. *Veterinary Parasitology* **117**, 37–42.

Lopez, R. (2002). Consideraciones epidemiológicas de la hidatidosis—echinococcosis en las provincias del norte Argentino. In: *Situación de la Hidatidosis en Argentina* (E. De Negri and A. Dopcich, eds), pp. 57–59. Buenos Aires: Sociedad Argentina de Parasitología.

Macpherson, C.N.L. (1981). *Epidemiology and strain differentiation of Echinococcus granulosus in Kenya.* Ph.D. Thesis, University of London.

Macpherson, C.N.L. (1983). An active intermediate host role for man in the life cycle of *Echinococcus granulosus* in Turkana, Kenya. *American Journal of Tropical Medicine and Hygiene* **32**, 397–404.

Macpherson, C.N.L., Bartholomot, B. and Frider, B. (2003). Application of ultrasound in diagnosis, treatment, epidemiology, public health and control of *Echinococcus granulosus* and *E. multilocularis. Parasitology* **127**, S21–S35.

Macpherson, C.N.L. and Craig, P.S. (1991). Echinococcosis—a plague on pastoralists. In: *Parasitic Helminths and Zoonoses in Africa* (C.N.L. Macpherson and P.S. Craig, eds), pp. 25–53. London: Unwin Hyman.

Macpherson, C.N.L., French, C.M., Stevenson, P., Karstad, L. and Arundel, J.H. (1985). Hydatid disease in the Turkana District of Kenya IV. The prevalence of *Echinococcus granulosus* infection in dogs, and observations on the role of the dog in the lifestyle of the Turkana. *Annals of Tropical Medicine and Parasitology* **79**, 51–61.

Macpherson, C.N.L. and Wachira, T.M. (1997). Cystic echinococcosis in Africa south of the Sahara. In: *Compendium on Cystic Echinococcosis in Africa and in Middle Eastern Countries with Special Reference to Morocco*

(F.L. Andersen, H. Ouhelli and M. Kachani, eds), pp. 245–277. Provo: Brigham Young University Print Services.

Macpherson, C.N.L., Wachira, T.M., Zeyhle, E. and Romig, T. (1986). Hydatid disease research and control in Turkana IV. The pilot control programme. *Transactions of the Royal Society of Tropical Medicine and Hygiene* **80**, 196–200.

Macpherson, C.N.L., Zeyhle, E. and Romig, T. (1984). An *Echinococcus* pilot control programme for north-west Turkana. *Annals of Tropical Medicine and Parasitology* **78**, 188–192.

Maggi, D. (1980). Mortalita per idatidosi. Analisi dei dati dal 1973 al 1977. *Il Medico d'Italia* **23**, 21–24.

McConnell, J.D. and Green, R.J. (1979). The control of hydatid disease in Tasmania. *Australian Veterinary Journal* **55**, 140–145.

McManus, D.P. and Thompson, R.C.A. (2003). Molecular epidemiology of cystic echinococcosis. *Parasitology* **127**, S37–S51.

McManus, D.P., Zhang, W., Li, J. and Bartley, P.B. (2003). Echinococcosis. *Lancet* **362**, 1295–1304.

Moro, P., Bonifacio, N., Gilman, R., Lopera, L., Silva, B., Takumoto, R., Verastegui, M. and Cabrera, L. (1999). Field diagnosis of *Echinococcus granulosus* infection among intermediate and definitive hosts in an endemic focus of human cystic echinococcosis. *Transactions of the Royal Society of Tropical Medicine and Hygiene* **91**, 611–615.

National Hydatids Council of New Zealand (1965). *Hydatids Eradication in Iceland*. Information Bulletin No. 15, Wellington.

National Hydatids Council of New Zealand (1980). Echinococcus granulosus in ewes and dogs. Twentieth Annual Report, Wellington.

Nelson, G.S. (1972). Human behaviour in the transmission of parasitic diseases. In: *Behavioural Aspects of Parasite Transmission* (E.U. Canning and C.A. Wright, eds), *Zoological Journal of the Linnean Society* **51**, supplement, 109–122.

Nelson, G.S. (1986). Hydatid disease: research and control in Turkana, Kenya 1. Epidemiological observations. *Transactions of the Royal Society of Tropical Medicine and Hygiene* **80**, 177–182.

Njoroge, E.M., Mbithi, P.M.F., Gathuma, J.M., Wachira, T.M., Magambo, J.K. and Zeyhle, E. (2000). Application of ultrasonography in prevalence studies of hydatid cysts in goats in northwestern Turkana, Kenya and Toposaland, southern Sudan. *Onderspoort Journal of Veterinary Research* **67**, 251–255.

Njoroge, E.M., Mbithi, P.M.F., Gathuma, J.M., Wachira, T.M., Magambo, J.K. and Zeyhle, E. (2002). A study of cystic echinococcosis in slaughter animals in three selected areas of northern Turkana, Kenya. *Veterinary Parasitology* **104**, 85–91.

Palmer, S.R., Biffin, A.H., Craig, P.S. and Walters, T.M. (1996). Control of hydatid disease in Wales. *British Medical Journal* **312**, 674–675.

Palsson, P.A. (1976). Echinococcosis and its elimination in Iceland. *Historia Medicinae Veterinariae* **1**, 4–10.

Pharo, H. (2002). New Zealand declares 'provisional freedom' from hydatids. *Surveillance* **29**, 3–7.

Polydorou, K. (1976). The control of the dog population as the first objective of the anti-echinococcus campaign in Cyprus. *Bulletin Office International Epizooties* **86**, 705–715.

Polydorou, K. (1993). Echinococcosis/hydatidosis eradication campaign in Cyprus. *Archivos Internacionales de la Hidatidosis* **31**, 67–68.

Purriel, P., Schantz, P.M., Beovide, H. and Menoza, G. (1973). Human echinococcosis (hydatidosis) in Uruguay: a comparison of indices of morbidity and mortality, 1962–71. *Bulletin of the World Health Organization* **49**, 395–402.

Rausch, R. (2003). Cystic echinococcosis in the Arctic and Sub-Arctic. *Parasitology* **127**, S73–S85.

Rausch, R.L. and D'Alessandro, A. (2002). The epidemiology of echinococcosis caused by *Echinococcus oligarthrus* and *E. vogeli* in the Neotropics. In: *Cestode Zoonoses: Echinococcosis and Cysticercosis. An Emergent and Global Problem* (P.S. Craig and Z. Pawlowski, eds), pp. 107–113. Amsterdam: IOS Press, NATO Science Series.

Rausch, R.L., Wilson, J.F. and Schantz, P.M. (1990). A programme to reduce the risk of infection by *Echinococcus multilocularis*: the use of praziquantel to control the cestode in a village in the hyperendemic region of Alaska. *Annals of Tropical Medicine and Parasitology* **84**, 239–250.

Reichel, M.P., Baber, D.J., Craig, P.S. and Gasser, R.B. (1996). Cystic echinococcosis in the Falkland islands. *Preventive Veterinary Medicine* **27**, 115–123.

Rickard, M.D. and Williams, J.F. (1982). Hydatidosis/cysticercosis: immune mechanisms and immunization against infection. *Advances in Parasitology* **21**, 229–296.

Romig, T., Zeyhle, E., Macpherson, C.N.L., Rees, P.H. and Were, J.B.O. (1986). Cyst growth and spontaneous cure in hydatid disease. *Lancet* **ii**, 861.

Rosenzvit, M., Zhang, L., Kamenetzky, L., Canova, S., Guarnera, E. and McManus, D. (1999). Genetic variation and epidemiology of *Echinococcus granulosus* in Argentina. *Parasitology* **118**, 523–530.

Ruiz, A., Schantz, P.M. and Arambulo, P. (1994). Proceedings of the Scientific Working Group on the Advances in the Prevention, Control and Treatment of Hydatidosis. Pan American Health Organization, PAHO/HCP/95/01, p. 306.

Scala, A., Garippa, G., Varcasia, A., Tranquillo, V.M. and Genchi, C. (2005). Cystic echinococcosis in slaughtered sheep in Sardinia (Italy). *Veterinary Parasitology* **135**, 33–38.

Schantz, P.M. (1997). Sources and uses of surveillance data for cystic echinococcosis. In: *Compendium on Cystic Echinococcosis in Africa and in Middle Eastern Countries with Special Reference to Morocco* (F.L. Andersen, H. Ouhelli and M. Kachani, eds), pp. 72–84. Provo: Brigham Young University Print Services.

Schwabe, C.W. (1979). Epidemiological aspects of the planning and evaluation of hydatid disease control. *Australian Veterinary Journal* **55**, 109–117.

Seimenis, A. (2003). Overview of the epidemiological situation on echinococcosis in the Mediterranean region. *Acta Tropica* **85**, 191–195.

Somocursio, J., Sanchez, E., Naquira, C., Schilder, J., Rojas, F., Chacon, I. and Yabar, A. (2004). First report of a human case of polycystic echinococcosis due to *Echinococcus vogeli* from neotropical area of Peru, South America. *Revista Instituto Tropicale Sao Paulo* **46**, 41–42.

Stallbaumer, M.F., Clarkson, M.J., Bailey, J.W. and Pritchard, J.E. (1986). The epidemiology of hydatid disease in England and Wales. *Journal of Hygiene* **96**, 121–127.

Stefanic, S., Shaikenov, B.S., Deplazes, P., Dinkel, A., Torgerson, P.R. and Mathis, A. (2004). Polymerase chain reaction for detection of patent infections of *Echinococcus granulosus* ("sheep strain") in naturally infected dogs. *Parasitology Research* **92**, 347–351.

Thompson, R.C.A. (1995). Biology and systematics of *Echinococcus*. In: *Echinococcus and Hydatid Disease* (R.C.A. Thompson and A.J. Lymbery, eds), pp. 1–50. Wallingford, UK: CAB International.

Torgerson, P.R. (2003). Economic effects of echinococcosis. *Acta Tropica* **85**, 113–118.

Torgerson, P. and Budke, C. (2004). Echinococcosis—an international public health challenge. *Research in Veterinary Science* **74**, 191–202.

Torgerson, P.R., Carmona, C. and Bonifacino, R. (2000). Estimating the economic effects of cystic echinococcosis: Uruguay, a developing country with upper-middle income. *Annals of Tropical Medicine and Parasitology* **94**, 703–713.

Torgerson, P.R. and Dowling, P.M. (2001). Estimating the economic effects of cystic echinococcosis. Part 2: an endemic region in the United Kingdom, a wealthy industrialized economy. *Annals of Tropical Medicine and Parasitology* **95**, 177–185.

Torgerson, P.R. and Heath, D.D. (2003). Transmission dynamics and control options for *Echinococcus granulosus*. *Parasitology* **127**, S143–S158.

Vidal, M. (1989). Control de la hidatidosis in Chile. *Archivos Internacionales de la Hidatidosis* **XXI**, 38.

Vidal, M., Bonilla, C., Jeria, E. and Gonzalez, C.G. (1994). Programa de control de hidatidosis el modelo Chileno. *Meeting of the Scientific Working Group on the Advances in Prevention, Control and Treatment of Hydatidosis*. Pan American Health Organization, Montevideo, 26–28 October.

Wachira, T.M., Bowles, J., Zeyhle, E. and McManus, D.P. (1993). Molecular examination of the sympatry and distribution of sheep and camel strains of *Echinococcus granulosus* in Kenya. *American Journal of Tropical Medicine and Hygiene* **48**, 473–479.

Walters, T.M.H. (1977). Hydatid disease in Wales. *Transactions of the Royal Society of Tropical Medicine and Hygiene* **71**, 105–108.

Walters, T.M.H. (1978). Hydatid disease in Wales: I. Epidemiology. *Veterinary Record* **102**, 257–259.

Walters, T.M.H. (1984). Hydatid control scheme in South Powys, Wales, UK. *Annals of Tropical Medicine and Parasitology* **78**, 183–187.

Walters, T.M.H. and Clarkson, M.J. (1980). The prevalence of *Echinococcus granulosus* in farm dogs in mid-Wales. *Veterinary Parasitology* **7**, 185–190.

Wen, H. and Ding, Z. (2000). *Altas of Echinococcosis*. Urumqi: Xinjiang Medical University, China.

Whitely, R.S. (1983). *Veterinary Research and Disease Control in the Falkland islands 1976–1983*. London: Overseas Development Administration.

WHO/OIE. (2001). In: *WHO/OIE Manual on Echinococcosis in Humans and Animals: A Public Health Problem of Global Concern* (J. Eckert, M.A. Gemmell, F.-X. Meslin and Z.S. Pawlowski, eds). Paris: World Health Organization for Animal Health.

Williams, B.M. (1976a). The epidemiology of larval (tissue) cestodes in Dyfed (UK). 1. The cestodes of farm dogs. *Veterinary Parasitology* **1**, 271–276.

Williams, B.M. (1976b). The epidemiology of larval (tissue) cestodes in Dyfed (UK). 2. The cestodes of foxhounds. *Veterinary Parasitology* **1**, 277–280.

Xu, M.Q. (1995). Imaging diagnosis with computerised tomography for human echinococcosis in liver. *Chinese Journal of Radiology* **29**, 612–615.

Yekutiel, P. (1980). Eradication of infectious diseases. In: *Contributions to Epidemiology and Biostsatistics* (M.A. Klinsberg, ed.), Vol. 2, p. 164. London: S. Karger.

Zinsstag, J. and Weiss, M.G. (2001). Livestock diseases and human health. *Science* **294**, 477.

Control of *Taenia solium* Cysticercosis/ Taeniosis

Arve Lee Willingham III[1] and Dirk Engels[2]

[1]*WHO/FAO Collaborating Center for Parasitic Zoonoses, Royal Veterinary and Agricultural University, Frederiksberg, Denmark and Human Health Impacts Operating Project, People, Livestock and the Environment Thematic Programme, International Livestock Research Institute, Nairobi, Kenya*
[2]*Coordinator, Preventive Chemotherapy and Transmission Control, Control of Neglected Tropical Diseases, World Health Organization, Geneva, Switzerland*

ABSTRACT

Cysticercosis is emerging as a serious public health and agricultural problem in many poorer countries of Latin America, Africa, and

ADVANCES IN PARASITOLOGY VOL 61
ISSN: 0065-308X
DOI: 10.1016/S0065-308X(05)61012-3

Asia. Caused by the pork tapeworm, *Taenia solium*, this zoonotic disease forms larval cysts in humans and pigs that can lead to epilepsy and death in humans, reduces the market value of pigs and makes pork unsafe to eat. It occurs where pigs range freely, sanitation is poor, and meat inspection is absent or inadequate, and is thus strongly associated with poverty and smallholder farming. Although theoretically easy to control and declared eradicable cysticercosis remains neglected in most endemic countries due to lack of information and awareness about the extent of the problem, suitable diagnostic and management capacity, and appropriate prevention and control strategies. Human neurocysticercosis occurs when the larval cysts develop in the brain. It is considered to be the most common parasitic infection of the human nervous system and the most frequent preventable cause of epilepsy in the developing world. Thus far the infection has not been eliminated from any region by a specific program, and no national control programs are yet in place. We consider the tools available for combating cysticercosis and suggest simple packages of interventions, which can be conducted utilizing existing services and structures in the endemic countries to provide appropriate and sustainable control of the disease.

1. INTRODUCTION

Cysticercosis is emerging as a serious public health and agricultural problem in lesser developed countries of Latin America, Africa, and Asia where pigs are raised for consumption under traditional pig husbandry practices. Caused by *Taenia solium*, the pork tapeworm, this zoonotic disease forms cysts in people and pigs that can lead to epilepsy and death in humans, reduces the market value of pigs and makes pork unsafe to eat. It occurs where pigs range freely, sanitation is poor, and meat inspection is absent or inadequate, and is thus strongly associated with poverty and smallholder farming. Although theoretically easy to control and declared eradicable (International Task Force for Disease Eradication (ITFDE), 1993) cysticercosis remains neglected in many endemic countries due to lack of information and awareness about the extent of the problem, suitable diagnostic and management capacity, and appropriate prevention and control strategies. The current state of knowledge concerning *T. solium* cysticercosis/taeniosis has recently been reviewed by Singh and Prabhakar (2002), Carpio (2002) and Garcia *et al.* (2003). Guidelines for surveillance, prevention and control of cysticercosis/taeniosis were first published more than 20 years ago by Gemmell *et al.* (1983) and have recently been revised (Murrell, 2005). The aim of this review is to further highlight opportunities related to improved surveillance, prevention and control of *T. solium* infections in light of recent scientific advances.

T. solium is a tapeworm (cestode) transmitted among humans and between humans and pigs or sometimes among humans to cause cysticercosis. Humans acquire taeniosis (tapeworm infection) when eating raw or undercooked pork meat infected with cysticerci, the larval form of *T. solium*. When ingested, the cysticerci migrate to the small intestine of humans where they evaginate, attach to the mucosa and within approximately two months develop into adult tapeworms, which can grow to more than 3 m long (Flisser, 1994). *T. solium* has a head (scolex) armed with a double row of hooks and four suckers. Its body (strobila) consists of several hundred segments or proglottids each containing about 50 000–60 000 eggs (Flisser, 1994; Pawlowski and Murrell, 2000). It has generally been accepted that a person is only parasitized by a single *T. solium* at any given time, hence the parasite's name, however, surveys involving treatment of tapeworm carriers and collection of their worms indicate that infections with multiple *T. solium* worms is possible (Jeri *et al.*, 2004).

The most distal proglottids (usually 1–5 daily) detach often in groups from the worm when their eggs have matured and pass out into the environment with the human host's faeces. These eggs can then in turn infect the same (autoinfection) or other humans as well as pigs if they are ingested following direct contact with tapeworm carriers or from consuming water or food contaminated with human faeces. In developing countries, pigs are often allowed to roam and eat human faeces that may contain tapeworm eggs though in some countries human faeces are fed directly to pigs (Flisser, 1988; Pouedet *et al.*, 2002; Shey-Njila *et al.*, 2003). Ingested eggs result in larval worms that migrate to different parts of the human and pig body

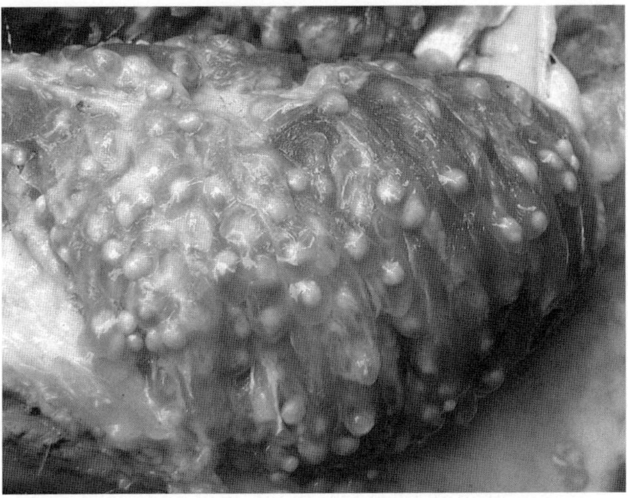

Figure 1   Taenia solium cysts in the masseter muscle of an adult pig. Each cyst contains a protoscolex (tapeworm head) which, when consumed by a human, can develop into a tapeworm. (Photo courtesy of A. Lee Willingham III)

(e.g. muscles, eyes and brain) via the circulatory system and form cysts resulting in cysticercosis (see Figure 1).

A principle site of migration in humans is the central nervous system and neurocysticercosis (NCC) occurs when the cysts develop in the brain leading to epileptic seizures, hydrocephalus and other neurological problems. The cysticercosis metacestode form infecting people and pigs is effective at avoiding complement activation and thus evading the hosts' immune system such that viable cysts with little or no inflammatory reaction are usually not associated with symptoms (White *et al.*, 1997). It is when cysts are recognized by the host following spontaneous degeneration or after drug treatment that an inflammatory reaction occurs usually resulting in clinical symptoms. Oedema around calcified cysticercal granulomas has also been found to cause symptoms (Nash and Patronas, 1999; Nash *et al.*, 2001, 2004). Unlike cysticercosis, taeniosis causes little if any disability and morbidity.

People who neither raise pigs nor consume pork are also at risk of cysticercosis if they ingest *T. solium* eggs after coming into direct or indirect contact with tapeworm carriers. For example, there have been reports of orthodox Jews in North America and Muslims in the Middle East, all banned from eating pork for religious reasons, being infected from their domestic helpers who were tapeworm carriers originally from endemic countries (Schantz *et al.*, 1992; Al Shahrani *et al.*, 2003; Hira *et al.*, 2004). Vegetarians in India have been found to be at high risk of infection from tapeworm-infected food preparers (Rajshekhar *et al.*, 2003) while in Vietnam, there have been reports suggesting a link between cysticercosis and the use of human faeces and 'wastewater' for fertilizing crops (Willingham *et al.*, 2003). *Taenia* spp. eggs have also been recovered from several varieties of vegetables and fruits available in local markets in endemic areas (Sorvillo *et al.*, 2004). Everyone in endemic areas should thus be concerned about cysticercosis irrespective of cultural, religious and/or consumption practices. Development workers from non-endemic countries sent to work in endemic countries have also become infected (Leutsher and Andriantsimahavandy, 2004). Although the life cycle of *T. solium* is generally considered to only involve humans and pigs, dogs have been found to harbour *T. solium* cysts and may possibly play a role in transmission in areas of the world where dog meat consumption is practiced (Jauregui and Marquez-Monter, 1977; Okolo, 1986a, b; Buback *et al.*, 1996; Ito *et al.*, 2002a, 2004).

2. DISEASE DISTRIBUTION AND BURDEN

2.1. Occurrence

Cysticercosis occurs worldwide primarily in lesser developed areas where pigs are raised, pork consumed and poor sanitation allows pigs access to human faeces. The global distribution of *T. solium* infections is presented in Figure 2. 'Hotspots' of the disease in the Western Hemisphere include Mexico and several countries in Central America such as Guatemala, Honduras and Nicaragua as well as the Andean countries of Ecuador, Peru and Bolivia, Colombia, Venezuela and northwestern Brazil in South America (Sarti *et al.*, 1994; Garcia-Noval *et al.*, 1996; Sanchez *et al.*, 1997, 1998; Sakai *et al.*, 1998; Rodriguez-Canul *et al.*, 1999; Carrique-Mas *et al.*, 2001; Flisser *et al.*,

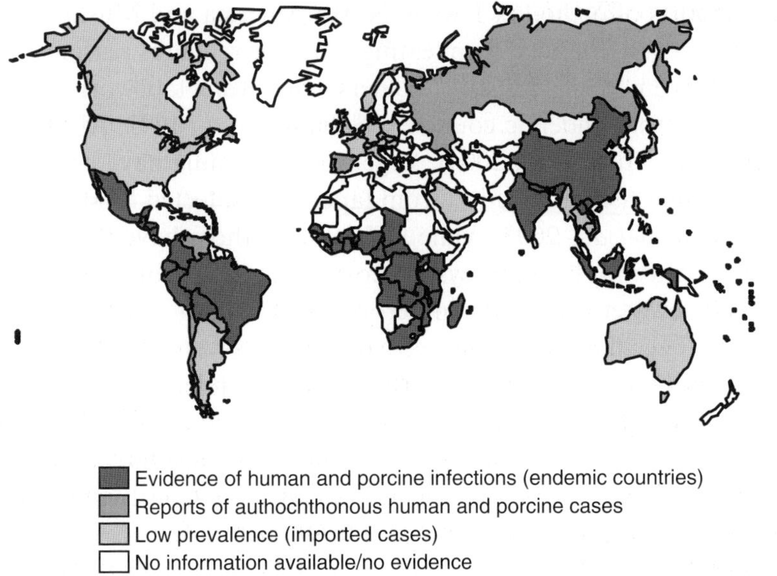

Figure 2 Map showing the global distribution of *Taenia solium* infections by country. (Adapted from: World Health Organization, 2003).

2003; Bucardo *et al.*, 2005). In South Asia, India, Nepal and Bhutan are known to be endemic while in Southeast Asia the disease has been found in Vietnam, Laos, China, parts of Indonesia (Papua) and the Philippines (Margono *et al.,* 2001; Erhart *et al.*, 2002; Ito *et al.*, 2003a, b; Rajshekhar *et al.*, 2003; Willingham *et al.*, 2003). *T. solium* is also found throughout much of sub-Saharan Africa and is emerging as a serious problem in that region related to the increasing popularity of raising pigs and consuming pork (Mafojane *et al.*, 2003; Phiri *et al.*, 2003; Zoli *et al.*, 2003; Preux and Druet-Cabanac, 2005). The occurrence of the disease in developing countries is expected to increase in relation to the growing demand for pork in those countries (Delgado, 2003). In connection with this phenomenon is the increase in transportation of infected pigs and migration of the human population from rural endemic sites to large urban centres. Cysticercosis is also found more and more in wealthier areas of the world as a result of immigration of infected persons from endemic areas and increased travel of persons from non-endemic to endemic areas (Schantz *et al.*, 1998).

2.2. Disease Burden

The World Health Organization (WHO) estimates that at least 50 million people in the world suffer from epilepsy with more than 80% of epileptics living in developing countries (WHO, 2000, 2001; Del Brutto *et al.*, 2001). NCC is considered to be the most frequent preventable cause of epilepsy in the developing world and the most common parasitic infection of the human nervous system (Román *et al.*, 2000; Del Brutto *et al.*, 2001). The disease is reported to cause between 20% and 50% of all late-onset epilepsy cases globally (Campbell and Farrell, 1987; Bern *et al.*, 1999; Carpio and Hauser, 2002; Nsengiyumva *et al.*, 2004; Del Brutto *et al.*, 2005; Preux and Druet-Cabanac, 2005) and is also reported to be a common cause of juvenile epilepsy in certain areas, in particular southern Africa (Shasha and Pammenter, 1991; Thomson, 1993; Grill *et al.*, 1996; Rosenfeld *et al.*, 1996; Mafojane *et al.*, 2003; Gaffo *et al.*, 2004). Initiatives are currently underway to better understand the burden of NCC in endemic countries of Africa, Asia and Latin America (Carabin *et al.*, 2005) as well as industrialized countries such as the USA where it is becoming a growing problem because of immigration of tapeworm carriers from areas of endemic disease (Schantz *et al.*, 1998).

The clinical manifestations of NCC vary and include asymptomatic infections, blindness from ophthalmic infections, brain parenchymal involvement mostly presenting as seizures, subarachnoid and ventricular involvement resulting in hydrocephalus, chronic meningitis and infarcts, and massive infection and encephalitis, resulting in substantial health care costs in relation to diagnosis and management. Epilepsy is a syndrome with considerable social, psychological, economic and social impact on a community, and patients with epilepsy suffer from a decreasing quality of life according to the frequency of their seizures (van Hout *et al.*, 1997). In endemic areas, 2–4% of the population may be affected by NCC (Goodman *et al.*, 1999) with 10% of acute neurological cases being NCC patients (Garcia *et al.*, 1995). It has been estimated that from 69% to 96% of symptomatic NCC cases develop epilepsy and that there are more than 400 000 symptomatic NCC cases in all of Latin America with nearly 10% of these cases residing in Peru (Bern *et al.*, 1999). In severe cases, NCC can be fatal and is noted increasingly as a cause of death of young adult Hispanics and Latinos in the USA (Richards *et al.*, 1985; Sorvillo *et al.*, 2004; Townes *et al.*, 2004).

In 1982 it was reported that in Mexico 5.4% of hospitalizations in the country were due to NCC, with NCC being the final diagnosis of 25% of individuals presenting for brain tumours and 10.3% of autopsies undertaken in the National Neurosurgical Institute reporting pathological evidence of NCC (Velasco-Suarez *et al.*, 1982). At that time the cost per NCC patient spent by public health institutions was estimated to be US $2173 whereas wage losses associated with NCC were estimated to be US $255 000 000 annually (Velasco-Suarez *et al.*, 1982). In 1994 treatment costs of NCC in Brazil were reported to be US $85 000 000 (Roberts *et al.*, 1994). In many African countries NCC patients often do not seek treatment and when they do they are not likely to be hospitalized (Zoli *et al.*, 2003). The health costs of NCC in Cameroon have been estimated at 13 520 000 euros based on 50% of active NCC cases seeking treatment (Nguekam, J.P. *et al.*, 2003). In the USA, total annual costs for hospitalization (US $6539 per case) and income loss (US $1416 per case) caused by NCC for an estimated 1100 cases were estimated to be US $8 750 490 per year (Roberts *et al.*, 1994). A study conducted in northeastern USA estimated that the annual cost for all medical services associated with one epilepsy case was US $9617 (Griffiths *et al.*, 1999).

Cysticercosis is considered to be one of the major parasitic diseases known to pose a serious public health threat, impairing development as well as the quality of life in endemic countries by being both a result of and contributor to poverty in endemic areas exacting a triple price by: (i) infection of humans affecting their health, social and family life and productivity, (ii) causing protein-energy malnutrition in nutritionally constrained settings due to poor pork meat quality and condemnation of pig carcasses and (iii) seriously reducing the household income of farmers, many of whom are women, as an obstacle to marketing of pigs and pork (Colley, 2000; Carabin *et al.*, 2005). Thus the disease is a serious constraint for improving the lives and livelihoods of especially smallholder farming communities. Social consequences of NCC, mostly as a result of seizures, include stigmatization and incapacitation leading to decreased work productivity (Campbell and Farrell, 1987; Brandt *et al.*, 1992; Thomas *et al.*, 2001; Boa *et al.*, 2002; Carpio, 2002; Carpio and Hauser, 2002; Carabin *et al.*, 2005). In many endemic countries, cysticercosis afflicts young adults representing a heavy toll among persons in young, highly productive age groups. Studies in India indicate that persons with epilepsy have an annual reduction in work productivity of up to 30% (Krishnan *et al.*, 2004).

When estimating the economic costs of epilepsy in relation to NCC one must consider other societal costs due to stigmatization, accidents and complications from 'traditional healing'. Communities may shun or cast out epileptics because it is considered a shameful and/or contagious disease resulting in epileptics often being isolated to prevent the spread of the ailment (Avodé *et al.*, 1996; Preux *et al.*, 2000). In West Cameroon it has been estimated that only 27% of epileptics marry and 39% fail to enter any professional activity (Preux *et al.*, 2000). Epileptics are also prone to accidents while having seizures such as serious burns from falling/rolling into fires, drowning from falling into water bodies and automobile accidents; these costs should be considered when estimating to the burden of NCC (Carabin *et al.*, 2005). In South Africa unqualified, self-taught healers use *Taenia* segments and their contents as treatment in cases of severe intestinal tapeworm infections whereby *Taenia* segments or their pulverized contents are added to medicinal mixtures, which can lead to high intensity infection with cysticercosis. Besides this practice, the malevolent use of *T. solium* by persons to punish their unfaithful spouses or lovers is also common, the contents of *T. solium* segments being added to beverages as punishment (Kriel and Joubert, 1996; Kriel, 1997). Certain other practices of traditional healers are also harmful to the patients-for example in Cameroon some epileptic patients are made to inhale smoke from burnt cola nut leaves and mistletoe as a form of treatment while others may be told to restrict certain foodstuffs, which may actually be highly nutritious foods (Zoli *et al.*, 2003).

There are also serious agricultural costs related to *T. solium* infection. Porcine cysticercosis often results in total condemnation of pig carcasses since pigs can harbour thousands of cysts making the meat unsafe to eat. Pig traders aware of the disease may detect infection during a pre-purchase examination and then refuse to buy a suspect pig. Farms and whole communities may become stigmatized when they are known for selling contaminated meat and/or infected pigs. In 1980 it was estimated that more than US $43 000 000 was lost in Mexico due to the rejection of infected pig carcasses at slaughter due to cysticercosis infection which was equivalent to two-thirds of the total investment in the nation's pig production at that time (Acevedo-Hernandez, 1982). More recently the annual losses due to porcine cysticercosis in 10 western and central African countries was estimated to be more than 25 000 000 euros (Zoli *et al.*, 2003). Due to lack of well-organized meat inspection and to common illegal slaughtering, partial or total condemnation of carcasses due to cysticercosis and their seizure in that region are rather exceptional and a high percentage of infected carcasses are marketed and/or consumed. Usually a pig carcass infected with cysticercosis is sold at a decreased price which can vary from 25% of the usual market price in Benin to 50% in Rwanda (Zoli *et al.*, 2003). Annual losses due to porcine cysticercosis in Cameroon alone have been estimated to be a minimum of 2 000 000 euros based on a loss of 30% of the value of the carcass. However in certain communities cysticercosis-infected meat is sometimes sold at a higher price than uninfected meat as it is considered to have a better flavour than healthy meat (Zoli and Tchoumboué, 1992). In China the amount of pork discarded in the whole country due to cysticercosis annually has been estimated at 200 000 000 kg with a value of more than US $120 000 000 (Ito *et al.*, 2003b).

The WHO has recently utilized decision tree analysis as an appropriate comprehensive method for assessing the burden of cysticercosis in endemic countries whereby both the health and agricultural impacts of the disease are given equal consideration (Carabin *et al.*, 2005). Decision tree analysis provides an organizational framework for information about population frequencies of infection types and frequencies of associated diseases and can then be complemented further by information about the average costs per case of each event represented by the branches which are then multiplied by the end probability of each branch (Haddix *et al.*, 2003). The sum of all of these values corresponds to the average cost per case of the disease of interest. Unfortunately for most endemic countries there is currently not enough quality epidemiological and cost data with which to conduct such an assessment and thus securing the evidence base on this issue remains a great need at the global level. Decision tree analysis has thus far been used to conduct a comprehensive estimate of the monetary burden of cysticercosis in only a few countries including hyperendemic Eastern Cape Province of South Africa. The overall monetary burden of cysticercosis in Eastern Cape Province was estimated at US $24.8 million to which the agricultural sector was found to contribute about one-third (average of $5.0 million) thus the human monetary burden alone is considerable ($19.8 million) (Carabin *et al.*, 2006). The monetary burden per capita was estimated at US $2.40, which is substantial when compared to annual health expenditures of US $41.26 for people living in poor dwellings in Eastern Cape Province (Statistics South Africa, 2004). The proportion of epilepsy cases attributable to NCC and the proportion of working time lost were found to have the most influence on the estimated monetary burden. These results for South Africa and in the future for other endemic nations should help guide stakeholders in deciding whether to invest their countries' scarce health and agricultural resources in combating cysticercosis.

3. DIAGNOSIS

3.1. Taeniosis

Identification of *Taenia* species infecting humans is usually based on a combination of comparative morphology and immunological and molecular diagnostic approaches (Wilkins *et al.*, 2002; Dorny *et al.*, 2003, 2005; Ito and Craig, 2003; McManus and Ito, 2005).

3.1.1. Questioning and Self-Detection

Questioning of tapeworm carriers as an auxiliary method for the diagnosis of *T. solium* taeniosis has not been considered reliable as *T. solium* proglottids are emerge passively with the host's faeces and thus the person infected is often unaware that they have a tapeworm (Allan *et al.*, 1996; Dorny *et al.*, 2005). This is in contrast to other *Taenia* tapeworms infecting humans (i.e. *T. saginata* and *T. s. asiatica*), which are more motile and will actively come out of the host's anus. Furthermore, patients may confuse nematodes such as *Enterobius vermicularis* and *Ascaris lumbricoides* as tapeworm proglottids leading to false positive reports (Dorny *et al.*, 2005). An awareness campaign aimed at educating physicians, nurses, animal health care practitioners and the general public about taeniosis and cysticercosis including the distribution of preserved tapeworm segments and guidelines for interviewing patients about tapeworm infection to clinical practitioners and identifying farms producing *T. solium* infected pigs has been found to increase the detection of tapeworm infections (Flisser *et al.*, 2005).

3.1.2. Stool Microscopy

Routine stool microscopy used for detecting parasite ova is known to have poor specificity and sensitivity for detecting *T. solium* taeniosis infections with yields ranging from 22.5% to 56% (Allan *et al.*, 1990, 1993; Willingham *et al.*, 2003). This method underestimates the prevalence of taeniosis because *Taenia* spp. eggs are excreted intermittently (Allan *et al.*, 1996). The test's efficacy can thus be improved by repeating it on different days (Hall *et al.*, 1981). Eggs of *T. solium* and that those of *T. saginata* as well as *T. s. asiatica* are morphologically similar so it is necessary to collect complete adult tapeworms or proglottids to determine the infecting species based on morphological characteristics. Mature or gravid proglottids of the tapeworm species can be differentiated on the basis of reproductive organs but need to be fixed and stained in order to facilitate this which is a laborious procedure (Morgan and Hawkins, 1949; Mayta *et al.*, 2000). Identification of *T. solium* is based on the observation of three ovarian lobes and the absence of a vaginal sphincter in mature proglottids and the presence of 7–16 unilateral uterine branches in gravid proglottids. Counting of the uterine branches can be facilitated by longitudinally sectioning the gravid proglottid, staining it with hematoxylin-eosin and then gently squashing it between glass slides or between the underside and the cover of a Petri dish before microscopic evaluation (Mayta *et al.*, 2000). Unfortunately some overlapping in the number of uterine branches may occur between *Taenia* species thus collection of the tapeworm to examine its scolex or molecular assays may be needed to differentiate the infecting species.

3.1.3. Peri-Anal Egg Detection

Graham's test which utilizes adhesive ('Scotch') tape for collecting *Taenia* spp. eggs sticking to the skin in the peri-anal region has been found to detect eggs of *T. solium* though its sensitivity for this *Taenia* species is questionable (Schantz and Sarti-Guttierez, 1989; de Kaminsky, 1991; Garcia *et al.*, 2003). The presence of eggs is determined by microscopic examination of the adhesive tape after using it to swab the peri-anal area.

3.1.4. Copro-Antigen Detection ELISA

The ability to parasitologically detect tapeworm carriers increased dramatically with the development of a test for *Taenia*-specific molecules in faecal samples (copro-antigens) (Allan *et al.*, 1990, 1996). The test is a polyclonal antibody-based sandwich enzyme-linked immunosorbent assay (ELISA) using antibodies obtained from hyperimmune rabbit sera against *T. solium* adult worm somatic antigens (Allan *et al.*, 1990). It has been found to have a sensitivity of about 95% and specificity greater than 99% (Allan *et al.*, 1996). A more rapid dipstick ELISA form of the copro-antigen test has been developed which requires minimal facilities making it a more appropriate option for epidemiological studies though it is less sensitive than the micro-plate assay (Allan *et al.*, 1993). Copro-antigens are detectable prior to patency and cease to be detectable within a week following treatment (Allan *et al.*, 1990). They are stable for weeks in unfixed faecal samples kept at room temperature and for years in frozen samples or in chemically fixed samples (e.g. formalin) kept at room temperature (Dorny *et al.*, 2005).

The copro-antigen ELISA is only genus specific, making it impossible to differentiate *T. solium* from *T. saginata* or *T. s. asiatica* infections. Determination of the tapeworm species infecting the host requires treating persons tested positive with niclosamide or praziquantel and collecting their worms following expulsion for morphological differentiation. If the tapeworm scolex is expelled it can be examined for hooklets to determine the species of infecting tapeworm as *T. saginata* and *T. s. asiatica* usually have no hooklets while *T. solium* usually has 22–32 hooklets on its scolex (Pawlowski, 2002). However, one should be aware when examining the scolex that due to morphological abnormalities the absence of hooklets may not automatically mean that the tapeworm is not *T. solium* (Rodriguez-Hidalgo *et al.*, 2002). Cleansing the intestine with an electrolyte-polyethyleneglycol salt (EPS) purge two hours before and again two hours after treatment with niclosamide/praziquantel improves the recovery of the scolex, as well as the quality of the expelled proglottids which facilitates species identification (Garcia *et al.*, 2003; Jeri *et al.*, 2004). Using a purge results in scolex recovery from only about one-third of tapeworm carriers however (Jeri *et al.*, 2004).

3.1.5. Copro-DNA Assays

Various molecular approaches have been developed to detect DNA of *Taenia* species in human faeces for diagnosis of taeniosis (McManus *et al.*, 1989; Nunes *et al.*, 2003; Ito and Craig, 2003; Yamasaki *et al.*, 2004; McManus, 2005; McManus and Ito, 2005). These techniques are highly sensitive and species-specific thus overcoming the limitations of differentiation of *Taenia* species based on morphology, however the expense and lack of capacity for utilizing these techniques currently limits their use in *T. solium* endemic countries. Molecular approaches for detecting taeniosis include polymerase chain reaction (PCR), PCR coupled to restriction fragment length polymorphism (RFLP) (Gonzalez *et al.*, 2000, 2002; Rodriguez-Hidalgo *et al.*, 2002) and multiplex-PCR (Yamasaki *et al.*, 2004). PCR with oligonucleotide primers derived from species-specific DNA probes provides a rapid and sensitive method of taeniosis diagnosis (Gonzalez *et al.*, 2000). PCR–RFLP and multiplex PCR permit differential diagnosis of the *Taenia* species without relying on the availability of intact mature or gravid proglottids. Multiplex PCR is an easy and time-saving technique for use on faeces and parasite specimens, does not require DNA sequencing and permits differential diagnosis of *Taenia* species by using a combination of different primer pairs in the same amplification reaction to produce species-specific sequences of mitochondrial DNA that can then be distinguished (Yamasaki *et al.*, 2002, 2004; Gonzalez *et al.*, 2003). In addition to differentiating between *Taenia* species infections it is valuable for molecular epidemiological studies concerning the genotypic variation in *T. solium* around the world (Okamoto *et al.*, 2001; Nakao *et al.*, 2002).

Adult proglottids expelled from human carriers, whole worms expelled after chemotherapy and eggs are all amenable to molecular identification. Parasite samples should be freshly obtained, rinsed several times in physiological saline solution and submitted for testing immediately or fixed in 75% ethanol or frozen as soon as possible (McManus and Ito, 2005). Faecal samples collected in endemic areas and kept frozen or fixed in ethanol are useful for DNA detection of worm carriers (Nunes *et al.*, 2003; Yamasaki *et al.*, 2004). Frozen faecal samples should be examined as soon as possible after collection within a maximum of 10 years (Yamasaki *et al.*, 2004). Fixing samples in 75% ethanol is the method of choice due to the convenience of transportation and ease of storage whereas formalin fixation/storage is not recommended due to the difficulties of DNA analysis on formalin-fixed samples (McManus and Ito, 2005).

3.1.6. Serology

A fingerstick *T. solium* taeniosis immunoblot assay (EITB-T) has recently been developed using copro-antigens of adult *T. solium* tapeworms for detection of human taeniosis (Wilkins *et al.*, 1999). The new serum *T. solium* taeniosis immunoblot is reported to be highly sensitive (95%) and specific (100%) compared to microscopy and copro-antigen detection (Wilkins *et al.*, 1999; Degiorgio *et al.*, 2005). A limitation of the EITB-T test is that since it is detecting antibodies to adult *T. solium* worms it informs about people with a history of tapeworm infection and not necessarily active infection and thus may result in false positives (Degiorgio *et al.*, 2005). Combination of the EITB-T and the copro-antigen ELISA may be a way of specifically detecting *T. solium* tapeworm carriers while avoiding the need for collecting and identifying the tapeworms from those identified.

3.2. Human Cysticercosis

Diagnosis of cysticercosis/NCC on clinical grounds can be difficult due to the non-specific signs and symptoms of the disease. A high proportion of people infected with NCC remain free of symptoms even when massively infected while others develop clinical manifestations many years after becoming infected (Garcia and Del Brutto, 1999). The most common clinical manifestation among those having symptoms is seizures while some NCC sufferers will have headache, increased intracranial pressure and hydrocephalus depending on the stage of the infection (Cruz *et al.*, 1995; Carpio, 2002; Garcia *et al.*, 2002a). The general opinion is that consistent and accurate diagnostic criteria of cysticercosis should be based on combined exposure history, clinical presentation, subcutaneous nodule biopsy, neuroimaging studies, serological tests and biopsy of subcutaneous nodules if present (Del Brutto *et al.*, 1996; White and Garcia, 1999).

3.2.1. Biopsy of Subcutaneous Nodules

Subcutaneous nodules, while rare in Latin America (Cruz *et al.*, 1994), are a distinctive sign of infection in Asia and parts of Africa prompting referral for treatment (Garcia *et al.*, 2003; Ito *et al.*, 2003a). They present as small, fluctuant, painless nodules that most commonly occur in the chest, arms and back (De *et al.*, 1998; Willingham *et al.*, 2003). People may have substantial numbers of subcutaneous nodules with cases having over 300 recorded (Lam and Tan, 1992). Biopsy or fine-needle cytology of the nodule is then conducted to confirm the cysticercosis diagnosis (Sahai *et al.*, 2002; Willingham *et al.*, 2003). Physical examination for detection of subcutaneous nodules is a simple method for detecting cysticercosis particularly in remote areas where more sophisticated techniques may not be available (Wandra *et al.*, 2003).

3.2.2. Imaging

Computerized tomography (CT) and magnetic resonance imaging (MRI) are used to identify cysticerci in the brain not only confirming the aetiology of the disease but also providing information on the intensity of infection, location of cysts and the stage of lesions (Flisser, 1994; Carpio, 2002). These imaging techniques provide a safe, precise, albeit expensive way of diagnosing cysticercosis but are scarce in many poor endemic areas of the world (Diop *et al.*, 2003). They are able to easily detect non-symptomatic cases of NCC and thus are helpful for conducting epidemiological surveys (Cruz *et al.*, 1999; Fleury *et al.*, 2003; Nash *et al.*, 2004). CT has been found to have sensitivity and specificity over 95% for the diagnosis of NCC and is more sensitive for detecting calcified cysts while MRI is considered to be the more accurate imaging technique for assessing the intensity of infection, the location and evolutionary stage of the cysts (Nash and Neva, 1984; Martinez *et al.*, 1989; Garcia *et al.*, 2003).

3.2.3. Immunodiagnosis

Immunodiagnosis of cysticercosis is useful for conducting surveillance, epidemiological surveys and community-based studies that contribute to a better understanding of the prevalence, burden and epidemiology of the infection, assisting in identifying endemic communities where prevention and control measures should be applied (Garcia-Noval *et al.*, 1996; Subahar *et al.*, 2001). Immunodiagnostic techniques can also be used to complement neuroimaging for the diagnosis of cysticercosis in individuals providing differential diagnosis of other 'cyst forming conditions' such as echinococcosis, tuberculosis and brain tumors (Chang *et al.*, 1988; Del Brutto *et al.*, 1996), however neuroimaging technology may not be accessible or affordable in rural populations at risk in many endemic countries in which case immunodiagnostic techniques may provide the only tool for diagnosis of cysticercosis. Immunodiagnosis is also useful for monitoring progress of individual treatment as well as community-based prevention and control programs (Garcia *et al.*, 2000; Sarti *et al.*, 2000; Vazquez-Flores *et al.*, 2001).

Immunodiagnostic techniques include detection methods for specific antibodies, which indicate present or past infection, and circulating parasite antigens, which indicate current infections, in serum as well as cerebrospinal fluid (CSF) (Correa *et al.*, 1989; Zini *et al.*, 1990). The use of fingerstick blood dried on filter paper for immunodiagnosis has recently been found to be an acceptable, convenient and economical way of transporting and storing field samples for epidemiologic surveys of cysticercosis in lesser developed endemic countries where cold-chain transport and maintenance of blood samples is problematic and people are often averse to venipuncture (Jafri *et al.*, 1998; Fleury *et al.*, 2001).

Antibody Detection. Infection with *T. solium* cysticercosis results in a specific antibody response, mainly of the IgG class (Carpio *et al.*, 1998). Detection of antibodies is confirmatory rather than decisive since they indicate prior exposure to infection and not necessarily current active infection with viable parasites. Currently the enzyme-linked immunoelectrotransfer blot (EITB) and ELISA are the antibody-detection assay formats most frequently used for diagnosis of cysticercosis (Brand and Tsang, 1989; Tsang *et al.*, 1989; Sciutto *et al.*, 1998; Sato *et al.*, 2003).

The EITB or Western Blot for cysticercosis, which uses seven purified glycoprotein antigens extracted from the *T. solium* cysticercus, has been a reliable serodiagnostic assay for cysticercosis since it was developed in 1989. The test is reported to have 100% specificity and a sensitivity of 98% with regard to parasitologically proven cases with two or more cysts (Tsang *et al.*, 1989). Its sensitivity drops to as low as 28% in patients with single lesions and the test is also less sensitive in patients with only calcified lesions (Wilson *et al.*, 1991). The EITB relies on acquisition and purification of native cyst material making it labor-intensive and costly and therefore not very suitable for conducting field studies or diagnosis in the many lesser developed countries where cysticercosis is endemic (Hancock *et al.*, 2003). The reliance of the EITB on parasite material is being changed by the development of synthetic and recombinant antigens giving similar sensitivity and specificity shown by the original native EITB (Hancock *et al.*, 2003, 2004; Scheel *et al.*, 2005).

Antibody-detecting ELISA technology is popular in developing countries because it is rapid, simple to perform, readily available and more affordable. The development of an antibody-detecting ELISA had been hindered by the presence of non-specific contaminants; however a new simple method for purifying *T. solium*-specific glyco-proteins fractionated from cysticerci cyst fluid has led to the production of highly specific antigens facilitating the development of an Antibody-ELISA with a reported specificity and sensitivity similar to that of the EITB (Ito *et al.*, 1998, 2002b). The Antibody-ELISA has been further refined through the production of recombinant antigens resulting in a test reported to have a sensitivity of 90% and specificity of 100% (Sako *et al.*, 2000).

A serious limitation of sero-prevalence field studies based on anti-body detection is the overestimation of active disease due to the occurrence of a transient antibody response whereby a large percentage of sero-positive people are found to be sero-negative upon repeat testing 1–3 years later (Garcia *et al.*, 2001). This may be due to exposure to *T. solium* eggs, which do not develop into a viable infection or as a result of self-cure (Garcia *et al.*, 2001). In addition antibodies may persist long after the parasite has been eliminated by immune mechanisms and/or drug therapy (Garcia *et al.*, 1997). The overestimation of active infection by detection of antibodies to *T. solium* must be considered when conducting community-based epidemiological studies. Active infection should be verified since it has relevance with regard to the need for individual administration of anti-parasitic treatment.

Antigen Detection. A monoclonal antibody-based ELISA has been found to be a sensitive and specific test for detecting circulating parasite antigens in people infected with cysticercosis (Garcia *et al.*, 1998; Brandt *et al.*, 1992). Antigen-ELISA only detects cases of active cysticercosis, i.e. the presence of living cysticerci, which may be helpful when making decisions as to whether or not anti-parasitic treatment should be provided since patients with only calcified cysts who would not benefit from anthelmintic treatment are consistently negative by the Antigen-ELISA (Erhart *et al.*, 2002; Nguekam, A. *et al.*, 2003). Antigen detection may be conducted on serum as well as on CSF (Choromanski *et al.*, 1990; Garcia *et al.*, 1998, 2000). Because of the localization of the cysts in the brain, antigen detection in CSF may be more appropriate for diagnosis than in serum, however sampling of CSF is more complicated and risky than blood sampling. The sensitivity of the Antigen-ELISA has been shown to be 85% with patients having only a single viable cyst or degenerating parasites giving false negative results while the specificity of the assay has been determined to be 92% (Garcia *et al.*, 2000). Antigen-ELISA, being much cheaper and more accessible than neuroimaging, is a useful tool for monitoring the success of anti-parasitic treatment of cysticercosis patients because of the good correlation between the presence of circulating antigen, biopsy of subcutaneous nodules and viable brain cysts (Garcia *et al.*, 2000; Erhart *et al.*, 2002). Results of the Antigen-ELISA usually become negative three months after the start of successful treatment (Garcia *et al.*, 2000; Dorny *et al.*, 2003).

3.3. Porcine Cysticercosis

Detection of porcine cysticercosis cases is important for determining whether a cysticercosis/taeniosis endemic situation exists and for monitoring any interventions undertaken. Methods for detecting cysticercosis in live pigs include tongue examination and serological testing as well as inspection of carcasses at slaughter.

3.3.1. Lingual Examination

Visual inspection and palpation for cysts on the ventral surface of the tongue is used by farmers and pig traders in endemic countries as an inexpensive and quick way of identifying pigs infected with *T. solium* cysticercosis (Figure 3). The specificity of the technique can be 100% if conducted by someone with experience (Gonzalez *et al.*, 1990; Dorny *et al.*, 2005).

The sensitivity of the technique depends very much on the intensity of infection of the animals and has reported to be as high as 71% in heavily infected pigs though considerably less in pigs with low intensities of infection (Gonzalez *et al.*, 1990; Sciutto *et al.*, 1998; Sato *et al.*, 2003; Dorny *et al.*, 2004, 2005). Thus this method of detection generally underestimates the prevalence of porcine cysticercosis.

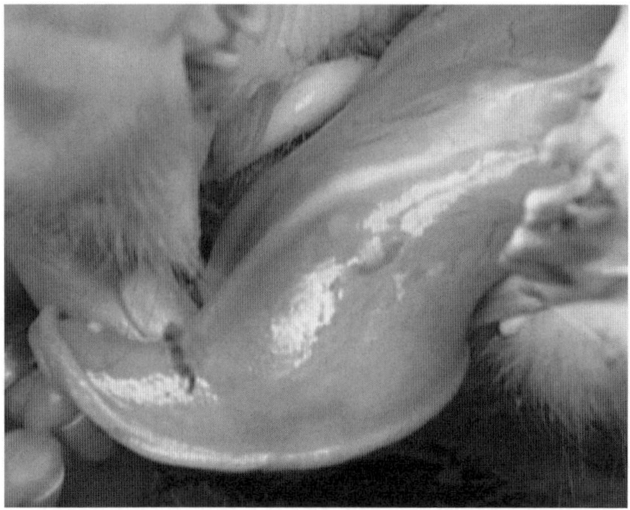

Figure 3   *Taenia solium* cysts on the ventral surface of a pig's tongue.

However, it can be a useful tool for rapid assessment of sites to determine and monitor endemic 'hot spots' and in countries where official meat inspection is minimal and capacity and/or funding for conducting immunodiagnosis absent it may be the only method available for detecting porcine cysticercosis.

3.3.2. Pig Carcass Inspection

Official guidelines and practices for the detection of *T. solium* cysticercosis during inspection of pig carcasses vary widely from one country to the another. In some countries only visual inspection is carried out on one or several selected muscle and organ sites, while in others incisions in some of these muscle groups may be required. The effectiveness of this method for detecting cases of porcine cysticercosis may be low depending on its thoroughness especially for pigs with low intensities of infection (Sciutto *et al.*, 1998; Boa *et al.*, 2002; Dorny *et al.*, 2004). Records from meat inspection while providing evidence on the presence of porcine cysticercosis are generally considered to underestimate the status of cysticercosis in the pig population due to the technique's low sensitivity as well as the fact that farmers and pig traders may avoid taking pigs to official slaughter establishments if they suspect that they are infected with *T. solium* (Gonzalez *et al.*, 1990). Meat inspection when conducted properly provides a useful tool for validating diagnostic methods and intervention strategies.

3.3.3. Immunodiagnosis

Immunodiagnosis in pigs provides an ante-mortem detection method more sensitive than lingual examination for use in prevalence and community-based surveys as well as intervention studies. Techniques developed for the diagnosis of cysticercosis in humans have also been adapted for use in detecting *T. solium* infection of pigs, including both antibody (EITB and Antibody-ELISA) (Gonzalez *et al.*, 1990; Tsang *et al.*, 1991; Ito *et al.*, 1999; Sato *et al.*, 2003) and antigen detection (Antigen-ELISA) (Erhart *et al.*, 2002; Phiri *et al.*, 2002; Pouedet *et al.*, 2002). It has been reported that the sensitivity of these available immunodiagnostic techniques is reduced in pigs with low intensities of infection (Sciutto *et al.*, 1998).

While the EITB and the newer formulations of Antibody-ELISA are popular tests for detecting porcine cysticercosis for both epidemiological studies and monitoring interventions care should taken with regard to the overestimation of infection due to the presence of antibodies in pigs in the absence of infection. Anti-cysticercal antibodies (IgG) are passively transferred from sows via colostrum to piglets and have been found to persist for more than six months after weaning (Gonzalez *et al.*, 1999). Considering that most pigs are taken to market at about 9–12 months they will maintain these antibodies for most of their lives whether infected or not. In addition, pigs may also develop a transient antibody response to *T. solium* infection without the establishment of a patent infection as seen in humans (Dorny *et al.*, 2003).

Logic suggests that the Antigen-ELISA would be the most appropriate immunodiagnostic test for detecting porcine cysticercosis since pigs usually do not live long enough for the *T. solium* metacestodes to die and thus would be expected to have active infection. It has been reported that the Antigen-ELISA is highly specific and sensitive, even detecting pigs harbouring one single *T. solium* cyst (Erhart *et al.*, 2002; Nguekam, A. *et al.*, 2003; Dorny *et al.*, 2004). The circulating antigens can be detected as early as two to six weeks post infection (Nguekam *et al.*, 2003). However, the genus specificity of the Antigen-ELISA test does not allow differentiation of larval *T. solium* infections from larval infections of other *Taenia* species such as *T. hydatigena* and possibly *T. saginata asiatica,* which becomes problematic in areas where these parasites co-exist (Dorny *et al.*, 2003, 2005). This species' specificity problem does not appear to be a problem of the Antibody-ELISA since pigs naturally infected with the metacestode stages of *T. hydatigena* are negative by that test (Sato *et al.*, 2003).

4. TREATMENT

4.1. Taeniosis

Treatment of tapeworm carriers is one of the key intervention points with regard to prevention and control of *T. solium* infections in humans. Niclosamide (2 g orally single dose) and praziquantel (5–10 mg/ kg orally single dose) are both considered to be more than 95% effective against *T. solium* tapeworm infection (Schantz *et al.*, 1998). Niclosamide, though not widely available in many *T. solium* endemic countries, is the preferred drug because it is not absorbed from the intestines and there have been reports of praziquantel treatment precipitating seizures, severe headache and other neurological symptoms in patients with asymptomatic NCC (Torres *et al.*, 1988; Flisser *et al.*, 1993). A pre- and post-niclosamide EPS purge (2 l orally before and after niclosamide treatment) has been found to greatly improve the recovery of tapeworm scolexes and gravid proglottids which indicates cure as well as provides parasite material for species identification of the infecting worm (Jeri *et al.*, 2004). If the scolex of the tapeworm is not expelled the worm can regenerate within two months.

4.2. Cysticercosis

4.2.1. Human Cysticercosis

Treatment of human cysticercosis cases helps reduce the burden of disease due to the substantial morbidity and mortality associated with

NCC but has no direct effect on control of *T. solium* infections at the household or community level since humans are a 'dead end' host for larval infection. However, a proportion of people with cysticercosis may also be *T. solium* tapeworm carriers (Gilman *et al.*, 2000; Willingham *et al.*, 2003). The management of NCC should be adapted to the individual based on the number, location, size and viability or stage of degeneration of the cysts in the nervous system and may involve antiparasitic drugs, steroids, antiepileptic drugs and surgery with symptomatic treatment very important as initial therapy (Garcia *et al.*, 2003; Maguire, 2004). The presentations of human NCC are classified into four major types: intraparenchymal disease, extraparenchymal disease, cerebrovascular complications and calcified lesions (Garcia *et al.*, 2005).

Both praziquantel (50–$100\,\mathrm{mg\,kg^{-1}\,mg^{-1}}$ orally, divided in three doses for 30 days for multiple cysts or single day treatment of three doses of $25\,\mathrm{mg/kg}$ given at two hour intervals for single or few cysts) and albendazole ($400\,\mathrm{mg}$ orally twice daily for 8–30 days repeated as needed; pediatric dosage $15\,\mathrm{mg/kg}$ daily up to a maximum of $800\,\mathrm{mg}$ split in two doses/day for 8–30 days repeated as needed) given simultaneously with steroids (dexamethasone at $0.1\,\mathrm{mg/kg/day}$ or, for long-term use, prednisone at $1\,\mathrm{mg/kg/day}$) have been found to be effective antiparasitic drugs for treating live *T. solium* cysts (Botero and Castano, 1982; Sotelo *et al.*, 1984, 1988, 1990; Escobedo *et al.*, 1987; Corona *et al.*, 1996; Garcia *et al.*, 2002a; The Medical Letter, Inc, 2004) however albendazole is generally considered the drug of choice since it has better penetration into the CSF and praziquantel interacts with steroids leading to a decrease in its serum concentrations hence may not be as effective against high intensities of cysts using the single day course of therapy (Vazquez *et al.*, 1987; Jung *et al.*, 1990; Pretell *et al.*, 2001). The use of antiparasitic drugs for cysticercosis is controversial since killing the larval parasites may cause an unnecessary increase in the inflammatory process thereby worsening neurological symptoms due to oedema and intracranial hypertension usually between the second and fifth day after antiparasitic therapy thus the reason for administering steroids simultaneously to reduce this inflammation (Carpio *et al.*, 1995; reviewed by Garcia *et al.*, 2003; Riley and White, 2003; Maguire, 2004). A recent controlled study has indicated that antiparasite therapy decreases the burden of parasites in patients with seizures due to viable parenchymal cysts and is safe and effective in reducing the number of generalized seizures (Garcia *et al.*, 2004). Antiparasitic treatment may be unnecessary or even contraindicated in some NCC patient subgroups (e.g. presence of only calcified cysts, spinal or ophthalmic cysticercosis and hydrocephalus with no viable cysts) while in others it may be beneficial and even lifesaving (e.g. giant growing cysts, subarachnoid cysts, hydrocephalus with viable cysts and chronic meningitis) (White, 2000; Proaño *et al.*, 2001; Garcia *et al.*, 2002a, b, 2003; Yancey *et al.*, 2005). There is increasing evidence that calcified *T. solium* cysts and associated perilesional oedema are a cause of seizures thus a better understanding of its development, role, prevention and treatment is needed (Nash *et al.*, 2004).

Antiepileptic drugs are the principal therapy for seizures associated with NCC and may eventually be tapered or even withdrawn with time. The presence of calcifications in the brain is a known risk factor for seizure relapse and the proportion of cysts calcifying may be higher in cysticercosis patients treated with antiparasitics (Del Brutto, 1994; Garcia *et al.*, 2004). In patients with intracranial hypertension secondary to NCC the priority is to manage the hypertension problem before considering any other form of therapy. Surgery is usually required for treating hydrocephalus secondary to NCC and is also appropriate for removal of ventricular, spinal or ophthalmic cysticerci (McCormick, 1985; White, 2000). Any cysticercocidal drug may cause irreparable damage when used to treat ocular or spinal cysts, even when corticosteroids are used. An ophthalmic examination of suspected or confirmed cysticercosis patients should always precede treatment to rule out intraocular cysts (The Medical Letter, Inc., 2004).

4.2.2. Porcine Cysticercosis

Both praziquantel and albendazole given orally have been found effective for treating porcine cysticercosis but involve multiple dosing making them impractical for large-scale control programs (Flisser *et al.*, 1990; Torres *et al.*, 1992; Gonzalez *et al.*, 1995; Kaur *et al.*, 1995). Treatment of pigs with albendazole has been found to result in side effects such as lethargy and anorexia (Gonzalez *et al.*, 1995). Subcutaneous injections of inexpensive albendazole sulphoxide, 15 mg/kg daily for eight days, has been found 100% effective for killing muscle cysts but less effective at killing brain cysts in pigs though again it requires multiple doses (Peniche-Cardeña *et al.*, 2002).

In contrast, an inexpensive veterinary benzimidazole, oxfendazole, has been found to be more than 95% effective in killing cysts in the pig when given in a single dose of 30 mg/kg and pigs may remain resistant to re-infection for at least three months after treatment (Gonzalez *et al.*, 1997, 2001). Brain cysts have been found to survive the single-dose therapy; however this may be inconsequential since pig brains are usually cooked for consumption (Gonzalez *et al.*, 1997). Infested meat in oxfendazole-treated pigs needs at least eight weeks for all the cysts to degenerate and up to 12 weeks to achieve a clear, acceptable appearance of the pork for human consumption thereby greatly increasing the meat's commercial value (Gonzalez *et al.*, 1998; Gonzalez, 2002). Oxfendazole was developed for use as an anthelmintic for ruminants and is administered to cattle at an oral dose of 4.5 mg/kg. The withdrawal time is seven days after treatment in cattle at this dosage whereby a cow is not slaughtered before this time as a safety precaution for beef consumers to ensure residual levels of the anthelmintic in the meat are safe (Fort Dodge Animal Health, Fort Dodge, IA, USA). The safety of oxfendazole for pigs as well as consumers at the much higher dosage needed to cure porcine cysticercosis remains to be examined. Oxfendazole has not yet been tested for treating human cysticercosis but has been found to be very effective for reducing the infectivity of larval cysts of the cestode *Echinococcus granulosus* infecting small ruminants (Blanton *et al.*, 1998; Dueger *et al.*, 1999; Njoroge *et al.*, 2005).

5. VACCINATION

Vaccination has been proposed as a key component of a 'best bet' integrated strategy for combating cysticercosis/taeniosis involving education and control of infection in both definitive and intermediate hosts (Lightowlers, 1999). Lowering the prevalence of porcine cysticercosis through effective vaccination would break the parasite's life cycle thereby blocking transmission to humans. Incorporation of an effective vaccine for prevention of infection in pigs would thus likely increase the effectiveness of *T. solium* disease control efforts and reduce the impact of incomplete chemotherapy coverage of human tapeworm carriers and reintroduction of disease transmission by immigration of human *T. solium* carriers into disease control areas by eliminating susceptible intermediate hosts, the source of human infections. Since the target population would be rural endemic villages in developing countries a vaccine would need to be low in cost to be acceptable and sustainable though being an international public good it may be appealing to international agencies such as the World Bank, regional development banks, the Global Alliance for Livestock Vaccines (GALV), etc., as a worthy cause for support due to the poverty alleviation aspects. The same vaccine could also be effective in humans but development of a human vaccine is hindered by the lack of cost–benefit studies justifying the substantial cost involved in undertaking clinical trials and in the manufacture of a vaccine suitable for use in humans rather than animals (Lightowlers, 2003). Several approaches are being examined towards development of vaccines against *T. solium*, including the application of recombinant oncosphere antigens and peptides (Sciutto *et al.*, 2002; Lightowlers, 2003, 2004).

Host-protective immune responses to taeniid cestodes are known to be directed towards the egg (oncosphere) in the early developing embryo (Rickard and Williams, 1982). Specific native oncosphere antigens have now been identified as a source of these host-protective responses and recombinant DNA techniques have been used to clone and express the genes encoding these antigens leading to vaccine candidate recombinant antigens (Gauci *et al.*, 1998; Gauci and Lightowlers, 2001). Two of the most promising recombinant *T. solium* oncosphere antigens, designated TSOL 18 and TSOL 45, have been evaluated in experimental vaccine trials in different countries and by groups in Latin America and Africa and have been shown to induce complete or near complete protection against experimental challenge infection in pigs (99.5–99.9% and 97–98.6%, respectively) (Flisser *et al.*, 2004; Gonzalez *et al.*, 2005). Various aspects of this oncosphere antigen subunit vaccine are currently being investigated before proceeding with controlled field trials.

A synthetic vaccine composed of three peptides has been developed in Mexico (Sciutto *et al.*, 2002), which is reported to be both preventative and therapeutic reducing the parasite load as well as the viability of cysticerci in pigs (Huerta *et al.*, 2000, 2002; de Aluja *et al.*, 2005). It apparently has a cysticidal effect on established metacestodes in vaccinated pigs thus lowering the number of viable cysticerci capable of transforming into tapeworms suggesting that people who ingest metacestodes in the meat of vaccinated pigs will be less at risk to develop intestinal taeniosis. In a field trial conducted in two rural endemic communities it was found that the peptide vaccine reduced by 52.6% the prevalence of naturally acquired porcine cysticercosis and reduced by 97.9% the total number of recovered cysticerci, with 80% of the cysts established in vaccinated pigs found damaged (Huerta *et al.*, 2002). Preliminary results thus suggest that immunization of pigs with the peptide vaccine can confer a high level of protection against an egg challenge while also inducing an immune response against the larvae, which are either destroyed or rendered non-infectious. Different methods of antigen production and delivery of the peptide vaccine are being explored to reduce the production costs of synthetic peptides and also improve their immunogenicity in order to increase the possibility of extensive application of the vaccine (Manoutcharian *et al.*, 2004).

Developers of *T. solium* vaccines for pigs face a serious challenge with regard to the persistence of porcine maternal antibodies and the relatively late development of the piglet's immune system. It is known that piglets in endemic villages may be exposed and infected with *T. solium* in the first few days after birth, as soon as they can follow their mothers searching for food (de Aluja *et al.*, 1998) and thus should already be protected at this time. However, pigs at a young age may not be able to mount an effective protective immune response to a vaccine at this time due to the immaturity of their immune system. In addition maternal antibodies may persist for six months or longer (Gonzalez *et al.*, 1999) which may inhibit responses by the piglet's own immune system. A vaccine trial with the peptide vaccine indicated that piglets immunized at 40 days had little or no immune response while those immunized at 70 days did (Huerta *et al.*, 2000). The pig's slow development of effective immunity against cysticerci, combined with the early exposure to the *T. solium* eggs, may warrant consideration of the development of a vaccine for pregnant sows that would promote passive transfer of antibodies against *T. solium* to neonate piglets via the mother's colostrum.

6. SURVEILLANCE AND REPORTING

One of the main obstacles to control and elimination of *T. solium* infections is the lack of reliable epidemiological data on cysticercosis/ taeniosis, which could be overcome through the institution of surveillance systems for the disease. Surveillance systems for cysticercosis have been implemented only rarely (e.g. Oregon and California in USA, Mexico, Kuwait and Ribeirã Preto Municipality in Brazil) (Ehnert *et al.*, 1992; Sorvillo *et al.*, 1992; Román *et al.*, 2000; Townes *et al.*, 2004). Results of a short-lived surveillance program in Los Angeles County, California, USA indicated that both travel- and locally acquired cysticercosis was more common than previously recognized (Sorvillo *et al.*, 1992).

Public health follow-up of cysticercosis cases, including screening of household contacts, can identify tapeworm carriers (transmission foci), who can be treated and removed as potential sources of further infection since epidemiological studies have demonstrated clustering of NCC cases around individuals infected with *T. solium* (Sarti *et al.*, 1992; Garcia *et al.*, 1999). The first step in tackling endemic cysticercosis/taeniosis could thus be to concentrate on NCC, its most important manifestation, or subcutaneous nodules where that manifestation is common, by implementing appropriate surveillance mechanisms such as case reporting.

An international group of neurologists have proposed upgrading the status of human cysticercosis to that of an international reportable disease as a first step necessary for the implementation of appropriate surveillance mechanisms for *T. solium* infections (Román *et al.*, 2002). However, taeniosis and cysticercosis do not lead to sudden large-scale international outbreaks of disease and therefore would not seem to constitute an appropriate subject for international notification. More appropriate would be for national authorities to establish national surveillance and reporting of cysticercosis/taeniosis as part of a routine system (WHO, 2003). Standardized criteria for differential diagnosis of epilepsy that are appropriate for peripheral health care structures in resource-poor areas remain to be established (Engels *et al.*, 2003).

Surveillance of cysticercosis in pigs has been proposed as a practical, inexpensive and sensitive method for indirectly assessing human risk and monitoring and evaluating the effectiveness of community-based control programs (Gonzalez, 2002). In endemic areas, many local pigs may not go through the formal slaughterhouse system, especially if the pig farmers screen them for cysticercosis by examining their tongues before taking them to the slaughterhouse; thus slaughterhouse prevalence statistics may grossly underestimate the real prevalence (Gonzalez *et al.*, 1990; Cysticercosis Working Group in Peru (CWGP), 1993). A more effective way to assess the changes in the intensity of environmental contamination with *T. solium* eggs is to bring in 'sentinel' pigs from non-endemic areas that can then be serologically tested periodically (Sarti *et al.*, 1997; Gonzalez, 2002).

7. PREVENTION AND CONTROL

As our understanding of the global burden of *T. solium* cysticercosis/taeniosis improves it becomes increasingly evident that the disease has a serious impact on the health and agricultural systems of pig producing/pork consuming countries in the developing world, contributing to rural poverty. Since cysticercosis is generally related to poverty and its associated manifestations, all strategies to control the disease must consider costs and locally available resources. *T. solium* is potentially eradicable through surveillance and available interventions, but such feasibility needs to be demonstrated over in a sizeable geographic area (ITFDE, 1993). Chief obstacles to eradication of *T. solium* cysticercosis/taeniosis include the need for simpler diagnostics for humans and pigs, lack of availability of drugs for treating human taeniosis and porcine cysticercosis (i.e. praziquantel, niclosamide and oxfendazole) in endemic areas, and a general lack of awareness and appreciation of the presence and impact of the disease by the affected communities as well as those in positions who could assist them in combating the problem. Thus far there is no evidence that eradication of *T. solium* is feasible within a reasonable time frame (Engels *et al.*, 2003). Alternatively, it is important to define a simple package of interventions, which can be routinely carried out by existing services and structures, and will give an optimal, long-term return in terms of reducing the burden of cysticercosis. Figure 4 gives an overview of various intervention measures at different points in the *T. solium* life cycle.

The following characteristics of *T. solium* make it vulnerable to eradication (ITFDE, 1993; Schantz *et al.*, 1993): (i) the life cycle

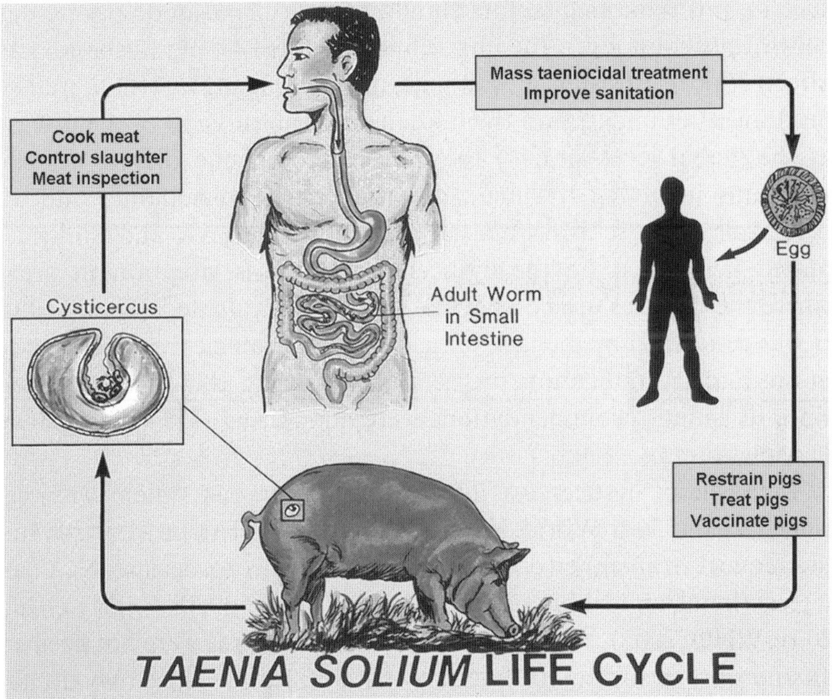

Figure 4 The life cycle of *Taenia solium* and different strategies for prevention and control of cysticercosis/taeniosis with regard to both the human and pig hosts. (Figure courtesy of U.S. Centers for Disease Control and Prevention, Atlanta, Georgia, U.S.A.)

requires humans as its definitive host, (ii) tapeworm infection in humans is the only source of infection for pigs, the natural intermediate hosts, (iii) domestic pigs, the intermediate hosts, can be managed, (iv) no significant wildlife reservoir exists and (v) practical intervention is available in the form of chemotherapy for human taeniosis and porcine cysticercosis with safe and effective drugs. In 2003 a reconvened ITFDE II met to consider the status of *T. solium* cysticercosis 10 years after initially targeting the disease as potentially eradicable. Recommendations of the ITFDE II include (ITFDE II, 2003): (i) demonstration of effective control or elimination of *T. solium* transmission on a national scale would probably be the greatest single stimulus to further action against cysticercosis/taeniosis, (ii) a program strategy that includes multiple interventions in flexible mass or targeted approaches would probably have the greatest chance of success, (iii) economic factors should be considered in designing any control program given the importance of domestic pig husbandry to affected local subsistence economies in endemic areas, (iv) there is a need to better understand the burden and transmission of the disease at the global level and (v) the impact of parasitic disease control programs involving the mass distribution of praziquantel and albendazole (e.g. schistosomiasis, lymphatic filariasis and soil-trasmitted helminths) on the cysticercosis/taeniosis situation in areas where the diseases are co-endemic should be evaluated. The ITFDE II was concerned by the lack of field-proven strategies and experience in large-scale eradication projects made during the 10-year period since its initial recommendations were announced (ITFDE II, 2003; Pawlowski *et al.*, 2005).

The issue of cysticercosis of the central nervous system was discussed at the 56th World Health Assembly (WHA) in May 2003 at the request of member countries following calls to declare NCC an international reportable disease (Román *et al.*, 2000; Engels *et al.*, 2003; WHO, 2003). While cysticercosis and taeniosis were not deemed an appropriate subject for international notification since they do not lead to sudden large-scale international outbreaks of disease, the WHA secretariat's report strongly encouraged national authorities to set up surveillance and reporting systems and adopt a more active approach towards prevention and control of the diseases (WHO,

2003). In addition, the report noted that control of human cysticercosis can be linked and actively promoted under the auspices of several international initiatives such as the Global Campaign against Epilepsy 'Out of the Shadows', the new initiative on 'Neglected Tropical Diseases', the Food Safety Programme and the Partnership for Parasite Control. An integrated, intersectoral approach to surveillance, prevention and control combining simple tools was promoted by the report for long-term success with regard to substantially reducing the disease burden in endemic areas as well as enhancing food safety and increasing economic benefits for smallholder pig farmers (WHO, 2003; Engels *et al.*, 2003).

Only tapeworm carriers and infected pigs are important in terms of transmission of *T. solium* infections and are thus the targets for prevention and control. Individuals with NCC are a health concern but not important for transmission unless they are also infected with an intestinal tapeworm. Thus to be effective and sustainable a practical, cost-effective combination of simple interventions targeting both the intermediate and definitive hosts should be considered (Lightowlers, 1999; Garcia, 2002). Any selected combination of interventions would need to ensure community cooperation and incorporate economic incentives to ensure sustainability. The appropriateness and justification for undertaking such interventions needs to first be verified through 'rapid epidemiological assessment' of the targeted communities to secure the evidence base on the public health and/or economic relevance of cysticercosis in order to ensure the commitment of local and national decision makers for implementing the proposed solutions (Engels *et al.*, 2003). Engagement of stakeholders from the various relevant sectors and interested parties including veterinary and medical workers should be promoted from the outset of activities to ensure success.

Sustainable control programs for *T. solium* infections must aim to both decrease the supply of infected meat to consumers and prevent environmental contamination with parasite eggs. *T. solium* carriers are extremely potent sources of cysticercosis, endangering everyone coming in contact with them including themselves. Reduction of human taeniosis by detection and treatment of human tapeworm carriers or by mass treatment of the whole population with praziquantel or niclosamide has proven effective for reducing environmental contamination of the parasite in the short-term, however these attempts have only had temporary success due to the continued presence of susceptible intermediate hosts and the movement of human tapeworm carriers into the targeted communities and thus would require continuous maintenance and intensive monitoring and surveillance to remain effective (Cruz *et al.*, 1989; Allan *et al.*, 1997; Garcia, 2002). Appropriate surveillance mechanisms should be implemented whereby new cases of NCC or porcine cysticercosis should be reported to national authorities to facilitate identifying and treating sources of tapeworm eggs, i.e. tapeworm carriers and any persons having close contact with them (Román *et al.*, 2000). There is a theoretical risk of a temporary increase in human and porcine cysticercosis infection during taeniosis treatment campaigns if disposal of human stools is not carefully controlled following treatment since *T. solium* worms and still infective eggs may be expelled. A study in Mexico found that porcine cysticercosis nearly doubled one year after mass human chemotherapy which did not take into consideration the need for safe disposal of faeces post-treatment (Keilbach *et al.*, 1989).

Local populations in endemic areas rarely understand the relationship between cysticercosis in pigs and taeniosis in humans and thus lack knowledge and incentive to change behaviour that fosters transmission. Efforts to educate communities via schools, village meetings and on an individual basis have been successful in terms of teaching villagers the life cycle of *T. solium*, the connection between infected pigs and themselves or others getting cysticercosis, and how to improve hygiene, sanitation and pig management practices to reduce the risk of infection (Keilbach *et al.*, 1989; Sarti *et al.*, 1997). However these initiatives solely based on education have not been shown to dramatically change behaviours affecting transmission and/ or risk factors, although in some situations environmental contamination appears to have decreased following educational campaigns (Sarti *et al.*, 1997). It is generally accepted that education should be an integral part of any control program due to the long-term effect of acquired knowledge on the sustainability of intervention efforts. Educational materials need to be designed in such a way to attract the reader and again with cysticercosis the economic issues involved should be exploited in order to relay the messages with maximum impact. For example in Tanzania a cysticercosis prevention brochure shows a farmer with a large healthy pig on the cover with the heading 'raise cysticercosis-free pigs—make more money!' while a children's colouring book informs about cysticercosis with the storyline that raising cysticercosis-free pigs enables the family to raise the children's school fees (H. Ngowi, Sokoine University of Agriculture, Tanzania). An awareness and prevention poster on *T. solium* cysticercosis recently produced in South Africa has been made available in different sizes for use as wall posters in medical, veterinary and livestock production establishments as well as inserts for local and farmer-related newspapers and is also available through the internet (see Figure 5). The poster is designed such that by changing the language and

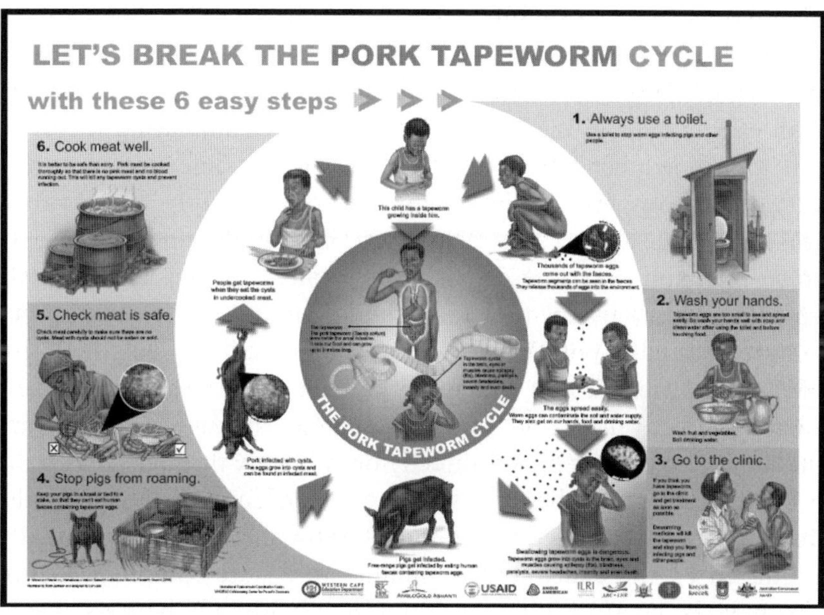

Figure 5 Cysticercosis awareness and prevention poster from South Africa designed to target various relevant stakeholder groups. The poster has been printed in various sizes for newspaper inserts as well as wall hangings. With a change in language and minimal alterations in illustrations it can be used throughout the Africa region. (figure courtesy of the Medical Research Council of South Africa, Krecek and Krecek cc and the International Livestock Research Institute)

making a few other small changes with regard to illustrations it can be used throughout Africa.

Interventions focused on the pig population will not only control any further infections of humans in the village, but also by increasing the value of the pigs will act as an economic incentive and lead to increased compliance with other control activities, such as human treatment and education. Intervention studies in Peru involving concurrent intensive chemotherapy of people and pigs indicate that it is possible to block transmission and eliminate the parasite from communities if the treatment regimen is maintained and a surveillance system is in place to counter the movement of human tapeworm carriers or infected swine into the treated communities (Garcia, 2002). Better market prices for treated pork and access to the formal marketing system will be strong incentives for farmers to treat their pigs, helping to ensure community cooperation. However, in order to improve the commercial value of pork its appearance should be clean and similar to non-infected meat; thus the availability of oxfendazole as an effective drug for curing pigs eventually eliminating the cysts with the added benefit of resistance to further infection provides strong incentives for small pork producers to comply with control measures (Gonzalez *et al.*, 1996, 1997, 2001). Vaccines against *T. solium* infection may one day make treatment of pigs unnecessary, providing a very useful tool for helping combat cysticercosis especially if they have both preventive and therapeutic effects (Sciutto, 2002; Lightowlers, 2003). An important factor with regard to their potential effectiveness and actual usefulness, the ability of the vaccines to protect young piglets directly or indirectly through sows prior to birth, is currently being assessed through controlled field trials. Much attention is needed with regard to how these tools can actually be utilized by the endemic communities to ensure compliance since they may not be affordable for many smallholder pig keepers. There again the economic incentives of prevention may overcome the compliance issue if the farmers are made aware of the benefits compared to the costs.

Transmission of *T. solium* infections can be blocked if the sale and consumption of infected pork is prevented by slaughterhouse meat inspection and confiscation of infected pig carcasses (Joshi *et al.*,

2003). Unfortunately in many endemic countries national pork inspection guidelines may be inadequate and little attention may be given to the porcine cysticercosis issue, thus leading to low detection of infected carcasses especially in countries where pig rearing and pork consumption have only recently become popular (Boa *et al.*, 2002; Phiri *et al.*, 2003). Policies concerning confiscation of infected pig carcasses must be strategic since confiscation without payment to the pig's owner may lead to the establishment of clandestine markets and unofficial slaughtering establishments for pigs infected with *T. solium*. In Peru where pigs are confiscated without payment to the pig's owner over 50% of the pigs are slaughtered illegally (CWGP, 1993). In addition to enforcing meat inspection, cooking and freezing of pork can also break the parasite's lifecycle. Cysticerci are killed best by cooking pork to at least 60 °C or until it loses its pink colour (Pawlowski and Murrell, 2000) or alternatively pork can be frozen at −5 °C for four days, −15 °C for three days or −24 °C for one day to kill the cysts (Sotelo *et al.*, 1986). Refrigeration of pork at temperatures about 0 °C does not affect the parasite however salt pickling for 12–24 hours has been found to kill *T. solium* cysticerci (Rodriguez-Canul *et al.*, 2002).

Targeting slaughterhouses as the primary intervention fails to influence the husbandry practices which occur before the pigs are brought to market (Lekule and Kyvsgaard, 2003). Pig keeping is popular among smallholder farmers in large part due to minimum inputs required in order to get a good return on their investment. By allowing a pig to roam it is able to supplement its diet with local garbage and human and other faeces thus helping to keep the community clean and saving the farmer from having to buy expensive feeds. Confining pigs results in major capital inputs from the farmers for proper housing and feeding. Control strategies must consider these potential costs and the economic incentives that will be required in order for different pig rearing practices to be adopted (Lekule and Kyvsgaard, 2003). There are instances of new crops being introduced into communities which made it economically advantageous to keep pigs confined or tethered in order to prevent them from consuming the crops, thereby reducing or eliminating the possibility of the pigs having access to human faeces and reducing the burden of cysticercosis in the pig population (Gonzalez *et al.*, 2003; M. E. Boa, Sokoine University of Agriculture, Tanzania).

8. CONCLUSIONS

Cysticercosis/taeniosis remains a serious neglected problem in marginalized communities in many developing countries mainly due to poverty and ignorance. The public health and economic relevance of cysticercosis needs to be better documented in order to convincingly bring it to the attention of affected communities, decision makers and potential investors. Aspects of the cysticercosis problem including the availability of appropriate tools, the combination of these tools and the ability to use them in an effective and cost-effective manner as well as the availability of sustained resources and the political will to undertake surveillance and control activities, must be considered in order to make a decision on whether and how to combat cysticercosis (Colley, 2000). Political will is a key factor for sustainability and depends on decision makers understanding the burden of cysticercosis, its impact on the health and agricultural systems, its impact overall on development and demand of the populations affected for action. It is the responsibility of all stakeholders involved to forge active links between the findings of researchers and those seeking to implement the appropriate resultant principles and methodologies in surveillance and control efforts. The creation of an enabling environment for integration of research activities with control needs will facilitate a thorough understanding and sustainable reduction of the burden of cysticercosis. Formation of regional working groups for combating cysticercosis is an effective way to bring together a variety of stakeholders to set regional priorities and help ensure that research activities are integrated with regional needs for surveillance and control.

A number of proven cost-effective intervention tools for combating cysticercosis/taeniosis appear to be available however from an operational standpoint several simple questions still need to be answered and the use of these tools in the field worked out. Some of the issues to be addressed are the need for an independent evaluation of the different diagnostic techniques as well as 'definitions' of the most simple epidemiological assessment tools, most cost-effective strategies to eliminate *T. solium* tapeworm carriers, optimal pig treatment strategies and the most effective, large-scale communication strategies (Engels *et al.*, 2003). Better documentation of the distribution, prevalence and economic impact of cysticercosis as well as a better understanding of the transmission dynamics of cysticercosis/taeniosis in the different endemic regions are also urgent needs. Advocacy efforts concerning the disease, its link with poverty and impact on endemic countries, and the possibilities for its elimination should hopefully instigate more involvement of international organizations, agencies and institutes with the issue and also lead to greater investment in cysticercosis research and control efforts by the endemic countries and international donor community.

ACKNOWLEDGEMENTS

The US Centers for Disease Control and Prevention, Krecek and Krecek cc, the Medical Research Council of South Africa and the International Livestock Research Institute are thanked for permission to use Figures 4 and 5.

REFERENCES

Acevedo-Hernandez, A. (1982). Economic impact of porcine cysticercosis. In: *Cysticercosis: Present State of Knowledge and Perspectives* (A. Flisser, K. Willms, J.P. Lacletter, C. Larralde, C. Ridaura and F. Beltran, eds), p. 63. New York: Academic Press.

Allan, J.C., Avila, G., Garcia-Noval, J., Flisser, A. and Craig, P.S. (1990). Immunodiagnosis of taeniasis by coproantigen detection. *Parasitology* **101**, 473–477.

Allan, J.C., Mencos, F., Garcia-Noval, J., Sarti, E. and Flisser, A. (1993). Dipstick dot ELISA for detection of *Taenia* coproantigens in humans. *Parasitology* **107**, 79–85.

Allan, J. C., Velasquez-Tohom, M., Fletes, C., Torres-Alvarez, R., Lopez-Virula, G., Yurrita, P., Soto de Alfaro, H., Rivera, A. and Garcia-Noval, J. (1997). Mass chemotherapy for intestinal *Taenia solium* infection: effect on prevalence in humans and pigs. *Transactions of the Royal Society of Tropical Medicine and Hygiene*, **91**, 595–598.

Allan, J.C., Velasquez-Tohom, M., Garcia-Noval, J., Torres-Alvarez, R., Yurrita, P., Fletes, C., de Mata, F., Soto de Alfaro, H. and Craig, P.S. (1996). Epidemiology of intestinal taeniasis in four rural Guatemalan communities. *Annals of Tropical Medicine and Parasitology* **90**, 157–165.

Al Shahrani, D., Frayha, H.H., Dabbagh, O. and Al Shail, E. (2003). First case of neurocysticercosis in Saudi Arabia. *Journal of Tropical Pediatrics* **49**, 58–60.

Avodé, D.G., Capo-Chichi, O.B., Gandaho, P., Bouteille, B. and Dumas, M. (1996). Epilepsie provoquée par la cysticercose. A propos d'une enquête sociologique et culturelle réalisée à Savalou au Bénin. *Bulletin de la Societe de Pathologie Exotique* **89**, 45–47.

Bern, C., Garcia, H.H., Evans, C., Gonzalez, A.E., Verastegui, M., Tsang, V.C.W. and Gilman, R.H. (1999). Magnitude of the disease burden from neurocysticercosis in a developing country. *Clinical Infectious Diseases* **29**, 1203–1209.

Blanton, R.E., Wachira, T.M., Zeyhle, E.E., Njoroge, E.M., Magambo, J.K. and Schantz, P.M. (1998). Oxfendazole treatment for cystic hydatid disease in naturally infected animals. *Antimicrobial Agents and Chemotherapy* **42**, 601–605.

Boa, M.E., Kassuku, A.A., Willingham, A.L., Keyyu, J.D., Phiri, I.K. and Nansen, P. (2002). Intensity, distribution and density of *Cysticercus cellulosae* by muscle groups and organs in naturally infected local slaughter pigs in Mbulu district of Tanzania. *Veterinary Parasitology* **106**, 155–164.

Botero, D. and Castano, S. (1982). Treatment of cysticercosis with praziquantel in Colombia. *American Journal of Tropical Medicine and Hygiene* **31**, 811–821.

Brand, J.A. and Tsang, V.C. (1989). A rapid immunoblot assay (Western blot) to detect specific antibodies for human immunodeficiency virus, *Schistosoma mansoni*, and *Taenia solium* (cysticercosis). *Journal of Immunoassay* **10**, 237–255.

Brandt, J.R., Geerts, S., De Deken, R., Kumar, V., Ceulemans, F., Brijs, L. and Falla, N. (1992). A monoclonal antibody-based ELISA for the detection of circulating excretory-secretory antigens in *Taenia saginata* cysticercosis. *International Journal for Parasitology* **22**, 471–477.

Buback, J.L., Schulz, K.S., Walker, M.A. and Snowden, K.F. (1996). Magnetic resonance imaging of the brain for diagnosis of neurocysticercosis in a dog. *Journal of the American Veterinary Medical Association* **208**, 1846–1848.

Bucardo, F., Meza-Lucas, A., Espinoza, F., Garcia-Jeronimo, R.C., Garcia-Rodea, R. and Correa, D. (2005). The seroprevalence of *Taenia solium* cysticercosis among epileptic patients in Leon, Nicaragua, as evaluated by ELISA and western blotting. *Annals of Tropical Medicine and Parasitology* **99**, 41–45.

Campbell, G.D. and Farrell, V.J. (1987). Brain scans, epilepsy and cerebral cysticercosis. *South African Medical Journal* **72**, 885–886.

Carabin, H., Budke, C.M., Cowan, L.D., Willingham, A.L., 3rd and Torgerson, P.R. (2005). Methods for assessing the burden of parasitic zoonoses: echinococcosis and cysticercosis. *Trends in Parasitology* **21**, 327–333.

Carabin, H., Krecek, R.C., Cowan, L.D., Michael, L., Foyaca-Sibat, H., Nash, T. and Willingham, A.L. (2006). Estimation of the monetary burden of *Taenia solium* cysticercosis in Eastern Cape Province, South Africa. *Tropical Medicine and International Health* (in press).

Carpio, A. (2002). Neurocysticercosis: an update. *Lancet Infectious Diseases* **2**, 751–762.

Carpio, A., Escobar, A. and Hauser, W.A. (1998). Cysticercosis and epilepsy: a critical review. *Epilepsia* **39**, 1025–1040.

Carpio, A. and Hauser, W.A. (2002). Prognosis for seizure recurrence in patients with newly diagnosed neurocysticercosis. *Neurology* **59**, 1730–1734.

Carpio, A., Santillan, F., Leon, P., Flores, C. and Hauser, W.A. (1995). Is the course of neurocysticercosis modified by treatment with antihelminthic agents? *Archives of Internal Medicine* **155**, 1982–1988.

Carrique-Mas, J., Iihoshi, N., Widdowson, M.A., Roca, Y., Morales, G., Quiroga, J., Cejas, F., Caihuara, M., Ibarra, R. and Edelsten, M. (2001). An epidemiological study of *Taenia solium* cysticercosis in a rural population in the Bolivian Chaco. *Acta Tropica* **80**, 229–235.

Chang, K.H., Kim, W.S., Cho, S.Y., Han, M.C. and Kim, C.W. (1988). Comparative evaluation of brain CT and ELISA in the diagnosis of neurocysticercosis. *American Journal of Neuroradiology* **9**, 125–130.

Choromanski, L., Estrada, J.J. and Kuhn, R.E. (1990). Detection of antigens of larval *Taenia solium* in the cerebrospinal fluid of patients with the use of HPLC and ELISA. *Journal of Parasitology* **76**, 69–73.

Colley, D. (2000). Parasitic diseases: opportunities and challenges in the 21st century. *Memorias de Instituto Oswaldo Cruz* **95**(supplement 1), 79–87.

Corona, T., Lugo, R., Medina, R. and Sotelo, J. (1996). Single-day praziquantel therapy for neurocysticercosis. *New England Journal of Medicine* **334**, 125.

Correa, D., Sandoval, M.A., Harrison, L.J., Parkhouse, R.M., Plancarte, A., Meza-Lucas, A. and Flisser, A. (1989). Human neurocysticercosis: comparison of enzyme immunoassay capture techniques based on monoclonal and polyclonal antibodies for the detection of parasite products in cerebrospinal fluid. *Transactions of the Royal Society of Tropical Medicine and Hygiene* **83**, 814–816.

Cruz, I., Cruz, M.E., Teran, W., Schantz, P.M., Tsang, V. and Barry, M. (1994). Human subcutaneous *Taenia solium* cysticercosis in an Andean population with neurocysticercosis. *American Journal of Tropical Medicine and Hygiene* **51**, 405–407.

Cruz, M., Davis, A., Dixon, H., Pawlowski, Z.S. and Porano, J. (1989). Operational studies on the control of *Taenia solium* taeniasis/cysticercosis in Ecuador. *Bulletin of World Health Organization* **67**, 401–407.

Cruz, M.E., Cruz, I., Preux, P.M., Schantz, P. and Dumas, M. (1995). Headache and cysticercosis in Ecuador, South America. *Headache* **35**, 93–97.

Cruz, M.E., Schantz, P.M., Cruz, I., Espinosa, P., Preux, P.M., Cruz, A., Benitez, W., Tsang, V.C.W., Fermoso, J. and Dumas, M. (1999). Epilepsy and neurocysticercosis in an Andean community. *International Journal of Epidemiology* **28**, 799–803.

Cysticercosis Working Group in Peru (CWGP). (1993). The marketing of cysticercotic pigs in the sierra of Peru. *Bulletin of the World Health Organization* **71**, 223–228.

de Aluja, A.S., Marinez, J.J. and Villalobos, A. (1998). *Taenia solium* cysticercosis in young pigs: age at first infection and histological characteristics. *Veterinary Parastiology* **76**, 71–79.

de Aluja, A.S., Villalobos, N.M., Nava, G., Toledo, A., Martínez, J.J., Plancarte, A., Rodarte, L.F., Fragoso, G. and Sciutto, E. (2005). Therapeutic capacity of the synthetic peptide-based vaccine against *Taenia solium* cysticercosis in pigs. *Vaccine* **23**, 4062–4069.

DeGiorgio, C., Pietsch-Escueta, S., Tsang, V., Corral-Leyva, G., Ng, L., Medina, M.T., Astudillo, S., Padilla, N., Leyva, P., Martinez, L., Noh, J., Levine, M., del Villasenor, R. and Sorvillo, F. (2005). Sero-prevalence of *Taenia solium* cysticercosis and *Taenia solium* taeniasis in California, USA. *Acta Neurologica Scandinavica* **111**, 84–88.

de Kaminsky, R.G. (1991). Albendazole treatment in human taeniasis. *Transactions of the Royal Society of Tropical Medicine and Hygiene* **85**, 648–650.

Del Brutto, O.H. (1994). Prognostic factors for seizure recurrence after withdrawal of antiepileptic drugs in patients with neurocysticercosis. *Neurology* **44**, 1706–1709.

Del Brutto, O.H., Rajshekar, V., White, A.C., Jr., Tsang, V.C., Nash, T.E., Takayanagui, O.M., Schantz, P.M., Evans, C.A., Flisser, A., Correa, D., Botero, D., Allan, J.C., Sarti, E., Gonzalez, A.E., Gilman, R.H. and Garcia, H.H. (2001). Proposed diagnostic criteria for neurocysticercosis. *Neurology* **57**, 177–183.

Del Brutto, O.H., Santibáñez, R., Hidrovo, L., Rodríguez, S., Dìaz-Calderón, E., Navas, C., Gilman, R.H., Cuesta, F., Mosquera, A., Gonzalez, A.E., Tsang, V.C.W. and Garcia, H.H. (2005). Epilepsy and neurocysticercosis in Atahualpa: a door-to-door survey in rural coastal Ecuador. *Epilepsia* **46**, 583–587.

Del Brutto, O.H., Wadia, N.H., Dumas, M., Cruz, M., Tsang, V.C. and Schantz, P.M. (1996). Proposal of diagnostic criteria for human cysticercosis and neurocysticercosis. *Journal of Neurolological Sciences* **142**, 1–6.

Delgado, C.L. (2003). Rising consumption of meat and milk in developing countries has created a food revolution. *Journal of Nutrition* **133**(11 supplement 2), 3907S–3910S.

De, N.V., Chau, L.V. and Dat, D.T. (1998). Infection of intestinal helminths in several places along the Srepok and Krongana rivers in Dak Lak Province. *Journal of Malaria and Parasite Diseases Control* **2**, 42–43.

Diop, A.G., de Boer, H.M., Mandlhate, C., Prilipko, L. and Meinardi, H. (2003). The global campaign against epilepsy in Africa. *Acta Tropica* **87**, 149–159.

Dorny, P., Brandt, J. and Geerts, S. (2005). Detection and diagnosis, In: *WHO/FAO/OIE Guidelines for the Surveillance, Prevention and Control of Taeniosis/Cysticercosis* (K.D. Murrell, ed.), pp. 45–52. Paris: Office International des Epizooties.

Dorny, P., Brandt, J., Zoli, A. and Geerts, S. (2003). Immunodiagnostic tools for human and porcine cysticercosis. *Acta Tropica* **87**, 79–86.

Dorny, P., Phiri, I.K., Vercruysse, J., Gabriel, S., Willingham, A.L., III, Brandt, J., Victor, B., Speybroeck, N. and Berkvens, D. (2004). A Bayesian approach for estimating values for prevalence and diagnostic test characteristics of porcine cysticercosis. *International Journal for Parasitology* **34**, 569–576.

Dueger, E.L., Moro, P.L. and Gilman, R.H. (1999). Oxfendazole treatment of sheep with naturally acquired hydatid disease. *Antimicrobial Agents and Chemotherapy* **43**, 2263–2267.

Ehnert, K.L., Roberto, R.R., Barrett, L., Sorvillo, F.J. and Rutherford, G.W., 3rd. (1992). Cysticercosis: first 12 months of reporting in California. *Bulletin of the Pan American Health Organization* **26**, 165–172.

Engels, D., Urbani, C., Belotto, A., Meslin, F. and Savioli, L. (2003). The control of human (neuro)cysticercosis: which way forward? *Acta Tropica* **87**, 177–182.

Erhart, A., Dorny, P., De, N.V., Vien, H.V., Thach, D.C., Toan, N.D., Cong, L.D., Geerts, S., Speybroeck, N., Berkvens, D. and Brandt, J. (2002). *Taenia solium* cysticercosis in a village in northern Vietnam: seroprevalence study using an ELISA for detecting circulating antigen. *Transactions of the Royal Society of Tropical Medicine and Hygiene* **96**, 270–272.

Escobedo, F., Penagos, P., Rodriguez, J. and Sotelo, J. (1987). Albendazole therapy for neurocysticercosis. *Archives of Internal Medicine* **147**, 738–741.

Fleury, A., Bouteille, B., Garcia, E., Marquez, C., Preux, P.M., Escobedo, F., Sotelo, J. and Dumas, M. (2001). Neurocysticercosis: validity of ELISA after storage of whole blood and cerebrospinal fluid on paper. *Tropical Medicine and International Health* **6**, 688–693.

Fleury, A., Gomez, T., Alvarez, I., Meza, D., Huerta, M., Chavarria, A., Carrillo-Mezo, R.A., Lloyd, C., Dessein, A., Preux, P.M., Dumas, M., Larralde, C., Sciutto, E. and Fragoso, G. (2003). High prevalence of calcified silent neurocysticercosis in a rural village of Mexico. *Neuroepidemiology* **22**, 139–145.

Flisser, A. (1988). Neurocysticercosis in Mexico. *Parasitology Today* **4**, 131–137.

Flisser, A. (1994). Taeniasis and cysticercosis due to *Taenia solium*. In: *Progress in Clinical Parasitology* (T. Sun, ed.), pp. 77–116. New York: CRC Press.

Flisser, A., Gonzalez, D., Shkurovich, M., Madrazo, I., Correa, D., Rodríguez-Carbajal, J., Cohen, S., Rodríguez del Rosal, E., Collado, M., Fernandez, B., Fernandez, F. and Aluja, A.S. (1990). Praziquantel treatment of porcine brain and muscle *Taenia solium* cysticercosis. I. Radiological, physiological and histopathological studies. *Parasitology Research* **76**, 263–269.

Flisser, A., Guaci, C.G., Zoli, A., Martinez-Ocaña, J., Garza-Rodriguez, A., Domínguez-Alpizar, J.L., Maravilla, P., Rodríguez-Canul, R., Avila, G., Aguilar-Vegas, L., Kyngdon, C., Geerts, S. and Lightowlers, M.W. (2004). Induction of protection against porcine cysticercosis by vaccination with recombinant oncosphere antigens. *Infection and Immunity* **72**, 5292–5297.

Flisser, A., Madrazo, I., Plancarte, A., Schantz, P., Allan, J., Craig, P. and Sarti, E. (1993). Neurological symptoms in occult neurocysticercosis alter single taeniacidal dose of praziquantel. *Lancet* **342**, 748.

Flisser, A., Sarti, E., Lightowlers, M. and Schantz, P. (2003). Neurocysticercosis: regional status, epidemiology, impact and control measures in the Americas. *Acta Tropica* **87**, 43–51.

Flisser, A., Vázquez-Mendoza, A., Martiñez-Ocaña, J., Gómez-Colín, E., Sánchez-Leyva, R. and Medina-Santillán, R. (2005). Short report: evaluation of a self-detection tool for tapeworm carriers for use in public health. *American Journal of Tropical Medicine and Health* **72**, 510–512.

Gaffo, A.L., Guillen-Pinto, D., Campos-Olazabal, P. and Burneo, J.G. (2004). Cysticercosis as the main cause of partial seizures in children in Peru. *Revista de Neurologia* **39**, 924–926 (Spanish).

Garcia, H.H. (2002). *Effectiveness of an interventional control program for human and porcine* Taenia solium *cysticercosis in field conditions*, p. 227. Thesis, Baltimore, Maryland: Johns Hopkins University.

Garcia, H.H. and del Brutto, O.H. (1999). Heavy nonencephalitic cerebral cysticercosis in tapeworm carriers. *Neurology* **53**, 1582–1584.

Garcia, H.H., Del Brutto, O.H., Nash, T.E., White, A.C., Jr., Tsang, V.C.W. and Gilman, R.H. (2005). New concepts in the diagnosis and management of neurocysticercosis (*Taenia solium*). *American Journal of Tropical Medicine and Hygiene* **72**, 3–9.

Garcia, H.H., Evans, C.A.W., Nash, T.E., Takayanagui, O.M., White, A.C., Jr., Botero, D., Rajshekhar, V., Tsang, V.C.W., Schantz, P.M., Allan, J.C., Flisser, A., Correa, D., Sarti, E., Friedland, J.S., Martinez, S.M., Gonzalez, A.E., Gilman, R.H. and del Brutto, O.H. (2002a). Current consensus guidelines for treatment of neurocysticercosis. *Clinical Microbiology Reviews* **15**, 747–756.

Garcia, H.H., Gilman, R.H., Catacora, M., Verastegui, M., Gonzalez, A.E. and Tsang, V.C. (1997). Serologic evolution of neurocysticercosis patients after antiparasitic therapy. *Journal of Infectious Diseases* **175**, 486–489.

Garcia, H.H., Gilman, R.H., Gonzalez, A.E., Pacheco, R., Verastegui, M. and Tsang, V.C. (1999). Human and Porcine *Taenia solium* infection in a village in the highlands of Cusco, Peru. *Acta Tropica* **73**, 31–36.

Garcia, H.H., Gilman, R.H., Tovar, M.A., Flores, E., Jo, R., Tsang, V.C., Diaz, F., Torres, P. and Miranda, E. (1995). Factors associated with *Taenia solium* cysticercosis analysis of nine hundred forty-six Peruvian neurologic patients. *American Journal of Tropical Medicine and Hygiene* **52**, 145–148.

Garcia, H.H., Gonzalez, A.E., Evans, C.A.W. and Gilman, R.H. (2003). *Taenia solium* cysticercosis. *Lancet* **362**, 547–556.

Garcia, H.H., Gonzalez, A.E., Gilman, R.H., Bernal, T., Rodríguez, S., Pretell, E.J., Azcurra, O., Parkhouse, R.M., Tsang, V.C., Harrison, L.J. and the Cysticercosis Working Group in Peru. (2002b). Circulating parasite antigen in patients with hydrocephalus secondary to neurocysticercosis. *American Journal of Tropical Medicine and Hygiene* **66**, 427–430.

Garcia, H.H., Gonzalez, A.E., Gilman, R.H., Palacios, L.G., Jiménez, I., Rodríguez, S., Verastegui, M., Wilkins, P., Tsang, V.C.W. and the Cysticercosis Working Group in Peru. (2001). Transient antibody response in *Taenia solium* infection in field conditions, a major contributor to high seroprevalence. *American Journal of Tropical Medicine and Hygiene* **65**, 31–34.

Garcia, H.H., Harrison, L.J.S., Parkhouse, R.M.E., Montenegro, T., Martinez, S.M., Tsang, V.C.W. and Gilman, R.H. (1998). A specific antigen-detection ELISA for the diagnosis of human neurocysticercosis. *Transactions of the Royal Society of Tropical Medicine and Hygiene* **92**, 411–414.

Garcia, H.H., Parkhouse, R.M.E., Gilman, R.H., Montenegro, T., Bernal, T., Martinez, S.M., Gonzalez, A.E., Tsang, V.C.W., Harrison, L.J.S. and the Cysticercosis Working Group in Peru. (2000). Serum antigen detection in the diagnosis, treatment and follow-up of neurocysticercosis patients. *Transactions of the Royal Society of Tropical Medicine and Hygiene* **94**, 673–676.

Garcia, H.H., Pretell, E.J., Gilman, R.H., Martinez, S.M., Moulton, L.H., Del Brutto, O.H., Genaro Herrera, M.D., Evans, C.A.W. and Gonazalez, A.E.

(2004). A trial of antiparasitic treatment to reduce the rate of seizures due to cerebral cysticercosis. *New England Journal of Medicine* **350**, 249–258.

Garcia-Noval, J., Allan, J.C., Fletes, C., Moreno, E., DeMata, F., Torres-Alvarez, R., Soto de Alfaro, H., Yurrita, P., Higueros-Morales, H., Mencos, F. and Craig, P.S. (1996). Epidemiology of *Taenia solium* taeniasis and cysticercosis in two rural Guatemalan communities. *American Journal of Tropical Medicine and Hygiene* **55**, 282–289.

Gauci, C.G.P., Flisser, A. and Lightowlers, M.W. (1998). A *Taenia solium* oncosphere protein homologous to host-protective *Taenia ovis* and *Taenia saginata* 18 kDa antigens. *International Journal for Parasitology* **28**, 757–760.

Gauci, C.G.P. and Lightowlers, M. (2001). Alternative splicing and sequence diversity of transcripts from the oncosphere stage of *Taenia solium* with homology to the 45W antigen of *Taenia ovis*. *Molecular Biochemistry and Parasitolgy* **112**, 173–181.

Gemmell, M., Matyas, Z., Pawlowski, Z., Soulsby, E.J.L., Larralde, C., Nelson, G.S. and Rosicky, B. (1983). *Guidelines for Surveillance, Prevention and Control of Taeniasis/Cysticercosis (VPH/83.49)*. Geneva: WHO.

Gilman, R.H., Del Brutto, O.H., Garcia, H.H. and Martinez, M. (2000). Prevalence of taeniosis among patients with neurocysticercosis is related to severity of infection. *Neurology* **55**, 1062.

Gonzalez, A.E. (2002). Control of *Taenia solium* with porcine chemotherapy. In: *Taenia solium Cysticercosis. From Basic to Clinical Science* (G. Singh and S. Prabhakar, eds), pp. 431–435. Wallingford, United Kingdom: CABI Publishing.

Gonzalez, A.E., Cama, V., Gilman, R.H., Tsang, V.C., Pilcher, J.B., Chavera, A., Castro, M., Montenegro, T., Verastegui, M., Miranda, E. and Bazalar, H. (1990). Prevalence and comparison of serologic assays, necropsy, and tongue examination for the diagnosis of porcine cysticercosis in Peru. *American Journal of Tropical Medicine and Hygiene* **43**, 194–199.

Gonzalez, A.E., Falcon, N., Gavidia, C., Garcia, H.H., Tsang, V.C., Bernal, T., Romero, M. and Gilman, R.H. (1997). Treatment of porcine cysticercosis with oxfendazole: a dose-response trial. *Veterinary Record* **141**, 420–422.

Gonzalez, A.E., Falcon, N., Gavidia, C., Garcia, H.H., Tsang, V.C., Bernal, T., Romero, M. and Gilman, R.H. (1998). Time–response curve of oxfendazole in the treatment of swine cysticercosis. *American Journal of Tropical Medicine and Hygiene* **59**, 832–836.

Gonzalez, A.E., Garcia, H.H., Gilman, R.H., Gavidia, C.M., Tsang, V.C., Bernal, T., Falcon, N., Romero, M. and Lopez-Urbina, M.T. (1996). Effective, single-dose treatment of porcine cysticercosis with oxfendazole. *American Journal of Tropical Medicine and Hygiene* **54**, 391–394.

Gonzalez, A.E., Garcia, H.H., Gilman, R.H., Lopez, M.T., Gavidia, C., McDonald, J., Pilcher, J.B. and Tsang, V.C. (1995). Treatment of porcine cysticercosis with albendazole. *American Journal of Tropical Medicine and Hygiene* **53**, 571–574.

Gonzalez, A.E., Garcia, H.H., Gilman, R.H. and Tsang, V.C. (2003). Control of Taenia solium. *Acta Tropica* **87**, 103–109.

Gonzalez, A.E., Gauci, C.G., Barber, D., Gilman, R.H., Tsang, V.C.W., Garcia, H.H., Verastegui, M. and Lightowlers, M.W. (2005). Short report: vaccination of pigs to control human neurocysticercosis. *American Journal of Tropical Medicine and Hygiene* **72**, 837–839.

Gonzalez, A.E., Gavidia, C., Falcon, N., Bernal, T., Verastegui, M., Garcia, H.H., Gilman, R.H., Tsang, V.C. and Cisticercosis Working Group in Peru (2001). Protection of pigs with cysticercosis from further infections after treatment with oxfendazole. *American Journal of Tropical Medicine and Hygiene* **65**, 15–18.

Gonzalez, L.M., Montero, E., Harrison, L.J.S., Parkhouse, R.M.E. and Gárate, T. (2000). Differential diagnosis of *Taenia saginata* and *Taenia solium* infection by PCR. *Journal of Clinical Microbiology* **38**, 737–744.

Gonzalez, L.M., Montero, E., Sciutto, E., Harrison, L.J., Parkhouse, R.M. and Garate, T. (2002). Differential diagnosis of *Taenia saginata* and *Taenia solium* infections: from DNA probes to polymerase chain reaction. *Transactions of the Royal Society of Tropical Medicine and Hygiene* **96**(supplement 1), S243–S250.

Gonzalez, A.E., Verastegui, M., Noh, J.C., Gaviria, C., Falcon, N., Bernal, T., Garcia, H.H., Tsang, V.C.W, Gilman, R.H., Wilkins, P.P. and the Cysticercosis Working Group in Peru. (1999). Persistence of passively transferred antibodies in porcine *Taenia solium* cysticercosis. *Veterinary Parasitology* **86**, 113–118.

Goodman, K.A., Ballagh, S.A. and Carpio, A. (1999). Case-control study of seropositivity for cysticercosis in Cuenca, Ecuador. *American Journal of Tropical Medicine and Hygiene* **60**, 70–74.

Griffiths, R.I., Schrammel, P.N., Morris, G.L., Wills, S.H., Labiner, D.M. and Strauss, M.J. (1999). Payer costs of patients diagnosed with epilepsy. *Epilepsia* **40**, 351–358.

Grill, J., Rakotomalala, W., Andriantsimahavandy, A., Boisier, P., Guyon, P., Roux, J. and Esterre, P. (1996). High prevalence of serological markers of cysticercosis among epileptic Malagasy children. *Annals of Tropical Paediatrics* **16**, 185–191.

Haddix, A.C., Teutsch, S. and Corso, P., eds. (2003). *Prevention Effectiveness. A Guide to Decision Analysis and Economic Evaluation*. Oxford, UK: Oxford University Press.

Hall, A., Latham, M.C., Crompton, D.W.T. and Stephenson, L.S. (1981). *Taenia saginata* (Cestoda) in western Kenya: the reliability of faecal examinations in diagnosis. *Parasitology* **83**, 91–101.

Hancock, K., Khan, A., Williams, F.B., Yushak, M.L., Pattabhi, S., Noh, J. and Tsang, V.C.W. (2003). Characterization of the 8-kilodalton antigens of *Taenia solium* metacestodes and evaluation of their use in an enzyme-linked immunosorbent assay for serodiagnosis. *Journal of Clinical Microbiology* **41**, 2577–2586.

Hancock, K., Pattabhi, S., Greene, R.M., Yushak, M.L., Williams, F., Khan, A., Priest, J.W., Levine, M.Z. and Tsang, V.C.W. (2004). Characterization and cloning of GP50, a *Taenia solium* antigen diagnostic for cysticercosis. *Molecular & Biochemical Parasitology* **133**, 115–124.

Hira, P.R., Francis, I., Abdella, N.A., Gupta, R., Ai-Ali, F.M., Grover, S., Khalid, N., Abdeen, S., Iqbal, J., Wilson, M. and Tsang, V.C. (2004). Cysticercosis: imported and autochthonous infections in Kuwait. *Transactions of the Royal Society of Tropical Medicine and Hygiene* **98**, 233–239.

Huerta, M., de Aluja, A.S., Fragoso, G., Toledo, A., Villalobos, N., Hernández, M., Gevorkian, G., Acero, G., Díaz, A., Alvarez, I., Avila, R., Beltrán, C., Garcia, G., Martinez, J.J., Sarralde, C. and Sciutto, E. (2002). Synthetic peptide vaccine against *Taenia solium* pig cysticercosis: successful vaccination in a controlled field trial in rural Mexico. *Vaccine* **20**, 262–266.

Huerta, M., Sciutto, E., Garcia, G., Villalobos, N., Hernández, M., Fragoso, G., Díaz, J., Díaz, A., Ramírez, R., Luna, S., Garcia, J., Aguilar, E., Espinoza, S., Castilla, G., Bobadilla, J.R., Avila, R., José, M.V., Larralde, C. and de Aluja, A.S. (2000). Vaccination against *Taenia solium* cysticercosis in underfed rustic pigs of México: roles of age, genetic background and antibody response. *Veterinary Parasitology* **90**, 209–219.

International Task Force for Disease Eradication (ITFDE) (1993). Recommendations of the International Task Force for Disease Eradication. *Morbidity and Mortality Weekly Report* **42**, RR-16, 1–46.

International Task Force for Disease Eradication II (ITFDE II) (2003). Summary of the Fourth Meeting of the ITFDE (II), April 16, 2003. http://www.cartercenter.org/documents/1367.pdf

Ito, A. and Craig, P.S. (2003). Immunodiagnosis and molecular approaches for the detection of taeniid cestode infections. *Trends in Parasitology* **19**, 377–381.

Ito, A., Nakao, M. and Wandra, T. (2003a). Human taeniasis and cysticercosis in Asia. *Lancet* **362**, 1918–1920.

Ito, A., Plancarte, A., Ma, L., Kong, Y., Flisser, A., Cho, S.Y., Liu, Y.H., Kamhawi, S., Lightowlers, M. and Schantz, P.M. (1998). Novel antigens for neurocysticercosis: simple method for preparation and evaluation for serodiagnosis. *American Journal of Tropical Medicine and Hygiene* **59**, 291–294.

Ito, A., Plancarte, A., Nakao, M., Nakaya, K., Ikejima, T., Piao, Z.X., Kanazawa, T. and Margono, S.S. (1999). ELISA and immunoblot using purified glycoproteins for serodiagnosis of cysticercosis in pigs naturally infected with *Taenia solium*. *Journal of Helminthology* **73**, 363–365.

Ito, A., Putra, M.I., Subahar, R., Sato, M.O., Okamoto, M., Sako, Y., Nakao, M., Yamasaki, H., Nakaya, K., Craig, P.S. and Margono, S.S. (2002a). Dogs as alternative intermediate hosts of *Taenia solium* in Papua (Irian Jaya), Indonesia confirmed by highly specific ELISA and immunoblot using native and recombinant antigens and mitochondrial DNA analysis. *Journal of Helminthology* **76**, 311–314.

Ito, A., Sako, Y., Nakao, M. and Nakaya, K. (2002b). Neurocysticercosis in Asia: serology/seroepidemiology in humans and pigs. In: *Cestode Zoonoses: Echinococcosis and Cysticercosis* (P. Craig and Z. Pawlowski, eds), pp. 25–31. Amsterdam: IOS Press.

Ito, A., Urbani, C., Qui, J.M., Vuitton, D.A., Qui, D.C., Heath, D.D., Craig, P.S., Zheng, F. and Schantz, P.M. (2003b). Control of echinococcosis and cysticercosis; a public health challenge to international cooperation in China. *Acta Tropica* **86**, 3–17.

Ito, A., Wandra, T., Yamasaki, H., Nakao, M., Sako, Y., Nakaya, K., Margono, S.S., Suroso, T., Gauci, C. and Lightowlers, M.W. (2004). Cysticercosis/taeniasis in Asia and the Pacific. *Vector-Borne and Zoonotic Diseases* **4**, 95–107.

Jafri, H.S., Torrico, F., Noh, J.C., Bryan, R.T., Balderrama, F., Pilcher, J.B. and Tsang, V.C. (1998). Application of the enzyme linked immunoelectrotransfer blot to paper blood spots to estimate seroprevalence of cysticercosis in Bolivia. *American Journal of Tropical Medicine and Hygiene* **58**, 313–315.

Jauregui, P.H. and Marquez-Monter, H. (1977). Cysticercosis of the brain in dogs in Mexico City. *American Journal of Veterinary Research* **38**, 1641–1642.

Jeri, C., Gilman, R.H., Lescano, A.G., Mayta, H., Ramirez, M.E., Gonzalez, A.E., Nazerali, R. and Garcia, H.H. (2004). Species identification after treatment for human taeniasis. *The Lancet* **363**, 949–950.

Joshi, D.D., Maharjan, M., Johansen, M.V., Willingham, A.L., 3rd and Sharma, M. (2003). Improving meat inspection and control in resource-poor communities: the Nepal example. *Acta Tropica* **87**, 119–127.

Jung, H., Hurtado, M., Sanchez, M., Medina, M.T. and Sotelo, J. (1990). Plasma and cerebrospinal fluid levels of albendazole and praziquantel in patients with neurocysticercosis. *Neuropharmacology* **13**, 559–564.

Kaur, M., Joshi, K., Ganguly, N.K., Mahajan, R.C. and Malla, N. (1995). Evaluation of the efficacy of albendazole against the larvae of *Taenia solium* in experimentally infected pigs, and kinetics of the immune response. *International Journal of Parasitology* **25**, 1443–1450.

Keilbach, N.M., de Aluja, A.S. and Sarti-Gutierrez, E. (1989). A programme to control taeniasis–cysticercosis (*T. solium*): experiences in a Mexican village. *Acta Leidensia* **57**, 181–189.

Kriel, J.D. (1997). *Taenia solium* in African *materiae medicae*: fact or fantasy. Report of an International Workshop on Cysticercosis. Agricultural Research Council, Onderstepoort Veterinary Institute, South Africa, 18–19 August 1997.

Kriel, J.D. and Joubert, J.J. (1996). African concepts of helminth infections: an anthropological perspective. *Journal of the South African Veterinary Association* **67**, 175.

Krishnan, A., Sahariah, S.U. and Kapoor, S.K. (2004). Cost of epilepsy in patients attending a secondary-level hospital in India. *Epilepsia* **45**, 289–291.

Lam, K.T. and Tan, N.T. (1992). Some comments on taeniasis and cysticercosis in several northern provinces of Vietnam. *Journal of Malaria and Parasitic Diseases Control* **4**, 39–44.

Lekule, F.P. and Kyvsgaard, N.C. (2003). Improving pig husbandry in tropical resource-poor communities and its potential to reduce risk of porcine cysticercosis. *Acta Tropica* **87**, 111–117.

Leutsher, P. and Andriantsimahavandy, A. (2004). Cysticercosis in Peace Corps Volunteers in Madagascar. *New England Journal of Medicine* **350**, 311–312.

Lightowlers, M. (2003). Vaccines for prevention of cysticercosis. *Acta Tropica* **87**, 129–135.

Lightowlers, M.W. (1999). Eradication of *Taenia solium* cysticercosis: a role for vaccination of pigs. *International Journal of Parasitology* **29**, 811–817.

Lightowlers, M.W. (2004). Vaccination for the prevention of cysticercosis. *Developments in Biologicals* **119**, 361–368.

Mafojane, N.A., Appleton, C.C., Krecek, R.C., Michael, L.M. and Willingham, A.L., 3rd. (2003). The current status of neurocysticercosis in eastern and southern Africa. *Acta Tropica* **87**, 25–33.

Maguire, J.H. (2004). Tapeworms and seizures – treatment and prevention. *New England Journal of Medicine* **350**, 215–217.

Manoutcharian, K., Díaz-Orea, A., Gevorkian, G., Fragoso, G., Acero, G., González, E., de Aluja, A., Villalobos, N., Gómez-Conde, E. and Sciutto, E. (2004). Recombinant bacteriophage-based multiepitope vaccine against *Taenia solium* pig cysticercosis. *Veterinary Immunology and Immunopathology* **99**, 11–24.

Margono, S.S., Subahar, R., Hamid, A., Wandra, T., Sudewi, S.S., Sutisna, P. and Ito, A. (2001). Cysticercosis in Indonesia: epidemiological aspects. *Southeast Asian Journal of Tropical Medicine and Public Health* **32**, 79–84.

Martinez, H.R., Rangel-Guerra, R., Elizondo, G., Gonzalez, J., Todd, L.E., Ancer, J. and Prakash, S. (1989). MR imaging in neurocysticercosis: a study of 56 cases. *American Journal of Neuroradiology* **10**, 1011–1019.

Mayta, H., Talley, A., Gilman, R.H., Jiménez, J., Verastegui, M., Ruiz, M., Garcia, H.H. and Gonzalez, A.E. (2000). Differentiating *Taenia solium* and *Taenia saginata* infections by simple hematoxylin–eosin staining and PCR-restriction enzyme analysis. *Journal of Clinical Microbiology* **38**, 1333–1337.

McCormick, G.F. (1985). Cysticercosis – review of 230 patients. *Bulletin of Clinical Neurosciences* **50**, 76–101.

McManus, D.P. (2005). Molecular discrimination of taeniid cestodes. *Parasitology International* (in press; December 5, 2005 electronic publication).

McManus, D.P., Garcia-Zepeda, E., Reid, A., Rishi, A.K. and Flisser, A. (1989). Human cysticercosis and taeniasis: molecular approaches for specific diagnosis and parasite identification. *Acta Leiden* **57**, 81–91.

McManus, D.P. and Ito, A. (2005). Application of molecular techniques for identification of the human *Taenia*, In: *WHO/FAO/OIE Guidelines for the Surveillance, Prevention and Control of Taeniosis/Cysticercosis*, (K.D. Murrell, ed.), pp. 52–55. Paris: Office International des Epizooties.

Morgan, B. and Hawkins, P. (1949). *Veterinary Helminthology*, p. 400. Minneapolis, MN: Burgess Publishing Company.

Murrell, K.D., ed. (2005). *WHO/FAO/OIE Guidelines for the Surveillance, Prevention and Control of Taeniosis/Cysticercosis*. Paris: Office International des Epizooties.

Nakao, M., Okamoto, M., Sako, Y., Yamasaki, H., Nakaya, K. and Ito, A. (2002). A phylogenic hypothesis for the distribution of two genotypes of the pork tapeworm *Taenia solium* worldwide. *Parasitology* **124**, 657–662.

Nash, T.E., Del Brutto, O.H., Butman, J.A., Corona, T., Delgado-Escueta, A., Duron, R.M., Evans, C.A., Gilman, R.H., Gonzalez, A.E., Loeb, J.A., Medina, M.T., Pietsch-Escueta, S., Pretell, E.J., Takayanagui, O.M., Theodore, W., Tsang, V.C. and Garcia, H.H. (2004). Calcific neurocysticercosis and epileptogenesis. *Neurology* **62**, 1934–1938.

Nash, T.E. and Neva, F.A. (1984). Recent advances in the diagnosis and treatment of cerebral cysticercosis. *New England Journal of Medicine* **311**, 1492–1496.

Nash, T.E. and Patronas, N.J. (1999). Edema associated with calcified lesions in neurocysticercosis. *Neurology* **53**, 777–781.

Nash, T.E., Pretell, J. and Garcia, H.H. (2001). Calcified cysticerci provoke perilesional edema and seizures. *Clinical Infectious Diseases* **33**, 1649–1653.

Nguekam, A., Zoli, A.P., Vondou, L., Pouedet, S.M., Assana, E., Dorny, P., Brandt, J., Losson, B. and Geerts, S. (2003). Kinetics of circulating antigens in pigs experimentally infected with *Taenia solium* eggs. *Tropical Medicine and International Health* **8**, 144–149.

Nguekam, J.P., Zoli, A.P., Zogo, P.O., Kamga, A.C.T., Speybroeck, N., Dorny, P., Brandt, J., Losson, B. and Geerts, S. (2003). A seroepidemiological study of human cysticercosis in West Cameroon. *Tropical Medicine and International Health* **8**, 144–149.

Njoroge, E., Mbithi, P., Wachira, T., Gathuma, J., Gathura, P., Maitho, T.E., Magambo, J. and Zeyhle, E. (2005). Comparative study of albendazole and oxfendazole in the treatment of cystic echinococcosis in sheep and goats. *International Journal of Applied Research in Veterinary Medicine* **3**, 97–1001.

Nsengiyumva, G., Druet-Cabanac, M., Nzisabira, L., Preux, P.M. and Vergnenègre, A. (2004). Economic evaluation of epilepsy in Kiremba (Burundi): a case-control study. *Epilepsia* **45**, 673–677.

Nunes, C.M., Lima, L.G., Manoel, C.S., Pereira, R.N., Nakano, M.M. and Garcia, J.F. (2003). *Taenia saginata*: polymerase chain reaction for taeniasis diagnosis in human fecal samples. *Experimental Parasitology* **104**, 67–69.

Okamoto, M., Nakao, M., Sako, Y. and Ito, A. (2001). Molecular variation of *Taenia solium* in the world. *Southeast Asian Journal of Tropical Medicine and Public Health* **32**(supplement 2), 90–93.

Okolo, M.I. (1986a). Cerebral cysticercosis in rural dogs. *Microbios* **47**, 189–191.

Okolo, M.I. (1986b). Observations on *Cysticercus cellulosae* in the flesh of rural dogs. *International Journal of Zoonoses* **13**, 286–289.

Pawlowski, Z., Allan, J. and Sarti, E. (2005). Control of *Taenia solium* taeniasis/cysticercosis: from research towards implementation. *International Journal of Parasitology* **35**, 1221–1232.

Pawlowski, Z. and Murrell, K.D. (2000). Taeniasis and cysticercosis. In: *Foodborne Disease Handbook (Second Edition), Volume 2: Viruses, Parasites, Pathogens and HAACP* (Y.H. Hui, S.A. Sattar, K.D. Murrell, W.K. Nip and P.S. Stanfield, eds), pp. 217–227. New York: Marcel Dekker, Inc.

Pawlowski, Z.S. (2002). *Taenia solium*: basic biology and transmission. In: *Taenia solium Cysticercosis. From Basic to Clinical Sciences* (G. Singh and S. Prabhakar, eds), pp. 1–14. Wallingford, United Kingdom: CABI Publishing.

Peniche-Cardeña, A., Dominguez-Alpizar, J.L., Sima-Alvarez, R., Argaez-Rodriguez, F., Fraser, A., Craig, P.S. and Rodríguez-Canul, R. (2002). Chemotherapy of porcine cysticercosis with albendazole sulphoxide. *Veterinary Parasitology* **108**, 63–73.

Phiri, I.K., Dorny, P., Gabriel, S., Willingham, A.L., III, Speybroeck, N. and Vercruysse, J. (2002). The prevalence of porcine cysticercosis in Eastern and Southern provinces of Zambia. *Veterinary Parasitology* **108**, 31–39.

Phiri, I.K., Ngowi, H., Afonso, S.M.S., Matenga, E., Boa, M., Mukaratirwa, S., Githigia, S.M., Saimo, M.K., Sikasunge, C.S., Maingi, N., Lubega, G.W., Kassuku, A., Michael, L.M., Siziya, S., Krecek, R.C., Noormahomed, E., Vilhena, M., Dorny, P. and Willingham, A.L., 3rd. (2003). The emergence of *Taenia solium* cysticercosis in Eastern and

Southern Africa as a serious agricultural problem and public health risk. *Acta Tropica* **87**, 13–23.

Pouedet, M.S.R., Zoli, A.P., Nguekam, L., Vondou, L., Assana, E., Speybroeck, N., Berkvens, D., Dorny, P., Brandt, J. and Geerts, S. (2002). Epidemiological survey of swine cysticercosis in two rural communities of West-Cameroon. *Veterinary Parasitology* **106**, 45–54.

Pretell, E.J., Garcia, H.H., Gilman, R.H., Saavedra, H. and Martinez, M. (2001). Failure of one-day praziquantel treatment in patients with multiple neurocysticercosis lesions. *Clinical Neurology and Neurosurgery* **103**, 175–177.

Preux, P.M. and Druet-Cabanac, M. (2005). Epidemiology and aetiology of epilepsy in sub-Saharan Africa. *Lancet Neurology* **4**, 21–31.

Preux, P.M., Thiemagni, F., Fodzo, L., Kandem, P., Ngouafong, P., Ndongo, F., Macharia, W., Dongmo, L. and Dumas, M. (2000). Anti-epileptic therapies in the Mifi Province in Cameroon. *Epilepsia* **41**, 432–439.

Proaño, J.V., Madrazo, I., Avelar, F., Lopez-Felix, B., Diaz, G. and Grijalva, I. (2001). Medical treatment for neurocysticercosis characterized by giant subarachnoid cysts. *New England Journal of Medicine* **345**, 879–885.

Rajshekhar, V., Joshi, D.D., Doanh, N.Q., De, N.V. and Zhou, X.N. (2003). *Taenia solium* taeniosis/cysticercosis in Asia: epidemiology, impact and issues. *Acta Tropica* **87**, 53–60.

Richards, F.O., Schantz, P.M., Ruiz-Tiben, E. and Sorvillo, F.J. (1985). Cysticercosis in Los Angeles County. *Journal of the American Medical Association* **254**, 3444–3448.

Rickard, M.D. and Williams, J.F. (1982). Hydatidosis/cysticercosis: immune mechanisms and immunization against infection. *Advances in Parasitology* **21**, 229–296.

Riley, T. and White, A.C., Jr. (2003). Management of neurocysticercosis. *CNS Drugs* **17**, 577–591.

Roberts, T., Murrell, K.D. and Marks, S. (1994). Economic losses caused by food-borne parasitic diseases. *Parasitology Today* **10**, 419–423.

Rodriguez-Canul, R., Argaez-Rodriguez, F., Pacheco de la Gala, D., Villegas-Perez, S., Fraser, A., Craig, P.S., Cob-Galera, L. and Domínguez-Alpizar, J.L. (2002). Taenia solium metacestode viability in infected pork after preparation with salt pickling or cooking methods common in Yucatán, México. *Journal of Food Protection* **65**, 666–669.

Rodriguez-Canul, R., Fraser, A., Allan, J.C., Dominguez-Alpizar, J.L., Argaez-Rodriguez, F. and Craig, P.S. (1999). Epidemiological study of *Taenia solium* taeniasis/cysticercosis in a rural village in Yucatan state, Mexico. *Annals of Tropical Medicine and Parasitology* **93**, 57–67.

Rodriguez-Hidalgo, R., Geysen, D., Benitez-Ortiz, W., Geerts, S. and Brandt, J. (2002). Comparison of conventional techniques to differentiate between *Taenia solium* and *Taenia saginata* and an improved polymerase chain reaction-restriction fragment length polymorphism assay using a mitochondrial 12S rDNA fragment. *Journal of Parasitology* **88**, 1007–1011.

Román, G., Sotelo, J., Del Brutto, O., Flisser, A., Dumas, M., Wadia, N., Botero, D., Cruz, M., Garcia, H., de Bittencourt, P.R.M., Trelles, L., Arriagada, C., Lorenzana, P., Nash, T.E. and Spina-França, A. (2000). A proposal to declare neurocysticercosis an international reportable disease. *Bulletin of the World Health Organization* **78**, 399–406.

Rosenfeld, E.A., Byrd, S.E. and Shulman, S.T. (1996). Neurocysticercosis among children in Chicago. *Clinical Infectious Diseases* **23**, 262–268.

Sahai, K., Kapila, K. and Verma, K. (2002). Parasites in fine needle breast aspirates-assessment of host tissue response. *Postgraduate Medical Journal* **78**, 165–167.

Sakai, H., Sone, M., Castro, D.M., Nonaka, N., Quan, D., Canales, M., Ljungstrom, I. and Sanchez, A.L. (1998). Seroprevalence of *Taenia solium* cysticercosis in pigs in a rural community of Honduras. *Veterinary Parasitology* **78**, 233–238.

Sako, Y., Nako, M., Ikejima, T., Piao, X.Z., Nakaya, K. and Ito, A. (2000). Molecular characterization and diagnostic value of *Taenia solium* low-molecular weight antigen genes. *Journal of Clinical Microbiology* **38**, 4439–4444.

Sanchez, A.L., Gomez, O., Allebeck, P., Cosenza, H. and Ljungstrom, L. (1997). Epidemiological study of *Taenia solium* infections in a rural village in Honduras. *Annals of Tropical Medicine and Parasitology* **91**, 163–171.

Sanchez, A.L., Medina, M.T. and Ljungstrom, I. (1998). Prevalence of taeniasis and cysticercosis in a population of urban residence in Honduras. *Acta Tropica* **69**, 141–149.

Sarti, E., Flisser, A., Schantz, P.M., Gleizer, M., Loya, M., Plancarte, A., Avila, G., Allan, J., Craig, P., Bronfman, M. and Wijeyaratne, P. (1997). Development and evaluation of a health education intervention against *Taenia solium* in a rural community in Mexico. *American Journal of Tropical Medicine and Hygiene* **56**, 127–132.

Sarti, E., Schantz, P.M., Avila, G., Ambrosio, J., Medina-Santillan, R. and Flisser, A. (2000). Mass treatment against human taeniasis for the control of cysticercosis: a population-based intervention study. *Transactions of the Royal Society of Tropical Medicine and Hygiene* **94**, 85–89.

Sarti, E., Schantz, P.M., Plancarte, A., Wilson, M., Gutierrez, I.O. and Lopez, A.S. (1992). Prevalence and risk factors for *Taenia solium* taeniasis and cysticercosis in humans and pigs in a village in Morelos, Mexico. *American Journal of Tropical Medicine and Hygiene* **46**, 677–685.

Sarti, E., Schantz, P.M., Plancarte, A., Wilson, M., Gutierrez, O.I., Aguilera, J., Roberts, J. and Flisser, A. (1994). Epidemiological investigation of *Taenia solium* taeniasis and cysticercosis in a rural village of Michoacan state, Mexico. *Transactions of the Royal Society for Tropical Medicine and Hygiene* **88**, 49–52.

Sato, M.O., Yamasaki, H., Sako, Y., Nakao, M., Nakaya, K., Plancarte, A., Kassuku, A.A., Dorny, P., Geerts, S., Benitez-Ortiz, W., Hashiguchi, Y. and Ito, A. (2003). Evaluation of tongue inspection and serology for diagnosis of *Taenia solium* cysticercosis in swine: usefulness of ELISA using purified glycoproteins and recombinant antigen. *Veterinary Parasitology* **111**, 309–322.

Schantz, P.M., Cruz, M., Sarti, E. and Pawlowski, Z. (1993). Potential eradicability of taeniasis and cysticercosis. *Bulletin of the Pan American Health Organization* **27**, 397–403.

Schantz, P.M., Moore, A.C., Munoz, J.L., Hartman, B.J., Schaefer, J.A., Aron, A.M., Persaud, D., Sarti, E., Wilson, M. and Flisser, A. (1992). Neurocysticercosis in an orthodox Jewish community in New York City. *New England Journal Medicine* **327**, 692–695.

Schantz, P.M. and Sarti-Guttierez, E. (1989). Diagnostic methods and epidemiologic surveillance of *Taenia solium* infection. *Acta Leidensia* **57**, 153–164.

Schantz, P.M., Wilkins, P.P. and Tsang, V.C.W. (1998). Immigrants, imaging and immunoblots: the emergence of neurocysticercosis as a significant public health problem. In: *Emerging Infections 2* (W.M. Scheld, W.A. Craig and J.M. Hughes, eds), pp. 213–241. Washington: ASM Press.

Scheel, C.M., Khan, A., Hancock, K., Garcia, H.H., Gonzalez, A.E., Gilman, R.H., Tsang, V.C.W. and the Cysticercosis Working Group in Peru. (2005). Serodiagnosis of neurocysticercosis using synthetic 8-kd proteins: comparison of assay formats. *American Journal of Tropical Medicine and Hygiene* **73**, 771–776.

Sciutto, E., Fragoso, G., Manoutcharian, K., Gevorkian, G., Rosas-Salgado, G., Hernández-Gonzalez, M., Herrera-Estrella, L., Cabrera-Ponce, J.L., López-Casillas, F., González-Bonilla, C., Santiago-Machuca, A., Ruíz-Pérez, F., Sánchez, J., Goldbaum, F., Aluja, A. and Larralde, C. (2002). New approaches to improve a peptide vaccine against porcine *Taenia solium* cysticercosis. *Archives of Medical Research* **33**, 371–378.

Sciutto, E., Martinez, J.J., Villalobos, N.M., Hernandez, M., Jose, M.V., Beltran, C., Rodarte, F., Flores, I., Bobadilla, J.R., Fragoso, G., Parkhouse, M.E., Harrison, L.J. and de Aluja, A.S. (1998). Limitations of current diagnostic procedures for the diagnosis of *Taenia solium* cysticercosis in rural pigs. *Veterinary Parasitology* **79**, 299–313.

Shasha, W. and Pammenter, M.D. (1991). Sero-epidemiological studies of cysticercosis in school children from two rural areas of Transkei, South Africa. *Annals of Tropical Medicine and Parasitology* **85**, 349–355.

Shey-Njila, O., Zoli, P.A., Awah-Ndukum, J., Nguekam, J.P., Assana, E., Byambas, P., Dorny, P., Brandt, J. and Geerts, S. (2003). Porcine cysticercosis in village pigs of northwest Cameroon. *Journal of Helminthology* **77**, 351–354.

Singh, G. and Prabhakar, S. (2002). *Taenia solium Cysticercosis. From Basic to Clinical Science*. Wallingford, United Kingdom: CABI Publishing.

Sorvillo, F.J., Portigal, L., DeGiorgio, C., Smith, L., Waterman, S.H., Berlin, G.W. and Ash, L.R. (2004). Cysticercosis mortality in California. *Emerging Infectious Diseases* **10**, 465–469.

Sorvillo, F.J., Waterman, S.H., Richards, F.O. and Schantz, P.M. (1992). Cysticercosis surveillance: locally acquired and travel-related infections and detection of intestinal tapeworm carriers in Los Angeles County. *American Journal of Tropical Medicine and Hygiene* **47**, 365–371.

Sotelo, J., del Brutto, O.H., Penagos, P., Escobedo, F., Torres, B. and Rodriguez-Carbajal, J. (1990). Comparison of therapeutic regimen of anti-cysticercal drugs for parenchymal brain cysticercosis. *Neurology* **237**, 69–72.

Sotelo, J., Escobedo, F. and Penagos, P. (1988). Albendazole vs praziquantel for therapy for neurocysticercosis: a controlled trial. *Archives of Neurology* **45**, 532–534.

Sotelo, J., Escobedo, F., Rodriguez-Carbajal, J., Torres, B. and Rubio-Donnadieu, F. (1984). Therapy of parenchymal brain cysticercosis with praziquantel. *New England Journal of Medicine* **310**, 1001–1007.

Sotelo, J., Rosas, N. and Palencia, G. (1986). Freezing of infested pork muscle kills cysticerci. *Journal of American Medical Association* **256**, 893–894.

Statistics South Africa (2004). Mid-year population estimates, South Africa 2004. Statistical Release P0302.

Subahar, R., Hamid, A., Purba, W., Sandra, T., Karma, C., Sako, Y., Margono, S.S., Craig, P.S. and Ito, A. (2001). *Taenia solium* infection in Irian Jaya (west Papua), Indonesia: a pilot serological survey of human and porcine cysticercosis in Jayawijaya District. *Transactions of the Royal Society of Tropical Medicine and Hygiene* **95**, 388–390.

The Medical Letter, Inc. (2004). Drugs for parasitic infections. In: *The Medical Letter on Drugs and Therapeutics, August 2004* (M. Abramowicz, ed.), p. 12. New York: The Medical Letter, Inc., www.medicalletter.org.

Thomas, S.V., Sarma, P.S., Alexander, M., Pandit, L., Shekhar, L., Trivedi, C. and Vengamma, B. (2001). Economic burden of epilepsy in India. *Epilepsia* **42**, 1052–1060.

Thomson, A.J.G. (1993). Neurocysticercosis – experience at the teaching hospitals of the University of Cape Town. *South African Medical Journal* **83**, 332–334.

Torres, A., Plancarte, A., Villalobos, A.N., de Aluja, A.S., Navarro, R. and Flisser, A. (1992). Praziquantel treatment of porcine brain and muscle *Taenia solium* cysticercosis. 3. Effect of 1-day treatment. *Parasitology Research* **78**, 161–164.

Torres, J.R., Noya, O., Noya, B.A. and Mondolfi, A.G. (1988). Seizures and praziquantel. A case report. *Revista do Instituto de Medicina Tropical de Sao Paulo* **30**, 433.

Townes, J.M., Hoffmann, C.J. and Kohn, M.A. (2004). Neurocysticercosis in Oregon, 1995–2000. *Emerging Infectious Diseases* **10**, 508–510.

Tsang, V.C., Brand, J.A. and Boyer, A.E. (1989). An enzyme-linked immunoelectrotransfer blot assay and glycoprotein antigens for diagnosing human cysticercosis (*Taenia solium*). *Journal of Infectious Diseases* **159**, 50–59.

Tsang, V.C., Pilcher, J.A., Zhou, W., Boyer, A.E., Kamango-Sollo, E.I., Rhoads, M.L., Murrell, K.D., Schantz, P.M. and Gilman, R.H. (1991). Efficacy of the immunoblot assay for cysticercosis in pigs and modulated expression of distinct IgM/IgG activities to *Taenia solium* antigens in experimental infections. *Veterinary Immunology and Immunopathology* **29**, 69–78.

van Hout, B., Gagnon, D., Souetre, E., Ried, S., Remy, C., Baker, G., Genton, P., Vespignani, H. and McNulty, P. (1997). Relationship between seizure frequency and costs and quality of life of outpatients with partial epilepsy in France, Germany, and the United Kingdom. *Epilepsia* **38**, 1221–1226.

Vazquez-Flores, S., Ballesteros-Rodea, G., Flisser, A. and Schantz, P.M. (2001). Hygiene and restraint of pigs is associated with absence of *Taenia solium* cysticercosis in a rural community of Mexico. *Salud Pública de México* **43**, 574–576.

Vazquez, M.L., Jung, H. and Sotelo, J. (1987). Plasma levels of praziquantel decrease when dexamethasone is given simultaneously. *Neurology* **37**, 1561–1562.

Velasco-Suarez, M., Bravo, M.A. and Quirasco, F. (1982). Human cysticercosis medical-social implications and economic impact. In: *Cysticercosis: Present State of Knowledge and Perspectives* (A. Flisser, K. Willms, J.P. Laclette, C. Larralde, C. Ridaura and F. Beltran, eds), pp. 47–51. New York: Academic Press.

Wandra, T., Ito, A., Yamasaki, H., Seroso, T. and Margono, S.S. (2003). *Taenia solium* cysticercosis, Irian Jaya, Indonesia. *Emerging Infectious Diseases* **9**, 884–885.

White, A.C., Jr. (2000). Neurocysticercosis: updates on epidemiology, pathogenesis, diagnosis and management. *Annual Review of Medicine* **51**, 187–206.

White, A.C. and Garcia, H.H. (1999). Recent developments in the epidemiology, diagnosis, treatment, and prevention of neurocysticercosis. *Current Infectious Diseases Report* **1**, 434–440.

White, A.C., Jr., Robinson, P. and Kuhn, R. (1997). *Taenia solium* cysticercosis: host-parasite interactions and the immune response. *Chemical Immunology* **66**, 209–230.

Wilkins, P.P., Allan, J.C., Verastegui, M., Acosta, M., Eason, A.G., Garcia, H.H., Gonzalez, A.E., Gilman, R.H. and Tsang, V.C. (1999). Development of a serologic assay to detect *Taenia solium* taeniasis. *American Journal of Tropical Medicine and Hygiene* **60**, 199–204.

Wilkins, P.P., Wilson, M., Allan, J.C. and Tsang, V.C.W. (2002). *Taenia solium* cysticercosis: immunodiagnosis of neurocysticercosis and taeniasis. In: *Taenia solium Cysticercosis: From Basic to Clinical Science* (G. Singh and S. Prabhakar, eds), pp. 329–341. Wallingford, United Kingdom: CABI Publishing.

Willingham, A.L., III, De, N.V., Doanh, N.Q., Cong, L.D., Dung, T.V., Dorny, P., Cam, P.D. and Dalsgaard, A. (2003). Current status of cysticercosis in Vietnam. *Southeast Asian Journal of Tropical Medicine and Public Health* **34**(supplement), 35–50.

Wilson, M., Bryan, R.T., Fried, J.A., Ware, D.A., Shantz, P.M., Pilcher, J.B. and Tsang, V.C. (1991). Clinical evaluation of the cysticercosis enzyme-linked immunoelectrotransfer blot in patients with neurocysticercosis. *Journal of Infectious Diseases* **164**, 1007–1009.

World Health Organization (WHO). (2000). *Bringing Epilepsy Out of the Shadows in Africa (Press Release, WHO 30, 4 May 2000)*. Geneva: World Health Organization.

World Health Organization (WHO). (2001). *Epilepsy: An Historical Overview. WHO Fact Sheet 168*. Geneva: World Health Organization.

World Health Organization (WHO) (2003). Control of neurocysticercosis. *Report of the Secretariat, Fifty-sixth World Health Assembly. Document A56/10*. Geneva: World Health Organization.

Yamasaki, H., Allan, J.C., Sato, M.O., Nakao, M., Sako, Y., Nakaya, K., Qiu, D., Mamuti, W., Craig, P.S. and Ito, A. (2004). DNA differential diagnosis of taeniasis/cysticercosis by multiplex PCR. *Journal of Clinical Microbiology* **42**, 548–553.

Yamasaki, H., Nakao, M., Sako, Y., Nakaya, K., Sato, M.O., Mamuti, W., Okamoto, M. and Ito, A. (2002). DNA differential diagnosis of human taeniid cestodes by base excision sequence scanning thymine-base reader analysis with mitochondrial genes. *Journal of Clinical Microbiology* **40**, 3818–3821.

Yancey, L.S., Diaz-Marchan, P.J. and White, A.C. (2005). Cysticercosis: recent advances in diagnosis and management of neurocysticercosis. *Current Infectious Disease Reports* **7**, 39–47.

Zini, D., Farrell, V.J.R. and Wadee, A.A. (1990). The relationship of antibody levels to the clinical spectrum of human neurocysticercosis. *Journal of Neurology, Neurosurgery and Psychiatry* **53**, 656–661.

Zoli, A., Shey-Njila, O., Assana, E., Nguekam, J.P., Dorny, P., Brandt, J. and Geerts, S. (2003). Regional status, epidemiology and impact of *Taenia solium* cysticercosis in Western and Central Africa. *Acta Tropica* **87**, 35–42.

Zoli, P.A. and Tchoumboué, J. (1992). Prevalence de la cysticercose porcine dans le Departement de la Menoua (Ouest-Cameroun). *Cameroon Bulletin of Animal Production* **1**, 42–47.

Implementation of Human Schistosomiasis Control: Challenges and Prospects

Alan Fenwick[1], David Rollinson[2] and Vaughan Southgate[2]

[1]*Schistosomiasis Control Initiative, Department of Infectious Disease Epidemiology, Imperial College, London W2 1PG, UK*
[2]*Wolfson Wellcome Biomedical Laboratories, Department of Zoology, The Natural History Museum, Cromwell Road, London SW7 5BD, UK*

ADVANCES IN PARASITOLOGY VOL 61
ISSN: 0065-308X
DOI: 10.1016/S0065-308X(05)61013-5

ABSTRACT

Schistosomiasis is a major disease of public health importance in humans occurring in over 70 countries of the tropics and sub-tropics. In this chapter, the history of the control of schistosomiasis is briefly discussed and current methods of control of schistosomiasis are reviewed; including mollusciciding, biological control of the intermediate snail hosts, the development of drugs to kill the adult worms, provision of clean water and health education, with a focus on the African situation. Since an effective vaccine against schistosomiasis is lacking, the emphasis today is placed on the drug praziquantel (PZQ). The marked reduction in the cost of PZQ together with the support of the Bill and Melinda Gates Foundation has enabled the drug to be used more widely in sub-Saharan Africa. Nevertheless, with the possibility of resistance to praziquantel emerging, the potential role of other drugs, such as artemether, in the control of schistosomiasis is examined. The World Health Organization (WHO) anticipates that at least 75% of all schoolchildren at risk of morbidity from schistosomiasis will be treated by 2010, with the aim of reversing morbidity. The importance of recent international initiatives such as the Schistosomiasis Control Initiative (SCI) working in Mali, Niger, Burkina Faso, Zambia, Tanzania and Uganda is recognised. There are benefits to integrating the control of schistosomiasis with other disease control programmes, such as gastrointestinal helminths and/or lymphatic filariasis (LF), since this markedly reduces the cost of delivery of the treatment. Countries that are situated on the perimeter of the distribution of schistosomiasis have either achieved or have made progress towards the elimination of the disease. For control programmes to be successful in areas such as sub-Saharan Africa, it is absolutely essential that these programmes are sustainable. Thus, it will be vital for Ministries of Health and Education to budget for the control of diseases of poverty in addition to school health, and to utilise funds from a range of sources, such as, government funds, pooled donor contributions, or bilateral and international agencies.

1. INTRODUCTION

1.1. Life History and Transmission—Breaking the Life Cycle

Around 200 million people are currently infected with schistosomiasis (Chitsulo *et al.*, 2000). This is ample proof of the success of the schistosome life cycle. Like all other trematodes, the schistosomes require a molluscan intermediate host in which to undergo development and freshwater snails from four different genera form an essential component in the life cycle of the four major schistosome species that are responsible for human schistosomiasis. This ties transmission of the disease to places where people and snails come together at the same water habitat. Hence, schistosomiasis tends to be commonly found in rural communities where contact with freshwater bodies can be a routine and inevitable occurrence. Everyday needs ensure that contact with freshwater is almost unavoidable in many situations. Collecting drinking water, washing of all kinds, bathing and playing bring people to the water, whilst many occupations, including fishing and agriculture, expose individuals to contaminated water on a regular basis.

The parasite relies on a basic behavioural characteristic of humans and that is the tendency to defecate and urinate in and around water. Much of the schistosome life cycle takes place in the aquatic environment and when eggs, which are excreted in large numbers with urine and/or faeces, reach freshwater, they hatch releasing a free-swimming larva or miracidium. The miracidium is a non-feeding, short-lived stage that attempts to seek out and penetrate a suitable intermediate snail host in which to continue development. Those eggs that do not reach water are soon desiccated and play no part in transmission. The most striking fact relevant to control is that if human behaviour could be changed to stop contamination of water bodies with urine and faeces containing schistosome eggs, then transmission of the parasite would cease. This fact is central to many longer-term control efforts, including the education of children, to reduce water contamination, together with the provision of piped water and better sanitation. In theory, the breaking of the schistosome life cycle is remarkably easy, whereas in practice, it is extremely difficult at the community level among poor and underserved populations.

Within the snail, the parasite develops and multiplies asexually. This allows the parasite to increase dramatically in numbers enhancing considerably the chances of reinfecting humans. The schistosome has an extremely specific and selective need at this stage in the cycle and will only develop successfully in certain snails (Rollinson and Southgate, 1987; Rollinson and Johnston, 1996). The main molluscan genera used by the human schistosomes are *Bulinus* (*Schistosoma haematobium*), *Biomphalaria* (*Schistosoma mansoni*), *Oncomelania* (*Schistosoma japonicum*) and *Neotricula* (*Schistosoma mekongi*). The global distribution of species that act as intermediate snail hosts reflects the distribution of human schistosomiasis. These snails, especially *Bulinus* and *Biomphalaria* thrive in areas frequented by man. Indeed certain species seem to favour habitats polluted with human excreta and the detritus of everyday living. The intricate relationship between snail and schistosome make this part of the life cycle vulnerable to control activities, and there is a long history of attempted snail control using chemicals (molluscicides) to kill snails (Paulini, 1958; Ferguson, 1961; Crossland, 1963; Gönnert, 1967; Barnish, 1970; Sturrock, 1995). Biological and environmental manipulation of the habitat to reduce numbers have been considered and targeting of specific intermediate snail hosts is a challenge for the future (Berg, 1973; Frandsen, 1987; Ault, 1994; Pointier and Jourdane, 2000; Pointier and David, 2004).

Snails have limited powers of dispersal and are unlikely to move far during their lifetime unless carried by freshwater currents. However, when they are introduced into favourable habitats, they colonise new water bodies quickly due to their large reproductive potential. Movement and spread of the parasite is much more likely due to the movement of infected people. Infection from snail to humans depends on water contact, the free-swimming larvae or cercariae released from the snail penetrating directly through areas of the skin in contact with water.

The adult worms which then mature in the human host are remarkable in many ways. Firstly, they live in the blood vessels of the infected host; an environment which, although food-rich, also exposes the parasite to the immunological onslaught of the host should they be detected. Nevertheless, evidence shows that schistosomes can and do survive for a number of years (Fulford *et al.*, 1995). Secondly, most unusually for trematodes, the majority of which are hermaphrodite, schistosomes are dioecious and males and females must pair in order to mature and mate and to locate to the blood systems in the body that allow the egress of eggs. Each female worm is capable of laying many hundreds of eggs on a daily basis (Loker, 1983) but many of the eggs fail to leave the body and get trapped in various tissues and organs; it is the eggs rather than the adult worms that are primarily responsible for the pathology associated with the disease. Eggs that escape through the bladder or intestine cause blood loss as capillaries are severed, and those that do not escape end up in organs and tissues such as the liver, causing long-term damage.

Thus the schistosome life cycle and the host parasite interactions involved are complex, involving the parasite moving, surviving, penetrating and developing in quite different environments: mammalian blood, water and intermediate snail hosts. The broad biological processes relating to the life cycle are now sufficiently well understood to help target efforts to control both the disease and its transmission.

1.2. Historical Perspective—Successes and Failures

Schistosomiasis presents a serious public health problem. The morbidity due to schistosomiasis has been underestimated, and for long periods there has been comparatively little in the way of control measures. This has been partly because of the high price of the commercially available drugs and molluscicides, and more recently because of the appearance of several acute emerging diseases, such as HIV/AIDS as well as the resurgence of malaria and TB, which have resulted in the already meagre resources being diverted from chronic diseases such as schistosomiasis to the more acute and fatal infections (King *et al.*, 2005).

The control of schistosomiasis has passed through a series of crests and troughs since the life cycle of the parasitic infection was first described. Egypt and Sudan were the first African countries in which control was attempted. In Egypt, Christopherson (1918) was the first to use antimonial drugs for treatment, and in Sudan, the planning of the Gezira irrigation scheme, which was built during the period 1915–1921 included the screening and treatment of Egyptian workers imported to dig the canals (El-Nagar, 1958).

Control measures in Egypt and Sudan moved from the use of the excruciating treatment of 21 injections using the antimony-based drugs pentostam and astiban to a hypothesis that possibly the snail was the weak link in the life cycle. To that end, copper sulphate was the first commercial molluscicide used, although its effectiveness in laboratory experiments did not transfer through to an equal effectiveness in natural water bodies.

Scientists began a search for other molluscicides: sodium pentachlorophenate (Klock *et al.*, 1957; Nasr, 1960; Dawood *et al.*, 1966) and N-tritylmorpholine (Frescon) (Amin, 1972; Duke and Moore, 1976) were the two almost taken to a commercial level, but their shortcomings were soon exposed. Then, during the 1960s, the pharmaceutical company Bayer discovered how effective niclosamide was against snails, and Bayluscide became the molluscicide of choice. This compound has been used extensively in Zimbabwe (Evans, 1983), Brazil (Katz *et al.*, 1980), St. Lucia (Prentice *et al.*, 1981), Egypt (Webbe and el Hak, 1990), Sudan (Meyerlassen, Daffalla, and Madsen, 1994) and elsewhere, in attempts to reduce levels of transmission, and hence to reduce levels of prevalence and intensity of infection in the human population. There is clear evidence that the population of snails can be much reduced, but this approach suffers from the fact that the molluscicide is not specific to killing molluscs. For example, fish are also killed, so the application of niclosamide has a deleterious impact on the environment and biodiversity. Unfortunately, the price of Bayluscide rocketed with the increase in price of petroleum during the 1970s, hence mollusciciding is a comparatively expensive operation, yet has to be sustained to be effective in the long term (Jobin,

1979). Once mollusciciding ceases, snail populations have the ability to breed and reach pre-control levels in a matter of two to three years. The high rate of increase of *Biomphalaria* spp. and *Bulinus* spp. is related to their ability to reproduce by both cross-fertilisation (outcrossing) and self-fertilisation (selfing) and their response to environmental stimuli (e.g. temperature, rainfall, etc.). Also, there must be question marks over the practicality of mollusciciding in large water bodies, such as the transmission foci on lakeshores, where it is inherently difficult to apply the chemical at the correct concentrations throughout the water body. It is probable that the most effective use of molluscicides is in small water bodies where the transmission foci are well defined in both geographical terms and periods of active transmission, such as found in Saudi Arabia (al-Madani, 1990).

Plant-derived molluscicides have an attraction in that they are theoretically less expensive and more readily available than synthetic molluscicides (Singh *et al.*, 1996) and can be produced in countries where schistosomiasis is endemic. The berries of endod, *Phytolacca dodecandra*, have perhaps been studied in greater detail than any other plant molluscicide (Lemma, 1971; Lemma *et al.*, 1972; Spielman and Lemma, 1973; Lemma and Yau, 1974a, b; Goll *et al.*, 1983; Lambert *et al.*, 1991; Madhina and Shiff, 1996; Erko *et al.*, 2002). Although some success has been reported in the reduction of infection rates in school children in Ethiopia, the lack of molluscan ovicidal activity and broad-spectrum faunal toxicity mitigate against a wider geographical application of this molluscicide.

The introduction of competitor freshwater snails (biological control) has been shown to be a successful strategy, particularly on many of the Caribbean islands, in either reducing snail numbers or indeed eliminating the schistosome intermediate host snails altogether (Prentice, 1983). The Louisiana red swamp crayfish, *Procambarus clarkii*, has been introduced into East Africa. The crayfish is able to reduce populations of the intermediate snail hosts through predatory and competitive interactions, and it has been demonstrated that re-infection rates in humans after chemotherapy can be slowed down in areas where crayfish are present because of their inhibitory effect on the intermediate snail hosts (Hofkin *et al.*, 1991; Mkoji *et al.*, 1999).

For the treatment of infection, which is the only control measure to bring relief to infected people, the early antimony-based treatments were improved upon by the discovery of ambilhar (Raffier, 1969; Arfaa *et al.*, 1970) and then hycanthone (Oostburg, 1972; Cook *et al.*, 1976). Ambilhar was used in several large-scale control campaigns, in particular, the Fayoum control programme in Egypt in the late 1970s (Abdel-Salam *et al.*, 1986) but with continued use more psychotic side effects were registered (Shekhar, 1991). Hycanthone use expanded because it was effective and had the advantage of being administered as a single injection but a number of unpredictable and unexplained deaths after injection caused it to be withdrawn from the market (Mengistu, 1982). Metrifonate was widely used against *S. haematobium* during 1970–1980 in Africa. Metrifonate had the advantage of being cheap and effective, but optimal results were obtained only with three treatments at weekly intervals and this proved to be too great a logistical obstacle for mass treatment in field conditions (Mgeni *et al.*, 1990). Metrifonate is no longer available and has been deleted from the WHO list of essential drugs (Fenwick *et al.*, 2003).

Oxamniquine, which is manufactured by Pfizer Ltd, is no longer available in Africa, but fortunately is more accessible in South America and has been extensively used as a chemotherapeutic weapon against *S. mansoni* in Brazil (Jewsbury, 1977). Resistance to oxamniquine has been reported from isolated villages in yet resistance to oxamniquine does not appear to have become a widespread problem in Brazil (Conceicao *et al.*, 1999). One of the probable reasons for this lack of spread of resistance may be associated with the fact that schistosomes resistant to oxamniquine are less fit than susceptible worms, for example, they are less infective to both intermediate and definitive hosts and are less fecund. Oxamniquine is being used less and less in South America as the price of praziquantel becomes comparatively cheaper (Beck *et al.*, 2001). There is some concern that the current lack of use of oxamniquine will lead to cessation of manufacture in the future. If so, this would leave praziquantel (PZQ) as the primary chemotherapeutic weapon against schistosomiasis with the obvious disastrous implications if resistance to that particular drug should develop and spread. Using a combination of oxamniquine and PZQ has been shown to be effective, but such a combination has never been adopted on any scale in the field (Creasey *et al.*, 1986; Zwingenberger *et al.*, 1987; Botros *et al.*, 1989).

By the mid-1970s, the effectiveness of the drug PZQ was being tested in multicentre trials worldwide under the auspices of WHO, and the drug originally owned by Merck but developed and subsequently marketed by Bayer appeared to be a very effective chemotherapeutic weapon against all species of schistosome (Davis *et al.*, 1979, 1981). It was shown to be extremely effective either as a split dose (20 mg/kg in the morning and again in the afternoon) but more importantly, it was effective when dispensed as a 40 mg/kg single dose (Kardaman *et al.*, 1983). Optimally, the drug must be given after food to increase absorption, but side effects have been few and far between and cure rates were excellent (Castro *et al.*, 2000). Even among those not cured, egg reduction after treatment was usually over 90% (Utzinger *et al.*, 2000). The drawback to PZQ was the price asked by Bayer—$1 per tablet, equivalent $4 for an adult dose. Since the health budget of most endemic countries was little over $1 per person per year, and incomes of infected people were usually around $1 per day, there was little chance that the treatment could be afforded, either by the governments or the individuals who required treatment. The only control programmes of any scale were donor funded by the German government and in Mali (Brinkmann *et al.*, 1988) the World Bank Egypt (Webbe and el Hak, 1990).

Control of schistosomiasis was revolutionised and mass treatment of schistosomiasis in Africa became a realistic possibility for the first time in the 1990s when, over a 10-year period, the price of praziquantel was reduced by over 90% (Savioli *et al.*, 2002; Fenwick *et al.*, 2003; Savioli *et al.*, 2004). This was made possible when Shin Poong, a South Korean pharmaceutical company, discovered a new method to synthesise PZQ. Within a few years, Shin Poong cornered the market, and schistosomiasis control programmes were implemented in Brazil, China, the Philippines and Egypt, all with World Bank funding. Notably, these countries were all wealthier than the developing countries of Africa, and also they considered schistosomiasis to be a high priority disease. Despite an estimated 180 million people being infected in sub-Saharan Africa, schistosomiasis remained mostly a neglected disease and was not considered worthy of a national control programme, partly because the infection was so focal. Some pilot control schemes were implemented in Cameroon, Malawi, Mali and Tanzania but, possibly because of the financial implications, these pilot schemes never translated into sustainable national programmes.

Despite its widespread use, the precise mechanism of action of PZQ is still not known, but clearly the drug causes tegumental damage to the parasite and paralytic muscular contraction, resulting in death and elimination of the schistosomula. The efficacy of PZQ appears to be related to the immune status of the host (Fallon *et al.*, 1995). The drug has a high level of efficacy against all species of adult schistosome, it has long shelf life (3 years), it is administered as a single oral dose, and clinical experience since the drug has been used in schistosomiasis control programmes has demonstrated that it is safe and well tolerated in both short- and long-term usage. The side effects that have been noted appear to be limited to abdominal pain, nausea, vomiting, anorexia and diarrhoea. Indeed, data that have been collated retrospectively, including the results of extensive risk/benefit analyses, indicate that it is safe to administer to pregnant and lactating women (Adam *et al.*, 2004). Notwithstanding this, WHO recommend that PZQ should be administered only in the second and third trimester. Women in developing countries may be pregnant or lactating for half of their reproductive lives, therefore the inclusion of this group of females in current control programmes is significant (Savioli *et al.*, 2003). The adverse effects caused by schistosome infection, such as anaemia and poor iron status, are relieved by treatment, and morbidity is reversed, all of which are beneficial to pregnant and lactating women. It is significant that the cost of PZQ has been reduced by about 90% of its original price now that other manufacturers can produce generic formulations, following expiry of the original patents.

One of the disadvantages of PZQ is that it is only effective against adult worms and schistosomula up to about two days of age; it is ineffective against schistosomula over two days of age and immature schistosomes. Depending on the maturation time for the different species of schistosome, this may be for a period between 4 and 8 weeks post-infection. This lack of activity against immature schistosomes possibly provided an explanation of the apparent ineffectiveness of the drug in areas of very high transmission rates, such as in the Senegal River Basin (SRB), although another interpretation at the time was the possible emergence of resistance (Fallon *et al.*, 1995; Stelma *et al.*, 1995; Gryseels *et al.*, 2001; Danso-Appiah and De Vlas, 2002). Indeed, there have been a number of documented cases where infected individuals have not responded to treatment with doses of PZQ at 40 mg/kg body weight (Ismail *et al.*, 1999; Lawn *et al.*, 2003). This has led to concerns as to whether the dose of 40 mg/kg is subcurative and will lead to the development of resistance (Doenhoff *et al.*, 2002). Resistance may be defined as a genetically transmitted loss of sensitivity in a parasite population that was previously sensitive to a given drug, whereas tolerance is an innate insusceptibility of a parasite to a drug, with the caveat that the parasite must have not been previously exposed to the drug (Fallon *et al.*, 1996). However, one aspect of control programmes for schistosomiasis, which mitigates against the development of resistance, is the fact that, simply for logistical reasons, control programmes are usually directed towards school children and high-risk groups, which inevitably means that a number of infected people are left untreated. Therefore, the worms infecting the untreated people are not subjected to selection pressure from PZQ. Subsequent generations from these worms will be able to interbreed with those offspring originating from the worms that have been subjected to PZQ and exhibited a degree of resistance to the drug. Hence, it could be argued that by default, this will slow down the development of resistance or the spread of resistance genes. The importance of leaving worms untreated (in refugia) has been demonstrated with parasites infecting domestic livestock (Coles, 2002a, b).

Interestingly, Botros *et al.* (2005a) returned to the five villages in the Nile Delta region where 1.6% of those infected with intestinal schistosomiasis had failed to respond to treatment with PZQ 10 years earlier. Despite the further 10 years of chemotherapeutic pressure on the schistosomes in these five villages, the survey carried out demonstrated normal cure rates of between 73.8% and 92.3% after one round of treatment with PZQ at 40 mg/kg, and after a further two rounds of treatment at 40 and 60 mg/kg, respectively, there were no uncured patients remaining in the study.

There was just one active national control programme in Africa in 2000, and that was in Egypt. It was very successful, and thanks to support from the World Bank and USAID, the prevalence of schistosomiasis, once over 60% in rural Egypt, was estimated by the Ministry of Health in 2002 to be below 5% although some independent researchers were still insisting prevalence was higher in 'hot spot villages' (Farag *et al.*, 1993; Barakat *et al.*, 2000). By 2002, schistosomiasis was no longer the number one public health problem in Egypt. It is probable that the building of the Aswan High Dam in 1960 changed the irrigation patterns in the Nile Delta, thus playing a part in the reduction of *S. haematobium* transmission and the concomitant increase in *S. mansoni* transmission (Webbe and el Hak, 1990). The decline in *S. haematobium* may have more to do with the changed habitat for *Bulinus* snails than chemotherapy (el Katsha and Watts, 1995; Morgan *et al.*, 2001). Treatment with PZQ from 1988 through to 2000 resulted in haematuria, previously a commonly accepted part of being a teenager, becoming a thing of the past. Squamous cell bladder cancer related to *S. haematobium* infection was in steep decline, and hepatomegaly, ascites and haematemesis due to *S. mansoni* were less common. Schistosomiasis in Egypt does seem to have been controlled, although many believe that vigilance is strongly advisable because conditions remain ripe for transmission to re-emerge once regular treatment is relaxed.

Sustained, versatile control activities in China have reduced the overall prevalence of human infection with *S. japonicum* by 90% from the level initially documented in the mid-1950s. Intersectoral collaboration and community participation ensured the sustained commitment of local resources. The control programme started with a strong focus on intermediate host snail control by means of environmental management but recently the emphasis moved to PZQ-based morbidity control funded by a 10-year World Bank Loan Project (Changsong *et al.*, 2002; Yuan *et al.*, 2002). New research is needed to sustain control and a new promising class of drugs, improved diagnostics, a potential vaccine development, and novel ways of disease risk prediction and transmission control using satellite-based remote sensing are all in the pipeline. There is an expectation that control activities should have the ultimate aim to eliminate schistosomiasis from the Chinese mainland (Utzinger *et al.*, 2005).

2. EPIDEMIOLOGY

2.1. Epidemiology and Distribution, GIS and Disease Prediction

One of the key factors for sustainable control is the ability to identify communities at highest risk of morbidity (Brooker *et al.*, 2005). In order to devise and target optimal intervention strategies, it is essential to know the distribution of schistosomiasis. There are a number of environmental factors that impact on the distribution of schistosomiasis, and coarse scale remote sensing and geographical information systems (GIS) can be of value in looking at distribution on a large spatial scale (Brooker *et al.*, 2000). Temperature, water body type, rainfall, water velocity and altitude can all have a significant effect on the schistosome life-cycle and survival of the intermediate snail host. For example, high temperatures may explain the absence of *Biomphalaria* spp. from coastal East Africa and the consequent absence of *S. mansoni* transmission (Sturrock, 1966). Similarly, high mortality of *B. pfeifferi* in South Africa is associated with periods of continuous high temperature (Appleton, 1977). In Uganda, GIS has been used to map the distribution of infection and to overlay parasitological data with interpolated environmental surfaces (Kabatereine *et al.*, 2004). Infection was shown to be widespread, with prevalence typically highest near the lakeshore and along rivers. Limits to transmission were identified as altitudes greater than 1400 m and areas where total annual rainfall was less than 900 mm. Hence, as well as excluding areas where *S. mansoni* is unlikely to be a problem, the results also identify those areas where the problem of *S. mansoni* is greatest. The analysis helps to estimate the population at risk, thus guiding implementation of intervention and effectively targeting resources (Brooker *et al.*, 2002).

A study in the Cote d'Ivoire shows the power of this approach for generating risk maps which can be used for the design and implementation of schistosomiasis control. Raso *et al.* (2005) collected socio-economic data from 3818 children, aged 6–16 years, from 55 schools and examined each child by the Kato Katz technique for the presence and intensity of *S. mansoni*. They also used remotely sensed environmental data from satellite imagery and digitised ground maps and combined the data sets to establish a comprehensive GIS. Bayesian variogram models were applied for spatial risk modelling and prediction. Interestingly, the goodness of fit of different spatial models revealed that age, sex and socio-economic status had a stronger influence on infection prevalence than environmental covariates.

Progress in China on developing prediction models using remote sensing, GIS and climate data with historical infection prevalence and malacology databases has been reviewed. One of the main issues concerns the effects of the Yangtze River Three Gorges Dam project on environmental changes that may impact on changes in the spatial and temporal distribution and abundance of *S. japonicum* in China, and thus on the future success of disease control programmes (Zhou *et al.*, 2001). Human and animal infection rates with *S. japonicum* have steadily declined in China over the last half-century, but the Three Gorges Dam may reverse this decline by creating new, or enlarging existing, ideal environments for the worm and its amphibious snail intermediate host. Seto *et al.* (2002a) have pointed out that the development of predictive models of the spatial distribution of schistosomiasis is hampered by the existence of different regional subspecies of the *Oncomelania hupensis* snails that serve as intermediate hosts for the disease in China. The habitats associated with these different subspecies vary considerably, with mountainous habitats in the west, and flood plain habitats in the east. Thus, the environmental changes resulting from the Three Gorges Dam and global warming are likely to result in an increase of the snail habitat. Hence with the limited public health resources it will be vital to map accurately and prioritize the areas at risk for schistosomiasis. Prediction of schistosomiasis risk using Landsat TM imagery to identify snail habitats in mountainous regions of Sichuan Province was complicated by the occurrence of seasonal flooding. It was suggested that the incorporation of soil maps may help to solve this complication (Seto *et al.*, 2002b).

A global network of collaborating health workers and earth scientists dedicated to the development of computer-based models that can be used to improve control programmes for schistosomiasis and other snail-borne diseases of medical and veterinary importance has been created (Malone *et al.*, 2001, and see www.gnosisGIS.org). The idea is for models to be assembled using GIS methods, global climate model data, sensor data from earth observing satellites, disease prevalence data, the distribution and abundance of snail hosts, and digital maps of key environmental factors that affect development and propagation of snail-borne disease agents. A work plan has been developed and agreement has been reached on the use of compatible GIS formats, software, methods and data resources, including the definition of a 'minimum medical database' to enable seamless incorporation of results from each regional GIS project into a global model. Gnosis will point users to a toolbox of common resources resident on computers at member organisations, provide assistance on routine use of GIS health maps in selected national disease control programmes and provide a forum for development of GIS models to predict the health impacts of water development projects and climate variation.

2.2. Water-Resource Developments

Plentiful freshwater supplies are essential for human and economic development. Developing countries faced with an increasing human population are required to expand agricultural production and in many areas this can only be achieved by intensification of water impoundment and irrigation. For example, in Africa, only 30% of the land is suitable for food crops if dependent on rainfall. However, by increasing the global area under surface irrigation, opportunities are created for greater food production and increased prosperity. The construction of water schemes to meet increasing agricultural and power requirements may have an unfortunate negative impact on health due to increases in water-borne diseases, especially schistosomiasis. The increase in freshwater habitats associated with dams, either in holding water bodies, irrigation canals or rivers, provides ideal conditions for intermediate snail hosts and facilitates greater water contact and transmission. On the positive side, water development activities such as sinking of wells, provision of clean tap water and adequate latrines, can play a major role in the reduction of transmission by reducing water contact (Jordan *et al.*, 1982).

There are many examples of increased transmission of schistosomiasis as a result of irrigation, the most dramatic being found along the Nile Valley in Egypt and Sudan and more recently along the SRB, where a serious outbreak of intestinal schistosomiasis in populations with no earlier experience of the disease was associated with a large water development programme (Picquet *et al.*, 1996; Southgate, 1997). The Diama Dam became operational in 1985 (Figure 1), approximately 40 km from the mouth of the river, and was constructed to prevent salt-water intrusion from the sea into the river at times of low water flow, and therefore create more freshwater for irrigation of rice and sugarcane cultivation. The Manantali Dam in Mali was completed in 1989 on the Bafing River (tributary of the

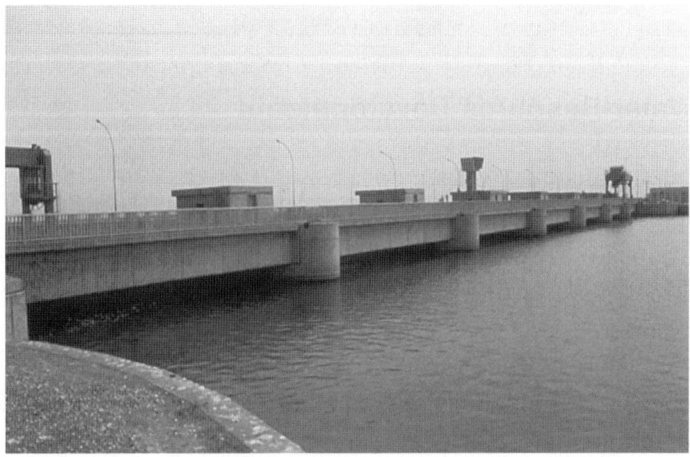

Figure 1 Major water development projects such as the Diama Dam in Senegal, built to prevent salt-water intrusion up the Senegal River, can have a major impact on schistosomiasis.

Senegal river), to provide hydroelectricity for the surrounding area, and to regulate the flow of water down the Senegal River. Prior to the water resource development, donor agencies assessed health risks but no means were provided for schistosomiasis control even though some studies warned of a possible extension of schistosomiasis in the SRB. The increase in prevalence and intensity of infection with *S. mansoni* was rapid. High prevalence of infection was observed in all age groups, suggesting that the infection was recent and that the population was immunologically naive. Intensity of infection, measured by the number of eggs per gram (epg) of faeces, was particularly high. In a cohort of 422 individuals in the town of Richard Toll, Senegal positive egg counts were found in 91% of the subjects, with a mean egg count of 646 epg. Forty-one per cent of the community excreted over 1000 epg and individual egg counts were as high as 24 000 epg (Gryseels *et al.*, 1994). *B. pfeifferi*, a snail which had previously been rare or absent in the lower SRB, rapidly colonised new water canals and proved to be highly compatible with the *S. mansoni* circulating in this region (Tchuem Tchuenté *et al.*, 1999).

During construction of large-scale water development programmes, simple engineering measures could often be taken to reduce the introduction and growth of snail populations and to provide safe and clean water for the local population. For example, concrete lining and covering of irrigation canals, altering the speed of water flow, regular drainage and reduction of water plants, can all help to minimise snail populations. Adequate piped water, washing areas and latrines need to be part of new and old settlements associated with any new water development projects in order to reduce dangerous water contact and contamination.

One example of implementing strategies preventing the spread of schistosomiasis transmission is associated with the building of the Ertan Dam in China (Gu *et al.*, 2001). Concrete irrigation canals and piping systems for the water supply were installed in order to eliminate the infection sources and *Oncomelania* snails. The immigrant workers were encouraged to build methane-generating tanks and improve sanitary facilities and conditions for the families who lived near the water-retaining line. In addition, 2360 people and 152 cattle were treated for schistosome infection and mollusciciding and environmental modification were carried out at an early stage. After three years of intervention, no infected snails were found and no infected people, cattle or wild rats were detected. The success of this project, where schistosomiasis control was financially supported right from the beginning of the Ertan Dam project, is an excellent model of what can be achieved. The authors recommend that continued surveillance of snails and infection sources should be carried out and suggest that the results provide the scientific basis for schistosomiasis control in the Three Gorges region, as well as other new projects of hydropower and water conservation in endemic areas.

There is no doubt that, with adequate planning, some potential problems associated with water developments can be avoided. Ghebreyesus *et al.*, (2002) suggest that the positioning of dams can be important. They assessed the impact of micro-dam construction in the northern Ethiopian highlands, in relation to possible increased risks of *S. mansoni* infection. They showed altitude and gender to be significant risk factors for infection, whereas proximity to a micro-dam was not significant, except possibly at very high altitudes. It was concluded that altitude was the major factor in this environment and that therefore, at least in terms of public health planning, micro-dams should be sited as high as local geography permits.

2.3. Infection, Re-infection and Genetic Factors

It has long been established that prevalence and intensity of infection change over the lifetime of an individual living in an endemic area. In established transmission foci, the peak of both prevalence and intensity is recorded around adolescence. Studies on treatment and rates of re-infection have shown that chemotherapy reduces egg excretion but children become rapidly re-infected. For example, Etard *et al.*, (1995) examined the effect of age, previous intensity of infection and exposure on rates of re-infection with *S. haematobium* after treatment in a cohort of 468 subjects six years of age and over, living within an irrigation scheme area in Mali. Prevalence and intensity of *S. haematobium* infection were measured each year between 1989 and 1991, but the re-infection study period was restricted to the last year of the follow-up. Observations were made at the principal water contact sites where the number of *Bulinus truncatus* shedding furcocercous cercariae was recorded. A cumulative index of exposure, taking into account time, duration, type of contact and malacological data, was calculated for each subject. Univariate analysis showed that the re-infection risk decreased with age and increased with exposure and pre-treatment intensity. These results were confirmed by fitting a logistic model that showed that this risk was seven times lower among those 15 years of age and older than among the 6–14-year-old children, while linear trends with exposure to infection and pre-treatment intensity were significant. The study supported the concept of an age-acquired resistance to re-infection and is in favour of a predisposition to infection thus raising the question of a genetic factor controlling susceptibility/resistance to *S. haematobium* infection.

The role of genetic factors in resistance to schistosomes has been the subject of numerous investigations. Abel *et al.*, (1991) investigated whether a major gene controls human susceptibility/resistance to infection by *S. mansoni*. Segregation analysis of infection intensities, adjusted for the factors relevant in schistosomiasis (water contact, age and sex), was performed on 20 Brazilian pedigrees (269 individuals), using both the unified mixed model and the regressive model of analysis. The results were consistent with the hypothesis that there is a co-dominant major gene controlling human susceptibility/resistance to infection by *S. mansoni*. Further work has identified the chromosome regions responsible and defined associations between particular human genotypes and infection status (Abel *et al.*, 2000; Quinnell, 2003; Kouriba *et al.*, 2005). The role that genetic factors might play in the development of pathology was examined by Kariuki *et al.*, (2001). Schistosomal fibrosis was identified during hepatic examination using ultrasound in a Kenyan population, and it was found that the peak prevalence of ultrasound proven fibrosis trailed 5–10 years behind the peak prevalence of infection, and declined sharply after age 50 years. This pattern was consistent with either resolution of severe fibrosis over 10–20 years or early death of those severely affected. Genetic predisposition appeared to be a weak factor in the development of severe disease in this population, since no household or familial aggregation could be identified.

3. CONTROL

3.1. Current Control Objectives and Strategies—Global Persuasion

There is no doubt that since 2000 there has been a greater interest in the health and well-being of Africans, with the result that today there are more and more national programmes to control schistosomiasis, mostly implemented within school health programmes and integrated with de-worming (removal of gastrointestinal helminths). The incentives for these programmes have been the reduction in the price of the drug praziquantel, funding from the Bill and Melinda Gates Foundation (www.gatesfoundation.org), the Millennium Development Goals (www.undp.org/mdg/), emphasis on reducing poverty and, more recently in 2005, the report of the Commission for Africa (www.commissionforafrica.org/) (Abugre *et al.*, 2005; Kiely, 2005).

At the 2001 Annual World Health Assembly, a strategy for control of schistosomiasis (and intestinal helminths) was approved, as summarised in the World Health Assembly resolution WHA 54.19 of May 2001.

The resolution urges Member States to ensure access to essential drugs against schistosomiasis and soil-transmitted helminthiasis in all health services in endemic areas for the treatment of clinical cases and groups at high risk of morbidity such as women and children. The aim is to attain a minimum target of regular administration of chemotherapy to at least 75% and up to 100% of all school-aged children at risk of morbidity by 2010. This policy is based on the evidence that morbidity can be controlled by periodic treatment of high-risk groups with anthelmintics.

Schistosomiasis, with its complicated life cycle sometimes including reservoir hosts is unlikely to be eradicated; any control programme should pre-determine its targets to avoid disappointment. Countries on the fringe of the endemic areas (e.g. Morocco), or countries with a high socio-economic development status (e.g. Puerto Rico) may target elimination. Only when water supplies and sanitation become universally available, and when improvements in education and socio-economic development have been achieved (as in Puerto Rico), can elimination of a water-borne disease such as schistosomiasis be contemplated. Therefore, in sub-Saharan Africa, where socio-economic development is slow, and provision of clean water and sanitation facilities are less than satisfactory, Ministries embarking on a disease control programme need to set realistic targets, first aiming for a reduction of morbidity by a treatment regime targeting heavily infected individuals as measured by egg output. A defined treatment strategy, either mass treatment of communities, mass treatment of school-aged children and or a 'selective population chemotherapy' targeting high-risk occupational groups should be selected according to baseline data.

Africa has not developed economically as much as Asia during the last 50 years, and so most of the poorest countries in the world are now on the African continent, and the poorest populations in those countries are either infected or at risk of schistosomiasis. The many millions of people infected deserve to be treated but cannot themselves afford to purchase the medication. Centrally funded control programmes are needed with the short-term objective of targeting the highly-risk populations in highly endemic areas with one, two or three treatments just to reduce worm burdens and reduce morbidity. Regular mass treatment of school-aged children, as a longer-term intervention would reduce the probability of morbidity developing in the future. Taking into account that in some countries, school attendance may not be high enough to guarantee adequate coverage, provision must be made to reach children who fail to attend school.

3.2. Current Strategies to Reduce and Reverse Morbidity using Praziquantel

The strategy for controlling morbidity due to schistosomiasis is based on chemotherapy using PZQ as defined in Table 1. The preferred methods for selecting the target populations to be treated are still under review.

WHO has generated, after a long process of consensus building, a strategy whereby most adults and children infected or at risk of

Table 1 WHO recommended treatment strategy for control of schistosomiasis

Community category	Prevalence in school survey	Strategy
High prevalence	>30% visible haematuria or	Access to PZQ for passive case treatment
Over 50% infection	>50% *S. mansoni* or *S. haematobium* by parasitology	Targeted mass treatment of school-aged children, once a year
		Offer Community Directed (mass) Treatment to high-risk groups
Moderate prevalence	<30% visible haematuria or	Access to PZQ for passive case treatment
10–50% infected	10–50% *S. mansoni* or *S. haematobium* by parasitology	Targeted mass treatment of school-aged children, annually or once every 2 years
Low prevalence	No visible haematuria	Access to PZQ for passive case treatment
Less than 10% infected	Or <10% *S. mansoni* or *S. haematobium* by parasitology	Targeted treatment of school-aged children, twice during primary schooling (once on entry, again on leaving)

developing morbidity will receive the treatment they need, and a sustainable programme of routine treatment of school-aged children will be introduced.

The number of PZQ tablets needed to treat any individual is dependent on the weight of the patient: the recommended dose is 40 mg/kg body weight. However, weighing scales are notoriously ineffective in Africa under conditions of heat, dust and uneven ground. Therefore an alternative measure has been developed which is the tablet pole: a wooden or even paper pole which is marked off in sections, where each section is a dose from one tablet rising by half tablets to four tablets (Figure 2). The dose pole has been validated in several countries for children, but may be less accurate for adults (Montresor *et al.*, 2001). The effectiveness of PZQ and its safety margins in dosage ensures that any source of error in using a pole is relatively unimportant.

It is recommended that the selection of the target population for mass treatment is based on Low Quality Assurance Sampling

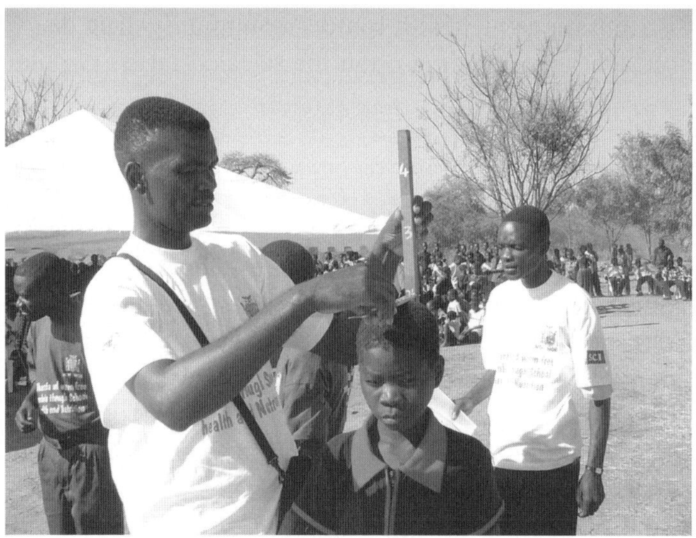

Figure 2 A wooden dose pole being used in Zambia.

(LQAS), which means that a small number of samples are examined and the results extrapolated to the larger population (Brooker *et al.*, 2005). For *S. haematobium*, the selected sample of individuals could be subjected to a questionnaire to determine reported blood in urine, and asked to provide a urine sample which could then be examined either microscopically, to identify at least one egg of the parasite, or by using a dipstick to detect blood which is taken as a marker for infection. Comparative studies have shown that the questionnaire approach underestimates the true prevalence by perhaps 30% and dipstick testing by 15% as compared to the more resource intensive but more accurate microscopic examination of urine (N'Goran *et al.*, 1998). Nevertheless, because these methods have been validated, they can substitute for the parasitological examination of urine. For *S. mansoni*, LQAS sampling can still be used, but the selected individuals must be asked to provide a stool sample, which is then examined under a microscope. A single slide from a stool sample examined will not identify all infections, especially when egg output is low. The mechanism selected for delivery of the drug to the target populations will depend on the local circumstances, but could be either distribution using health centres, community drug distributors, or schoolteachers, depending upon the selected target population.

3.3. Other Drugs

There has been considerable interest in the use of artemether, because this drug is more active than PZQ against the immature stages of schistosomes in the definitive host (Utzinger *et al.*, 2001, 2002). At the moment, the data are somewhat equivocal as to the benefits of using artemether with PZQ. Furthermore, because of the likelihood of the use of artemether as both a curative and prophylactic drug for malaria, it has been argued that it should not be used indiscriminately as a weapon against schistosomiasis, especially in areas where both malaria and schistosomiasis are sympatric. It has been demonstrated in a comparative study that the results obtained using PZQ were consistently better than those achieved with artesunate, an artemisin derivative, in the treatment of *S. haematobium* in primary school children in the villages of Lampsar and Makhana, in the delta of the SRB (De Clercq *et al.*, 2000, 2002).

Mirazid, an extract of myrrh, an aromatic gum resin derived from the plant *Commiphora molmol*, has been used extensively in Egypt as an alternative to PZQ. Mirazid has an attraction to both practitioners and patients because of its natural origin and price. However, recent data (Fenwick *et al.*, 2003; Botros *et al.*, 2004; Botros *et al.*, 2005b) question the usefulness of mirazid in the control of schistosomiasis, and their data contradict the claims (Sheir *et al.*, 2001; Abo-Madyan *et al.*, 2004) about the effectiveness of the drug in killing schistosomes. It may be helpful for an independent body, such as the World Health Organization, to organise some studies outside of Egypt to resolve this controversy about the effectiveness of mirazid once and for all.

3.4. Health Education

Schistosomiasis is regarded as a disease of poverty and is most prevalent in areas where supplies of clean water serving a community are

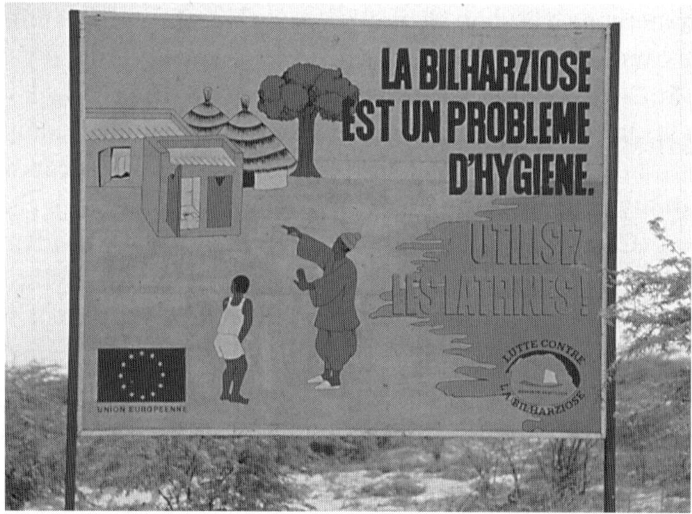

Figure 3   A road sign in Senegal contributing to health education.

either non-existent or at a minimal level. It is likely that as supplies of clean water become more available to communities living in endemic areas, periods of contact with natural, infected water bodies will be reduced, but health education should also be in place to improve people's knowledge of the causes, prevention and treatment of endemic diseases, including schistosomiasis. Health education can be incorporated into the Primary Health Care system (PHC), and also as part of control programmes in schools. Use of mass media, for example, radio, television, newspapers and posters, will facilitate health education of the adult population (Figure 3). It is hoped that the increase of knowledge and understanding of how schistosomiasis is transmitted, coupled with increases in standard of living, such as increases of supply of clean water, will eventually lead to changes of behaviour in the community, thus minimising contact with infected waters.

3.5. Vaccines

There is no doubt that an effective vaccine against human schistosomiasis would be a very effective control tool and an addition to current methods based on chemotherapy. Over the years, a number of vaccine candidates have been identified (e.g. paramysosin, irV-5, TPI, Sm23, Sm24 and glutathione-*S*-transferase (GST)). The lack of protection given by these vaccine candidates dashed initial optimism, but immunisation with GST showed a decrease in parasite fecundity and egg viability, and reduction in worm burden resulting from challenge infection (Capron *et al.*, 1992). However, despite these advances it seems that a major obstacle in vaccine development is the actual identification of antigens that mediate protection; the size of schistosome genome at 280 Mb DNA encoding up to 20 000 genes makes this task difficult, but the advances in both proteomics and the schistosomes genome project may make this task less forbidding in the future (Wilson *et al.*, 2004). Some researchers argue that a protective vaccine represents an essential component for the long-term control of schistosomiasis (McManus and Bartley, 2004). Bergquist *et al.*, (2005) suggest the combined use of chemotherapy and vaccination will serve as a basis for a novel, more versatile approach to control: a vaccine formulation based on novel adjuvants may improve the final outcome through selective manipulation of the immune response. Hagan and Sharaf (2003) emphasised the challenges in vaccine development against larger metazoan parasites such as schistosomes and the considerable difficulties reaching the stage of Phase 3 clinical trials.

4. SCHISTOSOMIASIS CONTROL INITIATIVE

4.1. Overview and Progress

The SCI is an African success story: successfully targeting morbidity due to schistosomiasis and intestinal worms using treatment, targeting children to improve their health and nutritional status, thus improving their chances of attending school and receiving a more effective education.

The SCI (www.schisto.org) was established in 2000 as a pilot programme to develop national strategies for a number of African countries, and in mid-2002 was awarded almost $30 million (US) funding from the Bill and Melinda Gates Foundation. The aim was to implement and evaluate, for the first time, six national control programmes to treat schistosomiasis in sub-Saharan Africa. However, what started as a single disease control programme has been expanded to integrate treatment of gastrointestinal helminths by co-administration of albendazole.

Administration of a single oral dose of praziquantel treats schistosomiasis and the addition of albendazole offers an effective and safe single oral treatment for the gastrointestinal helminths *Ascaris lumbricoides*, *Trichuris trichiura* and hookworm. One reason for this integration is that SCI monitors success by measuring changes in anaemia levels in children after treatment, and since hookworm and schistosomiasis co-exist, and both contribute to anaemia, it is logical to treat both infections concurrently. In 2005, the cost of a treatment with PZQ for a school child is approximately 20 US cents, and the albendazole costs less than an additional 2 US cents.

During the first three years of operation, SCI selected six countries to support from 12 applications. The selection criteria included the extent of the problem in the applicant countries, the strength of support from the government, the quality of staff available with whom to work, the probability of being able to make a difference, and the ability to carry out Monitoring and Evaluation (M&E) of the results. The six countries selected were Uganda (in 2002) and then Burkina Faso, Mali, Niger, United Republic of Tanzania and Zanzibar, and Zambia (in 2003) (Figure 4). With SCI support, the 6 countries have made the following progress. National plans have been developed; high level political commitment has been achieved and schistosomiasis control and school health have been placed in the Health Sector Strategic Plans; local government level administrators have been informed as to the effects of these infections and the value of treatment; teachers and community health workers have been trained to administer these drugs to selected populations; up to 1 million children and adults have been treated in three of the poorest countries in West Africa: Burkina Faso, Niger and Mali, and over 2 million people have been treated in Uganda; Uganda has commenced annual de-worming of children through 'health days' scheduled annually for October; pilot treatments have been carried out in conjunction with

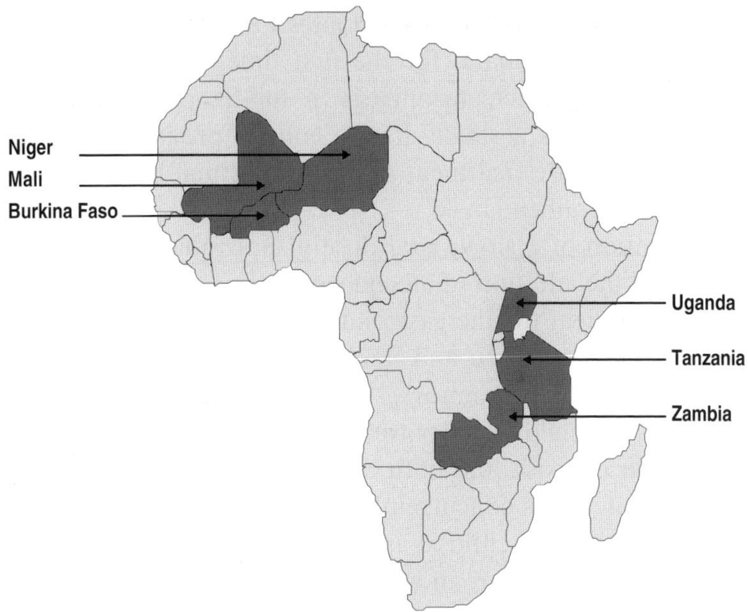

Figure 4 Map of Africa showing countries with schistosomiasis control programmes supported by SCI.

the World Food Programme in Tanzania and Zambia; large-scale treatment is planned for Tanzania and Zambia through school health programmes. Table 2 shows the current rate of treatment in the six countries supported by SCI. During 2005, the target population for treatment of 10 million individuals in the countries was reached and this number is set to double in 2006.

Not only is it cheap and easy to treat schistosomiasis and intestinal worms, but also the benefits are dramatic. Miguel *et al.*, (2004) have demonstrated that de-worming children reduces overall school absenteeism by 25%. Others have shown an immediate disappearance of blood in the urine and a reversal of liver pathology (Mahmoud *et al.*, 1983; Kheir *et al.*, 2000).

The Bill and Melinda Gates Foundation funding to SCI is due to finish in 2007, and by then SCI must ensure that the national programmes that have started have sustainable support to continue. Without new funding, the achievements of the countries and SCI will soon be reversed.

Table 2   The current rate of treatment in the six countries supported by SCI

	Launch date	Treated by June 2005	Total to be treated in 2005	Comments
Burkina Faso	May 2004	1.05 million children	2.5 million children	1 year follow up in 2005
Mali	November 2004	1.8 million	3.2 million	1 year follow up in 2006
Niger	October 2004	1.9 million	3.3 million	1 year follow up in 2006
Tanzania	July 2005	0.6 million	4 million children	1 year follow up in 2006
Uganda	March 2003	1.4 million adults and children (in 2004)	4 million	Three rounds to be completed in 2006/7
Zambia	June 2005	0.1 million	0.6 million children	1 year follow up in 2006
Totals		6.85 million	17.6 million	

Attitudes have changed, the perception of these diseases has changed and the knowledge of the damage caused by these infections has changed. The technology to treat schistosomiasis exists. The resources needed are minimal in a global context. What is now needed is a commitment by bi-lateral donors, international organisations and global funding sources to make the funds available. Perhaps after the G8 summit at Gleneagles, Scotland in 2005, the additional funding needed will materialise.

The SCI message is 'For an average of $0.50 per person treated per year, morbidity due to schistosomiasis and intestinal helminths could be reduced dramatically within five years. The infection would not be eliminated, but residual infections would be at low levels and of insignificant health importance. With an investment of $0.50 per child per year, all children in Africa could go to school, ready to face the day, feeling good, healthy and better nourished' (Fenwick *et al.*, 2005).

Soon after SCI was established, the 2001 World Health Assembly resolution 54.19 stated that all Member States in endemic areas should reach 75% of all school-aged children by the year 2010 with regular treatment for schistosomiasis and intestinal helminths. By assisting countries to target those at high risk of developing severe morbidity, especially school-aged children, women and those in high-risk occupations, SCI is improving the lives of the communities and creating the political momentum for change. It is hoped that successful national control programmes will create a demand for continued treatment within that country and other countries in Africa.

In each SCI supported country, a Memorandum of Understanding between the Government and Imperial College of Science, Technology and Medicine, London was developed to allow duty-free importation of essential drugs and equipment. Each government appoints National Co-ordinators and local administration staff. A conduit for funding is established in each country, which allows the co-ordinators to purchase essential equipment such as computers, communications, ultrasound machines, microscopes and vehicles. SCI provides technical assistance to each country until 2007, but to ensure that the programme remains country owned, no country-based expatriate staff are involved. Training courses are provided for local managers and administrators to ensure the required financial and management skills are available.

The treatment campaign in Uganda has been developed since 1999, but after training, implementation commenced in 2003, when the Vector Control Division of the Ministry of Health received supplies of PZQ and albendazole from SCI. In 2003, some 400 000 individuals including both adults and children were treated. In 2004, the same 400 000 were offered treatment again, and some 1 million people in the expanded area were offered a treatment for the first time. In 2005, the 400 000 received their third treatment, 1 million were treated for a second time and an extra 3 million received their first treatment. The SCI and the Ugandan scientists are working out what to do next, and how many treatments need to be carried out in relation to pre-treatment prevalence and intensity in order to reduce morbidity (Brooker *et al.*, 2004).

The Uganda Government has taken the first step towards integration (Ndyomugyenyi and Kabatereine, 2003) and, in November 2003, when a measles campaign was being organised by the Ministry of Health, WHO and UNICEF, it was decided that to make the package more attractive to parents, albendazole would be offered to children over five who presented for their measles vaccination. In one week, approximately 8 million children were de-wormed and received their measles vaccination, and this programme has become an annual event. The highest prevalence and intensity of schistosomiasis in Uganda is around the Lakes, but it is focal, which means that while countrywide the prevalence may be just over 10% in selected foci, there is almost 100% severe infection (Kabatereine *et al.*, 2004).

Results have shown that as a result of the National Control Programme in Uganda, awareness has increased many fold, prevalence of infection in the heavy infection group has been reduced, but most striking the prevalence of heavy intensity infections has fallen significantly. However, it is interesting to note that in an endemic area for *S. haematobium* in Burkina Faso, one round of treatment reduced prevalence from over 90% to less than 5% thus contrasting to the heavily endemic areas of *S. mansoni* (Fenwick, unpublished data). The explanation for these differences in reduction of prevalence may be linked with the differences in worms burden between *S. haematobium* and *S. mansoni*.

4.2. Political Commitment

SCI has recruited Ministerial and Presidential support for the control programmes, ensuring commitment and high visibility within each of the six countries. In Zanzibar, President Karume launched the national control programmes for the control of schistosomiasis and intestinal helminths on the islands of Unguja and Pemba on 18 October 2003 and 6 January 2004, respectively. In Burkina Faso, the programme was launched by the Minister of Health in the Kingdom of Ouahigouiya on 6 May 2004, in the presence of his Majesty the King. In Niger, the national programme was launched on 6 October 2004 by the Minister of Health. In Mali, the launch took place on 23 November 2004, under the patronage of the First Lady of Mali (Figure 5). In Zambia, the Minister of Education launched the programme on 21 June 2005. In Tanzania, the launch took place on 2 July 2005 and was attended by the Prime Minister and the Minister of

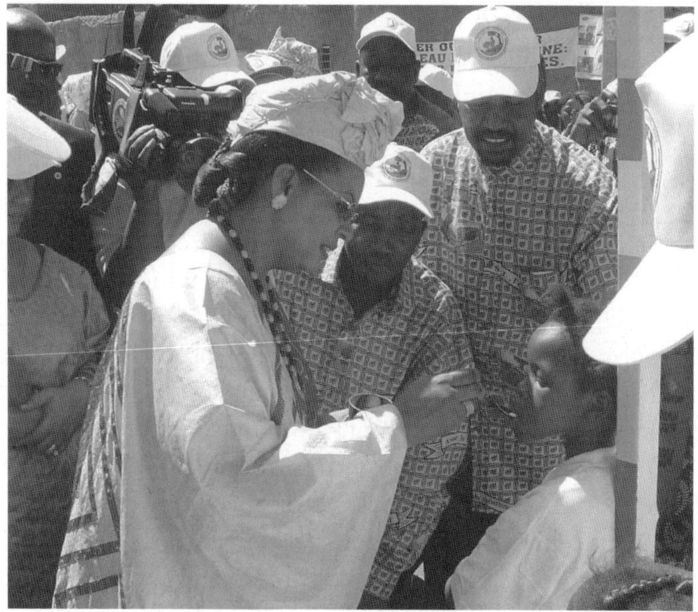

Figure 5   Launch of the National Schistosomiasis Control Programme in Mali, the first lady participates and treats a child.

Health. The launch preceded a national campaign to treat up to 4.5 million school aged children through the schools.

4.3. Procurement of Praziquantel and Albendazole

A major and practical role of SCI has been to provide funds for, and arrange procurement of, praziquantel and albendazole. Furthermore, SCI has endeavoured to ensure that the market could sustain the increased demand. In 2005, SCI encouraged two African-based manufacturers to formulate the drugs to international price and quality standards. An African disease can be treated with African formulated drugs. SCI has also initiated a donation programme to supplement the Gates Foundation funding, and Canadian donors working through MedPharm, an American pharmaceutical company, have responded with a supply of over 14 million tablets of praziquantel during 2004.

4.4. Future Strategies

Since 1999, there has been an expansion of the activities of several vertical disease control programmes, namely the International Trachoma Initiative (ITI) (www.trachoma.org), the Global Programme for the Elimination of Lymphatic Filariasis (GPELF) (www. filariasis.org) and the African Programme for Onchocerciasis Control (APOC). Since these programmes mostly target the same populations in Africa, their managers have started to work together to integrate each of their activities in several countries. These successful vertical programmes need to co-ordinate implementation activities to minimise duplication of effort and maximise possible synergies. SCI is trying to implement integration in different settings in Burkina Faso, Tanzania and Uganda (Ndyomugyenyi and Kabatereine, 2003).

By 2007, SCI should have facilitated treatment of over 30 million people, and many will have been treated more than once. The question is whether treating any individuals beyond three times is desirable, cost effective or necessary, and what should be the exit strategy—or long-term maintenance strategy? Also how can the success in six countries be expanded to the whole of sub-Saharan Africa, where it is estimated that the need is for 180 million people to be treated?

5. LOW TRANSMISSION AREAS

5.1. Towards Elimination of the Disease

Although schistosomiasis is found in approximately 76 countries of the tropics and sub-tropics, low transmission occurs in many of the countries on the periphery of the distribution of the disease. In April 2000, the World Health Organization hosted a consultation on schistosomiasis in low transmission areas in order to provide advice on control strategies for countries for example, Morocco, Oman, Mauritius and some of the Caribbean islands where elimination is considered feasible. In many cases, the low transmission of the disease is associated with implementation of control measures using chemotherapy, biological control and improvement of sanitation facilities. In some countries, there is always the constant problem of immigration of infected people from neighbouring endemic countries, and if snail control methods have either not been implemented or have been unsuccessful, it is understandable how easily transmission reappears after the disease has been eliminated.

From a clinical point of view, the indicators of interrupted transmission are the disappearance of typical symptoms and signs in the children born after the presumed date of eradication. Nevertheless, late stage syndromes and sequelae frequently persist in formerly infected individuals. Resurgence in an old focus is indicated by the occurrence of acute or early stage symptoms in the subjects who are younger than the interval since transmission has been interrupted (Andrade, 1998; Enk *et al.*, 2003; Bethony *et al.*, 2004).

Even in countries with very low transmission rates on the point of elimination of the disease, or indeed in those countries where transmission has been eliminated, it is essential that surveillance be continued, especially in known high-risk groups and in people living in specific risk areas/regions within the countries. In countries where schistosomiasis is on the point of elimination, case detection may be a problem because commonly used parasitological and clinical diagnostic procedures may not be sufficiently sensitive to detect people with light infections. In such situations, it may be more appropriate to utilise more sensitive diagnostic techniques, such as schistosome antigen assays. Experience from several countries is summarised below.

The well-managed control programme in Morocco reduced prevalence of *S. haematobium* from 10 645 cases in 1983 to 231 cases in 1999. In 2005, there was only a handful of cases in Tala province, and the disease is approaching elimination (Laamrani *et al.*, 2000a, b).

Both *S. haematobium* and *S. mansoni* are endemic in Saudi Arabia at levels of prevalence less than 1% as a result of a control strategy implemented in 1985 using chemotherapy, focal mollusciciding and health education. Prior to the control measures, prevalences of more than 40% were reported in several parts of the country (Arfaa, 1976). In the mid-1980s, the Ministry of Health recommended that schistosomiasis control operations should be integrated into the PHC system, which had more than 90% population coverage and therefore offered excellent opportunities to conduct chemotherapy programmes and to incorporate surveillance and maintenance operations. By the late 1980s, the goal of 1% prevalence was achieved, and has since been maintained, but at least 95% of the population have access to potable water, and the vast majority of vulnerable school children has access to schools. Therefore, the control teams that have worked in liaison with the Ministry of Education have had access to schoolchildren, a particularly vulnerable group. Today, about half of the people with schistosomiasis in Saudi Arabia are immigrants. The strategy for control of schistosomiasis has been integrated with other programmes, such as the control of gastrointestinal helminths, and these programmes are implemented through the PHC and field vector control stations. Indeed, integration of control programmes for different parasitic diseases is now a common strategy and reduces costs of drug delivery. Al Ghahtani and Amin (2005) reported on the successful elimination of *S. haematobium* from the Jazan region of Saudi Arabia with a strategy based on regular chemotherapy, snail control and health education, with screening at PHC centres by mobile teams and at diagnostic units. These authors suggest that total elimination in Saudi Arabia is possible if the health authorities in neighbouring areas can be persuaded to adopt a similar strategy of control.

The combined approach of selective chemotherapy, mollusciciding and additional provision of supplies of clean water in Iran reduced prevalence rates of *S. haematobium* in South-West Iran from 8.3% in 1970 to 0.01% by 1999 (Massoud, 2000). The incidence of infection between 1989 and 1999 was nil (Massoud, 2000).

Small numbers of people have been found infected with *S. mansoni* in the environs of Salalah, Oman, since 1979, but the quickly implemented government control programme comprising of mollusciciding, chemotherapy and health education has kept control of the situation although has yet to eliminate the disease from Oman (Idris *et al.*, 2003).

Mauritius is another example where urinary schistosomiasis is very close to elimination, and in 1993 the prevalence in the general population was 0.9%. There are only three endemic areas in Mauritius; Pamplemousses, Port Louis and Grand Port. The strategy for elimination in Mauritius consists of screening for microhaematuria and/or eggs in urine, chemotherapy, health education and mollusc-iciding (Dhunputh, 1994).

Infection with *S. mansoni* was historically one of the more serious public health problems in the Caribbean islands, but as a result of control programmes, including chemotherapy and biological control, intestinal schistosomiasis has either been eliminated or the prevalence has been markedly reduced. For example, the Dominican Republic is the northern limit for the extension of schistosomiasis in the Caribbean, and in the late 1980s, prevalence varied between 7.4%and 24.6% in different parts of the island. The competitive displacement of the intermediate host *B. glabrata* by two different species of freshwater snail, *Marisa cornuarietis* and *Tarebia granifera*, undoubtedly impinged on levels of transmission and has led to significantly lower levels of prevalence (Hillyer, 1983; Vargas *et al.*, 1987).

Similarly, in Puerto Rico, an epidemiological and malacological survey by Giboda *et al.* (1997) demonstrated a very low prevalence (0.6%) in the community, and the absence of *B. glabrata* was apparently primarily due to the invasion of the competitive snails, *M. cornuarietis* and *T. granifera* (Giboda *et al.*, 1997; Giboda and Bergquist, 2000).

In Martinique, the biological control programme, together with improved sanitation, has apparently interrupted transmission. However, in this case, another species of freshwater snail, *Melanoides tuberculata*, was successfully used as a competitor snail to replace *B. glabrata*. Consequently, there was a marked decline in disease prevalence in man between 1977 and 1996, and parasite transmission has now ceased (Schlegel *et al.*, 1997).

Guadeloupe presents a somewhat different situation because the rat, *Rattus rattus*, serves as a reservoir host for *S. mansoni* in the marshy forest area of Grand Terre island. Consequently the parasite is more difficult to eliminate from this part of Guadeloupe. Nevertheless, the integrated control programme has eliminated the parasite from Basse Terre island (Combes *et al.*, 1982).

In 1965, a research and control programme was initiated on the island of St. Lucia, where prevalence ranged between 22% and 57%. Several unique valleys were subjected to baseline data collection followed by different control interventions involving water supplies, chemotherapy, snail control, health education, etc. Prevalence had been reduced by the end of the project to levels between 4% and 14% (Dalton, 1976; Prentice *et al.*, 1981; Barnish *et al.*, 1982; Jordan *et al.*, 1982a, b). In the late 1970s, the introduction of *M. tuberculata* to the island had the effect of markedly reducing the populations of *B. glabrata*, thereby contributing to the control of the disease on the island through biological control (Prentice, 1983; Pointier and McCullough, 1989; Pointier and Jourdane, 2000).

Brazil is in a somewhat different situation from those countries that are on the verge of elimination of the disease. Notwithstanding that the success of morbidity control in Brazil by the Schistosomiasis Control Programme has been of great benefit to the population at large, nevertheless, it is estimated that about 2.5 million people remain infected currently, with an additional 25 million people at risk of infection. Approximately 19 of the country's 27 states remain endemic for schistosomiasis (da Silva *et al.*, 2002).

Japan is an example of a country where elimination has actually been achieved and there have been no new cases of schistosomiasis in Japan since 1977 (Hurter and Yokogawa, 1984).

6. INTEGRATION AND SUSTAINABILITY

6.1. Integration with other Health Programmes

In Africa today, there are a number of diseases of poverty, which are being tackled by vertical programmes using regular distribution of safe and effective chemotherapy, either aiming for elimination or morbidity control. Some programmes include more than just chemotherapy (e.g. trachoma and lymphatic filariasis (LF) have both a surgery and a hygiene component). In most countries, there are a number of international organisations and NGOs established, usually working independently of each other in the field of health. Each will have its own agenda, perhaps targeting pre-school-aged children or school children or other segments of the population, some on a large scale, but usually on a relatively small scale.

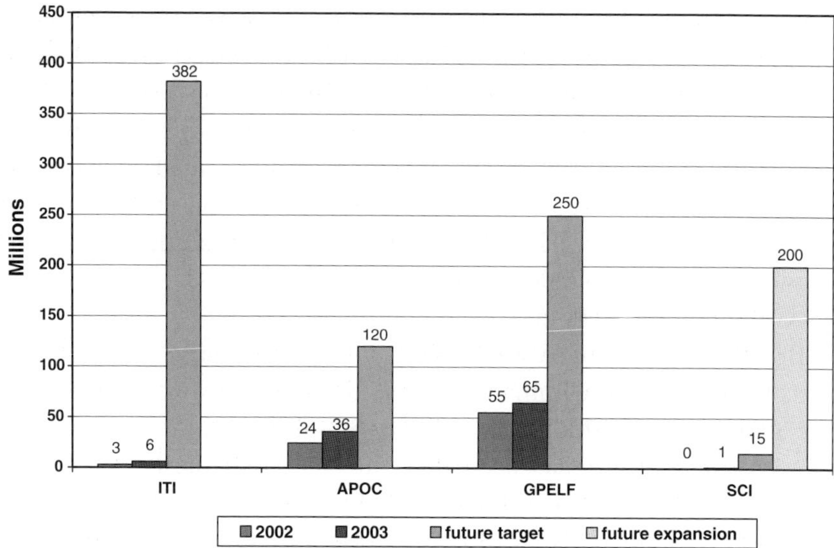

Figure 6 A chart showing past, present and future targets of major control initiatives (Fenwick, 2006).

Since the late 1990s, several global health partnerships targeting specific diseases have been established with the objectives of achieving global coverage and morbidity control or disease elimination for LF.

As shown in Figure 6, each of these programmes has plans to expand coverage almost exponentially. However, as they expand, the same poverty stricken poly-parasitised individuals are being targeted with a number of interventions. There is a danger of wasteful duplication of effort and overlapping of national programmes causing confusion among drug deliverers and recipients and even unnecessary treatments. It is therefore time for these vertical programmes to collaborate. The expansion of control programmes in Africa now requires development of an appropriate health package to be delivered under the co-ordination of government, identifying roles and responsibilities of the different partners and devolving resources and implementation responsibility to local levels. This can only be achieved by:

1. Improved communication and collaboration between donors and international programme managers (including African

Programme for Onchocerciasis Control (APOC), International Trachoma Initiative (ITI), (SCI), Global Alliance for the Elimination of Filariasis (GPELF) and international organisations such as WHO, World Food Programme (WFP) and UNICEF).
2. Improved communication in the individual country between decision makers in the Ministries of Health and Education, national disease control programme managers, NGOs and local representatives of WHO, WFP and UNICEF.
3. Strengthened health systems and linked control efforts within health sector frameworks against the diseases of poverty (schistosomiasis, intestinal helminths, LF, onchocerciasis, trachoma and malnutrition) to minimise duplication of effort.
4. Synergise intervention where possible (particularly with mapping, village census taking, training, health education and drug delivery) to optimise use of available human and financial resources.

In the 1990s, in the absence of any control measures, the prevalence of infectious and parasitic diseases in Africa was so high that almost every individual in rural Africa was infected with at least one parasite and many would have multiple infections. In 2005, an estimated 500 million people in Africa suffer from one or more of these infections—malaria (which kills one million children every year), schistosomiasis (bilharzia, 180 million infected), onchocerciasis (river blindness, 5 million infected), intestinal helminths (hookworm and round worm, 400 million infected), trachoma (preventable blindness, 84 million infected and over 8 million visually impaired) and LF (elephantiasis, 120 million infected in 83 countries) (Molyneux *et al.*, 2005). There are other parasitic diseases/infections, including leishmaniasis and trypanosomiasis (sleeping sickness) for which no easy and effective cure is currently available (Figure 7, which is Plate 13.7 in the separate colour plate section). While these parasitic diseases (with the exception of malaria) are rarely acute killers, they debilitate their hosts and leave them vulnerable to other infections.

It is estimated that malaria, HIV/AIDS and TB are responsible for 50% of all morbidity and mortality as measured by Disability Adjusted Life Years (DALYs) lost. However, the 12 parasitic and infectious diseases, which are known as 'neglected diseases' contribute 25% of the DALYs lost.

By 2004, a number of separate programmes had been launched using proven chemotherapeutic products. These programmes, mostly vertical public private partnerships, are based on multinational pharmaceutical company drug donations, local social mobilisation and drug delivery, using international expertise for management, M&E and parallel operational research.

The major programmes that are currently active include: the GPELF has overseen the treatment of some 80 million people with albendazole and either ivermectin (Mectizan®) or diethylcarbamazine (DEC) during 2003. Final GPELF targets are 1 billion worldwide, including 470 million people in Africa. The drugs are donated by Merck (Mectizan®) and GSK (albendazole).

The ITI has plans to target 200 million individuals for treatment with azithromycine (Zithromax® donated by Pfizer) to prevent blindness.

The APOC reaches 20 million people annually in 19 countries with Mectizan® (Merck) to control river blindness.

The SCI promotes implementation of national schistosomiasis and intestinal helminth control programmes using praziquantel and albendazole in six countries—over 15 million individuals will receive treatment by 2006. The drugs used by SCI have been purchased using funds donated by the Bill and Melinda Gates Foundation, supplemented by drug donations from the pharmaceutical company MedPharm using Canadian citizens' charitable donations.

De-worming and distribution of micro-nutrients to the under 5-year-olds is growing in Africa under the auspices of the Micro-nutrients Initiative (MI) and UNICEF, and WHO are currently negotiating with another multinational drug company for a sizable long-term donation of mebendazole for de-worming.

The SCI, GPELF, ITI, MI and APOC, plus the governments of Burkina Faso and Tanzania, partners such as WHO, WFP, UNICEF, NGOs including Save the Children, Catholic Relief Service (CRS), Helen Keller International (HKI) and Axios and the companies donating drugs (Merck, GSK, Pfizer and MedPharm) should examine the feasibility of integration of the current vertical programmes and develop a health package, which should be flexible enough to be a model for Africa. In so doing, they should address the policy, systems, technical, economic, social and political issues involved and subsequently evaluate the programmes.

6.2. The First Steps Towards Integration of Activities

The island of Pemba in Zanzibar has carried out annual treatment with Mectizan and albendazole since 2000 and plans to continue through 2007 to eliminate LF. The island also has a high schistosomiasis and hookworm prevalence, meriting annual treatment with PZQ and albendazole. The teams that treated the Pemba population for LF in October 2003 were given the task to reach the same population with PZQ and albendazole in May 2004. Pemba is a small island of less than 400 000 people, but the treatment programme worked smoothly, suggesting that on a larger scale, integration is feasible. In October 2004, the population of Tanga in Tanzania was treated for the first time with Mectizan® and albendazole against LF. School based treatment with PZQ was delivered in November 2005 and followed by community based treatment with Mectizan and albendazole in February 2006. Meanwhile, the LF and trachoma programmes have started to consider possible integration in Ghana and have planned the development of joint registers of communities prior to mass drug administration (MDA) and integrated training, case detection, social mobilisation and advocacy.

In Burkina Faso, the national co-ordinators of the schistosomiasis-helminth control programme (PNLSc) and the LF elimination programme (PELF) communicate and interact frequently under the Director for Disease Control. The treatment strategy is in both cases community based and the CSPS (Primary Health Care Dispensaries) are used as distribution points and focal points for mobile distribution teams. The PNLSc targets school-aged children (enrolled and non-enrolled) from 5 to 15 years of age; while the PELF targets any individual > 5 years old. Since an annual treatment with albendazole has been deemed sufficient to control soil-transmitted helminths (STH), the PNLSc distributes albendazole to the population aged

5–15 while the PELF distributes only to the population over 15 years old. The two programmes have therefore shared their drug resources. By the end of 2004, the PNLSc had covered about 1/3 of the country, treating about 1 million individuals, with further expansion planned for 2005. The PELF could cover the whole country if resources were available for drug delivery.

In Uganda, it has proved possible successfully to integrate de-worming with measles vaccination on a national scale, and 'health days' were held in October 2003, May and November 2004. In the past, vitamin A distribution was grafted onto 'polio days', but as these cease, child health days (or weeks) have become more frequent and vitamin A distribution is now linked to measles vaccination and de-worming (UNICEF).

6.3. Achieving Sustainability

The SCI funded control programmes in Tanzania and Burkina Faso hope to integrate the control of parasitic diseases, leading within 5 years to a low level sustainable maintenance phase of control to be funded by the governments.

In highly endemic countries, schistosomiasis control programmes require intensive mass treatment campaigns over several years to reduce prevalence and intensity of infection. However, after this intensive treatment, long-term control of morbidity may be achieved by routine and regular treatment of school-aged children, at intervals determined by prevalence and intensity of infection as determined by regular monitoring. If the initial implementation is donor funded, as is likely, then sustainability will depend on securing resources for implementation to continue uninterrupted for say 3–5 years, which has been estimated at $0.50 (US) per person to be treated per year. For Tanzania and Burkina Faso for example, with populations of approximately 30 and 11 million, respectively, a total of approximately $12 million and $4.40 million US $ per year will be needed. By the time the intervention treatment programme is complete, Tanzania and Burkina Faso should then each have in place a Ministry of Health budget and a Ministry of Education budget for diseases of poverty and school health, respectively, utilizing funds from the range of available resources: government budgets, pooled donor contributions (basket of currencies), bilateral and international agencies (the World Bank and the Global Fund). The national plan that will have been tried and tested, policy makers involved from the start and the proof of concept on integration of disease control can be used to make the case for these funds to be available for long-term control.

Transfer of the concepts to other countries will depend on the advocacy and publicity that is to be given to the success in Tanzania and Burkina Faso. Seminars, conferences and publication of results, mainly through the auspices of the WHO, will be a major part of this advocacy.

Chemotherapy remains the main control measure for the reduction of morbidity due to schistosomiasis in much of sub-Saharan Africa. However, in most endemic areas, in order to achieve long-term sustainable schistosomiasis control, it will be necessary to introduce other preventive measures focusing on clean water, adequate sanitation and health education to complement chemotherapy (Utzinger *et al.*, 2003), measures that will contribute to the reduction of transmission and help countries progress towards schistosomiasis elimination. The stage is set, with the political will and the necessary funding, existing tools and knowledge can be implemented to significantly reduce morbidity and transmission of schistosomiasis.

Since 2003, there has been a tremendous start to implementation of control of schistosomiasis and intestinal helminthes in sub Saharan Africa. As from 2006 there is an urgent need for further funding to continue the momentum in the countries already implementing control programmes and to encourage others to start. Foundations, International agencies and bilateral donors are all urged to collaborate to follow the recommendations of the Commission for Africa Report and assist the poor of Africa to attain the millennium Development Goals.

ACKNOWLEDGEMENTS

A.F. would like to express his appreciation to SCI Director of Monitoring and Evaluation, Joanne Webster, to the UK based SCI scientific staff (Yaobi Zhang, Russell Stothard, Artemis Koukounari, Elisa Bosque-Oliva, Albis Gabrielli, Fiona Fleming and Lynsey Blair) and the country co-ordinators, (Uganda: Narcis Kabatereine, Tanzania: Ursuline Nyandindi, Zanzibar: Hamadi Juma, Zambia: Faith Nchito and James Mwansa, Mali: Robert Dembele, Niger: Amadou Garba and Burkina Faso: Seydou Toure) for their work with SCI. SCI is supported by the Bill and Melinda Gates Foundation. DR would like to thank Fiona Allan for her help with the bibliography and acknowledges financial support from the Health Foundation.

REFERENCES

Abdel-Salam, E., Peters, P.A., Abdel Meguid, A.E., Abdel Meguid, A.A. and Mahmoud, A.A. (1986). Discrepancies in outcome of a control programme for schistosomiasis haematobia in Fayoum governorate, Egypt. *American Journal of Tropical Medicine and Hygiene* **35**, 786–790.

Abel, L., Demenais, F., Prata, A., Souza, A.E. and Dessein, A. (1991). Evidence for the segregation of a major gene in human susceptibility/resistance to infection by *Schistosoma mansoni. American Journal of Human Genetics* **48**, 959–970.

Abel, L., Marquet, S., Chevillard, C., elWali, N.E., Hillaire, D. and Dessein, A. (2000). Genetic predisposition to bilharziasis in humans: research methods and application to the study of *Schistosoma mansoni* infection. *Journal de la Societé de Biologie* **194**, 15–18.

Abo-Madyan, A.A., Morsy, T.A. and Motawea, S.M. (2004). Efficacy of myrrh in the treatment of schistosomiasis (*haematobium* and *mansoni*) in Ezbet El-Bakly, Tamyia Center, El-Fayoum Governorate, Egypt. *Journal of the Egyptian Society of Parasitology* **34**, 423–446.

Abugre, C., Baggaley, R. and Thomas, A. (2005). The commission for Africa: a recipe for success? *Lancet* **365**, 1461–1462.

Adam, I., Elwasila, E.T. and Homeida, M. (2004). Is praziquantel therapy safe during pregnancy? *Transactions of the Royal Society of Tropical Medicine and Hygiene* **98**, 540–543.

Al Ghahtani, A.G. and Amin, M.A. (2005). Progress achieved in the elimination of schistosomiasis from the Jazan region of Saudi Arabia. *Annals of Tropical Medicine and Parasitology* **99**, 483–490.

al-Madani, A.A. (1990). Schistosomiasis control in Saudi Arabia with special reference to the period 1983–1988. *Public Health* **104**, 261–266.

Amin, M.A. (1972). Large-scale assessment of the molluscicides copper sulphate and *N*-tritlymorpholine (Frescon) in the North Group of the

Gezira irrigated area, Sudan. *Journal of Tropical Medicine and Hygiene* **75**, 169–175.

Andrade, Z.A. (1998). The situation of hepatosplenic schistosomiasis in Brazil today. *Memorias Do Instituto Oswaldo Cruz* **93**(Suppl 1), 313–316.

Appleton, C.C. (1977). The influence of temperature on the life-cycle and distribution of *Biomphalaria pfeifferi* (Krauss, 1948) in South-Eastern Africa. *International Journal of Parasitology* **7**, 335–345.

Arfaa, F. (1976). Studies on schistosomiasis in Saudi Arabia. *American Journal of Tropical Medicine and Hygiene* **25**, 295–298.

Arfaa, F., Farahmandian, I. and Soleimani, M. (1970). Evaluation of the effect of mass chemotherapy with niridazole as a method of bilharziasis control in Iran. *Transactions of the Royal Society of Tropical Medicine and Hygiene* **64**, 130–133.

Ault, S.K. (1994). Environmental management: a re-emerging vector control strategy. *American Journal of Tropical Medicine and Hygiene* **50**, 35–49.

Barakat, R., Farghaly, A., El Masry, A.G., El-Sayed, M.K. and Hussein, M.H. (2000). The epidemiology of schistosomiasis in Egypt: patterns of *Schistosoma mansoni* infection and morbidity in Kafer El-Sheikh. *American Journal of Tropical Medicine and Hygiene* **62**, 21–27.

Barnish, G. (1970). The control of bilharziasis by the use of molluscicides. *Central African Journal of Medicine*, **16**(Suppl), 22–27.

Barnish, G., Jordan, P., Bartholomew, R.K. and Grist, E. (1982). Routine focal mollusciciding after chemotherapy to control *Schistosoma mansoni* in Cul de Sac valley, Saint Lucia. *Transactions of the Royal Society of Tropical Medicine and Hygiene* **76**, 602–609.

Beck, L., Favre, T.C., Pieri, O.S., Zani, L.C., Domas, G.G. and Barbosa, C.S. (2001). Replacing oxamniquine by praziquantel against *Schistosoma mansoni* infection in a rural community from the sugar-cane zone of Northeast Brazil: an epidemiological follow-up. *Memorias do Instituto Oswaldo Cruz* **96**, 165–167.

Berg, C.O. (1973). Biological control of snail-borne diseases: a review. *Experimental Parasitology* **33**, 318–330.

Bergquist, N.R., Leonardo, L.R. and Mitchell, G.F. (2005). Vaccine-linked chemotherapy: can schistosomiasis control benefit from an integrated approach? *Trends in Parasitology* **21**, 112–117.

Bethony, J., Williams, J.T., Brooker, S., Gazzinelli, A., Gazzinelli, M.F., LoVerde, P.T., Correa-Oliveira, R. and Kloos, H. (2004). Exposure to *Schistosoma mansoni* infection in a rural area in Brazil Part III: household aggregation of water-contact behaviour. *Tropical Medicine and International Health* **9**, 381–389.

Botros, S., Sayed, H., Amer, N., El-Ghannam, M., Bennett, J.L. and Day, T.A. (2005a). Current status of sensitivity to praziquantel in a focus of potential drug resistance in Egypt. *International Journal of Parasitology* **35**, 787–791.

Botros, S., Sayed, H., El-Dusoki, H., Sabry, H., Rabie, I., El-Ghannam, M., Hassanein, M., El-Wahab, Y.A. and Engels, D. (2005b). Efficacy of mirazid in comparison with praziquantel in Egyptian *Schistosoma mansoni*-infected school children and households. *American Journal of Tropical Medicine and Hygiene* **72**, 119–123.

Botros, S., Soliman, A., Elgawhary, N., Selim, M. and Guirguis, N. (1989). Effect of combined low-dose praziquantel and oxamniquine on different stages of schistosome maturity. *Transactions of the Royal Society of Tropical Medicine and Hygiene* **83**, 86–89.

Botros, S., William, S., Ebeid, F., Cioli, D., Katz, N., Day, T.A. and Bennett, J.L. (2004). Lack of evidence for an antischistosomal activity of myrrh in experimental animals. *American Journal of Tropical Medicine and Hygiene* **71**, 206–210.

Brinkmann, U.K., Werler, C., Traore, M. and Korte, R. (1988). The National Schistosomiasis Control Programme in Mali, objectives, organization, results. *Tropical Medicine and Parasitology* **39**, 157–161.

Brooker, S., Hay, S.I. and Bundy, D.A.P. (2002). Tools from ecology: useful for evaluating infection risk models? *Trends in Parasitology* **18**, 70–74.

Brooker, S., Kabatereine, N.B., Myatt, M., Russell Stothard, J. and Fenwick, A. (2005). Rapid assessment of *Schistosoma mansoni*: the validity, applicability and cost-effectiveness of the Lot Quality Assurance Sampling method in Uganda. *Tropical Medicine and International Health* **1**, 647–658.

Brooker, S., Rowlands, M., Haller, L., Savioli, L. and Bundy, D.A.P. (2000). Towards an atlas of human helminth infection in sub-Saharan Africa: the use of geographical information systems (GIS). *Parasitology Today* **16**, 303–307.

Brooker, S., Whawell, S., Kabatereine, N.B., Fenwick, A. and Anderson, R.M. (2004). Evaluating the epidemiological impact of national control programmes for helminths. *Trends in Parasitology* **20**, 537–545.

Capron, A., Dessaint, J.P., Capron, M. and Pierce, R.J. (1992). Vaccine strategies against schistosomiasis. *Immunobiology* **184**, 282–294.

Castro, N., Medina, R., Sotelo, J. and Jung, H. (2000). Bioavailability of praziquantel increases with concomitant administration of food. *Antimicrobial Agents and Chemotherapy* **44**, 2903–2904.

Changsong, S., Binggui, Y., Hongyi, L., Yuhai, D., Xu, X., Huiguo, Z. and Yong, J. (2002). Achievement of the World Bank loan project on schistosomiasis control (1992–2000) in Hubei province and the challenge in the future. *Acta Tropica* **82**, 169–174.

Chitsulo, L., Engels, D., Montresor, A. and Savioli, L. (2000). The global status of schistosomiasis and its control. *Acta Tropica* **77**, 41–51.

Christopherson, J.B. (1918). The successful use of antimony in *bilharziosis*. *Lancet* **2**, 325–327.

Coles, G.C. (2002a). Cattle nematodes resistant to anthelmintics: why so few cases? *Veterinary Research* **33**, 481–489.

Coles, G.C. (2002b). Sustainable use of anthelmintics in grazing animals. *Veterinary Record* **151**, 165–169.

Combes, C., Golvan, Y. and Salvat, B. (1982). Evaluation of 10 years of research on *S.mansoni* schistosomiasis A in the French West Indies. *Biomedicine and Pharmacotherapy,* **36**, 108–112.

Conceicao, M.J., Correa, A., Teixeira, A., Moura, D.C., Silva, O.C. and Silva, S.C. (1999). Partial lack of susceptibility to *Schistosoma mansoni* infection of *Biomphalaria glabrata* strains from Itanhomi (Minas Gerais, Brazil) after fourteen years of laboratory maintenance. *Memorias do Instituto Oswaldo Cruz* **94**, 425–426.

Cook, J.A., Jordan, P. and Armitage, P. (1976). Hycanthone dose–response in treatment of Schistosomiasis mansoni in St. Lucia. *American Journal of Tropical Medicine and Hygiene* **25**, 602–607.

Creasey, A.M., Taylor, P. and Thomas, J.E.P. (1986). Dosage trial of a combination of oxamniquine and praziquantel in the treatment of schistosomiasis in Zimbabwean schoolchildren. *Central African Journal of Medicine* **32**, 165–167.

Crossland, N.O. (1963). A large-scale experiment in the control of aquatic snails by the use of molluscicides on a sugar estate in the Northern Region of Tanganyika. *Bulletin of the World Health Organization* **29**, 515–524.

Dalton, P.R. (1976). A socioecological approach to the control of *Schistosoma mansoni* in St Lucia. *Bulletin of the World Health Organization* **54**, 587–595.

Danso-Appiah, A. and De Vlas, S.J. (2002). Interpreting low praziquantel cure rates of *Schistosoma mansoni* infections in Senegal. *Trends in Parasitology* **18**, 125–129.

da Silva, R.A., de Carvalho, M.E., Zacharias, F., de Lima, V.R. and Teles, H.M. (2002). *Schistosomiasis mansoni* in Bananal (state of Sao Paulo, Brazil): IV. Study on the public awareness of its risks in the Palha District. *Memorias do Instituto Oswaldo Cruz* **97**(Suppl 1), 15–18.

Davis, A., Biles, J.E. and Ulrich, A.M. (1979). Initial experiences with praziquantel in the treatment of human infections due to *Schistosoma haematobium. Bulletin of the World Health Organization* **57**, 773–779.

Davis, A., Biles, J.E., Ulrich, A.M. and Dixon, H. (1981). Tolerance and efficacy of praziquantel in phase-Iia and phase-Iib therapeutic trials in Zambian patients. *Arzneimittel-Forschung/Drug Research* **31**, 568–574.

Dawood, I.K., Dazo, B.C. and Farooq, M. (1966). Large-scale application of Bayluscide and sodium pentachlorophenate in the Egypt-49 project area. Evaluation of relative efficacy and comparative costs. *Bulletin of the World Health Organization* **35**, 357–367.

De Clercq, D., Vercruysse, J., Kongs, A., Verlé, P., Dompnier, J.P. and Faye, P.C. (2002). Efficacy of artesunate and praziquantel in *Schistosoma haematobium* infected schoolchildren. *Acta Tropica* **82**, 61–66.

De Clercq, D., Vercruysse, J., Verlé, P., Kongs, A. and Diop, M. (2000). What is the effect of combining artesunate and praziquantel in the treatment of *Schistosoma mansoni* infections. *Tropical Medicine and International Health* **5**, 744–746.

Dhunputh, J. (1994). Progress in the control of schistosomiasis in Mauritius. *Transactions of the Royal Society of Tropical Medicine and Hygiene* **88**, 507–509.

Doenhoff, M.J., Kusel, J.R., Coles, G.C. and Cioli, D. (2002). Resistance of *Schistosoma mansoni* to praziquantel: is there a problem? *Transactions of the Royal Society of Tropical Medicine and Hygiene* **96**, 465–469.

Duke, B.O.L. and Moore, P.J. (1976). The use of a molluscicide in conjunction with chemotherapy to control *Schistosoma haematobium* at the Barombi Lake foci in Cameroon. III. Conclusions and costs. *Tropenmedizin und Parasitologie* **27**, 505–508.

el Katsha, S. and Watts, S. (1995). The public health implications of the increasing predominance of Schistosoma mansoni in Egypt: a pilot study in the Nile delta. *Journal of Tropical Medicine and Hygiene* **98**, 136–140.

El-Nagar, H. (1958). Control of schistosomiasis in the Gezira, Sudan. *Journal of Tropical Medicine and Hygiene* **61**, 231–235.

Enk, M.J., Amorim, A. and Schall, V.T. (2003). Acute schistosomiasis outbreak in the metropolitan area of Belo Horizonte, Minas Gerais: alert about the risk of unnoticed transmission increased by growing rural tourism. *Memorias do Instituto Oswaldo Cruz* **98**, 745–750.

Erko, B., Abebe, F., Berhe, N., Medhin, G., Gebre-Michael, T., Gemetchu, T. and Gundersen, S.G. (2002). Control of *Schistosoma mansoni* by the soapberry Endod (*Phytolacca dodecandra*) in Wollo, northeastern Ethiopia: post-intervention prevalence. *East African Medical Journal* **79**, 198–201.

Etard, J.F., Audibert, M. and Dabo, A. (1995). Age-acquired resistance and predisposition to reinfection with *Schistosoma haematobium* after treatment with praziquantel in Mali. *American Journal of Tropical Medicine and Hygiene* **52**, 549–558.

Evans, A.C. (1983). Control of schistosomiasis in large irrigation schemes by use of niclosamide. A ten-year study in Zimbabwe. *American Journal of Tropical Medicine and Hygiene* **32**, 1029–1039.

Fallon, P.G., Sturrock, R.F., Niang, A.C. and Doenhoff, M.J. (1995). Short report: diminished susceptibility to praziquantel in a Senegal isolate of *Schistosoma mansoni*. *American Journal of Tropical Medicine and Hygiene* **53**, 61–62.

Fallon, P.G., Tao, L.F., Ismail, M.M. and Bennett, J.L. (1996). Schistosome resistance to praziquantel: fact or artifact? *Parasitology Today* **12**, 316–320.

Farag, M.K., el-Shazly, A.M., Khashaba, M.T. and Attia, R.A. (1993). Impact of the current National Bilharzia Control Programme on the epidemiology of Schistosomiasis mansoni in an Egyptian village. *Transactions of the Royal Society of Tropical Medicine and Hygiene* **87**, 250–253.

Fenwick, A. (2006). New initiatives against Africa's worms. *Transactions of the Royal Society of Tropical Medicine and Hygiene* **100**, 200–207.

Fenwick, A., Savioli, L., Engels, D., Bergquist, N.R. and Todd, M.H. (2003). Drugs for the control of parasitic diseases: current status and development in schistosomiasis. *Trends in Parasitology* **19**, 509–515.

Fenwick, A., Molyneux, D. and Nantulya, V. (2005). Achieving the millennium development goals. *Lancet* **365**, 1029–1030.

Ferguson, F.F. (1961). Use of molluscicides for bilharziasis control in Puerto Rico. *Bulletin of the World Health Organization* **25**, 721–723.

Frandsen, F. (1987). Control of schistosomiasis by use of biological control of snail hosts with special reference to competition. *Memorias do Instituto Oswaldo Cruz* **82**(Suppl 4), 129–133.

Fulford, A.J., Butterworth, A.E., Ouma, J.H. and Sturrock, R.F. (1995). A statistical approach to schistosome population dynamics and estimation of the life-span of *Schistosoma mansoni* in man. *Parasitology* **110**, 307–316.

Ghebreyesus, T.A., Witten, K.H., Getachew, A., Haile, M., Yohannes, M., Lindsay, S.W. and Byass, P. (2002). Schistosome transmission, water-resource development and altitude in northern Ethiopia. *Annals of Tropical Medicine and Parasitology* **96**, 489–495.

Giboda, M. and Bergquist, N. (2000). Post-transmission schistosomiasis: a new agenda. *Acta Tropica* **77**, 3–7.

Giboda, M., Malek, E.A. and Correa, R. (1997). Human Schistosomiasis in Puerto Rico: reduced prevalence rate and absence of *Biomphalaria glabrata*. *American Journal of Topical Medicine and Hygiene* **57**, 564–568.

Goll, P.H., Lemma, A., Duncan, J. and Mazengia, B. (1983). Control of schistosomiasis in Adwa, Ethiopia, using the plant molluscicide endod (*Phytolacca dodecandra*). *Tropenmedizin und Parasitologie* **34**, 177–183.

Gönnert, R. (1967). Experiences in the control of bilharziasis with molluscicides. *Annales de la Société Belge de Medecine Tropicale* **47**, 195–203.

Gryseels, B., Deelder, A.M. and Polderman, A.M. (1994). Schistosomiasis at the North Sea. *Tropical and Geographical Medicine* **46**, 195–196.

Gryseels, B., Mbaye, A., De Vlas, S.J., Stelma, F.F., Guisse, F., Van Lieshout, L., Faye, D., Diop, M., Ly, A., Tchuem-Tchuente, L.A., Engels, D. and Polman, K. (2001). Are poor responses to praziquantel for the treatment of *Schistosoma mansoni* infections in Senegal due to resistance?

An overview of the evidence. *Tropical Medicine and International Health* **6**, 864–873.

Gu, Y.G., Xia, L.F., Li, Z.W., Zhao, M.F., Yang, H.Y., Luo, Q.Y., Xia, W.H. and Feng, Q.Y. (2001). Study on schistosomiasis control strategy in Ertan reservoir. *Zhongguo Ji Sheng Chong Xue Yu Ji Sheng Chong Bing Za Zhi* **19**, 225–228.

Hagan, P. and Sharaf, S. (2003). Schistosomiasis vaccines. *Expert Opinion on Biological Therapy* **3**, 1271–1278.

Hillyer, G.V. (1983). Schistosomiasis in the Dominican Republic: a review. *Boletin de la Asociacion Medica de Puerto Rico* **75**, 114–117.

Hofkin, B.V., Mkoji, G.M., Koech, D.K. and Loker, E.S. (1991). Control of schistosome-transmitting snails in Kenya by the North-American Crayfish *Procambarus clarkii*. *American Journal of Tropical Medicine and Hygiene* **45**, 339–344.

Hurter, G.W. and Yokogawa, M. (1984). Control of schistosomiasis japonica in Japan. *Japanese Journal of Parasitology* **33**, 341–351.

Idris, M.A., Shaban, M., Richter, J., Moné, H., Mouahid, G. and Ruppel, A. (2003). Emergence of infections with *Schistosoma mansoni* in the Dhofar Governorate, Oman. *Acta Tropica* **88**, 137–144.

Ismail, M., Botros, S., Metwally, A., William, S., Farghally, A., Tao, L.F., Day, T.A. and Bennett, J.L. (1999). Resistance to praziquantel: direct evidence from *Schistosoma mansoni* isolated from Egyptian villagers. *American Journal of Tropical Medicine and Hygiene* **60**, 932–935.

Jewsbury, J.M. (1977). Oxamniquine in the prevention of bilharzial infection. *Central African Journal of Medicine* **23**, 18–20.

Jobin, W.R. (1979). Cost of snail control. *American Journal of Tropical Medicine and Hygiene* **28**, 142–154.

Jordan, P., Bartholomew, R.K., Grist, E. and Auguste, E. (1982a). Evaluation of chemotherapy in the control of *Schistosoma mansoni* in Marquis Valley, Saint Lucia. I. Results in humans. *American Journal of Tropical Medicine and Hygiene* **31**, 103–110.

Jordan, P., Unrau, G.O., Bartholomew, R.K., Cook, J.A. and Grist, E. (1982b). Value of individual household water supplies in the maintenance phase of a schistosomiasis control programme in Saint-Lucia, after chemotherapy. *Bulletin of the World Health Organization* **60**, 583–588.

Kabatereine, N.B., Brooker, S., Tukahebwa, E.M., Kazibwe, F. and Onapa, A.W. (2004). Epidemiology and geography of *Schistosoma mansoni* in Uganda: implications for planning control. *Tropical Medicine and International Health* **9**, 372–380.

Kardaman, M.W., Amin, M.A., Fenwick, A., Cheesmond, A.K. and Dixon, H.G. (1983). A field trial using praziquantel (Biltricide) to treat *Schistosoma mansoni* and *Schistosoma haematobium* infection in Gezira, Sudan. *Annals of Tropical Medicine and Parasitology* **77**, 297–304.

Kariuki, H.C., Mbugua, G., Magak, P., Bailey, J.A., Muchiri, E.M., Thiongo, F.W., King, C.H., Butterworth, A.E., Ouma, J.H. and Blanton, R.E. (2001). Prevalence and familial aggregation of schistosomal liver morbidity in Kenya: evaluation by new ultrasound criteria. *Journal of Infectious Diseases* **183**, 960–966.

Katz, N., Rocha, R.S. and Pereira, J.P. (1980). Schistosomiasis control in Peri–Peri (Minas Gerais, Brazil) by repeated clinical treatment and molluscicide application. *Revista Do Instituto De Medicina Tropical De Sao Paulo* **22**, 85–93 203–211.

Kheir, M.M., Baraka, O.Z., el-Tom, I.A., Mukhtar, M.M. and Homieda, M.M. (2000). Effects of single-dose praziquantel on morbidity and mortality resulting from intestinal schistosomiasis. *East Mediterranean Health Journal* **6**, 926–931.

Kiely, S. (2005). The commission for Africa: a recipe for success? *Lancet* **365**, 1461.

King, C.H., Dickman, K. and Tisch, D.J. (2005). Reassessment of the cost of chronic helmintic infection: a meta-analysis of disability-related outcomes in endemic schistosomiasis. *Lancet* **365**, 1561–1569.

Klock, J.W., Gerhardt, C.E., Ildefonso, V. and Serrano, J.M. (1957). Characteristics of sodium pentachlorophenate used against *Australorbis glabratus* in Puerto Rico. *Bulletin of the World Health Organization* **16**, 1189–1201.

Kouriba, B., Chevillard, C., Bream, J.H., Argiro, L., Dessein, H., Arnaud, V., Sangare, L., Dabo, A., Beavogui, A.H., Arama, C., Traore, H.A., Doumbo, O. and Dessein, A. (2005). Analysis of the 5q31-q33 locus shows an association between IL13-1055C/T IL-13-591A/G polymorphisms and *Schistosoma haematobium* infections. *Journal of Immunology* **174**, 6274–6281.

Laamrani, H., Khallaayoune, K., Madsen, H., Mahjour, J. and Gryseels, B. (2000a). New challenges in schistosomiasis control in Morocco. *Acta Tropica* **77**, 61–67.

Laamrani, H., Mahjour, J., Madsen, H., Khallaayoune, K. and Gryseels, B. (2000b). *Schistosoma haematobium* in Morocco: moving from control to elimination. *Parasitology Today* **16**, 257–260.

Lambert, J.D., Temmink, J.H., Marquis, J., Parkhurst, R.M., Lugt, C.B., Lemmich, E., Wolde-Yohannes, L. and de Savigny, D. (1991). Endod: safety evaluation of a plant molluscicide. *Regulatory Toxicology and Pharmacology* **14**, 189–201.

Lawn, S.D., Lucas, S.B. and Chiodini, P.L. (2003). Case report: *Schistosoma mansoni* infection: failure of standard treatment with praziquantel in a returned traveller. *Transactions of the Royal Society of Tropical Medicine and Hygiene* **97**, 100–101.

Lemma, A. (1971). Present status of endod as a molluscicide for the control of schistosomiasis. *Ethiopian Medical Journal* **9**, 113–118.

Lemma, A., Brody, G., Newell, G.W., Parkhurst, R.M. and Skinner, W.A. (1972). Studies on the molluscicidal properties of endod (*Phytolacca dodecandra*). I. Increased potency with butanol extraction. *Journal of Parasitology* **58**, 104–107.

Lemma, A. and Yau, P. (1974a). Studies on the molluscicidal properties of endod (*Phytolacca dodecandra*). III. Stability and potency under different environmental conditions. *Ethiopian Medical Journal* **12**, 115–124.

Lemma, A. and Yau, P. (1974b). Studies on the molluscicidal properties of endod (*Phytolacca dodecandra*): II. Comparative toxicity of various molluscicides to fish and snails. *Ethiopian Medical Journal* **12**, 109–114.

Loker, E.S. (1983). A comparative study of the life-histories of mammalian schistosomes. *Parasitology* **87**, 343–369.

Madhina, D. and Shiff, C. (1996). Prevention of snail miracidia interactions using *Phytolacca dodecandra* (L'Herit) (endod) as a miracidiacide: an alternative approach to the focal control of schistosomiasis. *Tropical Medicine and International Health* **1**, 221–226.

Mahmoud, A.A., Siongok, T.A., Ouma, J., Houser, H.B. and Warren, K.S. (1983). Effect of targeted mass treatment on intensity of infection and morbidity in *Schistosomiasis mansoni*. 3-year follow-up of a community in Machakos, Kenya. *Lancet* **16**, 849–851.

Malone, J.B., Bergquist, N.R., Huh, O.K., Bavia, M.E., Bernardi, M., El Bahy, M.M., Fuentes, M.V., Kristensen, T.K., McCarroll, J.C., Yilma, J.M. and Zhou, X.N. (2001). A global network for the control of snail-borne disease using satellite surveillance and geographic information systems. *Acta Tropica* **79**, 7–12.

Massoud, J. (2000). The control of schistosomiasis in the Islamic Republic of Iran. World Health Organization, Informal Consultation on Schistosomiasis in Low Transmission Areas: Control Strategies and Criteria for Elimination, London: pp. 1–7.

McManus, D.P. and Bartley, P.B. (2004). A vaccine against Asian schistosomiasis. *Parasitology International* **53**, 163–173.

Mengistu, M. (1982). Fatal liver toxicity due to hycanthone (Etrenol) in a patient with pre-existing liver disease: a case report. *Ethiopian Medical Journal* **20**, 145–147.

Meyerlassen, J., Daffalla, A.A. and Madsen, H. (1994). Evaluation of focal mollusciciding in the Rahad Irrigation Scheme, Sudan. *Acta Tropica* **58**, 229–241.

Mgeni, A.F., Kisumku, U.M., McCullough, F.S., Dixon, H., Yoon, S.S. and Mott, K.E. (1990). Metrifonate in the control of urinary schistosomiasis in Zanzibar. *Bulletin of the World Health Organization* **68**, 721–730.

Miguel, E. and Kremer, M. (2004). Worms: identifying impacts on education and health in the presence of treatment externalities. *Econometrica* **72**, 159–217.

Mkoji, G.M., Hofkin, B.V., Kuris, A.M., Stewart-Oaten, A., Mungai, B.N., Kihara, J.H., Mungai, F., Yundu, J., Mbui, J., Rashid, J.R., Kariuki, C.H., Ouma, J.H., Koech, D.K. and Loker, E.S. (1999). Impact of the crayfish *Procambarus clarkii* on *Schistosoma haematobium* transmission in Kenya. *American Journal of Tropical Medicine and Hygiene* **61**, 751–759.

Molyneux, D.H., Hotez, P.J. and Fenwick, A. (2005). "Rapid impact interventions": How a policy of integrated control for Africa's Neglected Tropical Diseases could benefit the Poor. *Public Library of Science (Medicine)* **2**, e336.

Montresor, A., Engels, D., Chitsulo, L., Bundy, D.A.P., Brooker, S. and Savioli, L. (2001). Development and validation of a 'tablet pole' for the administration of praziquantel in sub-Saharan Africa. *Transactions of the Royal Society of Tropical Medicine and Hygiene* **95**, 542–544.

Morgan, J.A., Dejong, R.J., Snyder, S.D., Mkoji, G.M. and Loker, E.S. (2001). *Schistosoma mansoni* and *Biomphalaria*: past history and future trends. *Parasitology* **123**(Suppl), S211–S228.

Nasr, T.S. (1960). Sodium pentachlorophenate as a molluscicide under Egyptian conditions. *Journal of the Egyptian Medical Association* **43**, 762–771.

Ndyomugyenyi, R. and Kabatereine, N. (2003). Integrated community-directed treatment for the control of onchocerciasis, schistosomiasis and intestinal helminths infections in Uganda: advantages and disadvantages. *Tropical Medicine and International Health* **8**, 997–1004.

N'Goran, E.K., Utzinger, J., Traoré, M., Lengeler, C. and Tanner, M. (1998). Use of a questionnaire for quick identification of the principal foci of urinary bilharziasis in central Ivory Coast. *Med Trop (Mars)* **58**, 253–260.

Oostburg, B.F. (1972). Clinical trial with hycanthone in *Schistosomiasis mansoni* in Surinam. *Tropical and Geographical Medicine* **24**, 148–151.

Paulini, E. (1958). Bilharziasis control by application of molluscicides; a review of its present status. *Bulletin of the World Health Organization* **18**, 975–988.

Picquet, M., Ernould, J.C., Vercruysse, J., Southgate, V.R., Mbaye, A., Sambou, B., Niang, M. and Rollinson, D. (1996). Royal Society of Tropical Medicine and Hygiene meeting at Manson House, London, 18 May 1995. The epidemiology of human schistosomiasis in the Senegal river basin. *Transactions of the Royal Society of Tropical Medicine and Hygiene* **90**, 340–346.

Pointier, J.P. and David, P. (2004). Biological control of *Biomphalaria glabrata*, the intermediate host of schistosomes, by *Marisa cornuarietis* in ponds of Guadeloupe: long-term impact on the local snail fauna and aquatic flora. *Biological Control* **29**, 81–89.

Pointier, J.P. and Jourdane, J. (2000). Biological control of the snail hosts of schistosomiasis in areas of low transmission: the example of the Caribbean area. *Acta Tropica* **77**, 53–60.

Pointier, J.P. and McCullough, F. (1989). Biological control of the snail hosts of *Schistosoma mansoni* in the Caribbean area using *Thiara* spp. *Acta Tropica* **46**, 147–155.

Prentice, M.A. (1983). Displacement of *Biomphalaria glabrata* by the snail *Thiara granifera* in field habitats in St. Lucia, West Indies. *Annals of Tropical Medicine and Parasitology* **77**, 51–59.

Prentice, M.A., Jordan, P., Bartholomew, R.K. and Grist, E. (1981). Reduction in transmission of *Schistosoma mansoni* by a four-year focal mollusciciding programme against *Biomphalaria glabrata* in Saint Lucia. *Transactions of the Royal Society of Tropical Medicine and Hygiene* **75**, 789–798.

Quinnell, R.J. (2003). Genetics of susceptibility to human helminth infection. *International Journal for Parasitology* **33**, 1219–1231.

Raffier, G. (1969). Activity of niridazole in urinary schistosomiasis: prophylaxis and principles of control. *Annals of Internal Medicine* **160**, 696–704.

Raso, G., Matthys, B., N'Goran, E.K., Tanner, M., Vounatsou, P. and Utzinger, J. (2005). Spatial risk prediction and mapping of *Schistosoma mansoni* infections among schoolchildren living in western Cote d'Ivoire. *Parasitology* **131**, 97–108.

Rollinson, D. and Johnston, D.A. (1996). Schistosomiasis—a persistent parasitic disease. *Interdisciplinary Science Reviews* **21**, 140–154.

Rollinson, D. and Southgate, V.R. (1987). The genus *Schistosoma*: a taxonomic appraisal. In: *The Biology of Schistosomes: From Genes to Latrines* (D. Rollinson and A.J.G. Simpson, eds), pp. 1–49. London: Academic Press.

Savioli, L., Albonico, M., Engels, D. and Montresor, A. (2004). Progress in the prevention and control of schistosomiasis and soil-transmitted helminthiasis. *Parasitology International* **53**, 103–113.

Savioli, L., Crompton, D.W.T. and Neira, M. (2003). Use of anthelminthic drugs during pregnancy. *American Journal of Obstetrics and Gynecology* **188**, 5–6.

Savioli, L., Stansfield, S., Bundy, D.A., Mitchell, A., Bhatia, R., Engels, D., Montresor, A., Neira, M. and Shein, A.M. (2002). Schistosomiasis and soil-transmitted helminth infections: forging control efforts. *Transactions of the Royal Society of Tropical Medicine and Hygiene* **96**, 577–579.

Schlegel, L., Pointier, J.P., Petitjean Roget, V., Nadeau, Y., Blateau, A. and Mansuy, J.M. (1997). The control of intestinal schistosomiasis from Martinique island. *Parasite-Journal de la Societé Francaise de Parasitologie* **4**, 217–225.

Seto, E., Xu, B., Liang, S., Gong, P., Wu, W.P., Davis, G., Qiu, D.C., Gu, X.G. and Spear, R. (2002a). The use of remote sensing for predictive modeling of schistosomiasis in China. *Photogrammetric Engineering and Remote Sensing* **68**, 167–174.

Seto, E.Y.W., Wu, W.P., Qiu, D.C., Liu, H.Y., Gu, X.G., Chen, H.G., Spear, R.C. and Davis, G.M. (2002b). Impact of soil chemistry on the distribution of *Oncomelania hupensis* (Gastropoda: Pomatiopsidae) in China. *Malacologia* **44**, 259–272.

Sheir, Z., Nasr, A.A., Massoud, A., Salama, O., Badra, G.A., El-Shennawy, H., Hassan, N. and Hammad, S.M. (2001). A safe, effective, herbal antischistosomal therapy derived from myrrh. *American Journal of Tropical Medicine and Hygiene* **65**, 700–704.

Shekhar, K.C. (1991). Schistosomiasis drug therapy and treatment considerations. *Drugs* **42**, 379–405.

Singh, A., Singh, D.K., Misra, T.N. and Agarwal, R.A. (1996). Molluscicides of plant origin. *Biological Agriculture and Horticulture* **13**, 205–252.

Southgate, V.R. (1997). Schistosomiasis in the Senegal River Basin: before and after the construction of the dams at Diama, Senegal and Manantali, Mali and future prospects. *Journal of Helminthology* **71**, 125–132.

Spielman, A. and Lemma, A. (1973). Endod extract, a plant-derived molluscicide: toxicity for mosquitoes. *American Journal of Tropical Medicine and Hygiene* **22**, 802–804.

Stelma, F.F., Talla, I., Sow, S., Kongs, A., Niang, M., Polman, K., Deelder, A.M. and Gryseels, B. (1995). Efficacy and side-effects of praziquantel in an epidemic focus of *Schistosoma mansoni*. *American Journal of Tropical Medicine and Hygiene* **53**, 167–170.

Sturrock, R.F. (1966). The influence of temperature on the biology of *Biomphalaria pfeifferi* (Krauss), an intermediate host of *Schistosoma mansoni*. *Annals of Tropical Medicine and Parasitology* **60**, 100–105.

Sturrock, R.F. (1995). Current concepts of snail control. *Memorias do Instituto Oswaldo Cruz* **90**, 241–248.

Tchuem Tchuenté, L.A., Southgate, V.R., Théron, A., Jourdane, J., Ly, A. and Gryseels, B. (1999). Compatibility of *Schistosoma mansoni* and *Biomphalaria pfeifferi* in northern Senegal. *Parasitology* **118**, 595–603.

Utzinger, J., Bergquist, R., Xiao, S.H., Singer, B.H. and Tanner, M. (2003). Sustainable schistosomiasis control—the way forward. *Lancet* **362**, 1932–1934.

Utzinger, J., Chollet, J., Tu, Z., Xiao, S. and Tanner, M. (2002). Comparative study of the effects of artemether and artesunate on juvenile and adult *Schistosoma mansoni* in experimentally infected mice. *Transactions of the Royal Society of Tropical Medicine and Hygiene* **96**, 318–323.

Utzinger, J., N'Goran, E.K., N'Dri, A., Lengeler, C. and Tanner, M. (2000). Efficacy of praziquantel against *Schistosoma mansoni* with particular consideration for intensity of infection. *Tropical Medicine and International Health* **5**, 771–778.

Utzinger, J., Xiao, S., N'Goran, E.K., Bergquist, R. and Tanner, M. (2001). The potential of artemether for the control of schistosomiasis. *International Journal for Parasitology* **31**, 1549–1562.

Utizinger, J., Zhou, X.N., Chen, M.G. and Bergquist, R. (2005). Conquering Schistosomiasis in China: the long march. *Acta tropica* **96**, 69–96.

Vargas, M., Gomez Perez, J. and Malek, E.A. (1987). *Schistosomiasis mansoni* in the Dominican Republic; prevalence and intensity in the city of Higuey by coprological and serological methods. *Tropical and Geographical Medicine* **39**, 244–250.

Webbe, G. and el Hak, S. (1990). Progress in the control of schistosomiasis in Egypt 1985–1988. *Transactions of the Royal Society of Tropical Medicine and Hygiene* **84**, 394–400.

Wilson, R.A., Curwen, R.S., Braschi, S., Hall, S.L., Coulson, P.S. and Ashton, P.D. (2004). From genomes to vaccines via the proteome. *Memorias do Instituto Oswaldo Cruz* **99**(Suppl), 45–50.

Yuan, H., Jiang, Q., Zhao, G. and He, N. (2002). Achievements of schistosomiasis control in China. *Memorias do Instituto Oswaldo Cruz* **97**(Suppl 1), 187–189.

Zhou, X.N., Malone, J.B., Kristensen, T.K. and Bergquist, N.R. (2001). Application of geographic information systems and remote sensing to schistosomiasis control in China. *Acta Tropica* **79**, 97–106.

Zwingenberger, K., Queiroz, J.A.N., Poggensee, U., Alencar, J.E., Valdegunas, J., Esmeralda, F. and Feldmeier, H. (1987). Efficacy of oxamniquine, praziquantel and a combination of both drugs in Schistosomiasis-Mansoni in Brazil. *Revista Do Instituto De Medicina Tropical De Sao Paulo* **29**, 305–311.

Index

ADVANCES IN PARASITOLOGY VOL 61
ISSN: 0065-308X $35.00
DOI: 10.1016/S0065-308X(05)61018-1

Contents of Volumes in This Series

Volume 41

Volume 42

ADVANCES IN PARASITOLOGY VOL 61
ISSN: 0065-308X
DOI: 10.1016/S0065-308X(05)61017-2

Volume 43

Volume 44

Volume 45

Volume 46

Volume 47

Volume 48

Volume 49

Volume 50

Volume 51

Volume 52

Volume 53

Volume 54

Volume 55 (Cumulative Subject Index – Vols. 28–52)

Volume 56

Volume 57

Volume 58

Volume 59

Volume 60

Colour Plate Section

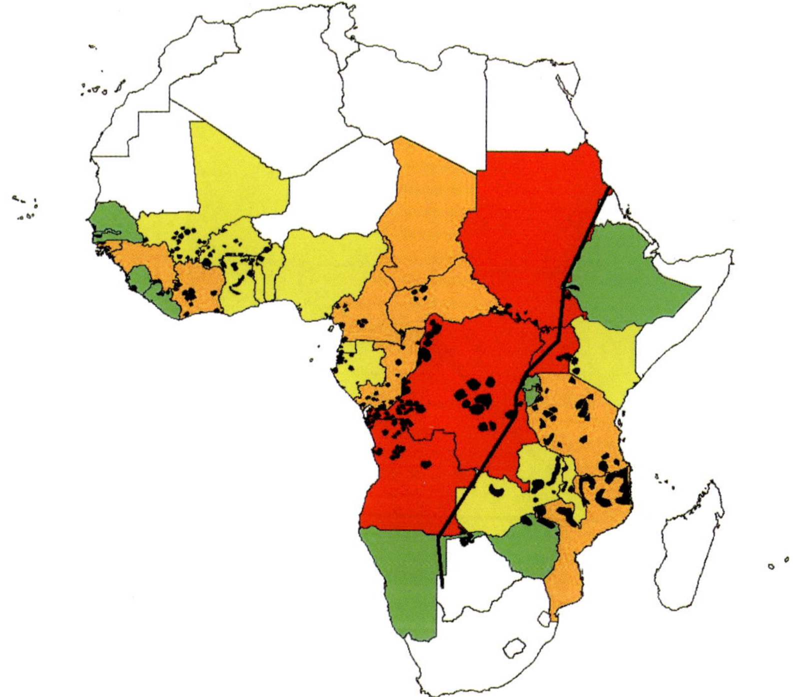

Plate 5.2 Map showing number of cases of human African trypano-somiasis in affected countries and the distribution of discrete foci. Red = very high; orange = high; yellow = low; green = sporadic. The black line denotes the boundary between *T.b. gambiense* (to the west) and *T.b. rhodesiense* (to the east)

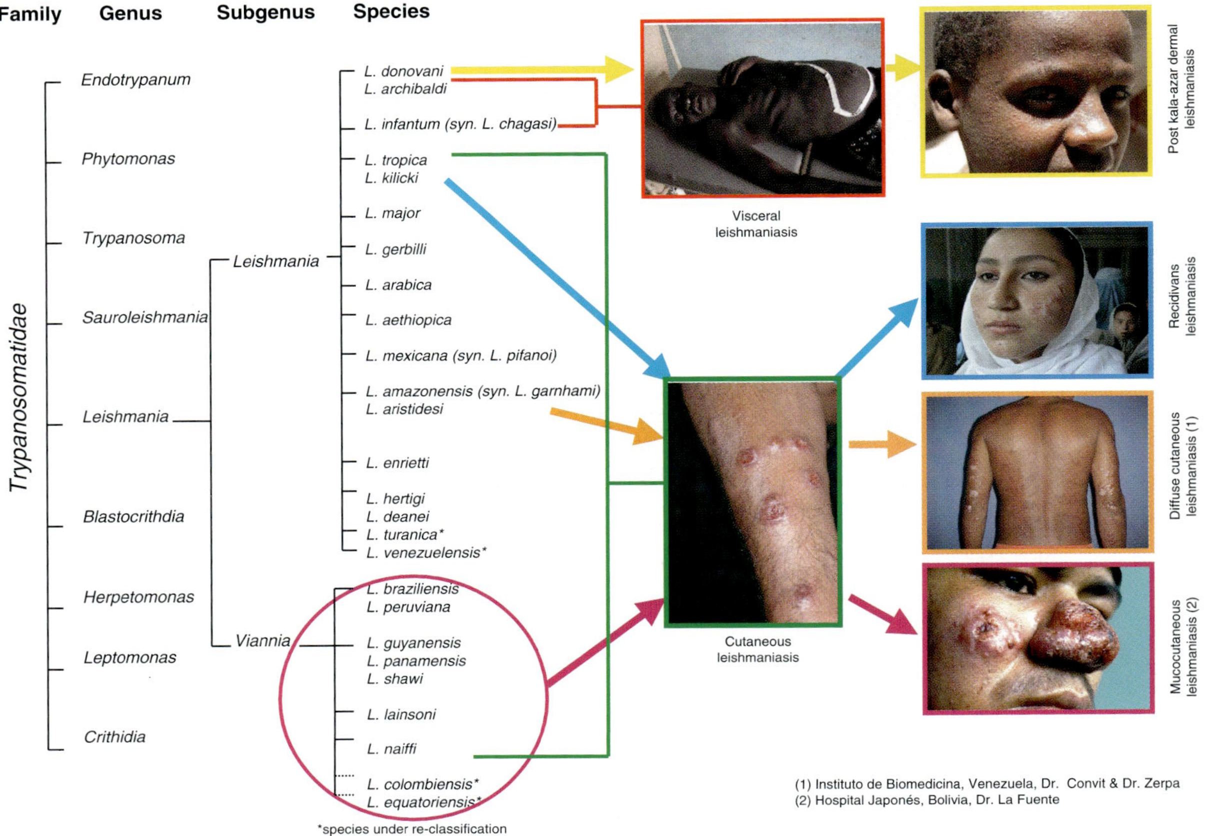

Plate 6.1   *Leishmania* species and resulting clinical presentations.

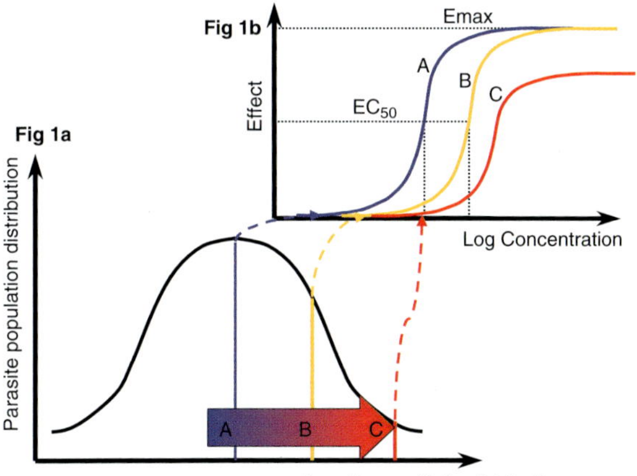

Plate 6.6 Visceral leishmaniasis: selection of resistant parasites under drug pressure. Although not well characterized, antimony resistance is likely to occur *in vivo* through the selection of naturally occurring mutants with survival advantages in the presence of the drug. Resistance can be visualized as a righward shift in the concentration–effect (dose–response) relationship. Historically, antimony has been used at low doses and unprotected. The analysis of clinical evidence from Bihar indicates that low dose single-agent antimony has selected a fraction of the original parasite population with lower sensitivity. Dose escalation over time on a parasite pool with reduced sensitivity has further selected parasites with increasing tolerance to higher drug levels, until such time that no dose can effectively control parasite growth (Olliaro *et al.*, 2005).

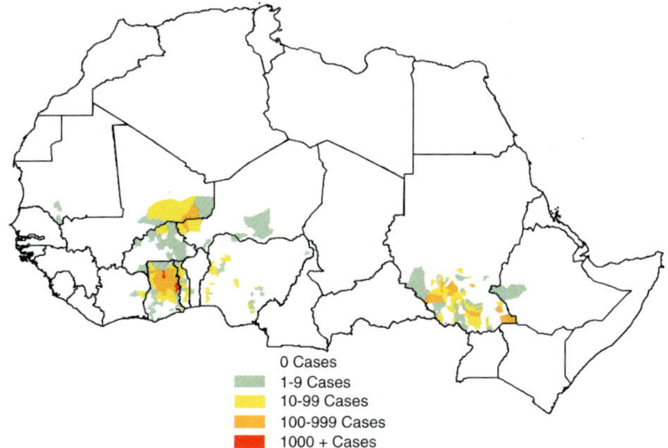

Plate 7.15 Districts in West Africa and states and region in Sudan and Ethiopia, respectively, reporting indigenous cases of dracunculiasis during 2004. WHO CCRTED archives.

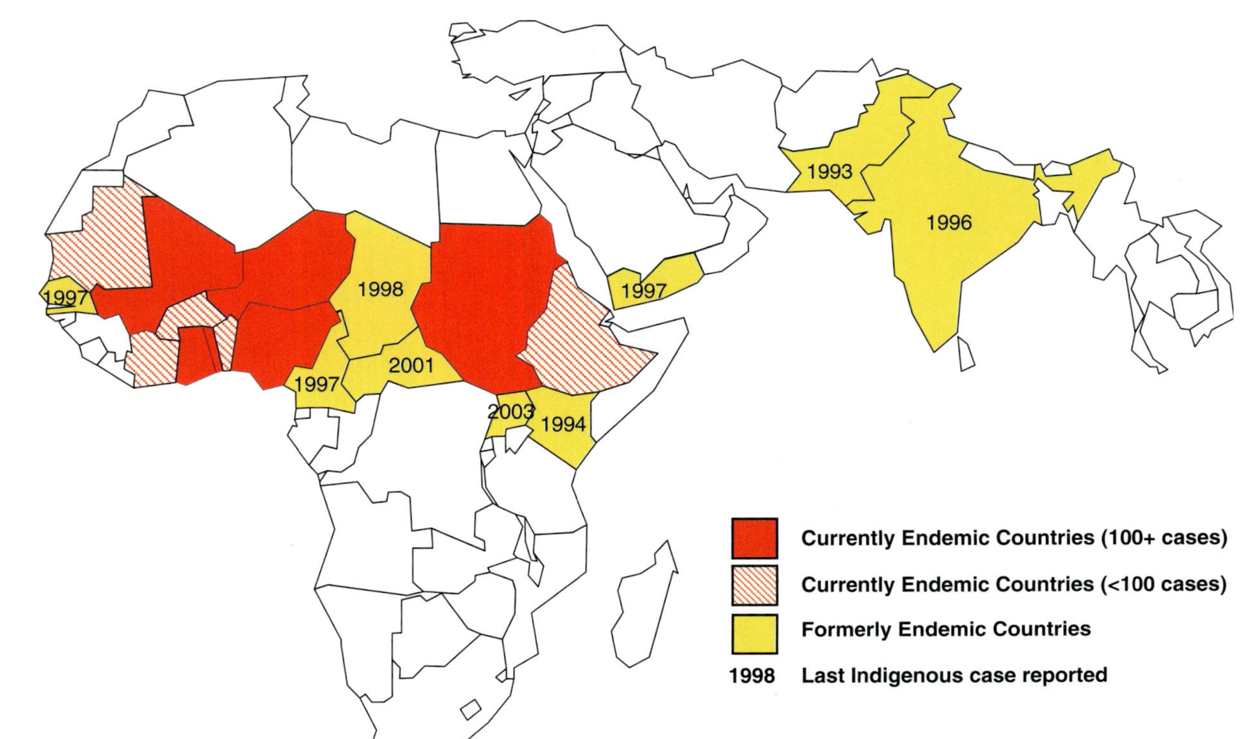

Plate 7.17   Dracunculiasis Eradication Programme: status of eradication efforts, 2004. WHO CCRTED archives.

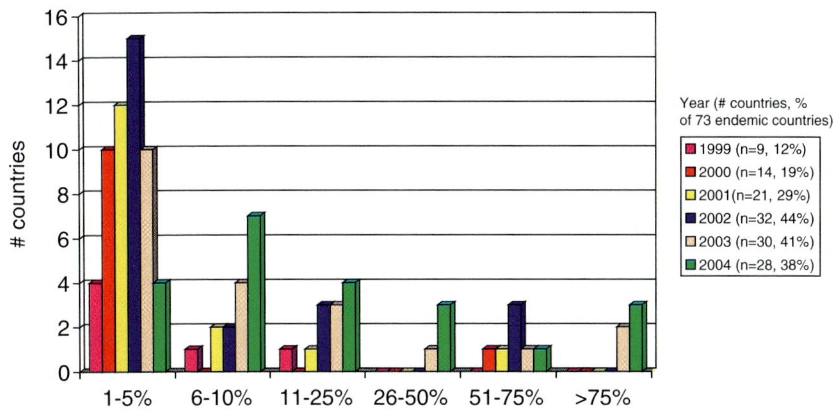

Plate 8.2   Global coverage of deworming treatment for soil-transmitted helminths, school-age children 1999–2004. Data from 73 endemic countries. (WHO, 2005.)

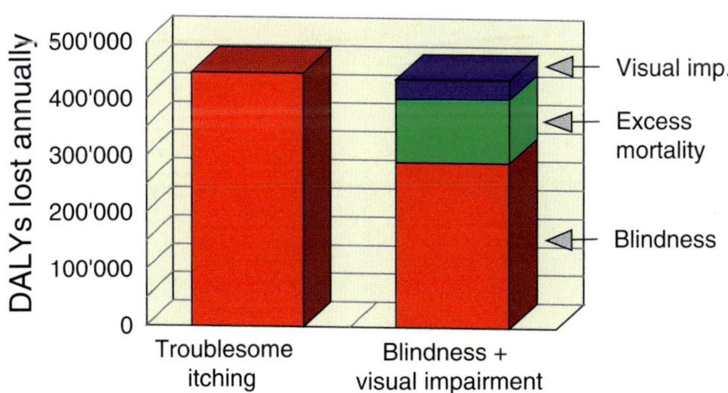

Plate 9.2   DALYs lost due to onchocerciasis. Results for 1990.

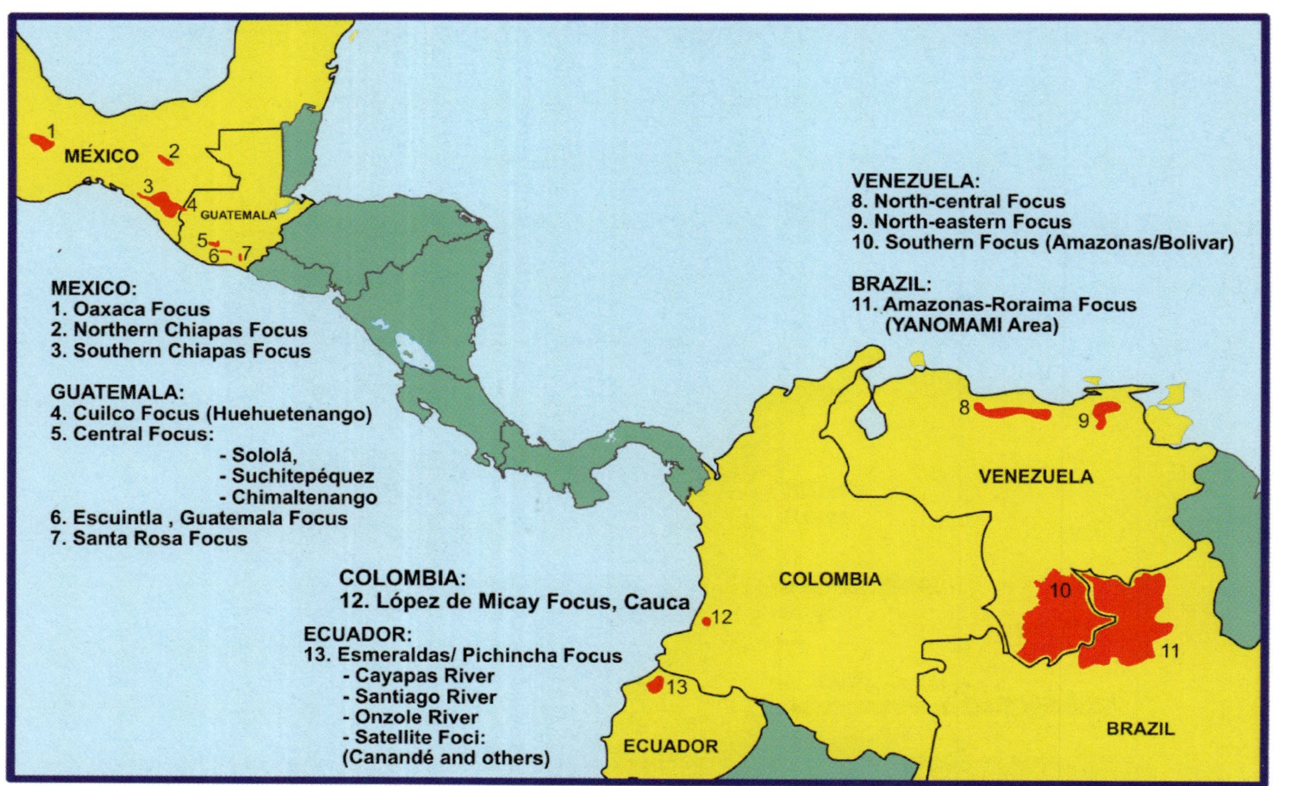

Plate 9.3 Geographic coverage of current regional onchocerciasis programmes (Americas).

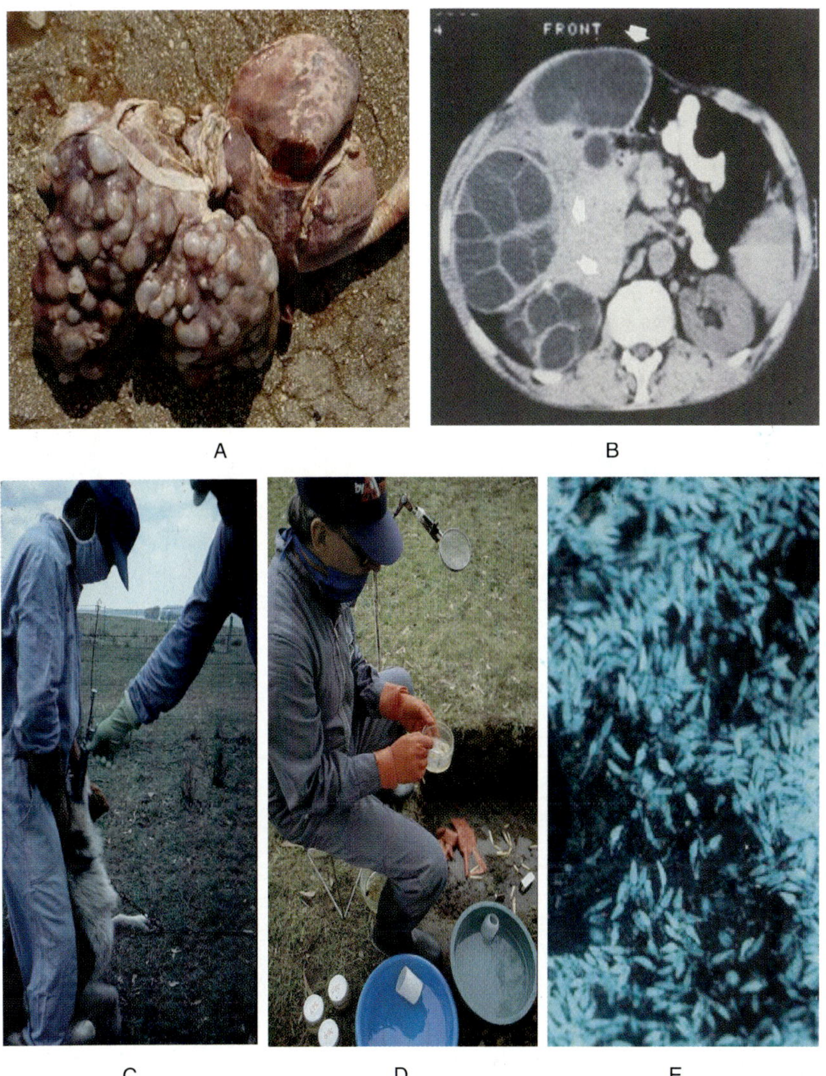

Plate 11.1 (A) Sheep liver and lungs infected with cystic echinococcosis at slaughter. (B) Abdominal CT scan of a Uruguayan hydatid patient with hepatic CE cysts (arrowed) showing presence of daughter cysts. (C) Dosing dogs with arecoline purgative in Uruguay (1990). (D) Field checking of purge samples for *Echinococcus granulosus* (Uruguay, 1990). (E) Large number of *Echinococcus granulosus* tapeworms under low magnification.

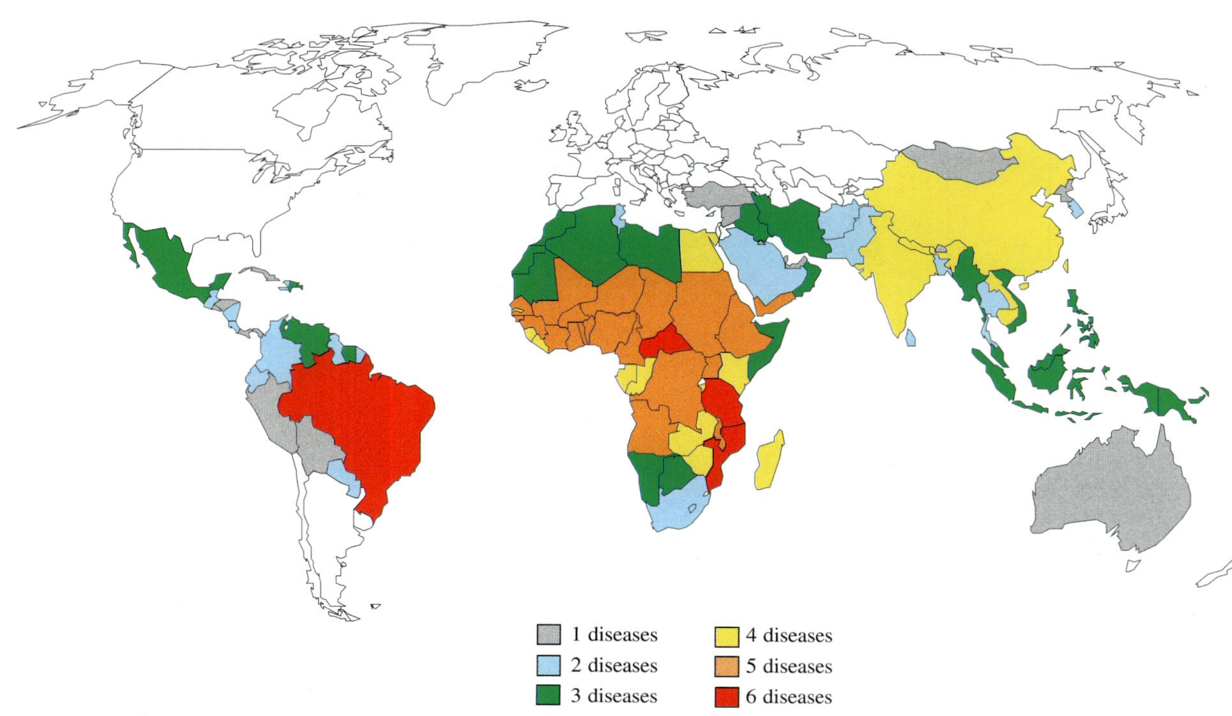

Plate 13.7 Global distribution map of polyparasitism (from Molyneux *et al.*, 2005).